QUANTITATIVE ANALYSIS OF DRUGS IN PHARMACEUTICAL FORMULATIONS

THIRD EDITION

Quantitative Analysis of Drugs in Pharmaceutical Formulations

Third Edition

Dr PD Sethi

MPharm, PhD

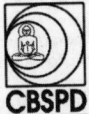

CBSPD

CBS Publishers & Distributors Pvt Ltd

New Delhi • Bengaluru • Chennai • Kochi • Kolkata • Lucknow • Mumbai
Hyderabad • Jharkhand • Nagpur • Patna • Pune • Uttarakhand

List of Contributors
1. Om Prakash BSc (Chem)
2. Dr Rajat Sethi M Pharm PhD (Manitoba, Canada)
3. Ms Deepa BSc (Hon)

Disclaimer
Science and technology are constantly changing fields. New research and experience broaden the scope of information and knowledge. The author has tried his best in giving information available to him while preparing the material for this book. Although all efforts have been made to ensure optimum accuracy of the material, yet it is quite possible some errors might have been left uncorrected. The publisher, printer and the author will not be held responsible for any inadvertent errors or inaccuracies.

Quantitative Analysis of Drugs in Pharmaceutical Formulations
Third Edition

ISBN: 978-81-239-0560-2

Copyright © PD Sethi

Third Edition: 1997
Reprint: 2003, 2004, 2005, 2008, 2010, 2011, 2015, 2019, 2023, **2025**

Published by **Satish Kumar Jain** and produced by **Varun Jain** for

CBS Publishers & Distributors Pvt Ltd
4819/XI Prahlad Street, 24 Ansari Road, Daryaganj, New Delhi 110 002, India.
Ph: 011-23266838, 23289259
Website: www.cbspd.com
e-mail: delhi@cbspd.com
Corporate Office: 204 FIE, Industrial Area, Patparganj, Delhi 110 092
Ph: 011-4934 4934
Fax: 011-4934 4935
e-mail: publishing@cbspd.com; publicity@cbspd.com

Branches

- **Bengaluru:** Seema House 2975, 17th Cross, KR Road, Banasankari 2nd Stage, Bengaluru 560 070, Karnataka, India
  Ph: +91-80-26771678/79   Fax: +91-80-26771680   e-mail: bangalore@cbspd.com
- **Chennai:** 18/8B, Subbarayan Street, Shenoy Nagar, Chennai 600 030, Tamil Nadu, India
  Ph: +91-44-42032115, 26681266
- **Kochi:** 42/1325, 1326, Power House Road, Opp KSEB, Power House, Ernakulum Kochi 682 018, Kerala, India
  Ph: +91-484-4059061-65,67   Fax: +91-484-4059065   e-mail: chennai@cbspd.com
  e-mail: kochi@cbspd.com
- **Kolkata:** 147, Hind Ceramics Compound, 1st Floor, Nilgunj Road, Belghoria, Kolkata-700056, West Bengal, India
  Ph: +033-25633055, 033-25633056   e-mail: kolkata@cbspd.com
- **Lucknow:** Basement, Khushnuma Complex, 7 Meerabai Marg (Behind Jawahar Bhawan), Lucknow-226001, UP, India
  Ph: +0522-4000032   e-mail: tiwari.lucknow@cbspd.com
- **Mumbai:** PWD Shed, Gala no 25/26, Ramchandra Bhatt Marg, Next to JJ Hospital Gate no. 2, Opp. Union Bank of India, Noorbaug, Mumbai-400009, Maharashtra, India
  Ph: 022-66661880/89
  e-mail: mumbai@cbspd.com

Representatives

- Hyderabad   0-9885175004
- Patna   0-9334159340
- Jharkhand   0-9811541605
- Pune   0-9664372571
- Nagpur   0-8692091830
- Uttarakhand   0-9716462459

Printed at Glorious Printer, Dilshad Garden, Delhi

Dedicated to fellow analysts
(Known and Unknown)

I have never used my knowledge as a vehicle but
only as means of sharing my experience with you.

Dear Analysts

Just because someone has developed the method and has claimed to have validated it in respect of various analytical parameters, does not simply imply that the method is reliable and can be directly applied. It has been found that most of the original research papers or their abstracts often do not provide adequate experimental details on LOD, LOQ, precision, accuracy, analytical range, reagents preparation and their storage, possible interference, or application of the described method in presence of other drug substances likely to be present in a multi-component formulation. Thus the reported method may have several weak spots which can give the method a kind of metastatic state. It may work one day but not the next. Although the analytical chemistry is based on reproduction of the method from written protocols as long as all the variables that can influence the reproducibility of the method are precisely controlled. However, skill obtained during development of the method cannot be simply transmitted via written description of the method. It is always preferable that you learn through your own experience as every described method may need some degree of optimisation. It is therefore desirable that any shortcoming in the method as and when observed or any practical suggestion about the method must be promptly brought to the notice of person authorized to make suitable changes in the method instead of wasting your time and your employer's resources collecting useless and unreliable analytical data.

Analytical procedures for currently available multi-component formulations included in this book have been described in sufficient details to be reproduced without difficulty, but some degree of optimization may be needed in certain procedures. It is my earnest feeling that with the sound knowledge of chemistry (inorganic/organic), equipped with special skill needed for analytical work and the information available in this book, you will be able to carry out the analysis of any viable combination of drugs either inadvertently escaped my attention or you may encounter in your analytical career. **Be determined that the method can and shall be devised, no analytical problem will ever defy solution.** You may even find better alternative method for your analytical problem than the one described in this book. If there is a better method of analysing your sample, follow it, it will give you considerable personal satisfaction. Without continuous improvement in skill you will become obsolete, most important thing to do is to develop life-time learning habit. However, if you are ever confronted with any analytical problem defying solution, discussion with the author will be rewarding and in mutual interest, as perfection for anyone is impossible to achieve. Your constructive criticism, comments and suggestions have always been source of inspiration to me. I shall feel obliged for sharing your practical experience with me.

Sincerely yours,

P.D. SETHI

"An analyst has to be in love with analysis without which it is virtually impossible to pass on the knowledge and experience one has to those wanting to learn."

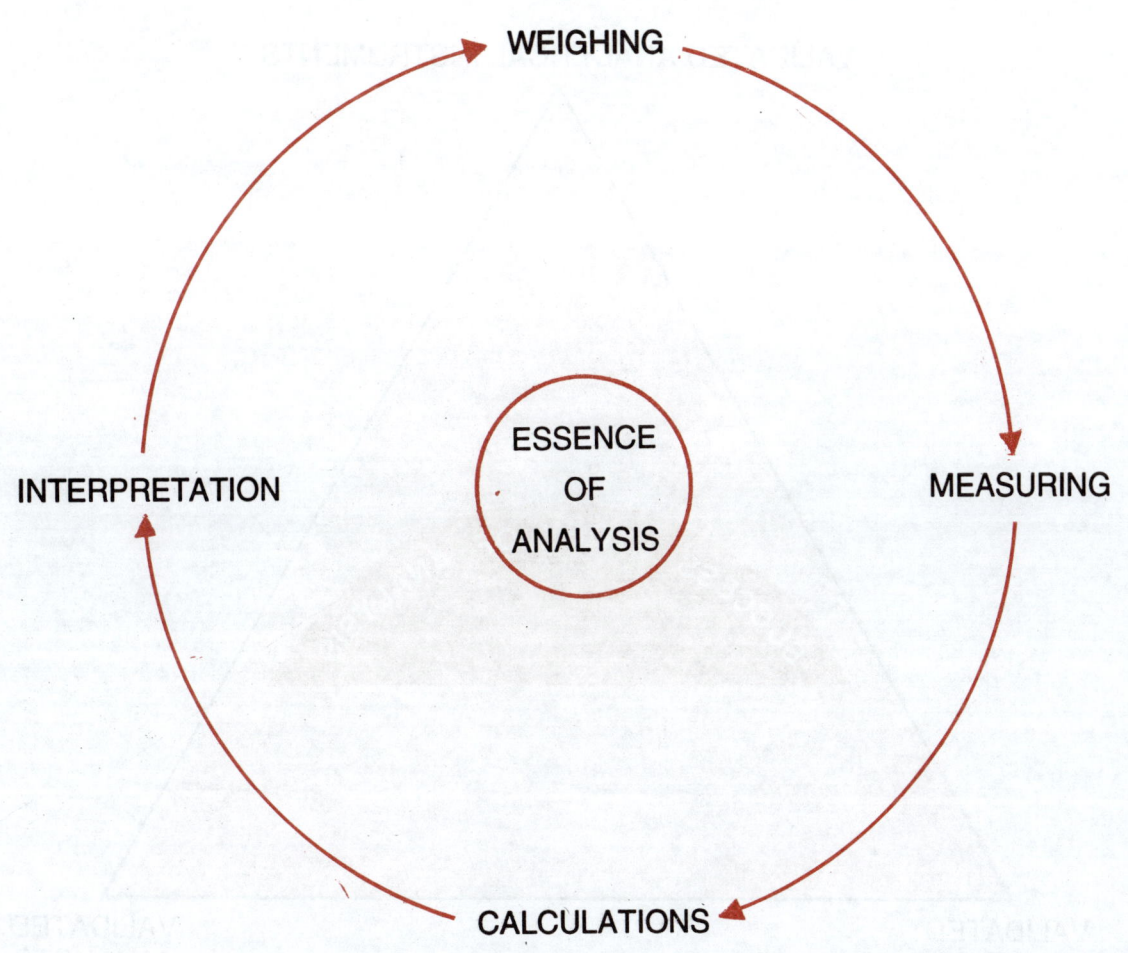

"If from any art, you take away which concerns weighing, measuring and arithmetic, how little is left of that art."

VALIDATED ANALYTICAL INSTRUMENTS

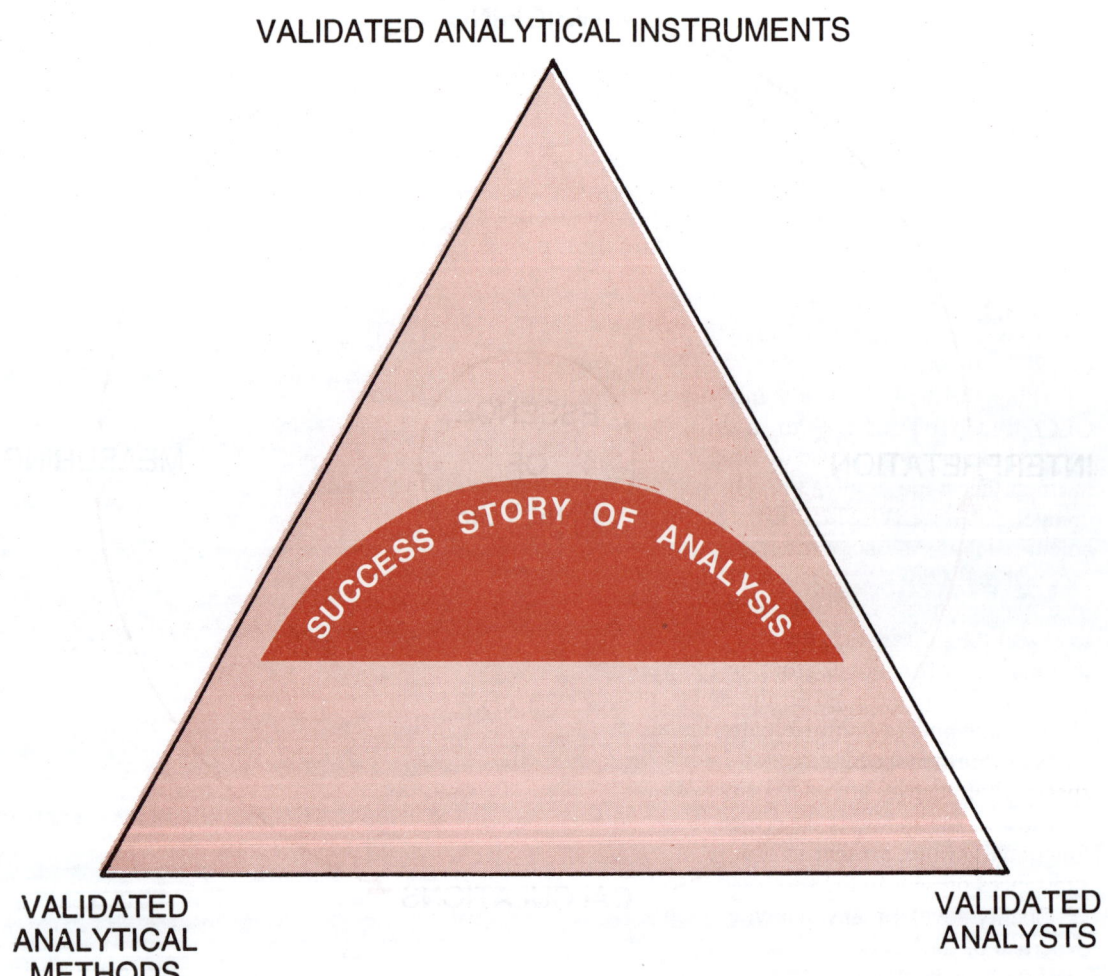

SUCCESS STORY OF ANALYSIS

VALIDATED
ANALYTICAL
METHODS

VALIDATED
ANALYSTS

"One of the most frustrating aspects for an analyst is working with an ill-defined, poorly designed and invalidated analytical method."

Preface to the Third Edition

Dog-eared and stained pages of earlier editions of this book often found at the laboratory benches are testimony to the practical usefulness of their contents. It is really a source of gratification to me that my contribution has found such a wider acceptance among my fellow analysts. Four years since the publication of the 2nd edition has brought about rapid emergence of quality culture among the pharmaceutical manufacturers primarily due to globilization.

Formulations containing two or more ingredients provide an unusual perplexity for identification and quantification of individual component. Methods may be available for analysis of such formulations, but most of them need verification. Further, requirements of specificity, precision, accuracy and degree of complexity in the analytical procedure vary considerably from task to task and therefore require a variety of analytical techniques to satisfy them which has resulted in a never-ending search for more accurate methods.

Although, there is steady increase in the use of advance physical methods of analysis such as GLC/HPLC/HPTLC/AAS to achieve highest specificity, precision and accuracy and one may be tempted to suggest that use of simple colorimetric methods based on colour reactions has diminished in importance and application. However, it is relevant to note that even the latest editions of various compendias (IP/BP/USP/JP/EP) contain identification tests for different drug substances based on the colour reactions of one or more specific functional groups present in the drug molecule. It is an accepted fact that real sample analysis is often too complex for direct analysis, no matter what new technology/ instrumentation are available. Selective chemical reactions provide the method to manipulate a sample to reveal the information desired. They also provide the means to increase the response of an analyte to a particular functional group or increase the selectivity of analysis by targeting certain components of the sample to respond to the selected reagents. As a matter of fact, most of the time, analytical chemist attempts to optimize compendial identification tests based on colour reactions for quantitative analysis. Further speed, simplicity and easy maintenance of such instruments (colorimeter, UV-visible spectrophotometric) are added advantages.

Most of the methods described in this revised edition are based on chemical reactions of specific functional groups present in a drug molecule, thus eliminating the possible interference due to other substances present in the formulation.

Quality level of any analytical work in a quality control laboratory primarily depends on the expertise of the analyst. Based on the level of skill, experience attained and functions performed, the analysts have been placed in five different grades. This is to help the quality control manager to assign duties. Some important and desirable qualities an analyst is ought to possess have been enumerated. The analyst can carry out self assessment periodically to maintain the highest standard of analytical work. The analyst must be fully aware how the results of analysis are affected by various steps in analytical methodology to enable him to control the quality of analysis by optimising important parameters. Estimation of individual drug in a multi-compound dosage form often remains a challenge for the analyst, who is almost every day confronted with the difficulty of selecting a most suitable method for a particular problem. It is rather impossible to familiarize oneself with all the possibilities by one's own experience or study, one is usually tempted to apply the methods those are well established. However, the choice may be more than often limited to facilities available in a laboratory such as type of instruments. While deciding to select a method, important analytical features of the method (limit of quantitative, sensitivity, precision, accuracy and possible interferences) must be considered and clearly identified. Analytical chemist too often seeks to achieve a quality of analytical results that are unnecessarily high. This stems from our early training when we are encouraged to produce the most accurate results possible. Such a strategy is appropriate for training students in skillful manipulation; in real-life, analysis is rarely germane for the purpose. The analyst must look for the method which is most specific for the drug under analysis, and has required accuracy and precision. The method so selected must be most productive, economical, convenient and amenable to routine use in the laboratory. It is important to emphasize that the method should be as accurate as required depending on the type of analysis and not as accurate as possible as then it may be difficult to control various parameters precisely. The methods included in this text have been extensively used in actual laboratory analysis and are reliable, speedy and uncomplicated, quite amenable and their results readily understood and best suited for routine quality control and are capable of being performed by personnel with minimum technical training/experience and under reasonable laboratory facilities. The premise has been to provide alternative analytical methods helping you to select and utilize the method best suited to your needs. However, as analytical chemists, we should never forget our fundamental training in chemistry and applying these principles to our day to day problems.

For equipping the laboratory with various analytical instruments, detailed guidelines for preparing specifications of the instruments and selection of vendors (scientific equipment supplier) have been compiled mainly based on personal experience. I am confident, these guidelines will help in selection of the instruments of correct specifications and from vendors of good reputation. Few laboratory layouts are proposed mainly suitable for small scale sector, however, much will depend on the availability of space and financial resources. For the convenience of analysts complete addresses of the agencies from whom reference substances can be procured are given. Interestingly for efficient storage of reference/ working standard a design of a laboratory table with special drawers is proposed.

Maintenance and calibration of the analytical instruments has been described with special reference to analytical balance and UV-visible spectrophotometer, the most important and most commonly used equipment in any analytical laboratory. Some common instruments such as analytical balance, UV-vis spectrophotometer, pH meter, potentiometric titrator, Karl-Fischer titrator, refrigerated centrifuge, polarimeter, m.p. apparatus, moisture balance of some leading manufacturers along with their local vendors will help in procuring the instruments.

Every effort has been made to scrutinize and update the text. Every chapter has been reviewed. Analytical methods for about 100 new formulations have been added, deleting the obsolete ones wherever necessary. The new format of the text is expected to be more convenient to read. The description of a method has been slightly rearranged to make it more presentable. Three additional chapters—Cardiac Drugs; Sedatives & Tranquillisers; and General Requirements, Quality Assurance and Accreditation of Calibration/Testing Laboratories (the latter being useful for laboratories seeking accreditation with "NABL", Deptt. of Science & Technology, Govt. of India)—have been added. The chapter on "Profile of a Quality Control Laboratory" has been elaborately re-written with several new features to meet the needs of laboratory analysts.

For any residual error, either of omission or commission which still remains, the responsibility rests with the author.

I place on record my most sincere appreciation of analysts (known and unknown) who have always been major source of my analytical knowledge. It is hoped that this revised (3rd) edition will meet aspirations of all the different grades of analysts, particularly the bench analysts and they will continue to share their practical experience with me.

I feel obliged to Dilip Charegaonkar, Managing Director, Anchrom Enterprises (I) Pvt. Ltd., Bombay for generously supporting all my scientific activities. Dr. Harish Nangia of Pharmaceutical Testing Laboratory, Ghaziabad (UP) was kind enough to provide several methods based on his own practical experience. The help provided by Shri K.K. Mandal of SICO Ltd. and Shri Bhupesh Pandey of Prime Communication, New Delhi in designing the cover is gratefully acknowledged.

Author wishes to express his sincere appreciation of Shri Satish K. Jain and Shri Vinod K. Jain for their courteous and helpful attitude during the publication of this book. Shri Dharmvir has provided most valuable suggestions in arranging the revised text. Author is indebted to his wife Usha in arranging the manuscript and going through the proofs at various stages and providing moral support for this difficult task.

New Delhi, India
1997

P.D. SETHI

Preface to the First Edition

Devising accurate assay procedures for each ingredient of complex dosage formulations containing several therapeutically and chemically compatible drugs with very similar chemical nature is a monumental undertaking. The very idea of separation, identification and estimation of each ingredient in such complex formulations would make the analyst's hair stand on end. Not only are the multiple active constituents present but they are usually there in widely divergent concentrations depending upon their relative potency and therapeutic need of the patient. The presence of additives, excipients and decomposition products further complicates the development of analytical procedures. Many of the classical tests long regarded as specific for certain substances are now answered by many more compounds. Nevertheless, the therapeutic advantage of such complex drug combinations should take precedence over any potential analytical problem which is ultimately the concern of the analyst. The increasing complexities of pharmaceutical preparations and the marked emphasis on quality control by the ethical manufacturers have placed greater load on the ingenuity of the quality control chemist.

An analyst who is in the need of an analytical method may be obliged to survey tremendous amount of literature in order to select one procedure which may appear to suit his need and facilities available, but when he subjects the selected procedure to actual test, he may find that he cannot reproduce the method. It is, therefore, essential that the practising analyst should have access to analytical procedures which are simple, reliable and workable under routine laboratory conditions.

Modern analytical techniques rely increasingly on complex techniques of analysis that require expensive equipments and highly specialized personnel. Such methods are not of much help in countries lacking these resources. For the most part, modern analytical techniques merely permit analysis to be carried out more rapidly than the conventional method of analysis, which though not bad are tedious and time-consuming. Even if a manufacturer is ready to procure and install modern instruments/ equipments, their maintenance in fittest condition is a herculean task. Non-availability of trained analytical personnel and precise, simple and suitable methods of analysis are major handicaps for pharmaceutical manufacturers in developing countries.

Taking into consideration the technical and economic constraints, it is necessary that the recommended methods should permit their use by drug laboratories located in developing countries. It is significant to stress that even simple instruments like colorimeter and spectrophotometer result in sensitive and accurate measurements with clear advantage of speed, simplicity and easy maintenance. The large volume of literature devoted to their application in almost every field of scientific research constitutes irrefutable evidence of their utility. It is, therefore, reasonable to assume that the analytical procedures involving the use of such simple instruments will find greater application. Selection of analytical method is a very critical point. The method must be accurate, sensitive, selective, reproducible and convenient.

In view of rapid advance during the last several years in the field of pharmaceutical analysis and marketing of ever increasing multi-component formulations, the available texts dealing in pharmaceutical analysis that have been written so far do not in general deal with the analysis of each component in wide range of complex pharmaceutical dosage formulations, particularly in presence of interfering substances. The official compendias are rarely of help in such formulations. To fill the existing gap in literature and keeping in view the economic and technical limitations of drug manufacturers, particularly in medium and small scale sector, it was felt that there exists a need to have a compilation of a simple, suitable and reliable methods for analysis of each ingredient of multi-component drug formulations.

This text, a maiden attempt, is meant to fulfill these needs. Analytical procedures for more than 200 drug formulations of divergent combinations have been compiled to serve as a convenient source of information for analysts and scientists engaged in the field. The focal point for this compilation is the presentation of practical aspect of the methodology using colorimeter and spectrophotometer as the main analytical tools.

For practical considerations, the drug formulations have been classified into 23 different categories based upon their common therapeutic uses as under :

1. Analgesics and antipyretics
2. Antacids and other ulcer healing drugs
3. Antacids, sedatives, antispasmodics
4. Anthelmintics
5. Anti-allergic drugs
6. Antibiotics
7. Anti-diarrhoeals
8. Anti-inflammatory drugs
9. Antimalarials
10. Anti-tuberculous drugs
11. Bronchospasm relaxants (anti-asthma)
12. Enzymes and digestives
13. Expectorants and cough suppressants
14. Eye, ear preparations
15. Keratolytics and cleansers
16. Laxatives, purgatives and lubricants
17. Nasal preparations
18. Oral rehydration salts
19. Rubefacients
20. Sedatives and tranquillisers
21. Topical antifungal, anti-infective preparations
22. Urinary anti-infective preparations
23. Vitamins, minerals and other nutritional additives.

For most of the formulations, several alternative methods have been described for a particular substance so that the analyst can intelligently select and apply the method to suit his need and the laboratory facilities available. Preliminary treatment of the sample for analysis utilizing conventional isolation and extraction procedures have been applied wherever necessary to eliminate the presence of potentially interfering substances. In other cases, the methods are sufficiently specific to permit the analysis of individual ingredients without pre-treatment. The procedures have been described in sufficient details highlighting the important steps in methodology so that these can be reproduced without much difficulty. Merits and demerits of each method and possibility of its application to other formulations have been discussed. To help the analyst and to enhance the book's usefulness, several worked out examples based on actual experimental data have been included. For drug manufacturers, who are interested to set up their independent quality control division, chapter on the profile of a quality control laboratory has been included giving brief outline of different sections.

Its importance for pharmaceutical teachers, students and institutions imparting special course in drug analysis cannot be overestimated. Science graduates interested in pursuing career as analytical chemist will find this compilation invaluable for daily use which will provide ready answers to most of their analytical problems. It is earnest feeling of the author that knowledge of the basic inorganic and organic chemistry tempered by judicious changes and the special skill needed in pharmaceutical analysis and the information included in this text will enable the analyst to overcome most specific problems and he will be able to analyse any viable combination of drug formulations he may encounter in future. It is pertinent to mention that analyst should cautiously choose the method and interpret the results carefully before certifying the product. It is hoped that this text will enable the analyst to take their rightful place in the pharmaceutical industry and in government laboratories concerned with the quality control of medicinal preparations.

The author is indebted to his wife, Usha for her moral support throughout his career.

The author wishes to express his sincere appreciation to Dr. O.P. Ghai, Professor and Head, Department of Pediatrics, All India Institute of Medical Sciences, New Delhi, for his helpful suggestions and guidance.

How far I have succeeded in my attempt, the decision is left to my fellow pharmacists and analysts.

P.D. SETHI

New Delhi, India
1985

Contents

Chapter 1

Introduction

"One of the most difficult situations that an analyst may be confronted with is the selection of suitable analytical method for a particular problem."

Introduction

Quality is important in every product or service but it is vital in medicine as it involves life. Unlike ordinary consumer goods there can be and there is no "second" quality in drugs. Quality control is a concept which strives to produce a perfect product by series of measures designed to prevent and eliminate errors at different stages of production. As a matter of fact, it is built in from the time of inception of the thought to make a product, to the time, it is finally made and sent out with an OK quality report. In popular practice, the quality of medicines or pharmaceutical products is assured through quality control. It is, therefore, essential that quality assurance department must adopt "Good Laboratory Practice" to ensure reliability and accuracy of results given out by them. The assurance of the quality and the reliability of pharmaceuticals, together with their careful control are our moral obligations arising from the humanism towards the sick human beings. Consequently, the manufacture and the control of drugs are very responsible tasks and they need substantial knowledge of the science.

The decision to release or reject a product is based upon one or two types of control actions or combination of both. If the product is a single entity of high purity, the analytical data is the basis for decision but most of the time, the formulation is a physical mixture of several potent drugs. With the growth of pharmaceutical industry during the last several years, there has been rapid progress in the field of pharmaceutical analysis involving complex instrumentations. Providing simple analytical procedures for complex formulations is a matter of foremost importance.

Preparation of samples

To enable to utilize any instrumental analysis to the full, sample should be optimally prepared. Only selective and specific sample preparations produce meaningful analysis and enable applications to be carried out in an economical and efficient manner.

It should ensure removal of interfering sample components and selective enrichment of substances to be analysed. As pharmaceutical analyst, one will be handling many type of formulations, hence proper sampling is extremely important for meaningful results. Since integrity of entire analytical results depends on the integrity of sample prior to analysis, the process used for proper sampling is important. Hence, primary goal of the analyst should be to ensure that the selected portion of the sample is true representative of the whole lot/batch or container and is homogeneous. The method followed for sampling different types of dosage formulation are :

(a) **Liquid samples :** Liquid samples, either solutions or suspensions, may be mixed thoroughly before sampling. Suspensions usually separate out quickly; to ensure homogeneity, the sample should be drawn as quickly as possible after mixing. Samples of low viscosity (injections, elixirs, syrups) are measured using pipette (to deliver type) and then diluting to volume with appropriate solvent. For more viscous samples, pipette to contain type or a Mohr wide-bore may be used. It is necessary to rinse the pipette with suitable solvent after draining major portion of the sample. If the samples are too viscous to be pipetted, weigh them and convert to volume using specific gravity of the sample.

(b) **Tablets :** Tablets should be powdered and passed through 40 mesh sieve. All grinding should be done in a hood to avoid possibility of inhaling any drug. To ensure complete extraction of the active drug substance from the tablet matrix, use of ultrasonic bath or hot water-bath may be necessary. After the solution is made up to volume, it should be filtered before resorting to further dilutions. Some tablet samples may create problems to analysts such as sugar-coated, enteric-coated or time-release tablets. Coloured sugar-coated tablets may have to be washed off to remove colour which may interfere in analysis and then dried before weighing and powdering.

(c) **Capsules :**

  (i) **Dry powder capsules :** Usually twenty capsules are accurately weighed and contents of each are emptied into a small beaker, shells are cleaned with small swab of cotton. The powder is mixed and reserved for analysis, whereas empty shells are weighed and average weight of the dry powder in each capsule is calculated.

  (ii) **Time-release capsules :** Handle as dry powder capsules, but shell need not be cleaned. The beaded material may be weighed and reduced to fine powder, sieved, mixed and used for analysis.

  (iii) **Soft gelatin capsules :** To remove the contents, each capsule is carefully sliced with a scalpel and liquid sample collected in a volumetric flask. Inside of the capsule is then rinsed with suitable solvent such as methyl alcohol by using a syringe with fine gauge needle. The rinsings are transferred to volumetric flask.

(d) **Miscellaneous :** Sampling from other formulations such as paste, ointment, cream, inhalators, implants, dermal patches may pose problems for analysts. In case of ointment and creams, the entire contents from the container should be removed, thoroughly mixed and then sample taken for analysis.

The sampling procedures described above are simply to make the analyst aware that it is imperative to obtain a homogeneous and representative sample for any meaningful analytical results.

Solvent

When name of the solvent is not indicated, it implies that water is the solvent. For preparation of the reagents or as diluent, distilled or deionised water of high quality should be used. It should be kept in mind that the demineralized water may dissolve organic impurities from the ion-exchange resin and is likely to contain dissolved gases. The term alcohol means ethyl alcohol (95 per cent v/v) and ethyl alcohol means absolute alcohol or dehydrated alcohol. Methyl alcohol may be substituted for ethyl alcohol wherever practical. Purity of solvents is critical in certain methods. While selecting a solvent for substances sensitive to oxidation use of n-hexane instead of ether is recommended; use of benzene should be discouraged.

Water-bath

Water-bath means boiling water-bath except when heating at some other temperature is indicated.

Extraction

Solubility characteristics of the substance to be extracted and its partition coefficient must be considered. Chloroform has the advantage that it is not inflammable and heavier than water, hence easy to separate. However, one may be confronted with emulsion formation while handling glanical or viscous formulations. Ether is lighter; separation is not time-consuming, but subsequent removal of ether is dangerous being highly inflammable. Further, separation can result in loss of active ingredients as after every extraction, one has to remove the aqueous (lower) layer to collect the ethereal extract. Peroxides present in ether can cause serious problems while dealing with extraction of vitamin A, D, phenothiazines and other substances prone to oxidation.

Chemicals and reagents

Reliability of the results does depend upon the quality of the reagents used in any assay procedure. The analysts should satisfy themselves that the impurities capable of interfering with accuracy of the method are not present. While making a reagent, it is assumed that unless stated specifically otherwise all the chemicals used are of analytical grade. Preparation of special reagents is described under each method, however, analyst may refer to official pharmacopoeia for preparation of common reagents and volumetric solutions.

Calculations

In all methods based on colour reactions, the calculations are based on comparison with working standards processed simultaneously. In method involving UV spectrophotometric measurement, value of A%, 1 cm has been employed, however, analysts should preferably use working standards for comparison to eliminate any experimental error.

Procedures

Quantity of the test sample should be weighed or measured accurately as specified under each method. Proportionately larger or smaller quantities than the one specified/suggested may be taken provided subsequent steps such as dilutions are adjusted to yield concentrations equivalent to those specified. Specific precautions given under a method should be adhered to for meaningful results.

Reference standard

It may be defined as drug substance of highest purity reasonably attainable, specifically prepared by independent synthesis or by further purification of existing production material and shown to be authentic material by an extensive set of analytical tests. The reference standard and substances are required to be maintained for judging the working standard.

Working standard

Defined as drug substance of established quality and purity as shown by comparison to the reference standard material and used as reference working substance for routine quality control. The analytical testing needed to document the suitability of reference standard is generally more extensive than that required by the bulk drug substance specifications. Appropriate testing procedures may include elemental analysis, chromatographic techniques (TLC/HPTLC, GLC/HPLC), infrared (IR), UV, NMR, MS, Optical Rotatory Dispersion (ORD), Circular Dichroism (CD), phase-solubility analysis, differential scanning colorimetry (DSC), differential thermal analysis (DTA), thermogravimetric analysis (TGA).

Drug product

Finished dosage form such as tablets, capsules, lotions, syrups contain a drug substance with or without association with one or more other ingredients.

Specific identification test(s)

Infrared, nuclear magnetic resonance (NMR) and mass spectrometry (MS) being specific tests should be capable of distinguishing the drug substance from related compounds. If only one specific identity test is to be performed, an IR spectrum (KBr pellet) is to be preferred. Chromatographic methods are considered confirmatory rather than specific. Doing additional confirmatory tests are encouraged, however doing several confirmatory tests cannot be a substitute for specific identity tests.

Impurity profile and limit

Tests to detect, identify and quantitate the presence of starting material and intermediate by-product, degradation products, solvents and other impurities as well as recommended limits of each of such impurities. The impurity should not only be detected, but be quantitated.

Major impurity

One that is important either because of quantity present or because of its toxicity.

Masking

Transformation of interfering species into a form that is not detected by the intended method.

Assay

The assay method for drug substance should be specific if possible as it can then only be used for stability indicating purpose. It may be possible to measure the drug substance and its impurities by the same procedure such as HPLC/HPTLC. When specific identity tests are performed and impurities are controlled by chromatographic methods such as TLC/HPTLC/GC/HPLC, other assay methods such as potentiometric titration may be employed.

Calibration

Defines instrument/component response according to prescribed test conditions versus accepted tolerance limits.

Standardisation

Defines entire system performance at the time of standardisation. Standardisation can normalize an instrument/component which is out of calibration. However it does not supersede calibration.

Quality control

It is primarily designed to detect and correct defects or checking to demonstrate whether the anticipated results are complied with.

Quality assurance

It is oriented towards preventing defects from occurring. "Prevention is better than cure." It is a managerial function which prevents problems by heading them off and by advising restraints and re-direction at the proper time and level.

Raw data

Defined as the first recorded representation of any information which is intended to support any decision-making activity. The raw data needs protection from alteration or any manipulation.

Phase separation filter (Whatman No. 1 PS)

It is a filter impregnated with water repellent (stable silicone) for effecting rapid separation of immisible mixture of aqueous and organic liquid on a laboratory scale. Since these filters are hydrophobic in character, organic liquids readily pass through the paper whereas aqueous liquid and solid are retained, thus rapid separation of two liquids is attained.

- Fold the paper in normal way and keep it in conical filter funnel.
- Pour mixed phases directly into the paper. It is not necessary to allow the phases to separate clearly before pouring.
- Allow the organic phase to filter completely through the paper, retained aqueous phase may be if

required washed with small volume of solvent. This is necessary particularly when separating phase which is lighter than water in order to clean the meniscus of aqueous phase.

• Do not allow the aqueous phase to remain on the filter paper for long time after phase separation as it will start seeping through because of evaporation of organic solvent from pores of filter paper, creating a local vacuum which in turn draws the water through—seeping process.

Generally acceptable specifications for drug products

(a) **Tablets :** Appearance, friability, hardness, colour, odour, moisture, strength, disintegration and dissolution.

(b) **Capsules :** Strength, moisture, colour, appearance, shape, brittleness and dissolution. For soft gelatin capsules, the fill medium should be examined for precipitate, cloudiness and pH.

(c) **Emulsions :** Appearance (such as phase separation), colour, odour, pH, viscosity and strength. Storage on the side or inverted is suggested for assessment of the closure systems. It is recommended that a heating/cooling cycle be employed (e.g. between 4°C and 45°C) to test physical stability.

(d) **Oral solutions and suspensions :** Appearance (precipitate, cloudiness), strength, pH, colour, odour, redispersibility, dissolution (suspensions), and clarity (solutions). Liquids and suspensions should be stored on their side or inverted in order to determine whether contact of the drug product with the closure system affects product integrity.

After storage, samples of suspensions should be prepared for assay according to the recommended labelling.

(e) **Oral powders :** Most oral powders are marketed for reconstitution prior to administration. The following characteristics of the powder should be examined : appearance, strength, colour, odour and moisture. The reconstituted product should be prepared according to the recommended labelling. Specific characteristics to be examined on the reconstituted material should include : appearance, pH, dispersibility and strength throughout the recommended storage period.

(f) **Metered-dose inhalation aerosols :** Strength, delivered dose per actuation, number of (metered) doses, colour, clarity (solutions), particle size distribution (suspensions), loss of propellant, pressure, valve corrosion, and spray pattern. Because the container contents are under pressure, filled containers must be checked for weight loss over the expiration dating period. For suspensions, aggregate (or solvate) formation may lead to clogged valves or to the delivery of a pharmacologically inactive dose. Corrosion of the metering valve or gasket deterioration may adversely affect the delivery of the correct amount of drug substance. If the drug product is intended for use in respiratory system, it is important to confirm that the initial release specifications are maintained to assure the absence of pathogenic organisms (e.g., *Staphylococcus aureus*, *Pseudomonas aeruginosa*, *Escherichia coli*, and *Salmonella* species) and the total microbial limit per canister.

(g) **Topical and ophthalmic preparations (ointments, creams, lotions, pastes, gels, solutions) :** Appearance, clarity, colour, homogeneity, odour, pH, resuspendibility (lotions), consistency, particle size distribution, strength and weight loss (plastic containers). The ophthalmic preparation needs test for sterility. Ointments, pastes and creams in containers larger than 3.5 grams should be assayed by sampling at the surface, middle, and bottom of the container. In addition, tubes should be sampled near the crimp.

Evaluation of nonmetered aerosols should include appearance, odour, strength, pressure, weight loss, net weight dispensed, delivery rate and spray pattern.

(h) **Small-volume parenterals (SVPs) :** SVPs include an extremely wide range of preparations. Evaluation of these drug products should include strength, appearance, colour, particulate matter, pH, sterility, and pyrogenicity (at reasonable intervals). Stability studies on powder products should demonstrate that the residual moisture content remains within acceptable limits and that the product is stable throughout the recommended storage period.

The stability of reconstituted products should also be determined after they are constituted according to the recommended labeling. Specific parameters to be examined at appropriate intervals throughout the maximum intended use period of the constituted drug product, stored under condition(s) recommended in labeling, should include appearance, odour, colour, pH, strength, dispersibility and particulate matter.

Continued assurance of sterility for all sterile products may be assessed by a variety of means, including evaluation of the container-closure integrity by appropriate challenge test(s), testing for preservatives (if present), and/or sterility testing.

For terminally sterilized drug products, a specification for maximum process parameters should be provided. Stability studies should evaluate and support the adequacy of the maximum release specification for process lethality.

Parenterals (except ampules) should be stored inverted or on their sides in order to determine, by comparison, whether contact of the drug product or solvent with the closure system affects product integrity or results in leaching of chemical substances from the closure material.

(i) **Large-volume parenterals (LVPs) :** Similar to those for SVPs, a minimum evaluation should include strength, appearance, colour, clarity, particulate matter, pH, volume (plastic containers), extractables (plastic containers), sterility and pyrogenicity (at reasonable intervals). Continued assurance of sterility for all sterile products may be assessed by a variety of means, including evaluation of the container-closure integrity by appropriate challenge test(s), by testing for preservatives (if present), or by sterility testing.

These products should be stored some inverted and some on their sides in order to determine whether contact of the drug product or solvent with the container-closure system affects product integrity, or results in leaching of chemical substances from the container-closure material.

(j) **Suppositories :** Suppositories should be evaluated for strength, softening range, appearance and dissolution. The effect of aging may also be observed from a hardening of the suppository and a polymorphic transformation of the drug substance; therefore, control and stability testing should include dissolution time at 37°C.

(k) **Drug additive :** For any drug product that is intended for use as an additive to another drug product, the possibility of incompatibilities exists. In such cases, the drug product labelled to be administered by addition to another drug product (e.g. parenterals, aerosols) should be studied for stability and compatibility in admixture with the other drug product.

A suggested stability protocol should provide for tests to be conducted at 0, 6 to 8 and 24 hour intervals, or as appropriate over the intended use period. These should include :

- Assay of the drug product and additive
- pH (especially for unbuffered LVPs), colour, clarity
- Particulate matter
- Interaction with the container

Analytical techniques

Some of the medicinal products are still being assayed by the time-tested procedures of gravimetric and titrimetric technique, though use of electronic balances and recording titrators have improved these classical procedures considerably. A wide diversity in the type of analytical technique has been characteristic of assay method for pharmaceuticals. Simple distillation is useful for determining alcohol contents of the glanicals, or other substances being volatile in current of steam such as menthol, thymol and even certain alkaloids such as ephedrine. Moisture contents have been determined by drying in a desiccator or in a heated oven. Use of moisture balance in which sample pan is directly heated by infrared lamp without removing the sample from the balance has been an innovation, though the most specific and convenient procedure being Karl-Fischer titration method, end point being detected manually or by electrometric with automatic titration. Separation techniques, particularly chromatographic method are valuable in analysis of pharmaceuticals. Modern spectrophotometer which incorporates features such as microprocessor control, diode array detector have become essential tools for analysis. Assay methods based on absorption in the ultraviolet and visible portion of electromagnetic spectra (Fig. 5.1) are used extensively. Some colourless substances required to be analysed are converted to a derivative having colour, the intensity of colour measured at suitable wavelength and compared with known amount of reference substance of known purity. The fluorometer measures fluorescence that may be present in the sample such as riboflavin or may be developed into the sample such as thiamine hydrochloride.

Solvents used for dilution for UV spectrophotometric assay require special purification which is often exacting and different from the requirement for other uses. It is preferable that blanks are run on the solvent and reagents used to obtain a correction for their inherent absorbances.

The following analytical techniques have been employed for estimation of different components in formulations included in the text.

1. Titrimetric and gravimetric.
2. Colorimetric and ultraviolet spectrophotometric.
3. Paper chromatography.
4. Preparative thin-layer chromatography.
5. Column chromatography.
6. Ion-exchange chromatography.
7. Flame photometry and atomic absorption spectrometry (AAS).

Filtration

In methods involving colour development, it is preferable to centrifuge the final coloured solution as use of filter paper or passing through layer of anhydrous sodium sulphate results in loss of colour intensity. In certain methods, use of glass sintered funnel is indicated, it must be adhered to.

Standard solution

The analyst shall maintain a record of normality/molarity of each standard solution. This record will indicate the normality that was measured when the solution was prepared and shall continue with the values obtained throughout its shelf life. The calculations should be checked by another chemist, usually the one who does calculation check for the sample.

When the standard solution is used regularly, measurements of its normality should be made once a week. If a standard solution is used less often than once a week, its normality should be measured and recorded each time it is used. If a standard solution is used in routine, titration analysis should be discarded if its normality changes by more than ± 1% of the initially determined value. Titrimetric standard solutions that exceed this limit within one week shall be standardized on the day of use.

Record of Titrimetric Standard Solution

Compound :	Date of preparation :
Method of preparation :	
Prepared by :	Standardized by :
Initial normality/molarity :	
Date : Normality/molarity :	Date : Normality/molarity :

1. Titrimetric methods
A. Acid-base titration
1. Direct titration
(a) Titration of an acid by a base
  (i) Titration of a liberated acid.

  (ii) Sorenson-Formol titration (free amino group present is first treated with formaldehyde to form a derivative methylamine, resulting in reduction in the basicity of amino group, to enable titration of free carboxylic group of the amino acid.

  (iii) Non-aqueous titration (Table 1.1) : Non-aqueous solvents have greater coefficient of expansion than water; even small difference in temperature during standardization and actual sample analysis can result in significant error. Further for non-aqueous titrations sample must be finely powdered and passed through sieve 100 before suspending it in glacial acetic acid. The coarse sample powder usually gives inconsistent end point and lower assay values as coarse particles do not disintegrate fully in non-aqueous medium to liberate the active drug for titration, hence leading to inconsistent end point.

Table 1.1. Experimental conditions for non-aqueous titration

Type of titration	Titration of bases and their salts	Titration of acids
Solvent	Glacial acetic acid	DMF
	Acetic anhydride	Pyridine
	Formic acid	n-butylamine
	Propionic acid	Ethylenediamine
Indicators	Crystal violet	Thymol blue
	Quinaldine red	Thymolphthalein
	p-Naphtholbenzein	Azo violet
	Malachite green	O-nitroaniline
Electrodes	Glass—calomel	Antimony-calomel
	Glass—Silver-silver chloride	Glass-calomel
		Platinum-calomel

Preparation of 0.1 N perchloric acid : Add slowly, keeping temperature below 20°C, 8.7 ml of perchloric acid to 1000 ml of glacial acetic acid. Allow the mixture to stand for about 1 hr. Determine quickly the moisture contents (% w/v) and designate this as 'A'. To the above solution add slowly $[(A - 0.03) \times 52.2]$ ml of acetic anhydride with shaking. Allow the solution to stand for 24 hrs and standardize with potassium hydrogen phthalate.

(b) Titration of a base by an acid
  (i) Titration of metal salts

  (ii) Non-aqueous titration.

2. Residual titrations
Titration of excess acid by a base

  (i) After distillation of a volatile base

  (ii) After addition to carbonate residue

  (iii) Alkaloidal assay.

B. Precipitation reactions
C. Redox titration
  (i) Cerric sulphate or cerric ammonium nitrate.

  (ii) Potassium permanganate.

  (iii) Dichlorophenol indophenol

    (iv) Potassium dichromate.
    (v) Ferrous ammonium sulphate.
    (vi) Potassium ferricyanide.
    (vii) Sodium nitrite.
    (viii) Iodometric and iodimetric.
  D. Complexation titration
    (i) EDTA
    (ii) Other miscellaneous titrants such as sodium lauryl sulphate.

2. Gravimetric method
  (i) Weigh drug after extraction.
  (ii) Weigh a derivative after separation.
  (iii) Weighing residue after ignition.

3. Spectrophotometric method
  (i) Dye complex method
  (ii) Colorimetric involving a chromogenic reagent
  (iii) Ultraviolet (UV) absorption
  (iv) Fluorimetry.
  (v) Flame photometry.
  (vi) Atomic absorption spectrometry

4. Electrochemical method
  (i) Potentiometry
Chromatographic method
  (i) Thin layer chromatography
  (ii) Paper chromatography
  (iii) Column chromatography

6. Miscellaneous
  (i) Optical
  (ii) Enzyme assay
  (iii) Differential solubility

In most of the spectrophotometric methods use of reference/working standard in conjunction with the sample under assay is recommended to avoid any error due to wavelength, or slit-width variations among various brands of spectrophotometers as well as to avoid error arising from differences in transmittance and placement of cells.

Ion-pair complex formation (Acid dye method)

Amines in their protonated state form a complex with an anionic species (acidic dye) to form natural ion-pair complexes which are distinguished by their solubility in organic solvents such as chloroform, benzene, dichloromethane. Thus by using a pairing agent, a coloured complex is produced and the amines can thus be measured colorimetrically. The equilibrium expression for ion-pair formation can be expressed as :

$$A^+_{aq} + D^-_{aq} \quad AD_{org}$$

A^+_{aq} is the protonated amine in aqueous phase, D^-_{aq} is the anionic pairing dye in aqueous phase and AD_{org} is the final ion-pair complex extractable into organic phase. These complexes are readily decomposed by extracting the complex with aqueous acid or alkali depending on the anion pairing dye.

The formation of neutral pair complex method has been extensively used in this text for estimation of several basic nitrogenous substances employing several anionic pairing ions (dyes). The relevant experimental conditions (pH of the buffer, extracting solvent and absorption maxima) for several compounds is given in Table 1.2.

Table 1.2.

Drug	Dye	Buffer (pH)	Extracting solvent	λ_{max} (nm)
Astemizole	BCG	2.5 (phosphate)	CHCl$_3$	424
	Tropeolin OOO	0.1 M HCl	CHCl$_3$	500
	Superchem violet 3B	1.3 (Glycine-HCl)	CHCl$_3$	590
Amitriptyline HCl	BTB	—	CHCl$_3$	620
Atropine SO$_4$	BTB	7.5 (phosphate buffer)	CHCl$_3$	450
Antazoline	MO	6.0 (phosphate buffer)	CHCl$_3$	420
	BCG	3.4	CHCl$_3$	420
	BPB	2.5		
	BTB	2.8-4.0		
Acebutalol	Orange-II	0.1 M HCl	CHCl$_3$	480
Amlodipine	Orange-II	—	CHCl$_3$	470
	BCG		CHCl$_3$	410
Amodiaquine	BPB	2.5	CHCl$_3$	420
	BCP	6.0.		415
Buspirone HCl	BCG	2.4		415
	BPB	3.4 (phthalate buffer)	CHCl$_3$	410
	BTB	2.6		415
	BCP	3.4		405
	MO	4.2	CHCl$_3$	450
Benzalkonium chloride	BTB	7.5 (phosphate)	H$_2$O	610
	MO	10 (KCl + NaOH)	CHCl$_3$ + HCl	510
Bromhexine HCl	BCP	Acidic	H$_2$O	410
Clidinium bromide	BCP	7.00	CHCl$_3$	420
Chlorhexidine gluconate	BCG	5.7 (citrate phosphate)	CHCl$_3$	410
	Alizarin yellow G	PO$_4$ buffer pH 7.6	CH$_2$Cl$_2$	405
Cyclomate Na$^+$	BTB	7.5 (phosphate)	H$_2$O	610
Chlordiazepoxide	Azure-A	5.8 (borate-PO$_4$)	CHCl$_3$	652
	Fast red-A	(acidic)	CHCl$_3$	515
	Orange-II	5.0 phthalate	CHCl$_3$	495
	Fast green FCF	5.0 phthalate	CHCl$_3$	630
Cimetidine	BTB	5.5 (citrate PO$_4$)	CHCl$_3$	420
Chloroquine PO$_4$	BTB	5.6 (citrate-PO$_4$)	CHCl$_3$	410
Ciprofloxacin	BCP	4.5 (phthalate)		
	BPB	2.5	CHCl$_3$	420

(Continued)

Drug	Dye	Buffer (pH)	Extracting solvent	λ_{max} (nm)
Clotrimazole	BPB	3.4 (phthalate)	$CHCl_3$	410
Codeine PO_4	CI and orange 4S	0.1 M citric acid	$CHCl_3$	422
	BPB/BTB	3.0	$CHCl_3$	420
	MO	3.5	$CHCl_3$	410
	BCG	3.8 (citrate–PO_4)	$CHCl_3$	418
Cisapride	Ergioglaucine A (EG-A)	—	$CHCl_3$	640
Celerazine HCl	MO	3.6	$CHCl_3$	423
Chlorpromazine HCl	SBT SDB FSB FF	2.0 3.0 4.0	$CHCl_3$	520
Cyclizine HCl	SBT SDB FSB FF	2.0 3.0 4.0	$CHCl_3$	520
Cyproheptadine HCl	SBT SDB FSB FF	2.0 3.0 4.0	$CHCl_3$	520
Clonidine HCl	BTB	7.6 (citrate–PO_4)	$CHCl_3$ + HCl	420
Domperidone	Metanil yellow	Dilute acetic acid	$CHCl_3$	530
	Suprachem violet 3B	1.3	$CHCl_3$	565
Diltiazem	Orange-II	0.1 N HCl	$CHCl_3$	490
	Alizarin red	0.1 N HCl	$CHCl_3$	440
Diazepam	Alizarin violet 3B	Glycine + HCl	$CHCl_3$	560
	Orange-II,	0.1 N HCl	$CHCl_3$	515
Diphenhydramine HCl	BCG	3.0 (phthalate)	$CHCl_3$	415
	BCG/BPB	4.4 (citrate–PO_4)	$CHCl_3$	412
	MO	5.0 (citrate–PO_4)	$CHCl_3$ + acidified CH_3OH	525
Doxepen HCl	MTB	4.0 (citrate–PO_4)	$CHCl_3$	413
Diclofenac Na^+	Methylene blue	6.8	$CHCl_3$	640
Dicyclomine HCl	Methylene blue	—	H_2O	590
Dextropropoxyphene HCl	BCG	4.0 (phthalate)	$CHCl_3$	420
Dextromethorphan HBr	BCP	4.0 5.3 citrate–PO_4	$CHCl_3$	415 420
Ephedrine HCl	BTB	7.5 (phosphate)	$CHCl_3$	405
Ethambutol HCl	BTB	7.0 (phosphate)	$CHCl_3$	425
	Alizarin violet 3B	2.0	$CHCl_3$	415
Emetine HCl	MO	5.0 (citrate–PO_4)	$CHCl_3$ + acidified CH_3OH	460

(Continued)

Drug	Dye	Buffer (pH)	Extracting solvent	λ_{max} (nm)
Enalapril	BCG	3.1	CHCl$_3$	413
Erythromycin	SBT	2.0 }	CHCl$_3$	520
	SDB	3.0		
	FSB FF	4.0		
Fluphenazine	Light green	5.0 (phthalate)	CHCl$_3$	635
Flunarizine	Orange G	0.1 M HCl	CHCl$_3$	560
	BCG	3.0 }	CHCl$_3$	415
	BCP	2.0		
	BPB	3.0		
	BTB	2.0		
Glycyrrhizin	Methylene blue	9.2 (citrate-PO$_4$-borate)	CHCl$_3$	640
Glibenclamide	BTB	5.6 (citrate-PO$_4$)	CHCl$_3$	410
Homatropine methyl bromide	BTB	10.5 (borate)	CHCl$_3$	420
Hydroxyzine HCl	BTB	7.5 (citrate-PO$_4$)	CHCl$_3$ + ammoniacal CH$_3$OH	420
	BPB	2.6	CHCl$_3$	420
	BCG	3.5		
	MO	4.5		
	SBT	2.0 }	CHCl$_3$	520
	SDB	3.0		
	FSB FF	4.0		
Hyoscyamine	BCP	2.5 (phosphate)	CHCl$_3$	440
Isopropamide	MO	10.2 (phosphate-bicarbonate)	CHCl$_3$ + HCl	510
Imipramine HCl	SBT	2.0 }	CHCl$_3$	520
	SDB	3.0		
	FSB FF	4.0		
	BCG	3.4 phthalate	CHCl$_3$	418
Ketotifen	BPB	3.2		416
	BTB	2.6 phthalate	CHCl$_3$	411
Ketoconazole	BCP	2.8		407
	BCG	2.5		420
	BCP	2.5	CHCl$_3$	420
	BPB	1.5		415
	MO	2.75		430
Loperamide	Tropeolin OO	3.0 (citrate-PO$_4$)	CHCl$_3$ + acidified CH$_3$OH	540
Lignocaine HCl	BCG	5.3 (citrate-PO$_4$)	CHCl$_3$	408
	BCG	4.2 (phthalate)	CH$_2$Cl$_2$	420

(Continued)

Drug	Dye	Buffer (pH)	Extracting solvent	λ_{max} (nm)
Lidocaine HCl	BCG	4.2 (phthalate)	CH_2Cl_2	420
	SBT	2.0	$CHCl_3$	520
	SDB	3.0		
	FSB FF	4.0		
Lomofloxacin	BTB	4.0	$CHCl_3$	410
	BCG	3.0		415
	BCP	3.0		405
	BPB	3.0		400
Miconazole NO_3	BCG	3.0 (citrate-PO_4)	$CHCl_3$	420
	Solochrome dark blue	4.0 (phthalate)	$CHCl_3$	530
Melclopamide	BTB	7.5 (citrate-PO_4)	$CHCl_3$	425
	BTB	5.7 (citrate-PO_4)		420
Metronidazole benzoate	BTB	4.4 (citrate-PO_4)	$CHCl_3$	430
Mebeverine HCl	BTB	—	$CHCl_3$	405
	Fast green FCF	—	$CHCl_3$	625
	Eriochrome black		$CHCl_3$	500
	Alizarin red	0.1 N HCl	$CHCl_3$	410
Methdilazine HCl	Brilliant blue		$CHCl_3$	420
Nifopam HCl	BCG	3.0		
	BPB	3.0 } phosphate	CHCl$_3$	410
	BTB	2.6		
	BCP	2.6		
Norfloxacin	BTB	2.0	$CHCl_3$	422
	Orange-II	5.0	$CHCl_3$	495
Nortriptyline HCl	Light green FCF	3.4	$CHCl_3$	630
Naphazoline NO_3	BCG	2.5/4.0		
	BPB	6.0	$CHCl_3$	420
	BTB	6.0 }		
	MO	2.0		
	SBT	3.0 }	$CHCl_3$	520
	SDB			
Noscapine	BCP	1.0 (NaCl + HCl)	Toluene	410
Oxymetazoline	BPB	2.5	$CHCl_3$	420
	BCG	3.4	CH_2Cl_2	

(Continued)

Drug	Dye	Buffer (pH)	Extracting solvent	λmax (nm)
Orphenadrine	BCG, BPB, MO	—	CHCl₃	430
Oxyfedrine HCl	BCG	3.5	CHCl₃	420
	BPB	2.5, 4.5		
	MO	2.0, 4.0	CHCl₃	520
Pentazocine HCl	Eriochrome black T, Solochrome dark blue	2 N HCl	CH₂Cl₂	625
Pilocarpine NO₃	Cobalt thiocyanate	6.0 (citrate-PO₄)	CHCl₃ + 0.1 N NaOH	580
Piperazine citrate	BCP	6.0		
	BTB	5.7 (phosphate)	CHCl₃	420
Procylidine HCl	BCG	3.5		
	BPB	2.5		
	BTB	2.8	CHCl₃	410
	MO	4.5		
	Solochrome black T	2.0		
	Solochrome dark blue	4.0	CHCl₃	520
Phenylbutazone	Basic fuchsin	7.8 (citrate-PO₄)	CHCl₃	545
Prazosin HCl	Orange-II	—	CHCl₃	490
	Alizarin violet 3B	—	CHCl₃	570
Promethazine HCl	BCG	2.8 (citrate-PO₄)	CHCl₃	415
	Sunset yellow	1.0	CHCl₃	480
	SBT	2.0		
	SDB	3.0	CHCl₃	520
	FSB FF4	4.0		
Pyrimethamine	BPB	2.5		
	BCP	3.5		
	BTB	3.8 (phthalate)	CHCl₃	420
	MO	4.5		
Probenecid	Basic fuchsin	7.0	CHCl₃	415
Quarternary ammonium salts	BCG	1.3	CH₂Cl₂	415
	MO	10.0 (KCl + HCl)	CH₂Cl₂	415
	BTB	7.5 (phosphate)	H₂O	610
Reserpine	Alizarin violet 3B, Alizarin brilliant violet B	1.2 (glycine + HCl)	CHCl₃	560

(Continued)

Drug	Dye	Buffer (pH)	Extracting solvent	λ_{max} (nm)
Sparteine	BCG	4.0	CHCl₃	420
Timolol	BCG	2.2	CHCl₃	410
	Solochrome black T	2.8		515
Tamoxifen	Alizarin	1.5 (glycine + HCl)	CHCl₃	440
Ticlopidine HCl	BCG	3.6		
	BPB	3.2 } phthalate	CHCl₃	415
	BTB	2.8		
	BCP	3.0		
Trimethoprim	BTB } BCG } BCP	4-6 (citrate-PO₄)	CH₂Cl₂	430
	BPB	3.2 (citrate-PO₄)	CHCl₃	418
Trihexyphenidyl	BCP	5.3 (PO₄)	CHCl₃	410
Tolazoline HCl	SBT	2.0		
	SDB	3.0	CHCl₃	520
	FSB FF	4.0		
Triprolidine HCl	SBT	2.0		
	SDB	3.0	CHCl₃	520
	FSBF	4.0		
Xylometazoline HCl	SBT	2.0		
	SDB	3.0	CHCl₃	520
	FSBF	4.0		
	BCG	3.4		
	BPB	2.5		
	BTB	3.8	CHCl₃	415
	MO	6.0		

BCG—Bromocresol green; BTB—Bromothymol blue; MO—Methyl orange; BPB—Bromophenol blue; BCP—Bromocresol purple; SBT—Solochrome black T; SDB—Solochrome dark blue; FSB FF—Fast sulphone black FF.

Theoretical conditions which help in choosing a rational system for a particular determination involves the knowledge of the dissociation constant of acidic dye and the basic compound and the pH dependence of the partition characteristics of the two substances and their addition product between aqueous and organic solvent. Since dyes are used in excess one of the basic requirements of this technique is that unreacted dye must be wholly retained in aqueous phase at the pH employed. If the initial partition coefficient of the dye (in acid form) is high, the pH of the buffer must be above the pKa of the dye. However, if acid form of the dye is insoluble in the organic phase, pH of the buffer may not have much role. As pH has no significant influence on partition characteristics of the dye above its pT, it is always advisable to explore the area between pK and pT (Table 1.3) to find out the most critical pH for a system i.e. the lowest pH at which the dye is wholly retained in the aqueous phase on shaking with an organic solvent.

Table 1.3.

Dye	pK	pT	pH	Organic solvent
Bromocresol purple	6.3	6.8	5.4	Benzene
Bromothymol blue	7.0	7.6	5.0	Toluene
Bromocresol green	4.7	5.4	6.6	Chloroform
Bromophenol blue	4.0	4.6	5.6	Chloroform
Bromochlorophenol blue	4.2	4.8	4.0	Benzene
Chlorophenol red	6.0	6.6	6.5	Benzene
Methyl orange	3.8	4.4	5.0	Ethylene dichloride/chloroform, benzene
Thymol blue	2.0	2.8	5.0	Chloroform
Tropaeolin	2.2	2.6	3.2	Chloroform

Most nitrogenous bases of pharmaceutical interest have pK between 4 and 8. Thus at a particular pH, the extent to which any base will exist in its free form will depend on its pKa value. The condition required is that the medium may not be too acidic so as to retain the base in the aqueous phase. It is sometimes necessary to operate at a pH somewhat higher than the pT of the indicator (dye). General guideline is that pH of the buffer chosen should be somewhat above the pKa of the base to be estimated and then select the dye for which this pH is optimum. For example, for methyl orange-chloroform system at pH 5.0, pKa of the base must be below 7.0.

The sensitivity of this method depends primarily on molar extinction coefficient of the dye in the medium in which the absorbance is measured. To increase the sensitivity of the method, the ion-pair complex so formed and extracted into organic layer, is brought back to aqueous layer (acidic or basic) by shaking the organic layer with 0.1 N HCl or 0.1 N NaOH depending on the dye initially used for complex formation. The dye used in the complex formation is quantitatively extracted with aqueous layer and the absorbance of the resultant aqueous solution is measured as is the case with clonidine and pilocarpine.

Note :   1.   Most of these complexes being yellow in colour absorb in far ultra-violet region in the range of 360-420 nm, the maxima is not sharp and difficult to locate.
2.   Reagent blank usually is very high.
3.   As formation of complexes is pH-specific, presence of other substances can effect the pH. For estimation of codeine in presence of aspirin, usually pH of higher value is required for formation of complex with methyl orange.

Colorimeter measurements

Colorimetric methods involving chemical reactions confer certain degree of specificity, thus other components present in the formulation do not interfere in the analysis, however the analyst should consider the following practical aspects while using colorimeter methods.

1.   Colour reagent should be selective for drug substance of interest to discriminate it from its degradation products, impurities and other excipients/matrix present in the formulation.

2. Effect of other parameters such as solvent, pH, reagent volume, order of adding reagent, age of reagent, reaction temperature, which may have bearing on the colour reaction should be identified and established.

3. Time required for optimum colour intensity.

4. Stability of chromophore formed.

Red or bathochromic shift : Shift in the peak position (λ_{max}) to a higher wavelength due to effect of substituents, solvents or molecular re-arrangement. This is often large (> 100 nm). This effect is exploited for quantitative and qualitative purpose.

Blue or hypsochromic shift : Shift in the peak position (λ_{max}) to a lower wavelength sometime as much as 30 nm.

Hyperchromic and hypochromic shift : Increase or decrease in the absorptivity value.

Bathochromic/hypsochromic shifts are usually accompanied with hyper- or hypochromic effects.

Isobestic (iso-absorption) point : The point (wavelength) at which molar absorptivity of different ionic species is identical. To determine this point, UV absorption spectra of different ionic species is scanned under identical conditions and concentrations. This property has been extensively used to develop analytical techniques for bi-component drug formulations. Certain methods described in the text are based on this technique.

Note : 1. Quantitative spectrophotometric analysis should preferably be carried out above 235 nm as in the range of 190-210 nm, special precautions are required to be observed.

2. Spectrophotometric measurements should be carried out at the peak of spectral absorption of the substance under estimation. It is always desirable to actually determine the peak wavelength of the compound in the instrument under use as minor variations in the apparent wavelength of the peak are observed from instrument to instrument.

3. Spectrophotometric measurements should usually be made first with the standard solution.

4. The concentration of sample and standard should be so chosen that the absorption value of final solution is in the range of 0.40 to 0.75 for least error.

5. When an assay is carried out with routine frequency, use of reference substance can be omitted and instead a suitable standard curve prepared with reference substance may be used.

6. When a new apparatus or new lot of reagents are used, standard curve needs confirmation.

7. In the event of uncertainty or dispute, direct comparison with the reference substance is necessary.

Ultraviolet and visible spectroscopy

Analytical absorption spectroscopy in ultraviolet and visible region of electromagnetic spectrum is widely used for quantitative analysis in the field of pharmaceutical and biomedical analysis. Since, this technique has been extensively used in this text while describing analytical procedures, it is appropriate that analyst is made conversant with some important and practical aspects of this technique.

The scope of absorption spectroscopy is further extended by use of colour reactions often with concomitant increase in sensitivity and/or selectivity. Such reactions are used to modify the spectrum of an absorbing molecule, so that it could be detected in visible region well separated from other interfering components. Chemical modification is also useful for transforming non-absorbing molecule to a stable derivative possessing significant absorption spectral behaviour. Selectivity can further be enhanced by number of chemical or instrumental techniques such as difference spectroscopy, derivative spectroscopy, derivative-difference spectroscopy and dual wavelength spectroscopy, however, such methods should be validated.

The prescribed unit used in UV-visible spectroscopy is wavelength expressed as nanometres (nm). The position of maximum absorbance of a peak is designated λ_{max}. The wavelength in this region is divided into two ranges i.e. 200-400 nm (ultraviolet region) and about 400-800 nm (visible region).

Outside these limits are designated as far ultraviolet (vacuum ultraviolet) and near infrared. The group in the molecule which is responsible for absorption is described as chromophore whereas group having little or no intrinsic absorption of its own, but modifies the absorption spectrum of the molecule is called auxochrome.

Measurement of chromophore in visible region has been extensively used. Most of the time, chemical species do not possess suitable chromogenic properties and are made to react with a suitable reagent giving rise to coloured species. Compounds having phenolic functional group with ortho or para position yield spectrophotometrically useful chromogens through nitrosation. The stability of nitroso-derivative is increased by addition of alcohol or alkalinization of the medium. Coordination of a transition metal with polydentate-ligand (ortho-nitroso-derivative) results in the formation of a stable water soluble metal chelate. Most of the drug substances with phenolic functions included in this text have been estimated either through their nitroso-derivative or metal chelate or both such as paracetamol, oxyphenbutazone, amoxycillin, salbutamol sulphate.

Ortho-nitroso-derivative (having para position occupied) are usually unstable in acidic medium, whereas para-nitroso-derivatives are stable in both the acidic and alkaline medium. Ortho-nitroso phenol derivations are capable of forming chelates with cobalt (II) ion, whereas para-nitroso derivatives do not form cobalt chelates. The cobalt chelate is sparingly soluble in water but easily extractable with organic solvents such as chloroform (yellow chromogen). Copper chelates are usually purple in colour.

The extent of absorption of radiation by a given absorbing system at a specific monochromatic wavelength is governed by two classical laws of absorptiometry.

Lambert's (Bougner's) law : At a given concentration (C) of a homogeneous absorbing system, the intensity of transmitted light decreases exponentially with increase in path light.

The complimentary Beer's law concerned with concentration (C) states that for a layer of defined path length, the intensity of transmitted light decreases exponentially with increase in concentration (C) of a homogeneous absorbing system. The combination of both these laws gives the popular law i.e. Beer-Lambert law i.e.

$$\log \frac{I_o}{I} = kcb$$

where k = absorptivity of the system.

When concentration is expressed in g/100 ml, k is described as specific absorption and is designated by the symbol $A_{1\,cm}^{1\%}$ or A (1%, 1 cm) i.e. absorbance of a 1% w/v solution of a substance in a cell of 1 cm path length. The term is also expressed as A_1^1 and is widely used in analytical chemistry.

$A_{1\,cm}^{1\%}$ values have been used in the text for calculating assay values, however, because of instrumental differences and possible effect of solvents, these values are subject to considerable variations. It is therefore advisable not to use these values where accurate assay is required or in case of dispute, use of reference substance is called for.

Molar absorptivity : Absorbance of a one molar solution in a cell of 1 cm path length. As per American convention absorptivity (a) is defined as absorption of 1 g/L solution of a substance in a cell of 1 cm path length.

$$\text{Absorptivity (a)} = \frac{A_1^1}{10} = \frac{\text{Value of A 1\%, 1 cm}}{10}$$

i.e. Absorptivity (a) is $1/10$th of specific absorption (A_1^1)

Example : Aspirin (Acetyl salicylic acid)

λ_{max} (acid) = 230 nm

A_1^1 (230 nm) = 466

Absorptivity (a) = 46.6

Molar absorptivity = 8397.32 (46.6 × 180.2)

Validity of Beer-Lambert law

The validity of the Beer-Lambert law is affected by number of factors. If the radiation is non-monochromatic the observed absorbance usually is lower than for monochromatic radiation. Thus sharp bands are more susceptible than broad bands to absorbance error on this account. Further if absorbing species undergoes association, dissociation, photodegradation, solvation, complexation or adsorption or emits fluorescence, then positive or negative derivations from the Beer's law may be observed. Stray light effects and the type of solvent used can also lead to non-compliance with the Beer's law.

For single-beam instruments the absorbance range for precise measurement should be below 0.3-0.6 absorbance units, the optimum range being 0.45 absorbance units. For double-beam spectrophotometry, the optimum range lies between 0.6 and 1.2 absorbance units. Five or more standard solutions whose absorbances are within working range should be measured in duplicate in a matched pair of cells against solvent as reference. The cell constant should be substituted for each individual measurement and needs to be checked regularly. If a graph absorbance (A) versus concentration (C) indicates any systematic (positive or negative) deviation, then additional points be inserted and working range estimated.

Practical application of absorbance values A_1^1 depends on various factors such as purity of substance, solvent used and precise conditions employed in the reference instrument and the type of instrument available. It is therefore desirable to ascertain the reported absorptivity data in one's own laboratory. It is advisable not to depend on reported absorptivity values when accurate assay values are required or in matter of dispute the use of reference substance for comparison is called for. The absorptivity values should be periodically determined if sufficient quantity of drug in pure form is available.

The validity of Beer-Lambert law should be established for each drug under the measurement conditions prevailing in the laboratory over the concentration range of interest. The reported range more than often is required to be re-established.

Instrumentation

Colorimeters : Employ tungsten radiation source and broad band (~ 300 nm) optical filters of nominal wavelength. It is usually difficult to establish linearity range in a colorimeter due to relatively broad spectral bandwidth employed. While employing colorimetric methods comparison with the standard is absolutely essential.

Spectrophotometer :

(a) Single beam spectrophotometer : Use prism or high quality diffraction grading monochromator and intense source of ultraviolet radiation—deuterium (hydrogen) lamp. As the sample and reference cells are manually moved in and out of radiation beam at each wavelength of interest, scanning of spectrum is not possible.

(b) Double beam spectrophotometer : Contain high quality optical components as in the case of single beam spectrophotometer but radiation in the monochromator splits into two identical beams, one passing through the sample and other through the reference cell, thus making scanning of spectra possible.

Absorption cells

For visible region (400-700 nm) matched pair of glass cell is used. For ultraviolet region, fused silica or quartz cells having high transmittance in the range of 190-1000 nm are employed (glass has poor transmission properly in the ultraviolet region). In routine analytical work, cells with 1 cm path length are used, however, cells of longer path length (up to 10 cm) are available and employed in case where the concentration of the substance to be determined is too low or the substance has low absorbance values. For estimation of ethinyloestradiol by colorimetric method employ glass cell of 5 cm path length whereas glass cell of 2 cm path length is used for assay of promethazine hydrochloride in elixir promethazine. Flow cells now available primarily to minimise the turbulent flow, through the cell are used for monitoring changes in the absorbance during a reaction dissolution studies or for HPLC. For enzymatic or temperature controlled studies, cells are provided with thermostatic control. Cells to be used for spectrophotometric analysis have optical surface opposite to each other whereas optical surface is at right angle to each other in case of fluorometric analysis.

Careful handling and care of cells is pre-requisite for precise and accurate measurements. The cells should be matched for absorbance of less than 1%. For correct identification, each pair of matched cells should be similarly marked i.e. more strongly absorbing cell as sample cell and other being coded as reference cell and this orientation should be maintained during actual analysis. This will ensure that cell constant is always possible and there is no oscillating error due to change in orientation (cell constant should be checked at wavelength of measurement or by scanning the baseline over the range of measurement).

Cleaning of cells : If the cell contained aqueous solutions, it can be rapidly cleaned by repeated rinsing with distilled water and then with methanol or ethanol. After day use, cell should be preferably soaked overnight in very dilute solution of detergents. Periodically the cells and stopper should be soaked in fresh solution of chromic acid followed by thorough rinsing with distilled water to restore their matched performance. Use of strong alkali or acid is not recommended and test solutions should be left in the cell for least possible time. Sharp glass or metal objects should not be introduced in the cell. Optical side of the cells should not be touched, preferably cleaned with soft muslin cloth or photographic lens tissue. Cells should be stored in pair in a closed protective container usually supplied by the manufacturer.

Solvents

Quality of spectral measurement is directly affected by the type and purity of solvent used. Each solvent has a cut-off wavelength (Table 1.4) and should not be used below its cut-off wavelength even if reference cell is used for compensation as there is greater risk of stray light effect.

Table 1.4. UV cut-off points for commonly used solvents (corresponding to about 10% transmittance)

Solvents	Wavelength (nm)	Solvents	Wavelength (nm)
Water (distilled)	190	Chloroform (stabilized)	245
Dilute inorganic acid	190	Carbon tetrachloride	265
Cyclohexane	210	Acetic acid glacial	250
Cyclopentane	210	n-butyl alcohol	215
Ethanol (96% v/v)	210	1,4-Dioxan	220
n-Heplane	210	Ethyl acetate	253
n-Hexane	210	Methyl ethyl ketone	330
Isopropyl alcohol	210	Iso-octane	210
Methanol	210	N,N-Dimethyl formamide	270
Ether	220	Benzene	280
Sodium hydroxide (0.2 M)	225	Pyridine	305
Ethylene dichloride	230	Acetone	330
Methylene chloride	235		

Distilled water, alcohol (methanol, ethanol), chloroform and dilute solutions of acid and alkali are most commonly used solvent for spectrophotometric analysis. The solvent should be free from UV absorbing contaminants and should not interact with the substance to be analysed. Analytical grade of solvents are usually suitable except in spectrophotofluorometric analysis.

It is preferable to use distilled water as deionised water may be contaminated with absorptive fragment of ion-exchange resin, or may contain bacterial metabolites contributing to non-specific absorbance. 95% alcohol should be used as dehydrated alcohol is likely to be contaminated with traces of benzene used to form azeotropic mixture for distillation. Acetone, usually used to clean the cell is highly absorptive and difficult to remove. Chloroform and carbon tetrachloride absorb around 250 nm and should be used above 280 nm. Ether, though transparent even down to 220 nm, has problem of volatility (inconsistent standard solution) and inflammability. Use of strong acids and alkalies should be avoided. Solvent so chosen should not interact with the substance to be analysed.

Variables in quantitative analysis

- Inhomogeneity of the medicament
- Sampling error
- Preparation of sample such as extraction
- Precision, accuracy and ruggedness of the method
- Random error including that of the operator

It is therefore essential that the analytical procedure must reasonably assess quality of the sample and should be capable of revealing inhomogeneity, suitability of the sampling procedure, precision and accuracy of the method and the extent of possible errors at different stages of the procedure.

Complementary colours

The accuracy will be improved if measurements are made at the wavelength which is being absorbed. The observed colour of the solution is due to the radiation which is not absorbed or the radiation which is transmitted by the coloured solution; the colour corresponding to this radiation is **complementary** to the colour corresponding to that of the radiation being absorbed.

Complementary colours

Wavelength (nm)	Hue (transmitted)	Complementary hue colour	Wavelength (nm)	Hue (transmitted)	Complementary hue colour
400-435	Violet	Yellowish-green	560-580	Yellowish-green	Violet
435-480	Blue	Yellow	580-595	Yellow	Blue
480-490	Greenish-blue	Orange	595-610	Orange	Greenish-blue
490-500	Bluish-green	Red	610-750	Red	Bluish-green
500-560	Green	Purple			

Common units of measurement

Units of length	Units of mass		Units of volume	
Metre (m)	Gram (g)		Litre (L)	
Centimetre (cm)	Milligram (mg)	10^{-3} g	Millilitre (ml)	10^{-3} L
Millimetre (mm)	Microgram (mcg)	10^{-6} g	Microlitre (μl)	10^{-6} L
Micrometre (μm)	Nanogram (ng)	10^{-9} g	**Units of time**	
Nanometre (nm)	Picogram (p)	10^{-12} g	Day (d)	
	Femto	10^{-15} g	Hour (h)	
	Atto	10^{-18} g	Minute (min)	
	Zepto	10^{-21} g	Second (s)	
	Yoeto	10^{-24} g	**Units of temperature**	
			Degree Celsius (°C)	

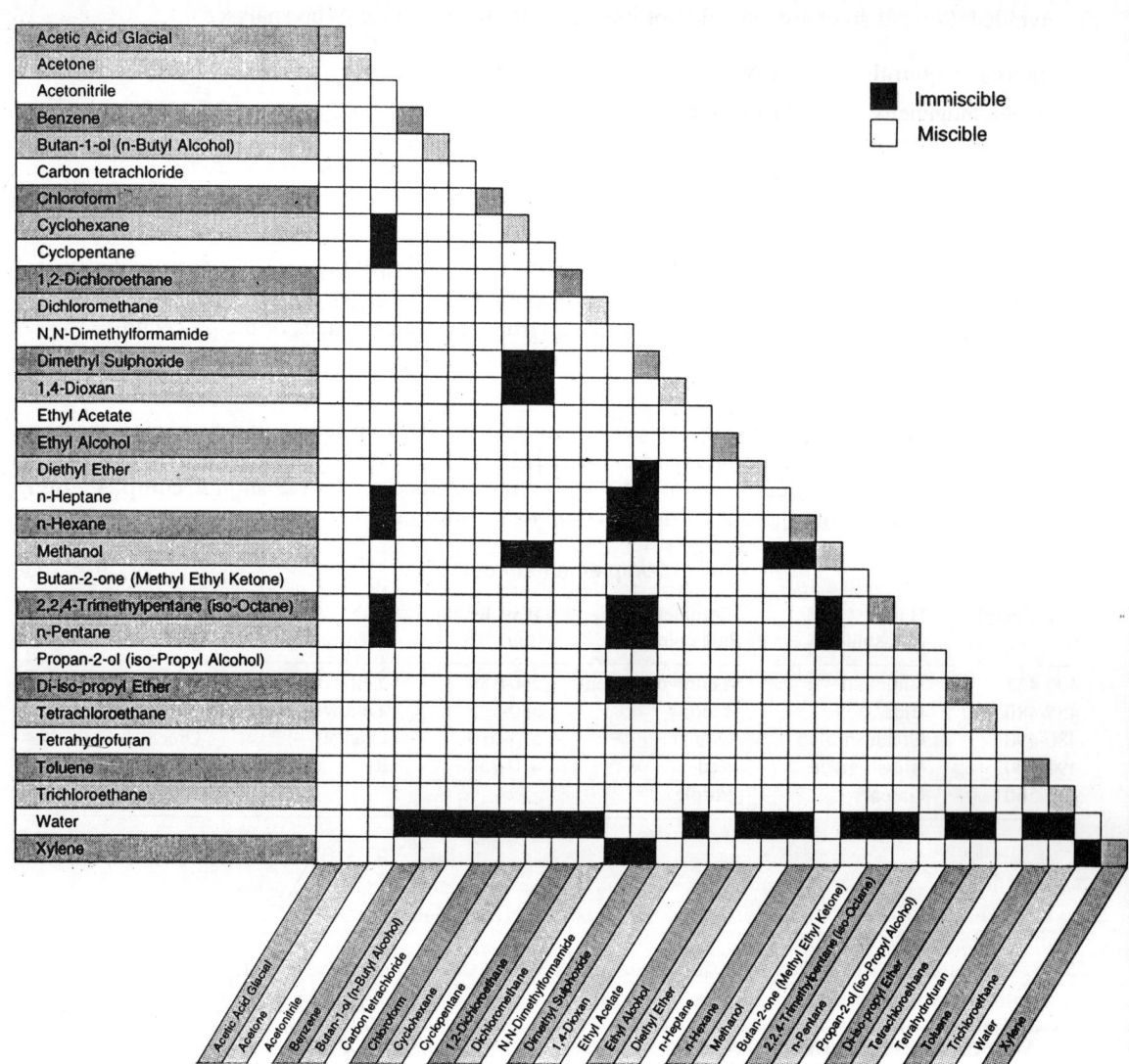

Miscibility characteristics of some common solvents.

Chapter 2

Good Laboratory Practices

"Would you trust the analytical results from your laboratory if your life depends on them."— Your answer should be emphatically YES.

Good laboratory practice (GLP) is concerned with the organisational processes and conditions with which the laboratory studies are planned, performed, monitored, recorded and reported. Adherence by laboratories to the principle of GLP ensures the proper planning of studies and the provision of adequate means to carry them out. It facilitate the proper planning of studies, promotes their full and accurate reporting and provides means whereby the integrity of the studies can be verified. The application of GLP to analysis assures the quality and integrity of data in taking final decision regarding quality of the drug.

Proper manufacture and quality control of pharmaceuticals is the vital segment of a strong primary health care programme in any country. Drugs more than any other manufactured commodity must comply with the regulations set forth by the authorities and there should be no room for substitution or variation. The quality of the drug is a degree of possession of all those characteristics designed and manufactured into it, which contribute to the performance of intended function, when the drug is used as directed. It is the total sum of all the factors which contribute directly or indirectly to the safety, efficacy or acceptability of the product. Quality must be built into the identity, strength, quality or purity of the drugs.

Undoubtedly, the Quality Control Laboratory is the most essential component of the drug industry. The trust and consistency of a laboratory's results are achieved by developing attitudes and environments that are based on proper management of human resources, ongoing controls (validation of materials, instruments and techniques) and successful communication. Of course, quality control may be easy for a well equipped and staffed enterprise, which has all the necessary facilities including sophisticated instruments like spectrophotometer, chromatographic apparatus etc., at their command, but the small enterprises may have some problems mainly due to financial constraints and the technical manpower. Such companies can engage the services of approved commercial testing laboratories to augment their testing capabilities. This policy is commonly being followed by many organisations. However the company must have a laboratory capable of performing in process controls not requiring sophisticated instruments such as infra-red spectrophotometer, high-performance liquid chromatography.

The establishment of any specifications, standards, sampling plan, test procedures or any other laboratory control procedures, including any change in such specifications should be finally reviewed and approved by the Quality Control Laboratory. The laboratory controls shall include the establishment of sound and appropriate specifications, standards and test procedures to assure that the final drug product conforms to the required standards of identity, strength, quality and purity. The Drug Control Authorities do have the interest in helping the industry to improve its quality control facilities to raise the quality assurance level of their products. The authorities should provide training and technical expertise to the industry in establishing their quality control laboratories. There exists some disagreement between the Regulated and the Regulators in this respect, but both the Drug Control Authorities and the Drug Industry are in agreement that consumer's interest is in everyone's best interest, because it is its mission and assignment both as a matter of conscience and business outlook.

For any discussion regarding Drug Control Laboratory, it is necessary to consider the specific functions of different kind of Laboratories. The Industrial Quality Control Laboratory is essentially concerned with routine examination of a limited range of raw material, intermediates and finished products. In a drug control laboratory owned by a company, the entire manufacturing history can be made available to the analyst. In contrast, the laboratory of a regulatory authority has to examine a much wider range of finished products about which very little background information is available. Other laboratories may be concerned solely with the developments of newer methods of analysis and analytical profile of new medicinal substances. The quality control laboratory has an important role to play in providing technical service leading to decisions as to the use or release for sale of material or to decision of legal nature. For such service to be efficient and effective, essential requirements are :

- Technical competence.
- Well equipped.
- Good internal organisation and co-ordination of the activities of the various sections of the laboratory.
- Co-ordination with other departments.

To inspire the confidence and respect that is so necessary for functioning of a laboratory, the above conditions are required to be fulfilled.

The laboratory is usually required to carry out the following type of testing :

Chemical, instrumental, general microbiological, sterility, microbiological assay (potency testing of antibiotics and vitamins), routine pharmacological. The division of the laboratory into sections may be based either on the main techniques used or on the type of products to be tested. However, care should be taken that the work load is evenly distributed among various sections and it should not restrict communication between the staff involved in testing of same sample.

The organisational setup of a laboratory usually depends on the work load, the nature and variety of the work, availability of trained personnel and equipments. The head of such organisation may be designated as Quality Assurance Manager who has the overall responsibility for all aspects of quality in the organisation. He must be satisfied that all key members of the laboratory staff have the requisite competence and matching responsibilities i.e. depending on the assignment, then, through a proportionate combination of education and experience, each person must have demonstrated competency for the responsibilities of that assignment.

Technical competence   The selection of the staff for this work is of prime importance. Not all graduates/post-graduates in pharmacy, chemistry or other allied sciences possess the aptitude and attitude of mind to become competent analysts. Patience, enthusiasm, determination, mental acuity and a critical approach to problems are most desirable characteristics for an analyst (*see* Desirable qualities of an analyst). The new graduates may acquire necessary knowledge and experience from training organised within the laboratory or by working under the directions of senior colleagues (*see* Grading of analysts). The training should not overlook the more basic procedures, the basic training should include exercises such as determination of moisture, sulphated ash, weight per millilitre, refractive index, total solids, alcohol contents, alkaloidal contents, melting point, boiling range, limit tests for heavy metals and specific rotation. The trainees should be encouraged to understand fully all calculation procedures and should avoid the application of arithmetical formulae without first understanding them. The more experienced staff should have an opportunity for specialised training in topics such as GLC, HPLC, HPTLC and IR spectrophotometry.

According to their qualifications and experience, the analysts fit into three general categories : Trainee/probationary, Experienced and Seniors. There can be overlap between these groups as senior analyst can be trainee in some new technique. However the skill attained and intended functions can help in grading the analysts. New analyst will require extensive training for procedures in use in the laboratory. The amount of time spent on training will vary depending on the background and previous experience of the individual analyst. With the increasing complexicity of analytical procedures and instrumentation, individual specialization cannot be avoided. Analyst at all levels should have the following minimum skill before he is allowed to handle the analysis of samples :

1. Knowledge of basic chemical principles, theories and laboratory techniques as gained through completion of degree course in pharmacy, chemistry or other allied sciences.
2. Use of common instruments like balance, UV, pH meter, polarimeter, melting point apparatus, refractometer required in compendial procedures.
3. Adequate knowledge of CGMP and CGLP.
4. Established laboratory safety procedures.
5. Communication of laboratory results in written reports.

Development of analytical procedures is an important function of the laboratory in which all analysts should be involved to some extent. It promotes job satisfaction and stimulates the critical attitude that is so necessary for an analyst.

GRADING OF ANALYSTS

This is primarily based on skill and functions, though there may be some overlapping.

Grade 1
1. Knowledge of basic chemical principles, theories and laboratory techniques as would be acquired through the successful completion of 4 year college course in Pharmacy, Chemistry.
2. Use of common instruments such as balances, pH meter, melting point apparatus, refractometer, colorimeter, polarimeter, moisture balance, required to be used in compendial methods in conformance with SOP.
3. Application of required quality assurance procedures.
4. Adherence to established laboratory safety procedures.
5. Communication of results in writing.
- Can analyse samples of pharmaceuticals (bulk and finished products) under guidance from supervisor or senior analyst.
- His work and analytical data needs to be discussed while in progress.

Grade 2
In addition to that of Grade 1, he should have attained :
1. Knowledge of use of more advanced instruments such as computer controlled HPLC/GC/IR, automated dissolution rate apparatus etc.
2. Knowledge of application of special techniques such as HPTLC/TA/Microscopy.
3. Knowledge of CGMP/CGLP.
- Can independently analyse samples using established and validated analytical procedures.
- His work is reviewed and discussed while in progress.

Grade 3
In addition to that of Grade 2, he should have :
1. Knowledge of agency's regulatory programme and objectives.
2. Experience in analysis of samples using compendial and manufacturer's method.
3. Previous experience or hands-on training with the instruments or techniques required by the method to be studied.
4. Knowledge of validation techniques and criteria for method acceptance.
5. Can select and apply the appropriate analytical method.
6. Can develop new methods or revise existing methods and validate the method so developed.
7. Participate in collaborative studies at inter- or intra-laboratory level.
- His work is discussed, if needed, otherwise be accepted.

Grade 4

In addition to Grade 1-3, the analyst should have :

1. Knowledge for use of advanced instruments such as FTIR, GC, Mass spectrometer and AA/MS.
2. Knowledge about validation of analytical procedures.
3. Planning of work for most efficient use of the resources.
4. Knowledge of statistical methods for data evaluation.
5. Leadership of a small group of analysts.

- He should be able to analyse samples (very difficult, complex, unusual and controversial), in addition to carry out check analysis or samples with doubtful results.
- Can evaluate methods submitted with NDA or ANDA.
- Can serve as a team leader for a project or study.
- Can supervise the proficiency testing of the analysts.
- His work is accepted as valid.

Grade 5

1. Expertise in operation and calibration of analytical instruments.

- Acts as a team leader.
- Conducts collaboration studies.
- Evaluates new laboratory methods.
- His work is considered as authoritative.

DESIRABLE QUALITIES OF AN ANALYST

1. Possesses aptitude and attitude of mind to become competent analyst.
2. Enjoys his assignment with pride.
3. Punctual and disciplined.
4. Has pleasant personality, is humane and modest.
5. Well organised and methodological.
6. Has initiative, drive, creative urge and ability to interact.
7. Flexible and appreciates other's view-point.
8. Imbibes confidence in his colleagues.
9. Able to work independently and as member of a team.
10. Plans his work for efficient use of time and resources.
11. Can complete his assignment (practical and written) in a given time frame.
12. Pays full attention to details (theoretical and practical).
13. Can identify the cause and solve the problem.
14. Able to think and evaluate scientifically and critically.
15. Questions what he is doing and why.
16. Always more than willing to improve upon quality of his work.
17. Possesses experimental skill.
18. Has sound knowledge of basic chemical principles and theory of laboratory techniques.
19. Able to follow oral and written instructions.
20. Good presentation and communication skill.
21. Sound knowledge of CGLP and CGMP.
22. Knowledge of method validation techniques as criteria for method acceptance.
23. Knowledge of basic statistical method for data evaluation.
24. Sound knowledge of common compendial procedures.
25. Knowledge in operation, calibration and maintenance of common analytical instruments.
26. Adheres to established laboratory safety procedures, while performing his analytical functions.

"Analysts are not merely the measuring-tape wielders but equal partners, often troublesome as their results cost money. Let the analysts be on guard against any analytical non-sense."

Even though the laboratory may have several specialised divisions or sections under the direction of competent staff, the ultimate responsibility rests with the quality assurance manager. It is, therefore, absolutely essential that he should have high professional standing and have had extensive experience in drug analysis and laboratory management in a quality control laboratory in the regulatory department or in industry and be conversant with the methods used in different sections of the laboratory and be aware of their capabilities and limitations. Head of the quality control who is ultimately responsible for final decision relating to the acceptability of the finished product should report to some higher level of authority other than the one directly responsible for producing the product. This will ensure independent function of both the divisions while taking ultimate decision on the acceptability or rejection of the products. It can be argued that a quality control unit might not have all the expertise required to carry out its responsibilities which include anything that may or may not have impact on drug quality. But the discipline of quality assurance includes the ability to ask proper questions about the functioning of various aspects of drug production in order to ensure quality. However judgement by a quality control unit must be based on facts and opinion which can be relied upon in reaching the conclusion.

Laboratory regulations should define procedures for sampling and distribution of samples within the laboratory, method of recording observations, checking of work sheets, transfer of technical information between sections, recording of technical data, care of apparatus, preparation and checking of standards solutions, keeping of reference sample, issue of reports and release notes. A convenient and well established basis for laboratory record of samples tested is the maintenance of log book of incoming samples in which all samples received for analysis are entered and given laboratory reference number. This reference number is to be used for all future work concerning that sample. The work sheets, reports and reference samples are filed in order of laboratory reference number to make it easily located when needed. The practical information and calculations recorded on work sheets may be brief but must include all essential observations and calculations including weights and dilutions. Every calculation should be checked to ensure that it is right in principle and correct arithmetically. A standard simple form of recording observations on report sheets should be adopted for all sections of the laboratory as defined in the material or product specifications. The analytical work sheet should preferably contain the following information :

- The registration number of the sample.
- The date of test request.
- The description of the sample received.
- The quality specifications to which the samples are tested (including any additional or special method employed, protocols of tests or analysis applied).
- The results obtained including calculations.
- The interpretation of the results and final conclusions.

It is important that instruments and other apparatus be regularly calibrated and maintained in working order. It is convenient to allocate responsibility to individual analyst and to fix a card to the instrument stating who is responsible so that all problems related to the instrument may be referred to that person.

In the entire analytical sequence, the personnel accountability should be documented and record should be maintained for each laboratory employee which should include :

1. Name
2. Academic qualification
3. Relevant experience with detail
4. Refresher courses and training undergone
5. Scientific publications
6. Responsibilities in the laboratory and the list of tests and assays the personnel is qualified to perform
7. Periodic validation of personnel.

It is preferable to segregate the work based on type of analysis with periodic change over to expose the analysts to different types of analysis.

When a person is being qualified to perform a particular assay method, there should be no access to verbal guidance from other laboratory staff, that is, the person being qualified must carry out the procedure as per written instructions only. If the written directions are not adequate, the individual will not be able to perform the test without additional instructions, reflecting the measure of method's transferability.

In pharmaceutical manufacturing organisation, the ideal quality control system is "tailor made" for that organisation. It is not adequate for the laboratory to examine the finished product for conformity with a pharmacopoeial specification. The laboratory must be concerned with a concerted quality control plan at all stages of material handling and processing. It is necessary to keep the following four questions always in mind :

1. What can possibly go wrong in the operation?
2. What can be done to prevent it going wrong?
3. If despite preventive measures, an error does occur, how can it be detected?
4. What is not going to go wrong in the process so that efforts should not be wasted?

To design an effective quality control system, the quality assurance manager must have free access to master formulae and be aware of the manufacturing process so that an appropriate sampling and testing scheme may be devised. It is logical to form a committee consisting of persons from production, product development and quality control to meet regularly for the purpose of establishing company specifications for new products. The major activity of the laboratory is normally routine examination of incoming material, intermediates (granules, uncoated tablets etc.) and finished products. This activity leads to the decision to accept for sale or to reject or possibility to require further processing.

The performance of a specific act must be documented at the time the act is performed. Strict interpretation would prevent the use of intermediate documents (which are later discarded) for the initial recording of the data or transfer of information. Intermediate documents such as a small notebook are generally used to record weighing or other information which is then transferred to more formal record which is signed and dated and kept as permanent record. Any deviation must not only be recorded and explained but must also be supported by sufficient reasons to show that it is needed and has no adverse impact on the drugs produced. Any unjustifiable deviation is violation of prescribed procedures. Specifications and test procedures are in many instances dictated by official compendias. The pharmaceutical manufacturers are allowed to substitute other procedures into analytical sequence as long as the results are comparable to those obtained using the official protocols. The new drug regulations restrict the methods to those which have been approved in the new drug application. But these methods are superseded when the drug is listed in an official compendia.

Internal quality control procedures facilitate correct operations. The use of control charts to record the analytical results for consecutive batches of a single product provide the means of detecting non-random variations and undesirable trends either in production or in the laboratory. Previously analysed samples and standard samples should be periodically submitted for re-analysis to check the accuracy of analytical procedures and performance of the quality control personnel. The services of a referral laboratory, if available, may be utilized where pre-analysed samples can be referred for post-testing auditing. This procedure should not be considered to have been simply designed to check the integrity of the analyst but in overall interest of the laboratory. Based on audit report, adequacy of existing staff, management and training programme of the analysts can be reviewed. It has been observed that errors mostly occur during preparatory work such as weighing, dilutions, quality of reagents (unsuitable or deteriorated), purity of reference drug substances, inappropriate methods (method which are difficult to reproduce) and variations in laboratory environments. The main cause of such errors is carelessness, fatigue, inadequate training and lack of aptitude and attitude in analytical work. The staff being assigned work beyond their level of competence should normally be avoided. The possibility of in-service training programmes should be explored to update professional competence and keep staff abreast of advances in analytical methods and instrumentation. For continuous automated analysis, standard should be assayed at regular intervals to correct for drift and to assure the accuracy of the results. Analytical method development units must develop and qualify and the quality control units must review and approve drug testing specifications for each component and raw material to be utilised in the product and its production. A representative sample from each assigned control number must meet the requirements of its protocols before the material can be released for use. The testing specifications established for each item should include the following data :

1. Product's name and number.
2. Required tests :
   (a) Refer to pharmacopoeial requirements or in-house specifications and should include amount of sample required for testing and retention for future analysis.
   (b) An amount of each reagent, buffer etc. necessary for various tests.
   (c) Equipment required.
   (d) Instrument required.
   (e) Personnel qualified for test.
   (f) Exact details of the testing procedures.
   (g) Procedure for computation of the results.
3. Tolerance allowable for each test : This should reflect pharmacopoeial requirements or in-house variance limits. It is preferable if the in-house tolerance limits are more stringent than the compendial limits to ensure that released product meets official requirements when subjected to regulatory inspection and testing.
4. Frequency for re-assaying each item.
5. A procedure for sampling protocols should be established and should include the following information :
   (i) Who has the responsibility and authority to draw sample from received goods.
   (ii) Number of units to be sampled based on the number of in-coming containers per control number.
   (iii) Method of selecting containers to be sampled.
   (iv) Size and distribution of sample from each container.
   (v) Entering sample information in the continuous log book maintained in the control laboratory.

The analyst must then determine what specification is to be used to assess the quality of the sample. If no suitable pharmacopoeial monograph exists, the analytical specifications and methods of analysis may be obtained from the manufacturer or drafted in the laboratory on the basis of published information or personal experience. Whatever may be the case, detailed note on the specifications adopted and method of analysis used must be recorded in the work sheet.

The testing specifications and sampling protocols are official master records and must be maintained in a secure storage area with limited access. The master record should be placed under the control of a single competent person with appropriate academic training and experience to make necessary and appropriate corrections, additions or deletions. The specifications of work in-process and finished products must meet the same stringent requirements as imposed on raw material. Calibration of instruments, apparatus, gauges and other recording devices at suitable intervals should be done in accordance with an established written programme containing specific directions, schedules, limits for accuracy and precision and provision for remedial action, in case accuracy and/or precision limits are not met. Instruments, apparatus, gauges and other recording devices not meeting the established specifications shall not be used. Even if the calibration of equipments has been contracted to outside agencies, the responsibility for the same must still rest with the analyst of the quality control department. The calibration procedures, acceptance criteria and the frequency must have his approval. It is not adequate to report that the equipment is acceptable, but calibration result must be recorded. Frequency of calibration is usually decided on the basis of experience and past performance of the equipment. It is always desirable that the analyst should always record the specific instrument and reference standard used in any analysis. This will narrow down the field of rechecking the analytical results in case of controversy. One can resort to mini calibration until and unless one has reasons to suspect about the satisfactory performance of the equipment. However, if a sample has been found not conforming to the prescribed specifications, the analysis should be repeated by another analyst using fresh lot of reference standard, chemicals and reagents.

Pharmacopoeial monographs describe tests for identity, limits for certain impurities, strength (per cent of active substance or biological potency) and also perhaps tests for stability or physical properties relevant to biopharmaceutical activity of the substance. The monographs generally include several tests for identity. Each individual test is not necessarily specific for the substance but may identify a certain chemical group or ion. A particular Rf value being selective is not a characteristic of one substance only. The intention of the monograph is that the qualitative and quantitative tests considered as a whole should provide adequate evidence as to identify. Pharmaceutical limits for impurities refer particularly to those substances whose presence might be expected from knowledge of the manufacturing process or decomposition route. However, the pharmacopoeia for example states in its general notices, "The requirements are not framed to provide against all possible impurities, it is not to be presumed, for example, that an unusual impurity is tolerated which is not precluded by the prescribed tests should rational consideration require that it be absent."

A problem arises when new routes are developed for the synthesis of a medicinal substance. The alternative routes may lead to impurities other than those limited by pharmacopoeial tests. For the licensing of a pharmaceutical formulation of a new medicinal substance, regulatory authorities normally require full details to be disclosed regarding the synthesis of that substance, likely impurities and control methods used to limit those impurities. However, for the manufacture of formulations of established drugs, there is generally no restriction on the source or method of manufacture of the ingredients. It appears that application of pharmacopoeial limit tests for impurities alone may sometimes be insufficient. As the suppliers of raw materials may be unwilling or unable to divulge the manufacturing process and the potential impurities, the problem is not easily resolvable. The pharmacopoeial requirement for potency or per cent purity is in some cases intended to allow for some deterioration on storage. Clearly then, when deterioration under normal storage conditions is to be expected, the raw material as purchased and the finished pharmaceutical product leaving the factory must be well above the minimum pharmacopoeial requirement. The pharmacopoeial limits are intended for application by the regulatory authority and make allowance for some decomposition during the shelf life of the product. The lower limit does, nevertheless seem very generous and the upper limit seems unnecessarily high. It is therefore, necessary for the company to set its own minimum standards.

It is a good general policy to examine representative samples submitted by potential suppliers of materials before deciding from which source to purchase.

Compendial monographs for sterility, dissolution test and content uniformity are quite specific. Achieving compliance with compendial requirements is considered as meeting a minimal quality criteria. The product manufacturers are required to ensure that quality of the product not only meets the labelled claim but also retains its potency throughout the shelf life within prescribed limits. The specifications for each product as developed and recorded is an official document and normally include the following data :

1. Product's name and number.
2. Required tests (compendial or in-house specifications) which include :
    (a) Potency test.
    (b) Identity test for ingredients, known contaminants and degradation products.
    (c) Hardness friability.
    (d) Dimension.
    (e) Colour determination.

    (f) Moisture determination.

    (g) pH determination.

    (h) Weight variation/content uniformity.

    (i) Disintegration time/dissolution time.

    (j) Visual defects (chipping, mottling, coating defects).

    (k) Abrasiveness or foreign material present in ophthalmic products.

    (l) Sterility.

    (m) Pyrogen.

3. Amount of drug and reagents required for each test.
4. Equipments and instruments required for each test.
5. Personnel qualified for the test.
6. Details of the exact test or assay procedures.
7. Permissible tolerance or variation for each test.
8. Recording of the analytical data.

Each batch of manufactured drug can be taken as homogeneous, if all the processing steps have been carefully designed, controlled and production sequences are uniform and followed identically. The laboratory test for the product under approval should be carried out at the batch level than for entire lot. The testing should be performed on samples which are withdrawn at intervals during processing. The sample being submitted to the quality control laboratory must be labelled to show :

1. Product's name and number.
2. Lot/batch number.
3. The date of manufacture.
4. Name of the operator and supervisor.
5. Name of the sampler.

The manufacturing protocols should be so devised so that movement of in-process production is co-ordinated with satisfactory completion of the testing required at each stage. This is economical as it will prevent subsequent reprocessing of defective material and recall of finished goods.

Specifications repository

Every Drug Control Laboratory must possess the correct edition of all the Pharmacopoeias official in the country including latest supplements, addendums and corrections. In addition, the laboratory should maintain a complete file of non-pharmacopoeial quality specifications for drugs to be tested for established specifications. All upgrading and correction should be noted in principal volumes of the pharmacopoeia to prevent any possibility of obsolete portion being used.

Central registry

It is part of supporting and coordinating sections of the laboratory. The Head of Central registry must be a person with wide experience in analysis and will be responsible for receiving all incoming samples and keeping constant check on the progress of analysis and final reporting. He will also supervise specification repository as well.

Reference materials

All the reference materials required to be used in the laboratory should be kept in a central register. The register should contain all details not only in respect of official reference substances and reference preparations but also of secondary reference materials and non-official materials prepared in the laboratory to be used as working standards. Each reference material should be assigned a separate number along with precise description of the material, its source, date of receipt, batch number and other identifying code, the purpose for which the material is intended to be used (infra-red reference material, impurity reference material, thin layer chromatography) and the storage conditions. In case of working standards, prepared in the laboratory, the information should include the results of all the tests and checks carried out to establish its purity. The laboratory identification number should be marked on each vial of the reference material and this must be mentioned by the analyst in the analytical work sheet every time the reference material is used. This will help in counter-checking the sample as and when required as the same reference material is required to be used.

A new number should be assigned to every new batch as soon as it is received or prepared. The reference materials should be inspected at regular intervals to ensure that they have not deteriorated and are being stored under appropriate conditions.

SAFETY GUIDELINES IN DRUG CONTROL LABORATORIES

Safety depends on the maintenance of laboratory discipline. Safety instructions, both general and specific, should be imparted to every new member of the staff and should be regularly supplemented. The general guidelines for safe working include :

1. Prevention of smoking, eating and drinking in the laboratory.
2. Knowledge about the use of fire fighting equipments and location of emergency exits.
3. Use of laboratory coats and other protective clothing including rubber gloves, ear plugs, safety shoes.
4. Full labelling of all containers of chemicals, warning to be included in case of poisonous and flammable chemicals.
5. Observation of safety rules in handling cylinders of compressed gases.
6. Provision of first-aid materials and instructions and use of antidotes.
7. Laboratory services (air, gas, water) should be turned off when not in use.
8. No one should work alone in the laboratory.
9. Unauthorized analysis or experiments should not be allowed in the laboratory.
10. When lifting heavy objects, use legs, instead of back.

The staff must be instructed to be cautious while handling flammable and oxidizing agents. While poisonous or hazardous products must be segregated, it should not be taken for granted that all other chemicals are safe. The contact with the reagents, solvents and their vapours should be avoided.

SYSTEMS AND PROCEDURES IN A QUALITY CONTROL LABORATORY

1. Good laboratory practices.
2. General procedures for analysis abstracted from IP/BP/USP.
3. Current approved and authorized specifications and standard test procedures.
4. Authorised documents for analysis.
5. Retention of analysed samples.
6. Reference substances and certified working standards and their periodic update.
7. Volumetric solutions and reagents and their standardization schedule.
8. Reporting system for each sample.
9. Analytical reference number.
10. Calibration of instrument, maintenance of log book and calibration schedule of each instrument.
11. Handling of product complaints.
12. Cleaning of laboratory glassware.
13. Records of temperature and humidity of critical areas of the laboratory.
14. Laboratory safety guidelines.
15. Opening and closing of the laboratory.
16. Validation (instruments, personnel and analytical procedures).
17. Regular job-based training and evaluation of quality control personnel.
18. Possible evidence that the systems continue to perform reliably and reproducibly.

19. Analyst data validation.
20. Periodic validation of analytical methods in use.
21. Periodic validation of analyst.
22. No dispatches without approval of quality control department.
23. Continuous upgrading of quality system.
24. Continuous upgrading of quality standards.

STEPS FOR SUCCESSFUL ANALYSIS

1. Working bench and apparatus should always be kept clean.
2. If glassware are to be kept in hot air oven, these should be rinsed with distilled or demineralized water. Inside of the glass should never be cleaned with cloth. Usually soap or detergent solution such as teepol is satisfactory for cleaning. If cleaning mixture (sodium dichromate in concentrated sulphuric acid) is employed, large volume of water shall be required for rinsing the wares. Glass apparatus (flasks, beakers etc.) should be kept in the hot air oven in inverted position to avoid deposit of any residue after evaporation of water.
3. Do not use broken or chipped glassware.
4. Graduated apparatus should neither be heated nor any hot liquid poured into it, because the apparatus will expand and may not contract to its initial volume on cooling to room temperature.
5. All reagent bottles must be returned to their correct position—reagent shelf—immediately after use.
6. Stopper of the reagent bottle must not be kept on bench, preferably held in left hand and replaced in the bottle as soon as the reagent has been used.
7. All reagent solutions should be labelled indicating identify, titre value or concentration and special storage condition, if any. If water bottle contains liquid other than water, it should be labelled appropriately (often for rinsing of cuvettes, methanol is introduced into water bottle).
8. In case of non-aqueous titrations, both standardization and sample analysis should be carried out at the same temperature as far as possible as non-aqueous solvents have greater coefficient of expansion than water so even small difference in temperature can result in significant error.
9. While taking out reagents, the position of the label on bottle should be on the top to avoid getting label spoiled.

PLANNING WORK IN THE LABORATORY

Often there is inordinate delay in reporting of samples; probably number of samples exceeds the analysis time, thereby causing analysis delay and cost. Following points may be of help to the analyst.

1. Proper selection of the method taking into consideration the nature and purpose of analysis and facilities available and to decide whether accuracy and precision are really important in given situation.
2. When a particular procedure fails, when should the analysis be terminated to try another method.
3. The samples may be grouped for analysis such as samples containing vitamins for high throughput.
4. Possible use of "Quick Assessment System" by which approximate idea about the quality of the drug (90-110% of claim) can be assessed.

For high throughput, the author has been using Quick Assessment Procedure for several years in respect of some commonly used drugs using semi-quantitative TLC.

STANDARDS OF TOTAL QUALITY MANAGEMENT

1. Commitment : Believe in the philosophy of quality and show constancy of purpose towards improvement of product and service if one wants to stay in the business for the foreseeable future.
2. Leadership : Show quality of leadership by example. Leadership is not the domain of managers only, but for everyone.
3. Customer orientation : It is entirely because of customers that you are here. Determine their needs and educate them for better understanding of their needs.
4. Team work : We are all in this together. Build yourself and the organisation on each other's ideas and strengths.
5. Communication : Always appreciate others' viewpoints. Communication is vital to business—national or international.
6. Empowerment : As a boss, take the blame and pass on the credit. Give people power, responsibility, pride of workmanship and recognition to the one who deserves; remove barriers to achieve this goal.
7. Training : Continuing education is important for continuous improvement. Build awareness of the need and opportunity for improvement.
8. Style : Believe in your own quality system. Learn from pioneers in the field, taking best from each to suit your system.
9. Pride of workmanship : Enjoy your work. You can hold your head high if you did the job right way and the quality way.
10. Drive out fear, so that every one may work effectively for the organisation. Do not be revengeful.
11. As we are in new economic age, one can no longer succeed with mistakes, defective material and defective workmanship.
12. Do not depend on mass inspection, build in the quality through evidence.
13. The characteristics that indicate quality and measurement of its success must be well defined. Critical quality problem be defined and the management must take the lead in solving them.
14. Quality is to be achieved by understanding and improving the system rather than reducing the defects through inspection and corrections.
15. Create a structure in the top management that should push everyone to improve.

Those who ignore "Total Quality Management Concept", do so at the peril of their future business. Charles Darwin's law of survival of the fittest, though a cruel law, and unrelenting, holds in the free enterprise. The only survivors will be the companies with constancy of purpose for quality, productivity and service.

RESPONSIBILITIES OF KEY PERSONNEL IN QUALITY CONTROL LABORATORY

As part of good laboratory practices, it should always be possible to trace who was responsible for certain results. Responsibility should be taken by people who should not only be trained to bear such responsibility but should have personality to cope with the responsibility in term of emotion, experience and knowledge. For this, the individual needs to have appropriate character, education, commitment, leadership and empowerment.

1. Approval or rejection of all raw materials, packaging materials, intermediate, bulk and finished products.
2. Evaluation of batch records.
3. Approval of sampling instructions, specification, test methods and other quality control procedures.
4. Checking the maintenance of laboratory premises and equipment including all instruments.
5. Ensuring initial and continuing training of quality control personnel relevant to their needs.
6. Ensuring validation/proficiency testing of analysts.
7. Ensuring validation of quality control procedures and calibration of equipments and maintenance of their records.
8. Setting up a system of quality assurance.
9. Preparing a quality control manual giving all details about the systems to be followed.

It is hoped that these guidelines will help in improving the quality control measures.

CRITERIA FOR ACCEPTANCE OR REJECTION OF ANALYTICAL RESULTS FOR PRODUCT RELEASE

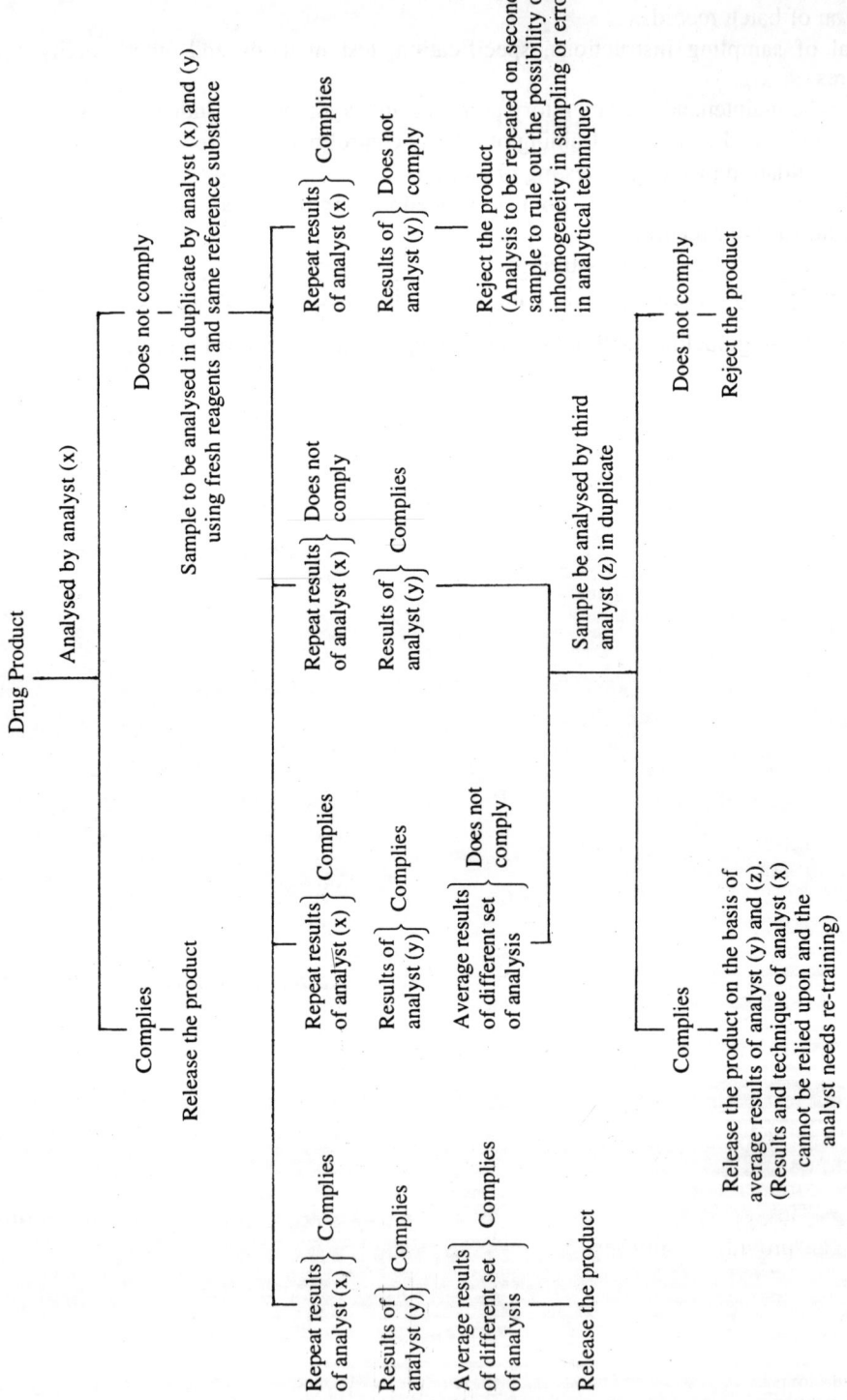

In case of non-compliance of analytical specifications, check for :

• The validity of analytical results including arithmetical calculations. • Any identifiable cause which could make the analytical results invalid. • Additional sampling and testing is called for before final decision about acceptance or rejection of product. • Identify the cause and initiate corrective measures to avoid re-occurrence. • Re-processed batch (if permissible by law) must conform to all the product specifications.

Note : The criteria is applicable only when validated analytical method has been used.

Chapter 3

General Requirements, Quality Assurance and Accreditation of Calibration / Testing Laboratories*

INTRODUCTION

In view of the changing national scenario in every field and public consciousness towards quality, the Indian industries have reached a critical stage and are poised to produce "quality" goods for domestic as well as for global markets. It can be stated without exaggeration that the rate of scientific and technical progress plays a crucial role in meeting the multiple objectives of quality assurance, consumer protection, export promotion and hence safety. Even a small unnoticed thing, for instance slight deviation from the optimum value of tyre pressure in the automobile, would result in a considerable amount of national loss in terms of consumption of petrol/diesel. Even in the world of domestic service, the pressure safety valve of pressure cooker or pan have got a tremendous impact on our day to day life. In medical fields, where detection of some of diseases largely depends on accurate measurements using medical equipments and also in simple to sophisticated surgical operation, small deviation in measurement can cause a havoc in human population. One can cite a large number of examples of critical usage of accurate measurements in every walk of our life. Hence people are now more conscious towards the kind of goods they are buying. That is why there is a significant rise in the number of premium goods with good brand name.

In order to produce a quality product by any industry, a need of laboratory is felt at every stage starting from selection of right type of raw materials to production of quality end product. One of the challenges any laboratory setting up a quality system is in establishing how it will meet all requirements for traceability. In this chapter we will discuss the general requirements for the competence and acceptance of calibration/testing laboratory, through **quality assurance** followed by **laboratory accreditation**.

GENERAL REQUIREMENTS

The function of any test house and laboratories which perform repetitive calibrations and/or tests in any field of testing/calibration viz. biological, chemical, electrical or mechanical etc. is to provide test or calibration data. On the basis of these data, decisions are made which affect all aspects of community life, health, safety, commerce, the environment etc. The need for reliable, competent testing has been recognised, therefore, for many years. There have always been problems, however, both in identifying laboratories that can provide quality testing services and in defining good laboratory management practice.

---

* Contributed by Shri T.R. Aggarwal, Senior Scientific Officer, Govt. of India, Deptt. of Science & Technology, M/O Science & Technology, New Delhi.

International Standards Organisation (ISO) and International Electro-technical Commission (IEC), on the basis of drafts prepared by International Laboratory Conference (ILAC) had first published a Guide-25 in 1978 followed by revised edition in 1982 when the concept of quality system was felt and introduced and guide's requirements were expanded. The latest edition of ISO-25 was published in 1990 and in this the guide was expanded to specifically include calibration laboratories.

The following requirements for a laboratory are based on ISO/IEC Guide-25 (1990), "General requirements for the competence of calibration and testing laboratories" together with the requirements of Europe as in EN 45001 (1989) and India NABL criteria 101 (1994).

Legal identity

1. The laboratory shall be legally identifiable.
2. If the laboratory is a part of a larger organisation, information on its relationship and ownership should be provided.

Organisation and management

1. The Laboratory shall be organised and operated in such a way that its permanent, temporary and mobile facilities meet the requirements of the criteria of any country's accreditation body.
2. The laboratory shall
   (a) have managerial staff with the authority and resources needed to discharge their duties;
   (b) specify and document the responsibility, authority and interrelation of all personnel who manage, perform or verify work affecting the quality of calibration and tests;
   (c) provide supervision by persons familiar with the calibration or test methods and procedures, the objective of the calibration or test and the assessment of the results (the ratio of supervisory to non-supervisory personnel shall be such as to ensure adequate supervision);
   (d) have a technical manager (however named) who has overall responsibility for the technical operations;
   (e) have a quality manager who has responsibility for the quality system and its implementation (the quality manager shall have a direct access to the highest level of management at which decisions are taken on laboratories' policy or resources and to the technical manager; in some laboratory, the quality manager may also be the technical manager or deputy technical manager);
   (f) nominate deputies in case of absence of the technical or quality manager.

Impartiality, confidentiality, independence and integrity

The laboratory shall
   (a) have arrangements to ensure that its personnel are free from any commercial, financial and other pressures which might adversely affect the quality of their work;
   (b) be organised in such a way that confidence in its independence of judgement and integrity is maintained at all times;
   (c) not engage in any activity that may endanger the trust in its independence of judgement and integrity in relation to its activities;
   (d) have documented policy and procedure, where relevant, to ensure the protection of clients' confidential information and proprietary rights;
   (e) ensure that the remuneration of the personnel engaged in testing activities shall not depend on the number of tests carried out nor on the results of such tests;
   (f) have provision for a clear preparation of different levels of responsibility and an appropriate statement shall be made when products are tested by bodies (e.g., manufacturers) who are concerned with their design, manufacture, or sale;

(g) ensure that the personnel of the testing laboratory observe professional secrecy with regard to all information gained in carrying out its tests; and

(h) observe terms and conditions to provide for confidentiality and security of its practices as required by the user of its services.

(i) reject requests to perform test according to test methods that are likely to endanger an objective result or have a low validity.

Quality system and quality manual

1. The laboratory shall establish and maintain a quality system appropriate to the type, range and volume of activities. The elements of this system shall be documented and it shall be made available for use to the laboratory personnel. The laboratory shall define and document its policies and objectives for, and its commitment to, good laboratory practice and quality of calibration or testing services. The laboratory management shall ensure that these policies and objectives are documented in a Quality Manual and communicated to, understood by and implemented by, all laboratory personnel concerned. The Quality Manual shall be maintained current.

2. The Quality Manual and related quality documents shall state the laboratory's policies, the established operational procedures and shall contain at least the following :

   (a) a quality policy statement, including objectives and commitments, by the top management;

   (b) the organisation and management structure of the laboratory, its place in any parent organisation and relevant organisational charts;

   (c) the relations between management, technical operations, support services and the quality system;

   (d) procedure for the control and maintenance of documentation;

   (e) procedure for the amendment of the quality system;

   (f) job descriptions of key staff and reference to the job description of other staff;

   (g) identification of the laboratory's approved signatories (where this concept is appropriate);

   (h) the laboratory's procedures for achieving traceability of measurements;

   (i) the laboratory's scope of calibrations and/or tests;

   (j) procedures for commencement of new work;

   (k) reference to the calibration, verification and/or test procedures used;

   (l) procedures for handling calibration items and test items;

   (m) reference to the major equipment and reference measurement standards used;

   (n) reference to procedures for calibration, verification and maintenance of test and measuring equipment;

   (o) reference to verification practices including interlaboratory comparisons, proficiency testing programmes, use of reference materials and internal quality control schemes;

   (p) procedures to be followed for feedback and corrective action whenever testing discrepancies are detected, or departures from documented policies and procedures occur;

   (q) the laboratory's management arrangements for making exceptions to permit departures from documented policies and procedures or from standard specifications;

   (r) procedures for dealing with complaints;

   (s) procedures for protecting confidential information and proprietary rights;

   (t) procedures for audit and review.

Audit, review and quality control

1. The laboratory shall arrange for audits of its activities at appropriate intervals to verify that its operations continue to comply with the requirements of the quality system. Such audits shall be carried out by trained and qualified staff who are, wherever possible, independent of the

activity being audited. Where the audit findings cast doubt on the correctness or validity of the laboratory's calibration or test results, the laboratory shall take immediate corrective action and shall immediately notify, in writing, any client whose work may have been affected.

2. The quality system adopted to satisfy the requirements of these criteria shall be reviewed at least once a year by the management to ensure its continuing suitability and effectiveness and to introduce any necessary changes or improvements.

3. All audit and review findings and any corrective actions that arise from them shall be documented. The person responsible for quality shall ensure that these actions are discharged within the agreed timeframe.

4. In addition to periodic audits the laboratory shall ensure the quality of the results provided to clients by implementing checks. These checks shall be reviewed and shall include, as appropriate, but not be limited to
   (a) internal quality control schemes using, whenever possible, statistical techniques;
   (b) participation in proficiency testing or other inter-laboratory comparisons;
   (c) regular use of certified reference materials and/or in-house quality control using secondary reference materials;
   (d) replicate testing, using the same or different methods;
   (e) re-testing of retained items;
   (f) correlation of results for different characteristics of an item.

Personnel

1. The laboratory shall have sufficient personnel, having the necessary education, training, technical knowledge and experience for their assigned functions.

2. The laboratory shall ensure that the training of its personnel is kept up-to-date.

3. Information on the relevant qualifications, training, status and experience of the technical personnel shall be maintained by the laboratory.

Accommodation and environment

1. Laboratory accommodation, calibration and test areas, energy sources, lighting, heating and ventilation shall be such as to facilitate proper performance of calibrations or tests.

2. The environment in which these activities are performed shall not invalidate the results or adversely affect the required accuracy of measurement. Particular care shall be taken when such activities are undertaken at sites other than the permanent laboratory premises.

3. The laboratory shall provide facilities for the effective monitoring, control and recording of environmental conditions as appropriate. Due attention shall be paid, for example, to biological sterility, dust, electromagnetic interference, humidity, mains voltage, temperature, sound and vibration levels, as appropriate to the calibration or test concerned.

4. There shall be effective separation between neighbouring areas when the activities therein are incompatible.

5. Access to and use of all areas affecting the quality of these activities shall be defined and controlled.

6. Adequate measures shall be taken to ensure good housekeeping in the laboratory.

Equipments and reference materials

1. The laboratory shall be furnished with all items of equipment (including reference materials) required for the correct performance of calibrations and tests. In those cases where the laboratory needs to use equipment outside its permanent control, it shall ensure that the relevant requirements are met.

2. All equipment shall be properly maintained. Maintenance procedures shall be documented. Any item of the equipment which has been subjected to overloading or mishandling or which gives suspect results, or has been shown by verification or otherwise to be defective, shall be taken out of service, clearly identified and stored at a specified place until it has been repaired and shown by calibration or test, to be performing satisfactorily. The laboratory shall examine the effect of this defect on previous calibration or tests.

3. Each item of equipment including reference materials shall, when appropriate, be labelled, identified to indicate its calibration status.

4. Records shall be maintained of each item of equipment and all reference materials significant to the calibrations or tests performed. The records shall include
   (a) the name of the item or equipment;
   (b) the manufacturer's name and type identification and serial number;
   (c) date of receipt and date placed in service;
   (d) current location;
   (e) condition when received (e.g., new, used, reconditioned);
   (f) copy of the manufacturer's instructions, where available;
   (g) dates and results of calibrations and/or verifications and the due date of next calibration and/or verification;
   (h) details of maintenance carried out to date and planned for the future;
   (i) history of any damage, malfunction, modification or repair and calibration.

Measurement, traceability and calibration

1. All measuring and testing equipment having an effect on the accuracy or validity of calibrations or test shall be calibrated and/or verified before putting into service. The laboratory shall have an established programme for the calibration and verification of its measuring and test equipment.

2. The overall programme of calibration and/or verification and validation of an equipment shall be so designed and operated as to ensure that, wherever applicable, measurements made by the laboratory are traceable to national and international standards of measurement and shall provide the measurement results and associated uncertainty of measurement and/or a statement of compliance with an identified meteorological specification.

3. Where traceability to national or international standards of measurement is not applicable, the laboratory shall provide satisfactory evidence of correlation of results, for example, by participation in a suitable programme of interlaboratory comparisons or proficiency testing.

4. Reference standards of measurement held by the laboratory shall be used for calibration only and for no other purpose.

5. Reference standards of measurement shall be calibrated by a competent body that can provide traceability to a national or international standard measurement. There shall be a programme of calibration and verification for reference standards.

6. Where relevant, reference standards and measuring and testing equipment shall be subjected to in-service checks between calibrations and verifications.

7. Reference materials shall, where possible, be traceable to national/international standard reference material.

8. Where automatic calibration techniques are used, the validity and security of the software should be ensured.

Working procedures (calibration and test methods)

1. The laboratory shall have documented instructions on the use and operation of all relevant equipment on the handing and preparation of items for calibrations and/or for testing. All instructions, standards, manuals and reference data relevant to the work of the laboratory shall be maintained up-to-date and be readily available to the staff.

2. The laboratory shall use appropriate methods and procedures for all calibrations and tests and related activities within its responsibility including sampling, handling, transport and storage, preparation of items, estimation of uncertainty of measurement and analysis of calibration and/or test data. They shall be consistent with the accuracy required and with any standard specifications relevant to the calibrations or tests concerned.

3. Where methods are not specified, the laboratory shall, wherever possible, select methods that have been published in international or national standards published by reputable technical organisations or in relevant scientific texts or journals.

4. Where it is necessary to employ methods that have not been established as standards, these shall be subject to agreement with the client, be fully documented and validated and be available to the client and other recipients of the relevant reports.

5. Where sampling is carried out as a part of the test method, the laboratory shall use documented procedures and appropriate statistical techniques to select samples.

6. Calculations and data transfers shall be subject to appropriate checks.

7. Where computers or automated equipments are used for the capture, processing, manipulation, recording, reporting, storage or retrieval of calibration or test data, the laboratory shall ensure that

   (a) the requirements of ISO/IEC Guide-25 are complied with;

   (b) computer software is documented and is adequate for use;

   (c) procedures are established and implemented for protecting the integrity of data (such procedures shall include, but not be limited to, integrity of data entry or capture, data storage, data transmission and data processing);

   (d) computer and automated equipments are maintained to ensure proper functioning and provided with the environmental and operating conditions necessary to maintain the integrity of calibration and test data;

   (e) it establishes and implements appropriate procedures for the maintenance of security of data including the prevention of unauthorised access to and the unauthorised amendment of, computer records.

8. Documented procedures shall exist for the purchase, reception and storage of consumable materials used for the technical operations of the laboratory.

Handling of calibration and test items

1. The laboratory shall have a documented system for identifying the items to be calibrated or tested, to ensure that there is no confusion regarding the identify of such items at any time.

2. Upon receipt, the condition of the calibration or test item, including any abnormalities or departures from standard condition as prescribed in the relevant calibration or test methods, shall be recorded. Where the item does not conform to the description provided, or where the calibration of test required is not fully specified, the laboratory shall consult the client for further instruction before proceeding. The laboratory shall establish whether the test item had received all necessary preparation, or whether the client requires preparation to be undertaken or arranged by the laboratory.

3. The laboratory shall have documented procedures and appropriate facilities to avoid deterioration or damage to the calibration or test item, during storage, handling, preparation, and calibration or test; any relevant instructions provided with the item shall be followed. Where items have to be stored or conditioned under specific environmental conditions, these conditions shall be maintained, monitored and recorded where necessary. Where a calibration or test item or portion of an item is to be held secure, the laboratory shall have storage and security arrangements that protect the condition and integrity of the secured items or portions concerned.

4. The laboratory shall have documented procedures for the receipt, retention or safe disposal of calibration or test item, including all provisions necessary to protect the integrity of the laboratory.

Certificates and reports

1. The results of each calibration, test or series of calibrations or tests carried out by the laboratory shall be recorded accurately, clearly, unambiguously and objectively, in accordance with any instructions in the calibration or test methods. The results should normally be reported in a calibration certificate, test report or test certificate and should include all the information necessary for the interpretation of the calibration or test results and all information required by the methods used.

2. Each certificate or report should include at least the following :
   (a) a title, e.g., "Calibration Certificate", "Test Report", or "Test Certificate";
   (b) name and address of the laboratory and location where the calibration or test was carried out if different from the address of the laboratory;
   (c) unique identification of the certificate or report (such as serial number) and of each page, and the total number of pages;
   (d) name and address of the client;
   (e) description and identification on the item calibrated or tested;
   (f) characterisation and condition of the calibration or test item;
   (g) date of receipt of calibration or test item and date(s) of performance of calibration or test, where appropriate;
   (h) identification of the calibration procedure or test method used, or of any non-standard method used;
   (i) reference of sampling procedure, where relevant;
   (j) any deviations, addition to or exclusions from the calibration procedures or test method and any other information relevant to a specific calibration or test, such as environmental conditions;
   (k) measurements, examination and derived results, supported by tables, graphs, sketches and photographs as appropriate and any failures identified;
   (l) a statement of the estimated uncertainty of the calibration or test result (where relevant);
   (m) a signature and designation or an approved seal of person(s) accepting responsibility for the content of the certificate or report and the date of issue;
   (n) a statement to the effect that the results relate only to the items calibrated or tested; and
   (o) a statement that the certificate or the report shall not be produced except in full, without the written approval of the laboratory.

3. Where the certificate or report contains results of calibrations or test performed by sub-contractors, these results be clearly identified.

4. Particular care and attention shall be paid to the arrangement of the certificate or report, especially on presentation of the calibration or test data and ease of assimilation by the reader. The format shall be carefully and especially designed for each type of calibration or test carried out, but headings etc. shall be standardised as far as possible.

5. Material amendments to a calibration certificate, test report or test certificate after issue shall be made only in the form of a supplementary document, or data transfer including the statement "Supplement to report or certificate number ..." or equivalent wording.

6. The laboratory shall notify clients promptly, in writing, of any event such as the identification of defective measuring or test equipment that casts doubt on the validity of results given in any calibration certificate, test report or test certificate, or amendment to a report or certificate.

7. The laboratory shall ensure that, where clients require transmission of calibration or test results by telephone, telex, facsimile or other electronic or electromagnetic means, staff will follow documented procedures which ensure that the requirements of ISO/IEC Guide-25 are met and that confidentiality is preserved.

Records

1. The laboratory shall maintain a record system to suit its particular circumstances and comply with any existing regulations. It shall retain on record all original observations, calculations and derived data, calibration records and a copy of the calibration certificate, or test report for an appropriate period. The records for each calibration and test shall contain sufficient information to permit their repetition. The records shall include the identity of personnel involved in sampling, preparation, calibration or testing.
2. All records shall be safely stored, held secure and in confidence to the client, unless otherwise required by law.

Subcontracting of calibration or testing

1. Where a laboratory subcontracts any part of the calibration or testing, this work shall be placed with a laboratory complying with these requirements. The laboratory shall ensure and be able to demonstrate that its subcontractors are competent to perform the activities in question and complies with the same criteria of competence as the laboratory in respect of the work being subcontracted. The laboratory shall advise the client in writing of its intention to subcontract any portion of testing to another party.
2. The laboratory shall record and retain details of its investigation of the competence and compliance of its subcontractors and maintain a register of all subcontracting.

Outside support services and supplies

1. Where the laboratory procures outside services and supplies, other than those referred to in this document, in support of calibration or tests, the laboratory shall use only those outside support services and supplies that are of adequate quality to sustain confidence in the laboratory's calibration or tests.
2. Where no independent assurance of the quality of the outside support services or supplies is available, the laboratory shall have procedures to ensure that purchased equipment, materials and services comply with specified requirements.
   The laboratory should, wherever possible, ensure that purchased equipment and consumable materials are not used until they have been inspected, calibrated or otherwise verified as complying with any standard specifications relevant to the calibrations or tests concerned.
3. The laboratory shall maintain records of all suppliers from whom it obtains support services or supplies required for calibrations or tests.

Complaints

1. The laboratory shall have documented policy and procedures for the resolution of complaints received from clients or other parties about the laboratory's activities. A record shall be maintained of all complaints and of the actions taken by the laboratory.
2. Where a complaint, or any other circumstance, raises doubt concerning the laboratory's compliance with its policies and procedures, or with the requirements of this document or otherwise concerning the quality of the calibrations or tests, the laboratory shall ensure that those areas of activity and responsibility involved are promptly audited in accordance with section "Audit, review and quality control" described above.

DEFINITIONS & TERMINOLOGY

For the purpose of above laboratory's requirements, the definitions of ISO/IEC Guide-2 (1986) are applicable : "General terms and their definitions concerning standardization and related activities".

Laboratory

Body that calibrates and/or tests.

Note : 1. In cases where a laboratory forms part of an organization that carries out other activities besides calibration and testing, the term "laboratory" refers only to those parts of that organisation that are involved in the calibration and testing process.

2. As used herein, the term "laboratory" refers to a body that carries out calibration or testing
    – at or from a permanent location,
    – at or from a temporary facility, or
    – in or from a mobile facility.

Testing laboratory

Laboratory that performs tests.

Calibration laboratory

Laboratory that performs calibration.

Calibration

The set of operations which establish, under specified conditions, the relationship between values indicated by a measuring instrument or measuring system, or values represented by a material measure, and the corresponding known value of measurand.

Note : 1. The result of a calibration permits the estimation of errors of indication of the measuring instrument, measuring system or material measure, or the assignment of values to marks on arbitrary scales.

2. A calibration may also determine other meteorological properties.

3. The result of a calibration may be recorded in a document, sometimes called a calibration certificate or a calibration report.

4. The result of a calibration is sometimes expressed as a calibration factor, or as a series of calibration factors often in the form of a calibration curve.

Test

A technical operation that consists of the determination of one or more characteristics or performance of a given product, material, equipment, organism, physical phenomenon, process or service according to a specified procedure.

Note : The result of a test is normally recorded in a document sometimes called a test report or a test certificate.

Calibration method

Defined technical procedure for performing a calibration.

Test method

Defined technical procedure for performing a test.

Verification

Confirmation by examination and provision of evidence that specified requirements have been met.

Note : In connection with the management of measuring equipment, verification provides a means for checking that the deviations between values indicated by a measuring instrument and corresponding known values of a measured quantity are consistently smaller than the maximum allowable error defined in a standard, regulation or specification peculiar to the management of the measuring equipment. The results of verification leads to a decision either to restore to service, or to perform adjustments, or to repair, or to downgrade, or to declare obsolete. In all cases it is required that a written trace of the verification performed be kept on the measuring instrument's individual record.

Quality system

The organizational structure, responsibilities, procedures, processes and resources for implementing quality management.

Quality manual

A document stating the quality policy, quality system and quality practices of an organization.

Note : The quality manual may call up other documentation relating to the laboratory's quality arrangements.

Reference standard

A material or substance, one or more properties of which are sufficiently well established, to be used for the calibration of an apparatus, the assessment of a measurement method, or for assigning values to materials.

Certified reference material (CRM)

A reference material, one or more of whose property values are certified by a technically valid procedure, accompanied by or traceable to a certificate or other documentation which is issued by a certifying body.

Traceability

The property of a result of a measurement whereby it can be related to appropriate standards, generally international or national standards, through an unbroken chain of comparisons.

Proficiency testing

Determination of the laboratory calibration or testing performance by means of interlaboratory comparisons.

Requirement

A translation of the needs into a set of individual quantified or descriptive specifications for the characteristics of an entity in order to enable its realization and examination.

QUALITY ASSURANCE

Recently, in response to 100 reports of children getting their hair and fingers caught in the doll's mouth, a big toy-making company, Mattel Inc., USA has withdrawn entire batch of their product when the cabbage patch kids snacktime kids dolls failed to turn up any indication of a safety hazard associated with the dolls. Testing was done by the company and Federal Consumers Product Safety Commission, USA (The Times of India, New Delhi dated 8th Jan. 1997). This indicates the awareness of the consumers, and the need for proper quality control and in-house testing. It is thus very essential to undergo rigorous quality checks to build consumers' confidence and maintain industry's reputation and eliminate financial loss.

In any analytical test laboratory, terms like **quality control** and **quality assurance** are frequently in use. In order to differentiate between the two, it is necessary to define each. Quality control is an operation undertaken in a laboratory to analyse a sample or material within the known probability limits of accuracy and precision. While quality assurance is defined as system through which laboratory conducts the analysis, the proof of which lies in documentation. Primarily documentation is designed to achieve following objectives :

1. As a proof that quality control operation or analysis is done. The details of analysis include specifications followed, calibration done, if any, or any other information relevant to work.
2. To ensure the accountability of data. It means that records indicate the results pertain to that sample only which customer has supplied.
3. To ensure traceability of the reported data without wasting time on a future date, if so required.
4. To ensure that adequate precautions are taken against the falsification of data i.e. data cannot be easily tampered. It calls for bounded notebook duly numbered and recording of raw data therein, instead of loose sheets.
5. Proper control of record book both after and during the use and its safe custody.
6. A proof of replacing testing, using the same or different methods to ensure the quality of the results provided to the clients by implementing checks.

LABORATORY ACCREDITATION

Laboratory accreditation is the formal recognition that a laboratory is technically competent to carry out specific calibrations/tests or type of calibrations/tests. Before going further it is essential to describe the terms Laboratory Accreditation System and Laboratory Accreditation Body. As per the international accepted definitions, laboratory accreditation system is a system that has its own rules of procedure and management for carrying out laboratory accreditation whereas laboratory accreditation body is a national body of any country that conducts and administers a laboratory accreditation system and grants accreditation. Laboratory accreditation was started in Australia as long back as 1947. Accreditation system of each country has been designed to meet particular national and local needs. Nevertheless they have in common the basic objectives of acceptance of the validity of test data, promoting confidence in test data, facilitating trade and commerce and making more efficient utilisation of testing facilities and resources. All countries are now following a uniform standards by which the competence of laboratory is judged. This is paving the way to recognise the laboratories that are capable of undertaking the types of tests for which they are accredited. The main purpose of national system is to accredit the laboratories and arrange for regular periodic surveillance. Some other countries like New Zealand (TELARC), USA (NVLAP), France (RNE), and UK (UKAS) started their own accreditation programme in 1973, 1976, 1979 and 1981 respectively in line with International Standards Organisation guidelines, ISO/IEC Guide-58 (1993) "Calibration and Testing Laboratories Accreditation System— general requirements for operation and recognition". The names of accreditation bodies of above countries are given in brackets.

The Indian national programme for accreditation of laboratories was formulated in 1982 by the Government of India, Department of Science & Technology under the name "National Coordination of Testing and Calibration Facilities (NCTCF). The programme became operational in 1989. Till 1992 it provided coordination and implementation of laboratories accreditation in various areas of testing and calibration, thus consistently updating a network of accredited laboratories. The laboratories were accredited as per criteria defined by ISO/IEC Guide-25 (1982) and 175 testing and calibration laboratories were accredited. A Quality Manual was not a mandatory requirement then. In 1992, the NCTCF was restructured under the name "National Accreditation Board for Testing and Calibration Laboratories" (NABL), in an endeavour to align the criteria with international requirements wherein all the applicant laboratories have to write a Quality Manual as a mandatory requirement. As a result the laboratories are now assessed for their compliance to NABL criteria 101 (1994) which are based on ISO Guide-25 (1990) and EN45001.

PROCEDURE FOR LABORATORY ACCREDITATION IN INDIA (NABL)

National Accreditation Board for Testing and Calibration Laboratories (NABL) under Government of India, Deptt. of Science & Technology (DST) is a national accreditation body to grant accreditation to testing and calibration laboratories. Laboratories desiring accreditation in the area of testing are to contact NABL Secretariat, DST and for calibration to NPL, New Delhi, which is a sister wing of NABL. The applications are required to be made on a proforma prescribed by NABL and submit to respective secretariat along with a copy of Quality Manual and application fee. The Quality Manual of a laboratory should portray a laboratory's quality system and measures employed to implement it primarily from the view point of laboratory personnel involved.

No quality manual, regardless of how well prepared, can serve a useful purpose unless the measures which it describes are actually followed on a day to day basis by any laboratory.

The guideline criteria applicable to the applicant laboratory is as per "NABL Criteria for Laboratory Accreditation (Second Edition) 1994" which are based on ISO/IEC Guide-25 (1990) and EN45001 as described above. The steps of procedure for accreditation are summarised in a flowchart as shown in Fig. 3.1.

The application, scope of testing/calibration and Quality Manual of the applicant laboratory, are examined by the NABL Secretariat and if some clarifications are required, it is sent back to applicant laboratory for improvement. After the documents are found to be in order, a lead assessor is appointed

PROCEDURE OF ACCREDITATION

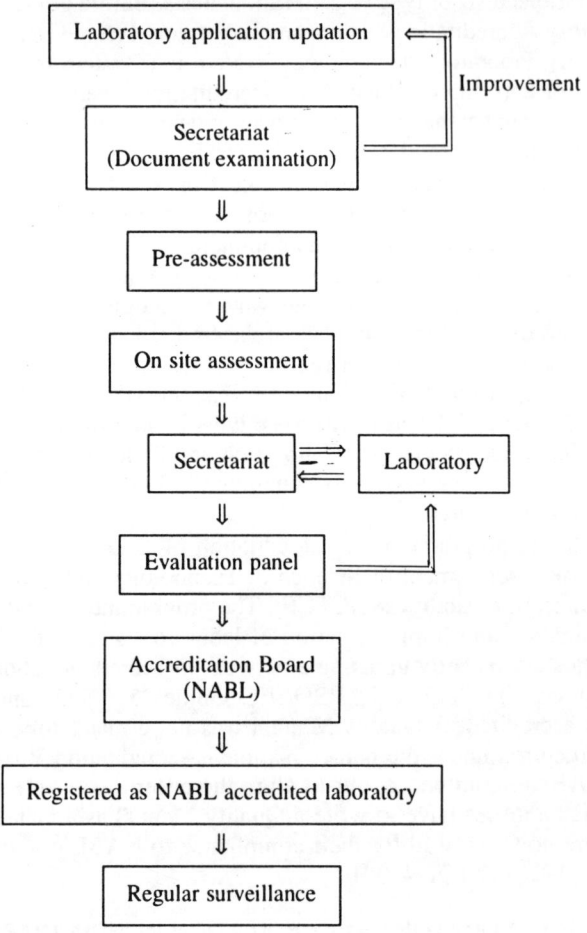

Fig. 3.1.

to examine the Quality Manual submitted by the applicant laboratory. Once the Quality Manual becomes in order, NABL arranges for on site pre-assessment/assessment.

A team of minimum two assessors (experts in the relevant areas of testing/calibration with one quality system expert) is to visit the laboratory to make on the spot assessment to see the compliance of NABL general and specific criteria of respective disciplines.

The lead assessor submits the assessment report to the NABL secretariat in prescribed format. The major and minor non-conformities observed during the assessment are communicated to the laboratory for rectification. After the rectification, a verification visit, if required, is made by one of the assessors. Final assessment report is then discussed by the experts of Evaluation Panel in respective disciplines of testing or calibration. The certificate of accreditation along with the details of test/parameter recommended by the evaluation panel and approved by the chairman of NABL is then issued. The accreditation is valid for a duration of three years. The performance of the accredited laboratories is monitored through regular yearly surveillance audits.

Application for renewal of accreditation is required to be submitted by the laboratory six months ahead of the date of expiry of validity of accreditation. NABL operates as per ISO Guide-58 (1993) "Calibration and Testing Accreditation System—general requirements for operation and recognition". NABL Board is the apex body of Indian Accreditation Programme of which the Secretary DST is the Chairman.

The scope of accreditation covers 10 identified fields of testing and 5 fields of calibration as shown below :

Testing laboratories	Calibration laboratories
1. Biological	1. Electro-technical measurements
2. Chemical	2. Fluid flow measurements
3. Electrical	3. Mechanical measurements
4. Electronics	4. Radiological measurements
5. Fluid flow	5. Thermal and optical measurements
6. Mechanical	
7. Non-destructive	
8. Optical/photometry	
9. Radiological	
10. Thermal	

For the benefits of applicant laboratory various NABL priced publications are available such as specific criteria of testing and calibration disciplines, guide for preparing a Quality Manual and a compendium of accredited NABL laboratories etc. Besides this, NABL is also regularly conducting training courses design for middle and senior level laboratory personnel involved in establishment and management of laboratory quality system.

BENEFITS OF LABORATORY ACCREDITATION

Formal recognition of competence by a third-party using internationally recognised accreditation criteria has many advantages :

1. Potential for increased business through greater user confidence.
2. Time and money saved through elimination of multiple assessment.
3. Better control of laboratory operations through assurance that quality procedures are in use.
4. Increased confidence of personnel in their work.
5. Users of laboratories can locate and identify with confidence the laboratories appropriate to their need from the Compendium of Accredited Laboratories.
6. Users of accredited laboratories would find greater market acceptability for their products when backed by the results from accredited laboratories.
7. To improve customer confidence in the calibration and testing reports issued by the laboratories so that all interested parties shall accept the report with confidence.
8. The recent liberalisation (of trade and industry) policy of the Government provides greater thrust for export. This makes it imperative for the laboratories where the products are assessed to be at international level of competence.

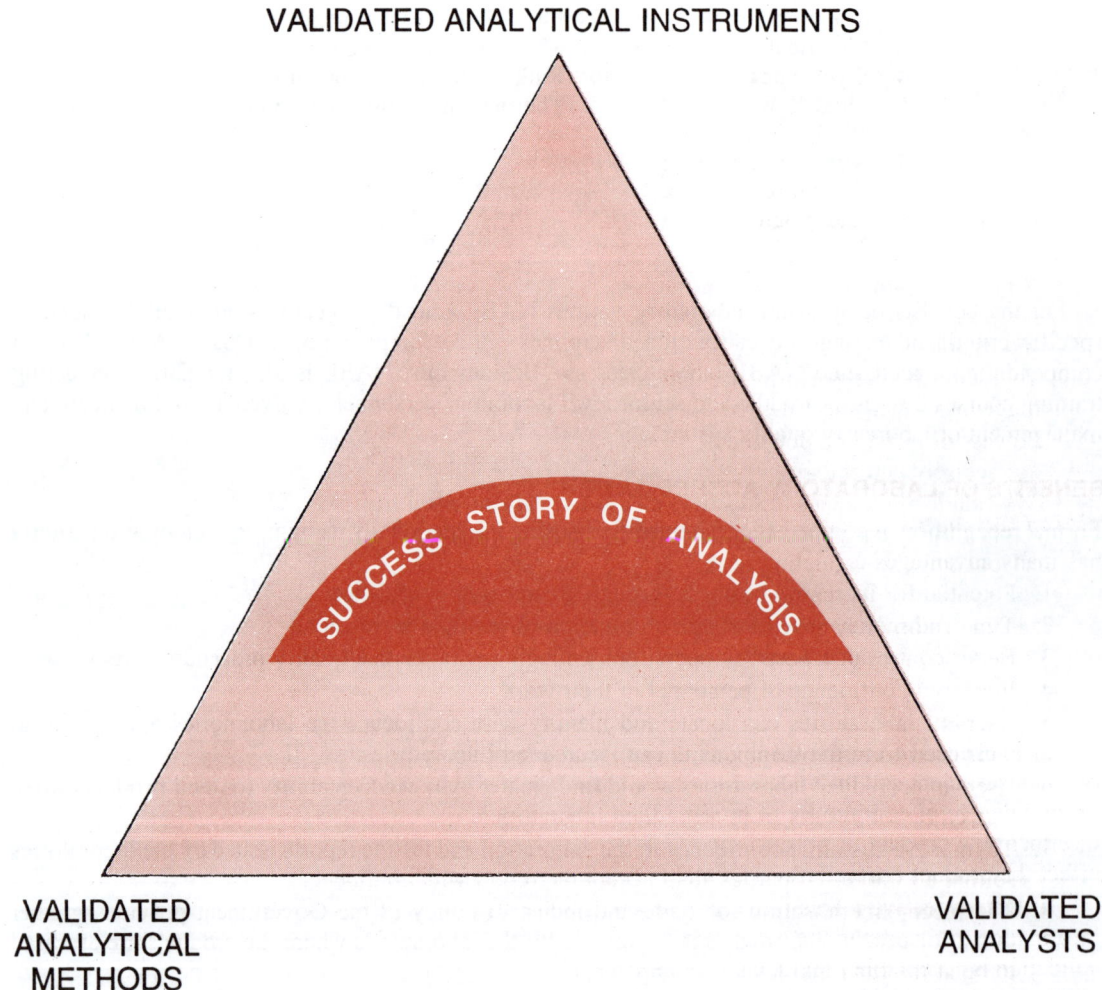

VALIDATED ANALYTICAL INSTRUMENTS

SUCCESS STORY OF ANALYSIS

VALIDATED
ANALYTICAL
METHODS

VALIDATED
ANALYSTS

**"One of the most frustrating aspects for an analyst is working with
an ill-defined, poorly designed and invalidated analytical method."**

Chapter 4

Analytical Procedures and Analyst Validation

To communicate effectively and purposefully on the subject like validation it helps if all can communicate from similar concept. It is hoped that this chapter will be useful to all those who are trying to understand this concept better. Attitude, proper management of human resources and communication skill are few inputs for validation of product/instruments/personnel/analytical methods.

VALIDATION

It may be defined in many ways, but most important point to emphasize is its practical application, concept, its significance and impact.

- A process involving confirmation or establishing by laboratory studies that a method/procedure/system/analyst give accurate and reproducible result for intended analytical application in a proven and established range.
- To establish that performance characteristics of the method (accuracy, precision, sensitivity, ruggedness, etc.) meet the requirements of intended analytical application.
- Process of providing documented evidence that the system/procedure does what it is intended to do precisely and reliably.
- Systematic approaches to identify, measure, evaluate, document, re-evaluate all the critical steps responsible to ensure qualitative/quantitative detection of analytes accurately and precisely before establishing the validation of the method under evaluation.
- Collection and evaluation in a documented form of repetitive evidence collected according to agreed protocols to provide high degree of assurance that the procedure under consideration will consistently produce a product meeting its pre-determined specifications or quality attributes.

Types of validation

(a) **Prospective validation :** This is employed when historical data of the product is not available or is not sufficient and in-process and finished product testing are not adequate to ensure reproducibility or high degree of compliance to product likely attributes. Such validation is conducted prior to release of either new product or product made under revised/new manufacturing process where revision may effect the product characters.

(b) **Retrospective :** This provides trend of comparative result i.e. review and evaluation of existing information for comparison when historical data is sufficient and readily available. Retrospective validation is acceptable provided specific test results generated by reliable analytical method on number of samples are available to allow statistical analysis. Simply pass/fail test results would not be accepted as part of retrospective validation—useful for trend setting.

(c) **Concurrent :** Based on information generated during implementation of a system. For this extensive testing and monitoring are performed as part of initial run of the method. Concurrent validation verifies the quality characteristics of a particular batch and provide assurance that the same quality would be attained again when subsequent batches are manufactured and analysed under similar conditions.

Analytical validation

Analytical monitoring of a pharmaceutical product or of specific ingredients within the product is necessary to ensure its safety/efficacy throughout all phases of its shelf life (storage, distribution and use). Such monitoring is in accordance with the specifications elaborated/validated during the product development. Analytical validation ensures that the selective analytical method will give reproducible and reliable results adequate for intended purpose. It is therefore necessary to define precisely both the conditions in which the procedure is to be used and the purpose for which it is intended. These principles are applicable both for pharmacopoeial and non-pharmacopoeial procedures being used. These guidelines are also applicable for examining physicochemical as well as biological procedures.

Reasons/purpose for validation

1. Enables scientists to communicate scientifically and effectively on technical matters.
2. Setting standards of evaluation procedures for checking compliance and taking remedial measures.
3. Economic : Reduction in cost associated with process sampling and testing. The consistency and reliability of validated analytical procedure is to produce a quality product with all the quality attributes, thus providing indirect cost saving from reduced testing or re-testing and elimination of product rejection.
4. As quality of the product cannot always be assured by routine quality control because of testing of statistically insignificant number of samples, the validation thus shall provide adequacy and reliability of a system or a procedure to meet the pre-determined criteria/attributes providing high degree of confidence that the same level of quality is consistently built into each unit of finished product from batch to batch.
5. Retrospective validation is useful for trend comparison of results compliance to CGMP/CGLP.
6. Closer interaction with pharmacopoeial forum to address analytical problems.
7. International pharmacopoeial harmonisation particularly in respect of impurities determination and their limits.
8. For taking appropriate action in case of non-compliance.

As quality control process is not static, some form of validation/verification should continue till the validated process is in use. It should not be the concept that once the procedure has been initially developed/validated and then forgotten. Pharmacopoeial methods are usually considered validated.

Selection of analytical method

One of the most difficult situations that an analyst may be confronted with is to select most suitable procedure for a particular problem. With ever increasing number of analytical methods being reported, it is impossible to familiarize with all the available methods. We are mostly relying on knowledge, experience, scanning of literature, dependent on habits/fashion—is that not muddling things. One is usually tempted to apply those methods which are well established or the analyst may have personal experience, though the choice is often limited because of laboratory facilities in term of instruments/personnel. In view of variables in quantitative analysis such as inhomogeneity, sampling error, random error (instruments/operator), the selected method must reveal all these variables. First stage in the selection or development of method is to establish what is to be measured and how accurately it should be measured. Unless one has series of methods at hand to assess quality of the product, validation programme may have limited validity. The selected method must have the following parameters :

1. As simple as possible.
2. Most specific.
3. Most productive, economical and convenient.
4. As accurate and precise as required.
5. Multiple source of key components (reagents, columns, TLC plates) should be avoided.

6. To be fully optimised before transfer for validation of its characteristics such as accuracy, precision, sensitivity, ruggedness etc.

Note : (a) Method validation for a particular analytical problem may not always be applicable in other situations due to interference of other ingredients present in the formulation.

(b) The method so developed must discriminate between the available for which it is designed, process contamination, decomposition products, related substances.

(c) Before finally selecting a method for application in a given case, trial run of the proposed method is advisable.

Type of analytical problems

1. It may be essentially a problem already solved and the earlier validated analytical procedure may be directly applied such as compendial procedures.
2. It may be related to earlier problem and the existing validation procedure may be applicable with some judicious changes/modifications.
3. It may altogether be a new problem, one might not have encountered or solved before. It is here that the experience/skill/expertise of the analyst is called for and the options are :
   (a) Use personal experience and knowledge of analytical chemistry.
   (b) Try out well-established procedures.
   (c) Survey the literature; unfortunately in most of the reported methods, the knowledge/ information about various parameters of the method (LOD, LOQ, precision, accuracy, range, interference) is often inadequate, and some degree of optimization is required.

Data for analytical procedures

(Before finalising the method, it is preferable to enlist the proposed analytical specifications to be applied to a particular substance or its dosage form.)

1. Justification for proposing an analytical procedure with comparison to other possible alternatives should be described.
2. Scientific basis i.e. the principle involved in the proposed procedure should be elaborated. If the proposed method is intended to replace the existing procedure comparative laboratory data including merits/demerits should be made available.
3. List of all necessary reagents, test solutions with directions for their preparation. Unstable reagents be identified, their storage conditions and usable shelf life be specified.
4. List of instruments required along with their parameters such as instrument type, cell dimensions, GLC/HPLC columns, TLC plates and sensitivity required.
5. Detailed step by step procedure along with equilibration, extraction and centrifugation time, system suitability parameters if required, preparation of sample, standard, use of blank and other procedural details as required.
6. Detailed complete formulae for calculation of analytical results with all terms/symbols defined along with representative calculations for each parameter.
7. Precautions or any other unusual hazards in carrying out the method be indicated.
8. It must be specified whether the method is capable of detecting decomposition products/ impurities/related substances or not.
9. Whether the proposed method is stability indicating or not.

Note : The proposed method must provide comprehensive details as deemed necessary to allow reasonably trained analyst to perform it in a reliable and reproducible manner.

Analytical parameters to be validated

- Accuracy
- Precision

- Selectivity (specificity)
- Linearity
- Range
- Sensitivity
- Limit of detection (LOD)
- Limit of quantitation (LOQ)
- Ruggedness
- Robustness

Accuracy

It relates to the closeness of test results to true value i.e. measure of exactness of analytical method. It is expressed as % recovery by the assay of known/added amount of analyte in the linearity range.

One can design experiments for recovery of known or spiked samples (usually ± 10% of the claim) in presence of expected matrix, keeping the matrix constant. Accuracy can also be determined by comparing the results with those obtained using an alternative method which has already been validated.

Precision

It expresses as degree of agreement among individual test results when procedure/method is applied to an homogeneous sample—usually expressed as SD/RSD. It is a measure of degree of repeatability or reproducibility under normal conditions.

(a) Repeatability (under same conditions)

Precision of the method when repeated by the same analyst, same test method and under same set of laboratory conditions (reagent, equipments etc.) within a short interval of time, the only difference being the sample. The repeatability of any test procedure is required to be assured by carrying out complete separate determination on separate sample of the same homogeneous batch of material under normal laboratory conditions. This is the criteria of concern for compendial assay procedures.

(b) Reproducibility (under different conditions)

When the subject method is carried out by different analysts in different laboratories, using different equipments, reagents and laboratory settings and on different days—variability of analytical results as function of analyst, day-to-day, laboratory-to-laboratory, equipment-to-equipment etc. using the samples from same homogeneous batch. Problems connected with reproducibility of the test results are naturally compounded when tests are performed in different countries. When discussing confidence in test results, a major concern is assuring a sufficient degree of reproducibility. Ideally all test methods should produce accurate results with high degree of precision and be described in such a way as to ensure high levels of repeatability and reproducibility. Unfortunately, test methods possessing all these characteristics are rare and considerable efforts are required in this direction.

In terms of international trade, problems with reproducibility often lead to serious disputes.

Reproducibility of test results requires :

(a) Inter-laboratory trials (proficiency tests) are required on a continuing basis to ensure that laboratories are maintaining satisfactory level of performance and may be used to generate reliable reproducibility data.

(b) The tests must be based on test methods which do not allow different procedures or interpretation.

(c) The accuracy and/or precision of the test methods must be known in advance. This requires the adoption of test methods which have been properly validated.

(d) Technical competence of the laboratory must be demonstrated which requires some kind of evaluation.

Solution to most of these problems can only be provided through better standard methods of testing, regular assessment and evaluation of the laboratories.

(c) Intermediate precision

Within the same laboratory but different days, analysts, equipments and reagents.

Specificity/selectivity

Ability of the method to measure accurately and specifically the analyte of interest in presence of matrix and other components likely to be present in the sample matrix and impurities, degradation products and other related substances. For this, one may compare the test results of analysis of samples containing other ingredients/impurities/degradation products/related substances/placebo ingredients with those obtained from analysis of sample without these, i.e., the method must allow distinct analytical measurement of analyte of interest and exclusion of all other relevant interferences. If the impurities/ degradation products or potential contaminants are not available, one can apply a proposed method to the strained and stressed (heat, light, humidity) samples. Degree of agreement among results will explain specificity of the method.

If the impurities/degradation products are not available, one may carry out additional purity tests by chromatography—HPLC/HPTLC.

Linearity and range

Linearity : Ability of the method to elicit test results that are directly proportional to the concentration of analyte.

Range : Lowest and highest level of analyte that the method can determine with reasonable accuracy and precision in the range of 80/100/120% of the claim.

- Use of reference standard
- Analysis in duplicate.
- Determination by least square method/regression line, slope of curve will provide rsd.
- Response-concentration curve on graph paper to establish Beer's law—response to be linear on at least 5-6 points.

Note : Extrapolation of the curve at either end is not desirable.

Three point linearity curve in the concentration range of 80-120% of the claim gives an error of ± 1.0% and may be resorted to.

Slope of regression line—measure of linearity.

Y intercept—measure of potential assay bias.

Limit of detection (LOD)

Lowest concentration of the analyte in the sample that the method can detect but not necessarily quantify under the stated experimental conditions simply indicates that the sample is below or above certain level. Limit test prescribed as percentage or as parts per million (ppm—mcg/ml). The LOD will not only depend on the procedure of analysis but also on the type of instrument.

A. Instrumental

(a) S/N 2 : 1 or 3 : 1

(b) 2-3 times of SD of blank response

B. Non-instrumental : One has to establish the minimum level at which analyte can be reliably detected—usually LOD is 2-3 times lower than LOQ.

Obviously LOD is influenced by absolute value of the blank and SD of the method of analysis.

Limit of quantitation (LOQ)

It is defined as the lowest concentration of the substance (analyte) in a sample that can be estimated

Analytical data required for assay validation

Parameters	Type of analysis			
	1	2		3
	Assay	QT	QL	Assay
Accuracy	Yes	Yes	—	—
Precision	Yes	Yes	No	Yes
Specificity	Yes	Yes	Yes	—
LOD	No	No	Yes	—
LOQ	No	Yes	No	—
Linearity	Yes	Yes	No	—
Range	Yes	Yes	—	—
Ruggedness	Yes	Yes	Yes	Yes

quantitatively with acceptable precision, accuracy and reliability by a given method under stated experimental conditions. The procedure usually followed is to analyse samples containing decreasing known quantity of the analyte and determine the lowest level at which acceptable level of accuracy/precision is attained. However, it is preferable to validate the method at or near LOQ.

- Instrumental—Usually 10 times of standard deviation of blank response; 2-3 times higher than LOD.
- Non-instrumental—One has to establish the level experimentally depending on the method of analysis employed.

Ruggedness

Degree of reproducibility of test results obtained by analysing the same sample under variety of normal test conditions such as different

- Analysts
- Instruments
- Days
- Reagents
- Columns and TLC plates

i.e., lack of influence of environmental variables on the method. Comparison of reproducibility of test results to the precision of assay is the direct measure of ruggedness of the method.

Robustness

It is the measure of the capacity of the analytical method to remain unaffected by small but deliberate variations in procedure. It provides an indication about variability of the method during normal laboratory conditions.

Sensitivity

Capacity of the test procedure to record small variations in concentrations.

Transferability

It is ability of the method to be used correctly by others without recourse to additional information. It is one of the important parameters of a method in addition to accuracy and precision.

Information

Defined as difference in uncertainty before and after experimented data.

Traceability

All aspects of the procedure including calibration, specifications of the reagents and other operational parameters are well defined. The measurement should be on sound chemical and physical principles described in the literature and thoroughly tested. It should always be possible to trace back all the relevant information about a pre-tested sample as and when necessary. Traceability is the most prominent concept used by analytical chemist to characterize quality of measurements. It is the chain of comparison from measurements back to the standard of some kind by reference to which one can estimate the uncertainty of the results.

Summary of validation procedure

Type of validation	Test for
Specificity	Interference
Accuracy	Recovery; Linearity
Sensitivity	Limit of detection; Limit of quantitation
Precision	Repeatability; Reproducibility; Ruggedness
Personnel	Qualifications; Experience; Responsibility; Proficiency
Equipment	Specifications; Vendor; Calibration; Maintenance
Service	Sanitation; Water, waste disposal

It is better to do a modest amount of validation work on as many cases as possible rather than do an exhaustive job on few and no work on other.

Steps for validation procedures

1. Establish validation of proposed protocols.
2. Perform experimental studies.
3. Evaluate the analytical results.
4. Carry out statistical evaluation.
5. Prepare the report documenting all the results.

Scope for application of validation

1. Manufacturing process control (raw material).
2. Pre-formulation evaluation of dosage forms.
3. Stability studies.
4. Environmental control/checks.
5. Cleaning controls (contamination).

Information supporting the suitability of analytical method for dosage form

1. Data demonstrating accuracy, precision and linearity of the method over 80-120% of the labelled claim.

2. Data demonstrating the specificity of the method and its suitability for determining the limits of known/unknown impurities, degradation products, related substances and other drug substances likely to be present in the finished product (multiple component formulations).
3. Data demonstrating recoveries from sample matrix.
4. Data demonstrating that neither the fresh nor degraded placebo interferes with the proposed method.
5. Data demonstrating the stability of the analyte during purification, extraction, assay.
6. LOD and LOQ to be established and documented.
7. Degradation scheme (acid/base hydrolysis, temperature degradation, photolysis and oxidation) of active ingredients.
8. If the method is not stability indicating, then limit test for degradation product must be included for assessing quality of the product.
9. System suitability test (for chromatographic assays) and standardization of dissolution test apparatus may be carried out and documented.
10. While analysing samples often overages are required to be added due to stability problem, data about repeatability parameter should be available.
11. Ruggedness data (reproducibility of results by analysis of same sample i.e. day-to-day, lab-to-lab, analyst-to-analyst, instruments-to-instrument, different time, different lots of reagents) to confirm lack of operational variables should be documented.
12. Legible reproduction of representative instrumental records/chromatogram.

Revalidation

As the method under validation is required to be used as written, any modification (given below) requires revalidation.

- One may be required to quantify additional components.
- Method simplification or improvement.
- Safety concern (such as use of benzene is no more recommended).
- Changes in manufacturing process.
- Economic consideration.
- Sample throughput.
- Complexity of the method (method simplification/improvement).
- Change of column/TLC plates due to manufacturer.
- FDA guidelines/requirements.

Note : There has to be a formal monitoring system by which qualified representatives of the AMD or QCL review the proposed or actual changes that may affect the validated status of the method and cause corrective measures/actions to be taken to ensure that the analytical method retains its validated status during use.

Following examples call for revalidation :

1. Change of sample preparation.
2. Change in dilution steps.
3. Change of chromatographic column.
1. Sample preparation (whole tablets vs. powdered composite)

   Recovery ⎫
   Linearity ⎬ To be revalidated
   Precision ⎭

2. Dilution steps
   A. Same analyte concentration and identical solvent ratio. Precision to be revalidated.
   B. Different solvent ratio. Linearity and precision to be revalidated.
   C. Different analyte concentration. Linearity, precision, specificity to be revalidated.

3. Change of chromatographic column or brand of TLC plates

$$\left.\begin{array}{l}\text{Precision}\\\text{Specificity}\\\text{Resolution}\\\text{Recovery}\end{array}\right\}\quad\text{To be revalidated}$$

Essential principles of method transfer (intra-transfer)

Most of the pharmaceutical houses usually have two independent laboratories

A. This laboratory (designated as R&D lab or AMD lab) is assigned the function of developing analytical procedure and its validation.
   - This is well-equipped (instruments/personnel skill and experience and numbers) with sophisticated analytical instruments, high level of technical expertise required.
   - Not working under pressure for batch release.

B. QCL : Where the methods so developed and validated are routinely used.

It is this transfer of analytical methodologies which presents a formidable challenge for obtaining validated results during routine use.

AMD laboratory should take care of major problem area which might have caused difficulties while developing the method before transfer to QCL.

1. Should discuss all practical aspects with authorized personnel from QCL before transfer.
2. Should provide written protocols with all details which defines the basis of acceptance of an analytical method.
3. Background information on the method.
4. Should set up method transfer protocols and performance of testing.
5. Difficulties encountered.
6. Suggested precautions.
7. All critical steps in methodology that may require special attention.

Note : Review the data for conformance and arrange follow-up with AMD laboratory if needed. Before transfer it is preferable that an analyst from QCL is sent to AMDL to observe the more experienced analyst of AMDL run the actual test or may be allowed to run the test under close supervision of experienced analyst. This creates mutual faith.

Note :
1. If the analytical method is found not to be optimum or if any deficiency and difficulty are observed during application, the method should be returned to the originating chemist for re-evaluation.
2. It is absolutely essential that AMD laboratory is aware of the facilities and conditions to which the method is to be sent for actual quality control use.
3. Validation procedures usually consist of exhaustive comparative study between QCL and AMD laboratory. This study consists of both laboratories arranging three different lots of drug products with 10 samples being assay from each lot.

Method transfer protocols

1. Linearity
2. Recovery
3. Precision
4. Statistical analysis
5. Representative batch testing

Method transfer study design

1. Analyst to analyst
2. Day-to-day
3. Lab to lab

Minimum requirements are :

(a) Triplicate samples of distinct lots
(b) Six replicates
(c) Single analyst
(d) Single day

Acceptance criteria for method transfer

- Compare accuracy (bias) and precision.
- Have pass/fail limits agreed by AMD and QC laboratories.
- Carry out statistical tests.

Collaborative studies

It provides unbiased information on the performance of the analytical method. These are usually indicated when variability in analyst to analyst, instrument to instrument is high. A detailed protocol for the conduct of collaborative studies has been published by IUPAC, 1988 (Harmonised protocols for the design, conduct and interpretation of collaborative studies, W Horwitz (Ed.) Pure and Applied Chem., 1988, 60, 855-864). Regulatory authorities invariably require the use of validated methods. The validation process produces performance data which is then evaluated by analysts to determine "fitness of purpose" before use in the laboratory. The candidate methods are first evaluated in a single laboratory to ascertain satisfactory repeatability data and robustness. Replication experiments also serve to highlight problems caused by heterogeneous distribution of analyte in the sample matrix. The method should then be tested in a properly organised collaborative study indicating a minimum of eight participating laboratories. Careful thought will need to be given to the material to be tested and the level of analyte present. Mode of incorporating analyte into the matrix is critical. Usually the mean of all acceptable results obtained in the collaborative study is acceptable. Confirmation of these values could be achieved by analysis using other analytical techniques. Recovery studies can help in confirming the results. However, the possibility of matrix-analyte interaction in real sample which could effect the applicability and performance of the method must be considered.

The data received from laboratories participating in the collaborative studies should be scrutinised for obvious discrepancies. Any such result should be referred back to the originator for checking or remedial purpose on technical grounds. The remaining results are then subjected to statistical evaluation and in particular, the removal of outliner using Cochran and Grubbs tests. IUPAC recommendations permit the removal of up to 22% of the participants in this way—it obviously implies that more than 78% of the participants ought to be able to obtain satisfactory results with a properly validated method as participating laboratories are normally at their "best behaviour" while taking part in such collaborative studies. On the other hand it may indicate that these laboratories were unfamiliar with the method or technique involved.

Analysis today is so complex that few workers would guarantee obtaining a correct result first time. This highlights the need to ensure that the method is indeed written up in sufficient details that the analysts who had not been involved in its development can obtain satisfactory results.

The analyst must be careful not to use such a method outside its tested range and field of application without checking that the data obtained are equally valid.

Procedural details for collaborative studies :

1. The method should be clearly and precisely written (no ambiguity).
2. The method so chosen must be demonstrated to apply to concentration of analyte of interest in presence of matrices.

3. All the critical variables and their effect on the results must have been determined and the need and the way for their control must be emphasized.
4. The method should provide full written details by the leader of the team and preferably tested by junior analyst or an analyst who does not have background of the method.
5. All the reagents, equipments including unusual ones should be located and available from common supplier to make collaborating laboratories to procure the same. Alternatively sufficient quantity should be procured and supplied to the collaborating laboratories.
6. The samples must be identical and homogeneous to keep sampling error to minimum.
7. For inter-laboratory collaborative studies, at least 8 laboratories should participate to analyse sufficient samples to generate minimum of 40 point data.
8. Samples must be stable to withstand stress and strain of transport/storage.
9. Reserve samples (to replace lost sample or for re-analysis of sample—to evaluate the cause in case of abnormal results).
10. Instructions for carrying out collaborative studies should be clear and reviewed by personnel not associated with study.
11. If the analyte is not very stable, all participants should start analysis at the same time.
12. Practice samples to be provided for establishing recovery, repeatability of the methodology.

Advantages
1. Regulatory credibility for method validation.
2. Best estimate for reproducibility.
3. Best way to test that the method works as written.
4. Well-defined guidelines.

Disadvantages
1. Time and resources required for conducting the study.
2. Employment of highly qualified and experienced personnel.
3. Usually large number (8) of laboratories are required to obtain a good reproducibility estimate.

Collaborative study design
1. Triplicate samples (distinct lots)
2. Six replicates
3. Single analyst
4. Single day
5. Analyst to analyst
6. Day to day
7. Lot to lot.

Documentation

"DO AS WRITTEN & WRITE AS DONE."

Good documentation is an essential part of CGMP/CGLP. Its aim is to define the specification for all the materials and method of analysis and control, so that all personnel concerned with quality control know what to do and when to do, so that authorized persons have all the information necessary to decide whether or not to release a batch for sale, to provide an audit tract that to permit investigation of history of any suspected defective batch. The design and use of documents depends on the manufacturer.

General information
1. The document should be designed, prepared, reviewed and distributed with care. They shall comply with relevant part of the manufacturing process (manufacture, QC, marketing authorization).

2. Documents should be approved, signed and dated by appropriate authorized persons. No document should be changed without authorization.

3. Documents should have unambiguous contents i.e. title, nature and purpose should be clearly stated.

4. Documents should be regularly reviewed and kept up-to-date. When a document is revised, a system should be available to prevent inadvertent use of the superseded version of the method.

5. Any alteration made in a document should be signed and dated. The alteration should permit the reading of original information. Where appropriate, the reason for alteration should be recorded.

6. Records should be made or completed when any action is taken, so that all significant activities are traceable.

7. Data may be recorded by electronic data-processing system/photographic or other reliable means. If documentation is handled by electronic data-processing method, only authorized persons should be able to enter/modify/delete the data.

Stability studies

1. Quality control (QC) department should evaluate the quality and stability of the finished pharmaceutical product if necessary of starting material/intermediate product.

2. QC department should establish expiry dates and shelf life specifications on the basis of stability tests related to storage conditions.

3. A written programme for ongoing stability determination should be developed and implemented. Elements are :
   (a) Complete description of the drug involved in the study.
   (b) Complete testing protocols/parameters and method describing all tests to check potency, purity, physical characteristics with documented evidence that these protocols will indicate stability.
   (c) Provision for inclusion of adequate number of batches.
   (d) Testing schedule for each drug.
   (e) Provision of special storage conditions.
   (f) Provision for sample retention.
   (g) Summary of all experimental data generated, its evaluation and conclusion of the study.

Stability of the product should be determined prior to marketing following any significant changes in process, equipment or packing material.

Criteria for stability indicating method

The proposed method must be capable of discriminating between principal compound and other :
   1. Known impurities
   2. Active degradation products oxidation/hydrolysis
   3. Placebo degradation products
   4. Excipients, preservatives

Methods usually employed are TLC/HPTLC/GC/HPLC.

Personal validation

In addition to in-house audit programme, there should be a proven basis of evidence for reviewing the performance of an analyst called "proficiency testing".
   1. Analysis of pre-analysed samples in respect of potency/assay/impurities.
   2. Analysis of standard samples prepared for validation purpose.
   3. Analysis of samples in replicate and measure of SD/RSD.
   4. Analysis of samples for recovery studies after spiking the pre-analysed samples.

5. Services of a referral laboratory may be obtained for post-testing audit.
6. Corrective action based on validation report.

Common problems for successful validation

1. Failure to include sample of critical impurity, degradation product or internal standard necessary to assess the adequacy of the method.
2. Failure to list complete specifications of the method.
3. Selection of unsuitable specifications such as those which do not account for assay building.
4. Failure to provide sufficient details of reagent preparation or equipment parameters.
5. Use of arbitrary arithmetic correction.
6. Use of single source of equipment or reagent without full specifications.
7. Use of specialized tools, equipments not commercially available.
8. Use of internal standard or any other reagent which is not commercially available.
9. Failure to provide fully characterized reference standard.
10. Failure to submit complete, legible data and labelled chromatographs and spectra.

Future of validation

In spite of the advances in analytical technology offering newer methods of analysis which are more accurate and precise, the need for validation shall always remain.

It is better to do modest amount of validation work on as many assays/products as possible rather than do an exhaustive job for few and no work on others.

As quality control process is not static, some form of validation/verification should continue till the validated procedure is in use. It should not be a concept that once the method is initially developed and validated, it is forgotten.

Responsibility

For validation work, one may require personnel with specialized training/qualifications beyond that usually required for routine quality control. Such personnel should not only bear the responsibility but should have personally to cope with the responsibility in term of emotion, experience and knowledge for which individual needs to have appropriate character i.e. education, commitment, leadership and empowerment.

It is advisable to get this work done from consultants under contractual obligations instead of hiring specialized personnel and facilities.

Consultant

Consultants are individuals or a group of persons hired by a company or organisation on a contractual basis. The advantages and disadvantages of having a work performed by consultants are the same in any given situation.

Consultants are able to review the present protocols and are in a position to apply experience gained in other organisations and field to problems that the personnel within the hiring company might not have anticipated. This has definite advantages as the hiring company need not go through potentially time-consuming and arduous task of recruiting technical personnel with specialized talent for particular job. This is more economically viable as work is taken up under contractual agreement with predetermined cost and completion schedule.

Precaution : Since such works are time and cost bound, the initial contract must clearly spell completion schedule of the project and the overall cost.

Essential requirements of analytical measurements

1. Analytical measurements should be made to satisfy the desired and agreed parameters.
2. Analytical measurements should be made using methods, protocols and equipments which have been tested and validated to ensure that they are fit for intended measurements.
3. Personnel making analytical measurements should be professionally qualified and competent to undertake the analysis.
4. Technical performance of the laboratory should be regularly assessed by an independent authority.
5. Analytical data obtained in one location should be consistent with those elsewhere—reproducibility.
6. The laboratory should have well-defined quality control and quality assurance procedures.

Chapter 5

Profile of a Quality Control Laboratory for Pharmaceutical Units

A laboratory can only be for analysing samples or an institution for investigation, creativity, development, training and education in addition to a trusted testing site. Reliability and consistency of results depend on overall environment and attitude of management and employees in addition to instruments and techniques employed for analysis.

Safety, potency and efficacy are the three aspects of drug quality. All the quality control tests are primarily designed to evaluate these aspects. The principal task of a control laboratory is to carry out tests to establish whether the sample of a drug conforms to appropriate specifications. The tests used for drug quality assessment require various analytical methods such as chemical, physicochemical, microbiological, biochemical and biological. A laboratory equipped for performing tests requiring chemical and physicochemical techniques are able to assess the quality of a considerable number of drugs. The Pharmaceutical Quality Control Laboratory is composed of several divisions/sections for carrying out various tests requiring different analytical techniques.

Premises

A medium size quality control laboratory will require working floor area of about 200 square metres. The premises should meet the specific need for proper functioning of the different divisions. All laboratory rooms should be provided with utilities like running water, drainage and electrical power. Each specialised unit should be provided with rooms equipped for its specific requirements. An adequate control on the temperature and humidity conditions of a part of the laboratory area is important in warmer climate and decisive in the tropical one to carry out some special tests like thin layer chromatography, otherwise no reliable analytical results can be obtained (see layouts of the laboratory).

Technical personnel

Drugs control laboratory should preferably be headed by a pharmacist familiar with many facets of drug quality assessment and should have demonstrated ability to work independently. The analysts should be selected among graduates in pharmacy, analytical chemistry, biochemistry or microbiology as required for specific task.

The various divisions are :
1. Chemical
2. Physico-chemical
3. Biochemical
4. Microbiology
5. Pharmacology
6. Instrumentation (central instrument room)
7. Animal house
8. Reference standard, specification repository
9. Central registry.

Chemical division

All pharmaceutical units need a chemical laboratory for evaluation of raw material and finished products. A room of about 10 × 6 metres with proper cross ventilation and exhaust arrangement is suitable for a chemical laboratory. A smaller room may be a health hazard in view of fumes and vapours of organic solvents, common feature in chemical laboratory. The laboratory may be provided with standard laboratory benches, sinks, fumes hood, shelves for keeping daily use reagents, storage cabinet for solvents, a suitable space (with marble table top) for placing analytical balance. Suitable placement of laboratory equipments/instruments is necessary for efficient use of the available space.

A chemical laboratory can undertake majority of the tests for raw material, finished products and packing material. Tests like solubility, identification reaction, melting and boiling range, loss on drying, ash contents, limit tests for arsenic, heavy metals, lead, chloride and sulphate, optical rotation, specific gravity, total solids, refractive index, alcohol contents, alkaloidal assay, nitrogen estimation and pH can be carried out with little investment.

List of equipments for central instrument room

- Double beam UV-visible spectrophotometer
- FTIR spectrophotometer (may require controlled humidity)
- High performance liquid chromatograph (HPLC)
- HPTLC scanner with accessories
- Gas liquid chromatograph (GLC)
- Spectrophotoflourimeter
- Atomic absorption spectrometer (AAS); requires separate room
- Polarimeter (digital)
- Polarograph
- Analytical balance with printer
- pH meter
- Potentiometric titrator (auto-titrator) with printer
- Moisture balance with printer
- Computer with printer

All these instruments should be provided with fully stabilized electric current and housed in air-conditioned room.

Common equipments required for chemical. physicochemical and biochemical analysis

1. Ammonia distillation apparatus
2. Balance, analytical
3. Top-pan balance
4. Boiling-range apparatus
5. Constant temperature water-bath (thermostatically controlled)
6. Centrifuge (rectangular with head to hold 15 ml and 50 ml tubes)
7. Disintegration test machine
8. Dissolution test apparatus
9. Flourimeter
10. Heating mantles (different capacity)
11. Hot plate
12. Karl-Fischer titrator
13. Magnetic stirrer
14. Melting-range apparatus
15. Muffle furnace

16. Nesslers' cylinders
17. Oven, drying
18. pH meter
19. Polarimeter
20. Refractometer
21. Refrigerator
22. Semi-microbalance
23. Sieves (set)
24. Flame photometer
25. Spectrophotometer (visible and UV)
26. TLC kit including accessories
27. UV viewing cabinet (short and long)
28. Vacuum oven
29. Vacuum pump
30. All glass water distillation assembly (single and double)
31. Hot-air oven
32. Vortex mixer
33. Sonicator with heating assembly
34. Deep freezer
35. Potentiometric titrator
36. Oxygen flask combustion apparatus
37. Fuming chamber
38. Infrared moisture balance
39. Bulk density apparatus
40. Refrigerated centrifuge
41. Particle size analyser
42. Viscometer
43. Magnetic stirrer with hot plate
44. Vacuum (rotary) evaporator (film flash evaporator)
45. Hot and cold air blower
46. Rotary shaking machine
47. Grinder mixer
48. Soxhet extraction apparatus
49. Dessicator (plain and vacuum type)

Note : Specific equipments shall be required to undertake the testing of any specific material such as sutures, surgicals, condoms, disposable/non-disposable syringes, needles, blood bags, etc.

No listing of chemicals, reagents, glassware and general laboratory implements is given, as such lists can easily be compiled at the laboratory. Specific equipments will depend on the number and types of various units and sample to be analysed. However, it has to be stressed that sufficient glassware be kept in stock in the laboratory to allow for possible breakage in use, especially in situation where long lead times are needed to get replacements. This should pertain to items of every day use like burettes, pipettes, separating funnels, conical and volumetric flasks and graduated cylinders.

Microbiology division

The main activities of the division are antibiotic and vitamin analysis, sterility testing, and microbial limit test for non-sterile products. Separate rooms should be assigned for antibiotic and vitamin analysis. The area for sterility testing should be under positive pressure with satisfactory locking system.

Common equipments required for microbiological analysis

1. Antibiotic zone reader
2. Autoclave (horizontal)
3. Colony counter with magnifier (table model)
4. UV-visible spectrophotometer
5. Deep freezer
6. B.O.D. incubator
7. Laminar flow, bench type
8. Membrane filtration assembly (both single and three stage)
9. Microbalance/analytical balance
10. Microscope (binocular)
11. Hot air sterilizer/oven
12. pH meter
13. Refrigerator
14. Water-bath (thermostatically controlled)
15. Sonicator
16. Centrifuge
17. Hot plate
18. Magnetic stirrer with hot plate
19. Vacuum pump
20. Vacuum oven
21. Top-pan loading balance
22. Vial decapping machine
23. All glass double water distillation assembly
24. Fluorescence microscope

General chemicals, reagents and glassware may be compiled in the laboratory itself.

Pharmacology division

Pharmacological testing of drugs and pharmaceutical formulations is one of the most important aspects of quality control. Pharmacological analysis primarily involves :

1. Pyrogen test
   (a) Using rabbit
   (b) LAL/bacterial endotoxin test
2. Toxicity test
3. Test for histamine-like substances

Common equipments required for pharmacological evaluation

1. Isolated organ bath
2. Kymograph complete with operation table, respiration pump
3. Manometer
4. Hot air oven/sterilizer
5. Oxygen cylinder
6. Pyrothermometer with 6 probes or precise rectal thermometer
7. Self-indicating balance to weigh animals
8. Analytical balance
9. Rabbit restraint boxes
10. Animal cages, suitable for rats, mice and rabbits

11. BOD incubator
12. pH meter
13. Top-pan loading balance
14. Refrigerator
15. Centrifuge
16. Vial decapping machine
17. Microscope
18. UV-visible spectrophotometer
19. Water-bath
20. Water-bath thermostatically controlled
21. Magnetic stirrer with hot plate
22. Shadowless lamp
23. Facilities for conducting LAL/bacterial endotoxin test
24. Hot plate
25. All glass double water distillation assembly

List of glassware, syringes, surgical equipments and other accessories may be compiled.

Instruments

A separate instrument room, so-called central instrument room, is preferred, otherwise serious corrosion may spoil the costly instruments. Electric supply to the instruments should be controlled by suitable voltage stabilizer. While selecting major pieces of instruments, it should be ensured that facilities for their maintenance (after-sale service) are available. It may be of advantage to confer with laboratories located in the region on the choice of instruments for purchase (see selection of vendors). Central instrument room should preferably be air-conditioned. The room housing infrared spectrophotometer should be fitted with dehumidifier. Regular calibration of all the instruments used to measure the physical properties of drug substances or their dosage forms is absolutely essential and a specific schedule should be established for each type of instrument. Standard operating procedure should be placed besides the complicated instruments along with the schedule for calibration. A separate log book should be maintained for each instrument which should include : when the instrument was last used, who had used it and the purpose for which it was used. Pharmacopoeial monographs on dissolution test clearly envisage the calibration of the required apparatus. It is interesting to note that a disintegration test apparatus which is so commonly used is given least attention; also requires calibration for its upward-downward movements.

Maintenance and calibration of instruments and apparatus

It is primarily responsibility of the analyst who operates the instrument to ensure that the instrument is of appropriate design, adequate capacity to perform intended functions consistently and precisely. Obviously, ultimate responsibility for accuracy and precision of an instrument and data it generates is with the analyst using the equipment. It is therefore essential that instruments be inspected, cleaned and adequately maintained. The need for calibration and/or standardization of the instruments is well recognised among scientific community for obtaining analytical data to be subjected to validation process. The laboratory should establish schedules for each instrument based on the recommendations of the manufacturer or based on own laboratory experience.

Note : No instrument will be used until and unless calibrated or checked for its performance while undertaking the development of a new method.

Calibration : Comparison with standard measurement or instrument of a known accuracy to detect, co-relate or eliminate by adjustment any variation in the accuracy of the instrument being compared.

Standardization : Comparison with a standard of known and accepted value such as use of standard weights in calibration of analytical balances.

Every laboratory instrument should comply with :

(a) Installation qualification : Checking of instrument against standard of operating environments, physical connections, safety parameters and functional parameters prior to the initial utilisation of the system. It will confirm that the system is correctly installed.

(b) Operational qualifications : It is the process to ensure that the instrument performs consistently as specified over all the intended operating ranges.

(c) Performance qualification : It is the process of testing normal operations and requires continuing evidence that the system is in control such as by generating control charts with calibrating data.

Since **analytical balance** is the most important instrument employed in any analytical laboratory and may contribute significantly to any analytical error, the detailed procedure for its use, maintenance and calibration is described for guidance of analysts particularly the newer ones.

Factors influencing the accuracy of a weighing balance

It is presumed that the analysts are well acquainted with the principles of weighing and its use in weighing. Weighing accuracy is usually not indicated in the protocols of an analytical procedure. Accuracy (agreement between weighing results and actual mass of the sample) largely depends on the analyst who weighs the sample and the environment rather than the BALANCE. Validity of any analytical work depends on how accurately the sample has been weighed and if the weighing is not accurate, the validity of analytical result will always remain questionable.

Following points are intended to draw attention to certain important practical aspects to ensure accuracy of the balance and consequent weighing.

- Sample must not be weighed directly on the balance pans.
- Hot objects must be cooled to room temperature before introducing into the balance. If the sample is warm relative to the balance, convection currents cause the pan to be buoyed up; weighing results will be unstable and non-reproducible, hence weigh the sample at ambient temperature neither cold nor hot.
- Some samples may take up water or carbon dioxide from the air during weighing or lose weight even at room temperature due to volatile nature. For meaningful results, the sample must be handled and weighed in a sealed, capped bottle.
- Liquid samples should always be weighed in a suitable stoppered container—weighing bottle—to avoid spilling of material on the balance pan or inside the case of balance.
- A sample carrying a charge of static electricity is attracted to various parts of the balance or has tendency to jump when handled with a spatula tip, leading to erratic, non-repeatable weighing results. This can easily be overcome by controlling the humidity to constant level, i.e., above 30% RH or static electricity may be discharged with anti-static gun if available.
- As a rule finer the readability of a balance, the more critical is the choice of location. Preferably analytical balance should be kept away from air current such as windows, doors, heat, air-conditioning outlets. Exposure to strong radiant heat source such as direct sunlight, ovens, hot water-baths should be avoided.
- Never locate the electronic balance in the main chemical laboratory or near water taps, wash basin.
- Instrument room housing electronic equipments should have no water connection; any waste may be collected in a suitable container and disposed of outside.
- The balance should preferably be installed on a vibration proof table, stone tables are preferred (balances are affected by vibrations—from rotating machines, elevators, slamming doors, nearby road traffic). Electronic balances are less prone to the effect of vibrations than the mechanical balances.
- Balance should not share the same powerline circuit with another equipment as it may cause interference. A powerline filter is usually recommended.
- Zero point and calibration of the balance are affected by variations in temperature. Normal indoor

laboratory conditions are adequate. Since electronic balances produce heat (10-20 W), it is desirable that the balance is left constantly under power in order to avoid warming off drift at the beginning of any weighing. It is for these reasons that in most of the electronic balances "ON-OFF" is for turning off the display, but keeps power "ON" for rest of the system.

- Allow the balance to stabilize before making any weighing, preferably leave the balance turned on permanently.
- Keep the balance chamber closed at all times except when adding or removing the objects to be weighed as changes in temperature, humidity, air current, vibrations will alter the readings.
- Handle all the containers or objects with either tweezers or tongs. Handling with fingers can change the temperature or leave grease smudge that will obviously alter the weight; to handle tared apparatus, make use of finger cots or gloves.
- Make readings without delay, allow enough time for sample to come to an equilibrium and the display to stabilize.

  Note : It may not be necessary to weigh the sample to a degree of accuracy if same level of accuracy cannot be achieved in subsequent steps of analysis. In volumetric work, the accuracy of the apparatus (volumetric flasks, pipettes) is about $\pm 0.2\%$, therefore for weighing 1 g of the sample up to ± 0.0001 g is not necessary as it will give an error of only $\pm 0.01\%$ in weighing.

- Since electronic balances read the weight directly, the analyst is likely to become complacent and may assume that all readings are correct at all times—*it is not so*. Balances need frequent calibration—for this a calibrated 100 mg weight can serve as a useful daily check on balance and gives confidence in balance reading.
- To clean the weighing pan and housing, a soft cloth with a mild detergent is sufficient. Do not use any strong solvent for the purpose. To remove solid residue use of nylon brush is suggested.
- Small bags containing dried silica gel (indicating type) should be kept inside the chamber of the balance. When silica gel turns pink, it may be regenerated by heating in an oven at 105°C till it acquires uniform blue colour.
- In balances having built-in calibration facility, manufacturing tolerance is usually 100 ± 0.0002 g. This small uncertainty is of no significant value in practical applications. However, serious problem often confronted is that due to surface contamination, the built-in weight may change. It is therefore desirable that occasionally calibration must be checked with a reliable standard mass—a certified weight.
- There are deviations in weighing results when the sample is kept in the middle and then in other position on weighing pan. This kind of error is usually small, however, weighing load should never be kept off centre.
- Balance doors must be closed when final weighing is done. Balances with facility for auto opening-closing of doors are now available.

Note : Minimum sample weight should be at least 3000 times the standard deviation of the balance.

General precautions for weighing the sample

- In case of samples being hygroscopic, or deliquescent, the exposure to atmosphere be reduced to minimum.
- If the sample is to be transferred to a vessel with narrow aperture, make use of funnel.
- Ensure that mouth of the vessel to which sample is being transferred is absolutely dry.
- Do not return any sample to weighing bottle after it has been transferred to receiving vessel.
- Weighing vessel should not be too large to avoid any changes due to absorption of moisture and also avoid exceeding the capacity of the balance.

Standard operating procedure and calibration of analytical balances

Weighing is the single most used step in all analytical procedures. Most common problem encountered during weighing is the balance drift, the primary causes for the same are :

1. Improper leveling of balance.
2. Balance doors not closed while weighing.
3. Vibration from other operations in the laboratory.
4. Balance not located in suitable laboratory area.
5. Temperature variations in balance housing and the sample.

Before weighing any sample these causes should be eliminated. All direct reading electronic balances should be left with power 'ON' as electricity consumption is negligible. This will ensure that balance has temperature equilibrium while weighing. Alternatively, at least 1 hour is recommended for equilibrium (microbalances even may need 24 hours to reach equilibrium).

Note : Balance drift, if any, can be determined by weighing a fixed weight on daily basis.

The following guidelines are intended to ensure that the weighing, the most common source of error, is correct and reliable.

1. Check power and position of the level bubble.
2. Calibrate with internal 20 g weight for analytical balance and with 100 mg as a microbalance before making any weighing.
3. Do not depend on any prior calibration.
4. Each day, a fixed weight stored in the balance housing should be weighed and any deviation of more than one in the place indicated below for the particular balance should be reported.
   (a) Analytical balance : Use 20 g weight; there should be no variation in the observed weight in the first four places to the right of decimal.
   (b) Microbalance : Use 100 mg weight; there should be no variation in the first three places to the right of decimal.

   Note : Accuracy of weight (20 g or 100 mg) is not important, aim of above check is to find out if any drift has been there. Weighing of fixed weights will determine whether the knife edge is defective or not. If there is no drift, there will be no variation in the observed weight in the first four or three places as the case may be.

5. Weigh the samples when they are at the same temperature as the balance.
6. Record the weight after the reading is stable for at least few seconds. Do not allow the sample to remain on the balance for longer period as there can be change in weight due to humidity.
7. If the sample has been stored in refrigerator allow sufficient time for the sample and the container to attain temperature as that of balance.
8. Do not open the container until sample and container are at equilibrium to prevent condensation of moisture in the sample.
9. Weights or samples should be just placed (not dropped) on the pan to avoid damage to the balance.

Note : The above procedure will eliminate or reduce the errors. The extra time required for checking will be compensated by improved accuracy of the results.

Calibration of Sartorius BP series analytical balances

- Ensure that the balance has been checked for any drift and is placed on vibration-free surface.
- Handle weights only with non-scratching forceps.
- Use only certified weights.
- Allow at least 30 min time for initial warm up.
- If necessary, remove the pan and clean with fibre-free cloth and alcohol.
- Calibration may be done at least at four months interval.

A. Accuracy and precision for higher range (110/210 g)

(a) Low-load test
1. Set the balance for appropriate range—110 or 210 g.

2. Place 10 g weight in the middle of pan and tare the balance to read zero.
3. Add 1 g weight to this pan and record the readings.
4. Remove 1 g weight, the balance which had earlier been tared with respect to 10 g weight should show zero reading.
5. Repeat the step (3) and (4) to get five values.
6. Calculate mean and standard deviations of five values, apply correction if 1 g weight used differs from the actual standard weight. The balance complies with specifications if the corrected mean value is 1.0 g $\pm$ 0.00021 g with standard deviation of 1.4×10^{-4} g.

(b) High-load test

1. Place 105 g (100 + 5) weights on the pan and tare the balance to read zero.
2. Carry out the steps 2 to 5 as above.

The balance complies with specifications if the corrected mean value is 1.0 g $\pm$ 0.00033 g with standard deviation of 2.2×10^{-4} g.

B. Accuracy and precision of lower range (30/60 g)

1. Carry out the above steps using initially 5 g (low-load test) or 25 g (5 + 20) (high-load test).
2. Corrected mean values are 1.0 g $\pm$ 0.000042 g (Sd—2.8×10^{-5} g) for low-load and 1.0 g $\pm$ 0.000054 g (Sd—3.6×10^{-5} g) for high-load test.

Note :   1. Usually the manufacturers provide details about accuracy and precision of a balance which is the guiding factor for calibration of a balance.
2. In general, the performance of the balance can be checked by using fixed weight procedure as described above.

Calibration of UV-visible spectrophotometer

One of the most important part of any validation plan is the procedures put in place to ensure that the instrument systems are in calibration as calibration is one of the fundamental building blocks that ensure compliance. For calibration of UV-visible spectrophotometer many methods have been suggested each having its problems and limitations. Various parameters to be validated are absorbance accuracy, wavelength accuracy, stray light (220 nm and 340 nm), drift and noise.

Most commonly recommended method for checking absorbance accuracy is to use solution of potassium dichromate (6.006 mg/100 ml in 0.005 N sulphuric acid). It exhibits characteristic spectral graph having minima (valley) at 235 and 313 nm and maxima at 257 and 350 nm (Fig. 5.2). In addition to resulting process errors that arise from making up the solutions, potassium dichromate is a notorious oxidizing agent resulting in very poor stability of the solution. Off-the-shelf made up solutions have their merits but their stability cannot be guaranteed once the bottle has been opened. Many customers use filters those having calibration traceable to international standards. Filter tolerances have to be taken into account but these errors are consistent for a given set of conditions. Usually, a set of four neutral density filters are available. Holmium filler for absorbance accuracy, Didymium filter for wavelength accuracy and two filters designed to assess stray light at 220 nm and 340 nm. One can use 1.2% solution of potassium chloride to check the level of stray light. Fig. 5.3 shows the typical spectral graph with Holmium oxide glass filter with characteristic maxima at 241.5, 287.5, 360.9, 445.2, 460.5 and 536.2 nm.

Note :   1. For calibration of wavelength, tolerance of $\pm$ 1 nm in the range of 200-400 nm and $\pm$ 3 nm in visible range is usually recommended.
2. Level of stray light increases with the age of instrument.

Indian pharmacopoeia recommends the use of holmium perchloride solution, the emission lines of deuterium lamp or the lines of mercury vapour lamp. Using the emission lines from deuterium lamp has the benefit as the source is present in the instrument. However, this source has only two useful wavelengths i.e. 656.1 nm and 486.0 nm (Fig. 5.4), hence the complete wavelength range especially the UV region cannot be checked. Incidentally, most of the drug substances absorb in UV region. Recently, new models of UV-visible spectrophotometer having mercury vapour lamp have been introduced. The emission lines of mercury vapour lamp covers the entire wavelength range (Fig. 5.5).

Table 5.1. Absorbance accuracy of UV-visible spectrophotometers using 60.0 mg/litre of potassium dichromate solution in 0.005 M sulphuric acid

Wavelength (nm)	A 1%, 1 cm	Absorbance
235 nm (minima/valley)	124.54	0.748 (0.740-0.756)
257 (maxima)	144.02	0.865 (0.856-0.894)
313 nm (minima/valley)	48.62	0.292 (0.289-0.295)
350 (maxima)	106.56	0.640 (0.634-0.646)

Typical Calibration/Validation Sheet of an Instrument

Name of the Section/Division

Name of the instrument and manufacturer   Date of validation

Calibration standard

Result   Tolerance limit

Next date of calibration/validation

Remarks

Signature of validation analyst

Calibration/validation record of UV-visible spectrophotometer

Name of the manufacturer ....   Model No. and year of manufacture ....
Division of the laboratory where installed and Lab. No. ....
Date of installation ....   Previous calibration date ....
Re-calibration date ....
Date of test ....

Parameter validated	Status
Absorbance accuracy	Passes
Wavelength accuracy	Passes
Linearity check	Passes
Drift	Passes
Noise (0A/2A)	Passes
Stray light (220/340 nm)	Passes

Comments : On this day, the instrument identified above has been calibrated/validated and meets the manufacturer's specifications.

(Name & signature of calibrating analyst)

Schedule for calibration/inspection of some major instruments

Instrument	Interval (months)
UV-visible spectrophotometer	6
Infrared spectrophotometer	4
NMR spectrometer	6
Thermogravimetric analyser	6
Polarimeter	6
Fluorimeter	4
pH meter	6
Dissolution test apparatus	3
Disintegration test apparatus	6
Ultrasonic water-bath	6
Heating baths (constant temperature)	4
Analytical balance	3 (Fixed weight calibration on daily basis)

This schedule helps in service contract with the manufacturer/distributor.

SELECTION OF VENDOR (SCIENTIFIC EQUIPMENT SUPPLIER)

"Certification and qualification of vendors/suppliers of raw material, instruments and other inventories should be the responsibility of quality control department and be part of pre-approval programme of all potential vendors/suppliers."

One of the most difficult task in choosing an instrument is selecting a vendor because human interaction, personalities and emotions come into the picture. It is advisable to make several contacts with one or more vendors' representatives before selecting an instrument as people will be your main source of information about the product and the manufacturer. You should feel comfortable while speaking with them, asking them questions and hearing their advice. Try calling the technical support line and see how quickly and accurately they answer your questions. The best measure of a vendor is the satisfaction of the current users of the product you are planning to purchase. Most vendors will supply you the names, addresses and telephone numbers of only selected users, who are almost always happy with the product and after-sale service. To get less biased evaluation of a vendor, it is preferable if you can find users through other channels such as professional societies, scientific seminars/conferences and other professional contacts. However, it is preferable that the vendor (SES) should have greater expertise than the customer on the technique and the instrument being offered.

To help the analysts to select the vendors, and procurement of instrument with required specifications, some important guidelines have been compiled.

CRITERIA FOR PREPARING SPECIFICATIONS AND CONFIGURATIONS OF ANALYTICAL INSTRUMENTS
(Validated analytical procedures to be followed only in the laboratory)

1. Nature of analytical work (quality control, R & D, in-process control).
2. Is the analysis required qualitative, semi-quantitative or quantitative?
3. Are the reference standards available for comparison?
4. What is the degree of analytical precision and accuracy required?
5. What is the expected range of analyte concentration?
6. What is the quantity of sample usually available for each analysis?
7. What is the probable sample matrix and which component of the matrix is likely to interfere in the analysis?
8. Are you required to follow only compendial (USP/BP/IP/EP/JP) methods or alternative methods of analysis can also be employed?

9. Pre-installation requirements.
10. What safety practices are required?
11. Number of samples to be analysed per day (throughput per day).
12. How quickly the results are required?
13. Is automation required? If so, to what extent?
14. Do you plan to upgrade the instrument at later date to meet future requirements?
15. Are measurements to be done in a laboratory, plant or at field site?
16. What type of instruments are being used in other laboratories engaged in similar analytical work?
17. Spares and consumables.
18. Are there any economic constraints?
19. Academic qualifications and training level of the personnel who will handle the instruments.

Note : Usually some degree of compromise is necessary; high throughput is not usually compatible with precision. One must assign priorities to various factors considering the ultimate objective of analysis and future planning.

"Do not hesitate to consult fellow analysts before final decision."

GUIDELINES FOR SELECTION OF VENDOR FOR PURCHASE OF ANALYTICAL INSTRUMENTS

Vendor : Scientific equipment supplier (SES)

1. Is the vendor specialized in the analytical field or is just a trader?
2. Is the vendor dedicated to selling analytical instruments only or is just a small part of a big organisation?
3. What is the financial status of the vendor?
4. For how long the vendor has been in the field of selling analytical instruments (vendor's previous experience)?
5. Vendor's familiarity with CGMP and CGLP?
6. For how long the vendor has been exclusive selling agent or authorised dealer for various companies manufacturing analytical instruments?
7. Has the vendor lost any dealership or agency of any manufacturer in the last two years? If so, what were the reasons?
8. Does the vendor has the list of customers particularly in your region to whom he has supplied the instruments in the last two years?
9. Can the vendor provide the list of customers whose instrument has not broken down for more than five years?
10. Can the vendor establish that the instruments under consideration are proven to operate satisfactorily in Indian conditions?
11. Will the vendor carry out after-sale service of the instrument? Has he the facilities for annual service contract? If so, what will be the charges?
12. Before finalising the purchase, can the vendor arrange practical demonstration of the instrument with actual sample analysis of your field?
13. Is the vendor equipped with application laboratory and trained technical personnel?
14. Will the vendor provide necessary help and guidance in developing and validating method of analysis?
15. Does the vendor support the customer for training including the level of training in his application laboratory? If so, are there any financial effects?
16. Will the vendor import the instrument and supply you in Indian Rupee?
17. Will the vendor assist you in getting various formalities including custom clearance completed in case you want to import yourself?

18. Does the vendor usually stock substantial amount of consumables required for maintenance and after-sale service of the instrument?
19. Does the vendor has the facilities for updating the knowledge of your analysts from time to time with application notes?
20. Will the vendor be arranging workshop/seminars from time to time? If so, what shall be the charges for participating in them?
21. Has he informed you the additional facilities required in your laboratory for installation and operation of the said instrument and has your laboratory been adequately equipped as suggested?
22. Have you any previous experience with the vendor either directly or through knowledge gained from other laboratories? If so, how do you assess his general performance particularly in respect of after-sale service and your own confidence in vendor's ability?
23. Have you prepared the detailed specifications of the instrument you are looking for, considering the requirements of your laboratory before making trade enquiries?
24. Have you consulted your fellow analysts in the field known to you before making final choice of the instrument?
25. Are you satisfied that the instrument to be procured shall meet your present requirements and can be updated to meet future requirements?
26. If you are duplicating the instrument, take into consideration the past performance of the existing one.
27. Is the investment justified taking into consideration the nature and load of work in your laboratory?
28. While making budgetary provisions for the purchase of an instrument, consider procurement of consumable spares at least for two years.
29. Carry out comparative evaluation of technical and financial aspects of various marketed brands of the instrument meeting your specifications before making the final choice.
30. Has any of your technical personnel been trained in the operation and maintenance of different analytical instruments including the one under consideration for purchase?

Note : 1. Although technical and economic factors have significant bearing on the selection of vendor, however final decision should be made after properly assessing each prospective vendor's capabilities in respect of above factors. This will help you in short-listing the vendors.
2. Strong relationship with fewer but better suppliers is mutually beneficial to facilitate improvement in quality, cost and overall responsiveness.
3. Once the vendor is chosen, he should be considered important player of your team. The vendor should provide all the possible assistance in establishing the equipment validation. The vendor will carry out normal operations checks for its pre-qualification acceptability criteria.
4. Once the vendor has demonstrated the equipment validation, optimal limitation of the instrument should clearly be understood by the analytical chemist.

If you are not happy with your decision of selecting the vendor you will probably be reminded of it almost every day.

Animal house

With greatest stress on the use of analytical techniques not involving animals such as LALs/bacterial endotoxin test, for pyrogens, comparatively smaller animal house is required. (Interestingly, more than 90% of LVP/SVP are now required to be tested for pyrogens by LALs/bacterial endotoxin test as compared to use of rabbit as test animal.)

Animal house should be located in quiet atmosphere and be kept tidy and clean. Separate room for each species, breeding and experimental purpose are preferable. It should preferably be air-conditioned. Animal used in testing components, in-process materials or drug products for compliance with established specifications shall be maintained and controlled in a manner that assures their suitability for intended use. They shall be identified and adequate record be maintained showing the history of their use. Record requirement is necessary to maintain control of their use in experimentation, testing or assay procedures, record should include :

1. Identification code
2. Description of animal, such as its weight, sex, etc.
3. Source
4. Date of arrival
5. Age at time of arrival
6. Details about its use in testing with dates and nature of test.

If the animal is to be used for repeated assay procedures, i.e., pyrogen testing, toxicity test, a time period sufficient for complete clearance of the drug is necessary. Animal area should be as far as possible segregated from all other manufacturing and analytical activities and should have limited access. Animals such as rabbits are likely to develop immunity on repeated use such as in pyrogen test. Age of rabbits to be used in pyrogen test is important as older animals are rather immune.

REFERENCE STANDARDS

Any person engaged in the quality assurance of drugs and pharmaceuticals must be fully aware of the need of reference material with which the test material is to be compared before deciding about its quality. Various tests like identification by UV absorption spectrophotometry or determining the presence and/or absence of impurities/decomposition products/related substances or determination of potency/strength, one would need the use of reference material of known purity or potency. The use of such reference standards during determination of individual ingredient in multi-drug formulations needs no emphasis with respect to accuracy and ease of such determinations.

In India, Central Drugs Laboratory, Calcutta is presently responsible for making available only IP reference standards to the drugs manufacturers as well as to approved drug testing laboratories, but all the required reference standards may not be available. Further, most of the related substances/decomposition products for which pharmacopoeial limits are prescribed are usually not available thus jeopardising the very purity of drug substances. It will be appropriate if the regulatory authorities attend to this problem on priority to explore the possibilities of alternative sources of supply of reference material.

This problem has now been partially solved as two organisations at present are distributing USP reference standards in India after procuring them from the international official agencies.

1. M/s E. Merck (India) Ltd., Shiv Sagar Estate, Dr. Annie Besant Road, Worli, Mumbai - 400019. Tel. 4964855-59.
2. M/s Promochem (India) Pvt. Ltd., P. Box No. 416A, Basavangudi, Bangalore - 560004. Tel. 621253.

The other alternative suggestions are :

(a) Government of India may set up a reference standard centre for making available not only IP standards but other reference standards such as USP/BP/EP reference standards. For this, three well-equipped regional drug testing laboratories proposed to be set up under the control of Government of India can be assigned collaborative work for reference standards. The centre can then price the reference standards for distribution to enable the centre to be self-sufficient.

(b) The Association of Drug Manufacturers in India such as IDMA may establish a centre with the approval of Drug Controller General of India for preparing certified reference standards. This centre could procure primary reference standards from various official agencies and calibrate the substances against them to prepare certified reference standards and then could distribute on payment.

(c) The approved drug testing laboratories in India may jointly undertake such an exercise to supply certified working standards.

Since primary reference standards are available in small quantities and are very expensive, it is desirable that working reference standards should be prepared and used for day to day analysis. The bulk drug substances may be obtained from the manufacturers of basic drugs and then standardized as per method below :

1. Collect the suitable pure chemical substance about 5 to 50 g in quantity and store it in a sealed large glass ampoules at a temperature of about 6-10°C. Certain substances may require even a lower temperature.

2. Test the bulk chemical substance as per pharmacopoeia requirements for all tests.

3. Determine the content/potency, the content/potency should be determined by three experienced analysts independently and average taken for computation of content, if the results obtained from these three analysts are very close.

4. Transfer the standardised working reference standard in amber coloured small ampoules each containing about 50 to 100 mg in quantity and seal the ampoule. The ampoule should be sealed in nitrogen environment, if possible. Label each ampoule with potency and the date after which it should not be used. Such ampoules should be stored in a refrigerator between 6-10°C.

REFERENCE SUBSTANCES AND INFRARED REFERENCE SPECTRA FOR PHARMACOPOEIAL ANALYSIS

Addresses for the purchase of reference substances

International chemical reference substances (ICRS)

WHO Collaborating Centre for Chemical Reference Substances, Apoteksbolaget AB, Centrallaboratoriet, S-105 14 Stockholm, Sweden, Telex : 115 53 APOBOL S; Fax : 46 8 740 60 40.

Reference materials from pharmacopoeial and other sources

- Central Drug Laboratory, Calcutta for chemical substances and Central Research Institute, Kasauli for biological preparations of Indian Pharmacopoeia.

- ASEAN Reference Substances (ARS) issued under ASEAN TCDC Programme on Pharmaceuticals; available at individual participating laboratories :

1. National Quality Control Laboratory of Drug and Food, Jl. Percetakan Negara No. 23, Jakarta, Indonesia; Telephone : (021) 41 507; Fax : (021) 4201 427.

2. National Pharmaceutical Control Bureau, Ministry of Health, Jalan Universiti, P.O. Box 319, 46730 Petaling Jaya, Malaysia; Telephone : (603) 7573611; Fax : (603) 7562924.

3. Bureau of Food and Drugs, D.O.H. Compound, Alabang, Muntinlupa, Metro Manila, Philippines; Telephone : (632) 8422213; Fax : (632) 8424603.

4. Institute of Science and Forensic Medicine, Outram Road, Singapore 0316; Telephone : (065) 2216800; Fax : (065) 2290749.

5. Drug Analysis Division, Department of Medical Sciences, Ministry of Public Health, Tiwanon Road, Nonthaburi 11000, Thailand; Telephone : (662) 5915233; Fax : (662) 5910203.

- British Pharmacopoeia Chemical Reference Substances (BPCRS), Medicines Control Agency Laboratory, Government Buildings, (Block 2) Honeypot Lane, Stanmore HA7 1AY, UK; Telephone : +44 (0) 171-972 3608; Fax : +44 (0) 181 951 3069; Telex : 940 16760 BPC LG.

- Comitè Mexicano de Sustancias Farmacèuticas de Referencia, Av. Cuauhtèmoc No. 1481 Sta Cruz Atoyac, Deleg-Benito Juàrez 03310 Mexico, D.F., Mexico, Telephone : 688-9817, 688-9530; Fax : 604-9808.

- European Pharmacopoeia Commission Secretariat (EPCRS), Council of Europe, B P 907, F 67029 Strasbourg Cedex 1 France; Telephone : (88) 41 28 52; Fax : (88) 41 27 71.

- French Pharmacopoeia Reference Substances (FPRS), Agence du Medicament, 14, rue Ecole de Pharmacie, 34000 Montpellier, France; Telephone : 67 02 31 31; Fax : 67 60 78 84.
- Japanese Pharmacopoeia Reference Substances (JPRS).
  1. National Institute of Hygienic Sciences, Osaka Branch, 1-1-43, Hoensaka, Chuo-ku, Osaka 540, Japan; Telephone : +81-6-941-1533; Fax : +6-942-0716.
  2. The Society of Japanese Pharmacopoeia, 2-12-15, Shibuya-ku, Tokyo 150, Japan; Telephone : +81-3-3400-5634; Fax : +81-3-3400-3158.
- Mexican Pharmacopoeia Reference Substances (MXPRS), Laboratorio Nacional de Salud Publica, Secretaria de Salud, Mexico D.F., Mexico X.
- Laboratory of Antibiotic Drugs, Department of Biological and Blood Products, The National Institute of Health, 4-7-1, Gakuen, Musahimurayama City, Tokyo 208, Japan; Telephone : (0425) 61-0771.
- National Institute for Standards and Technology (NIST), Office of Standard Reference Materials, Room B311, Chemistry Building, Gathersburg, MD 20899, USA.
- Office of Reference Materials (ORM), Laboratory of the Government Chemist, Teddington, TW11 OLW, UK.
- Swiss Pharmacopoeia Reference Substances (SPCR), Office federal de la sante publique, Laboratoire federal de la pharmacopee, Case postale, 3001 Beme, Switzerland.
- U.S. Pharmacopoeial Convention, Inc. Reference Standards Order Department, 12601 Twinbrook parkway, Rockville, Maryland 20852, USA.

There are certain other materials which may not be required in analysis of drugs but pharmaceutical manufacturers may require them for associated testing like test for pesticides in herbal medicines, test for environmental pollution control. For such testing Certified Reference Materials (CRM) are available from some well established institutions.

Sources for other certified reference materials

1. Institute for Reference Materials & Measurements (IRMM), Retieseweg, B-2440 Geel, Belgium.
2. Reidel-de Ha'en Aktiengesellschaft Wunstorfer Straße 40, P.O. Box D-30918; Seelze. (Outside Germany represented by Hoechst AG).
3. Institute for Environmental Research & Technology; National Research Council of Canada, Montreal Road, Ottawa, Ontario, Canada K1A0R6.
4. Bureau of Analysed Samples Ltd. (BAS); Newham Hall, Newby Middlesbrough Cleveland, England TS8 9EA.
5. The Office of Reference Materials, Laboratory of the Govt. Chemist, Queens Road, Teddington; Middlesex TW11 OLY, UK.

Preparation, maintenance and storage of working standards

Difficulty is always experienced by Analytical Laboratories or Quality Control Department to procure reference standards from official sources within the country or outside. It has been common practice with the Laboratories to use working standards, either prepared in the Laboratory or procured from basic material supplier. Prior to accepting a standard for use, it is necessary to generate an elaborate analytical data on working standard which is to be accepted as reference standard. The data should primarily comprise of (i) evidence of chemical structure (UV and IR, TLC, Optical rotation), (ii) Assay (UV), (iii) Purity (total solid impurities, specific impurities (TLC, HPLC). A material conforming to above tests and showing results within the acceptable limits can be accepted as a satisfactory working standard. The summary of this data can either be stored electronically or on card. Cards have been observed to be more convenient and handy for recording of data on subsequent dates. Other methods such as TGA/NMR can be employed for characterisation.

Maintenance of convenient quantity of standards also requires stability studies to be conducted on prepared/procured standards. The selection of analytical methods to be used for stability monitoring requires careful consideration. The. choice of method, of course, much depends on the nature of the substance concerned. However, a generally applicable guiding principle is to use methods of high reproducibility and to stick as closely to the same methods and the same experimental conditions for re-examination of reference materials, as was used for initial analysis. This reduces the chance of analytical error and facilitate early detection of degradation of the material. The progress in analytical chemistry and introduction of new methods may be adopted from time to time if they are considered to be more informative and/or more convenient. However, the responsibility for assessing the suitability of the standard will rest with the user. As a general principle, it is recommended to store these standards protected from light and moisture, and preferably at a temperature between 15-25°C. Special storage conditions whenever required are to be mentioned on the label. Retesting data may include IR, TLC, MP, LOD, Light Absorption and HPLC.

An example of contents of analytical report generated in addition to routine pharmacopoeial tests is given here.

Infrared spectrum	To be concordant with the reference spectrum published or spectrum obtained from reference standard.
Selectivity test	In case, IR Spectrum is not considered a suitable identification method, complementary methods such as TLC and HPLC are recommended for identification.
UV spectrum	Maximas to be indicated.
Assay	Chemical assay data, microbiological assay data, if any, the data obtained from manufacture of substance and laboratory findings compared.
Purity	TLC—Generally two different solvent systems are to be used and spots identified and compared for total impurities/specific impurities. HPLC—Two different systems to be used and selection depending on a greater separation efficiency.
Other characteristics	LOD, water (KF), Specific Optical Rotation, any specific limit test characteristic to the product.
Stability of known hygroscopic substances	In case the information is available about the hygroscopic nature of the substance to be accepted as working standard, the percentage of water (H_2O) preferably by Karl Fischer is to be tested by exposing the substance for 24 hours to uncontrolled room temperature, controlled conditions (desiccate) and 70-80% Rh and readings noted.
Storage	Conditions of storage to be mentioned. (Quantity in a container should be as little as practicable to avoid repeated opening and exposure of working standard.) For efficient storage of standards, design of a table is described in Figs. 5.8A & B and 5.25. Each drawer can accommodate 36-48 vials depending on the size of table and rack. This table can be kept in central instruments room which is normally air-conditioned. All the working standards should preferably be stored in airtight amber-coloured bottles to avoid any effect of light and air.

SUGGESTED LABORATORY LAYOUTS

The laboratory must be designed to ensure maximum efficiency, safety and security considering the local climate and other factors. The cost of establishing a laboratory will vary from region to region depending on the local building codes and on the nature and specifications of construction materials. In general, the layout design should provide for adequate space and for such services as electricity, water, gas, ventilation and waste drain lines. Provision should be made for fumes cupboards as well as vibration-free area for analytical balances. Volatile solvents should be stored in a separate and adequately ventilated room, fitted with spark-free electrical sockets and well insulated explosion-proof light bulbs. The drain lines and working benches/experimental table tops should be acid-resistant. Emergency showers, eye and face wash fountain and fire extinguishers should be installed.

A quality control laboratory usually consists of following areas :

1. Chemical analysis
2. Physical testing
3. Hot room/fumes cupboard etc.
4. Microbiological testing
5. Sterility testing
6. Central instruments room
7. Pharmacology laboratory along with animal house
8. Central sample storage
9. Laboratory chemical/reagents/acid/solvent storage
10. Glassware storage
11. Washing
    (a) General glassware
    (b) Microbiology
12. Documents and record
13. Library
14. Administrative office
15. OIC, laboratory.

Few layouts (Figs. 5.6 and 5.7) for chemical laboratory for testing of drugs are suggested which may be helpful in planning a laboratory.

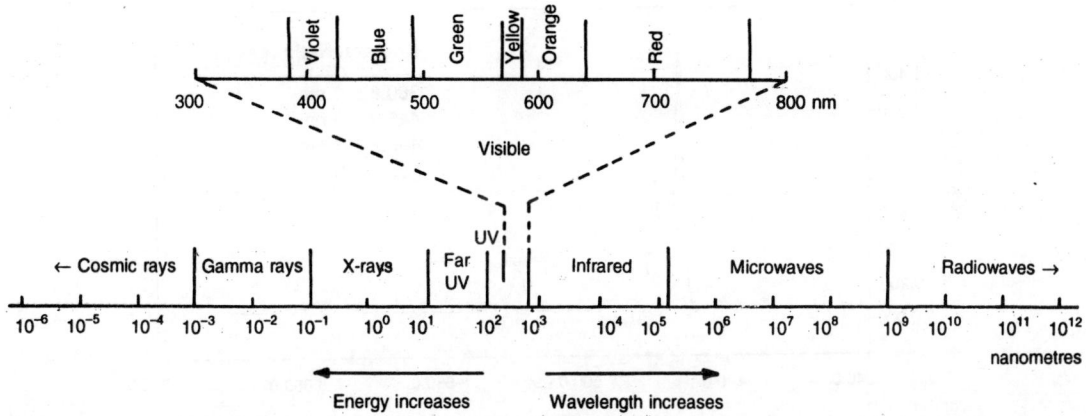

Region	Wavelength (nm)
Far ultraviolet	10-200
Near ultraviolet	200-380
Visible	380-780
Near infrared	780-3,000
Middle infrared	3,000-30,000
Far infrared	30,000-300,000
Microwave	300,000-1,000,000,000

The human eye is only sensitive to a tiny proportion of the total electromagnetic spectrum between approximately 380 and 780 nm and within this area we perceive the colours of the rainbow from violet through to red. If the full electromagnetic spectrum shown in the figure was redrawn on a linear scale and the visible region was represented by the length of one centimetre, then the boundary between radio and microwaves would have to be drawn approximately 25 kilometres away!

Fig. 5.1. The electromagnetic spectrum. (*Courtesy :* "Application Laboratory (Spectrometer), Unicam", 206 York Street, Cambridge, U.K.)

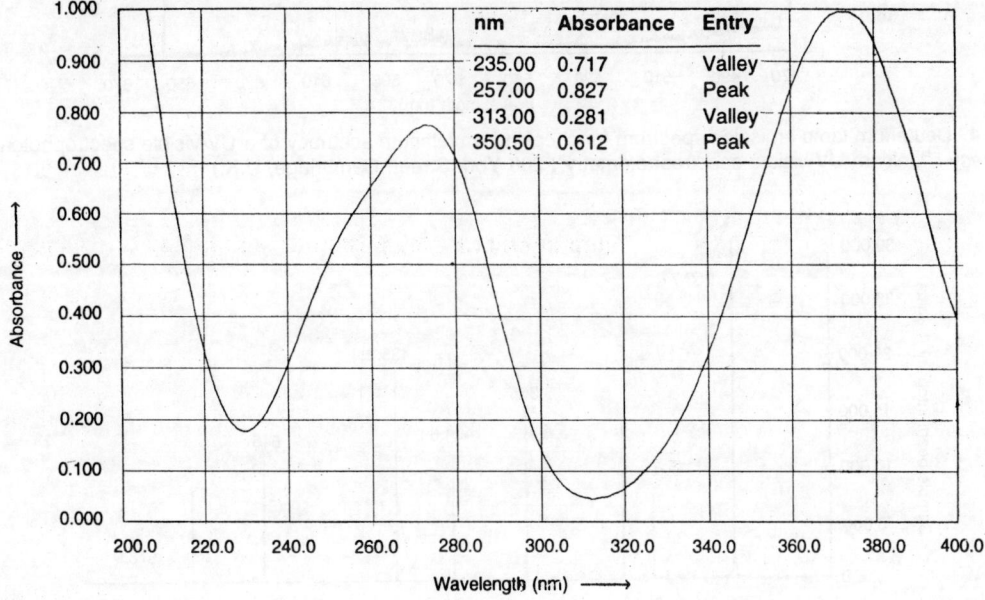

nm	Absorbance	Entry
235.00	0.717	Valley
257.00	0.827	Peak
313.00	0.281	Valley
350.50	0.612	Peak

Fig. 5.2. Typical spectrum of potassium chromate solution in 0.01 N sulphuric acid for checking absorbance accuracy of UV-visible spectrophotometer. (*Courtesy :* "Unicam UV-visible spectrophotometry", 206 York Street, Cambridge, U.K.)

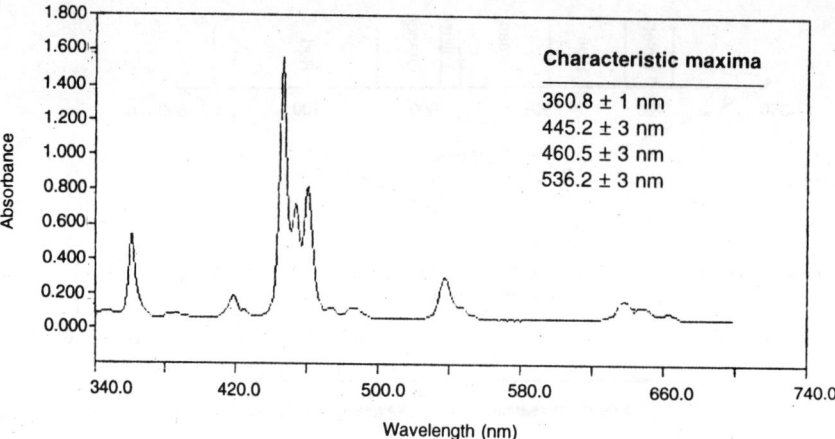

Fig. 5.3. Typical spectrum using calibrated holmium oxide glass filter for checking wavelength accuracy of a UV-visible spectrophotometer.

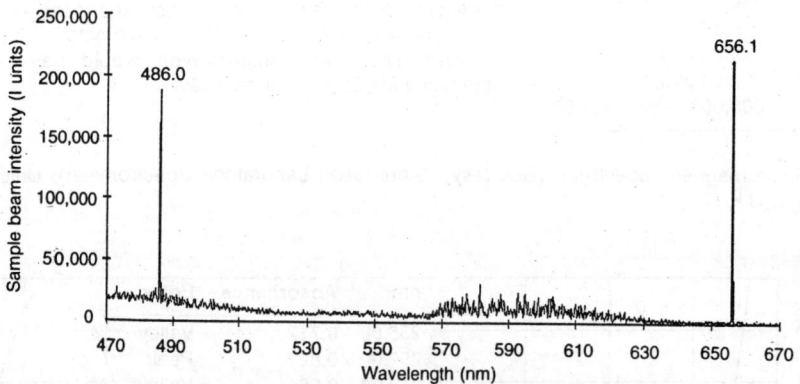

Fig. 5.4. Deuterium lamp emission spectrum for checking wavelength accuracy of a UV-visible spectrophotometer. (*Courtesy :* "Unicam UV-visible spectrophotometry", 206 York Street, Cambridge, U.K.)

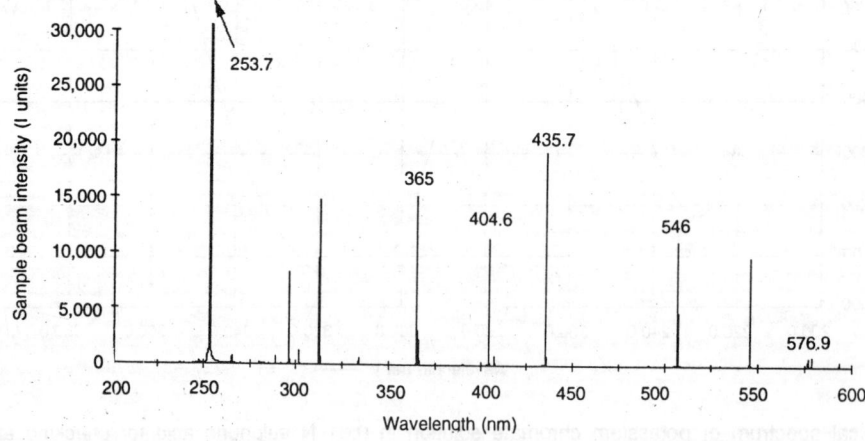

Fig. 5.5. Typical mercury lamp emission spectrum for checking wavelength accuracy of a UV-visible spectrophotometer. (*Courtesy :* "Unicam UV-visible spectrophotometry", 206 York Street, Cambridge, U.K.)

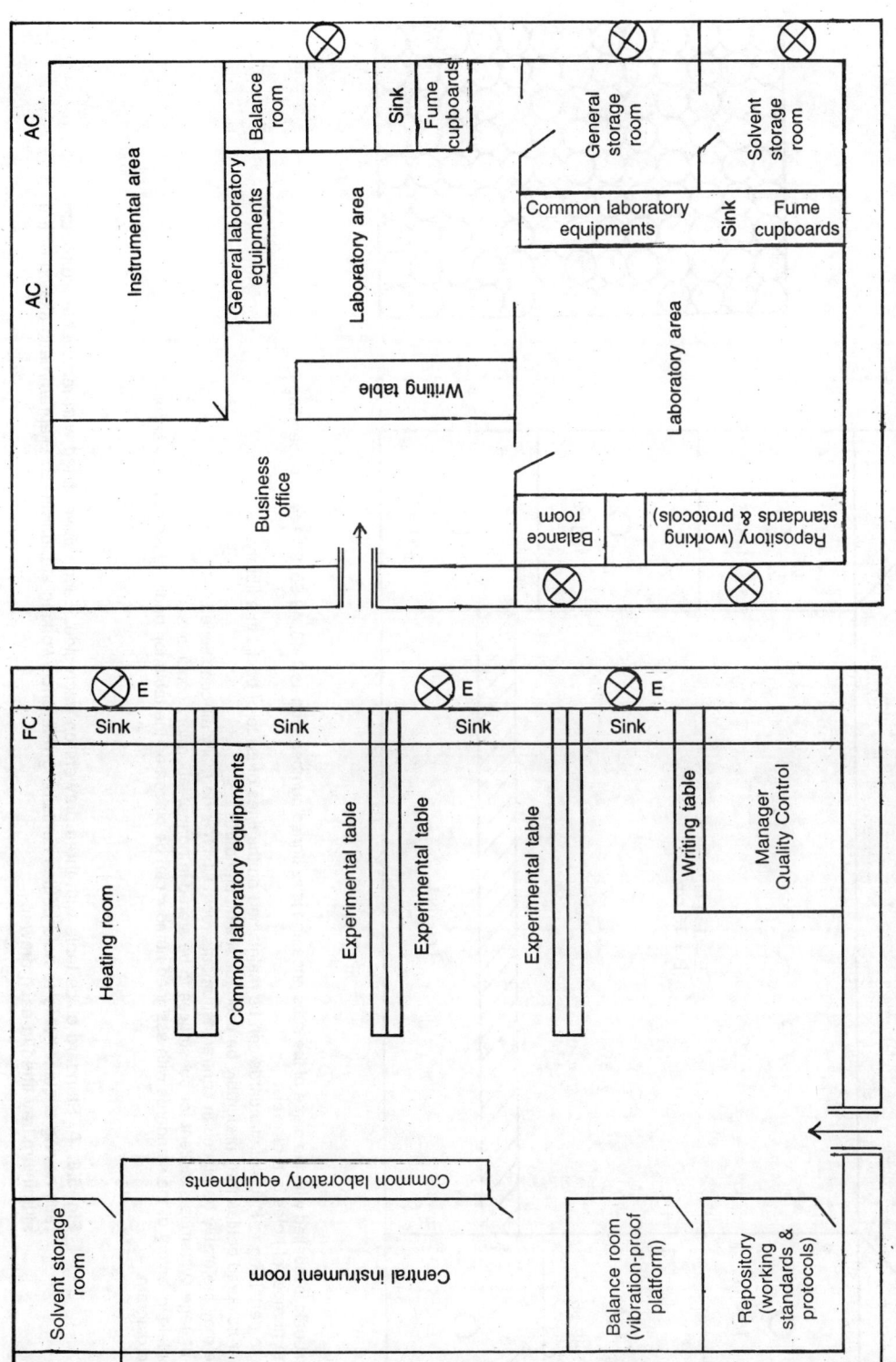

Fig. 5.6. Suggested layout of a chemical laboratory for testing of drugs.

Fig. 5.7. Suggested layout for a chemical laboratory.

- Experimental table/working benches should have acid-proof table tops.
- 2-3 tier racks above experimental table for storing reagents, glassware of daily use.
- Cupboards below the working tables for storing chemicals, glassware for frequent replacement.

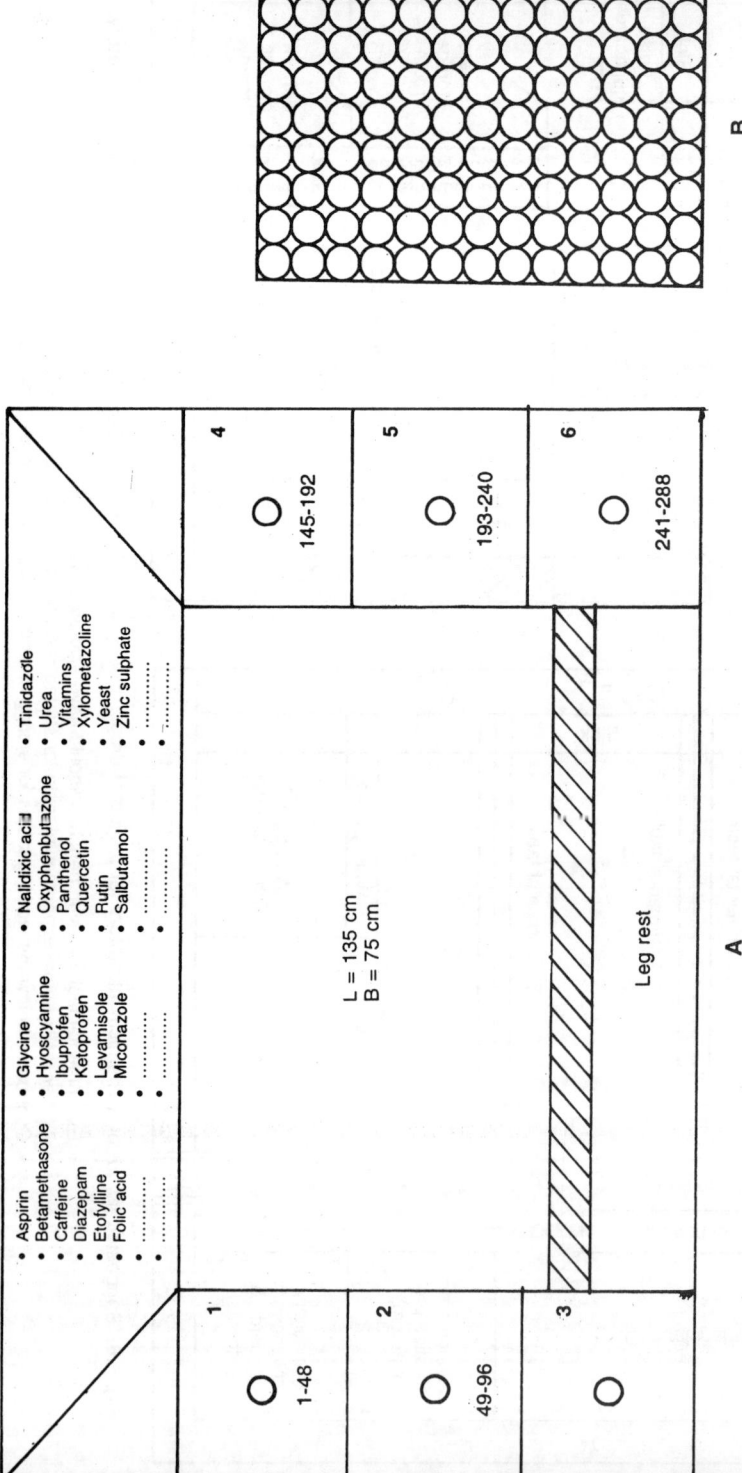

- Aspirin
- Betamethasone
- Caffeine
- Diazepam
- Etofylline
- Folic acid
- ....

- Glycine
- Hyoscyamine
- Ibuprofen
- Ketoprofen
- Levamisole
- Miconazole
- ....

- Nalidixic acid
- Oxyphenbutazone
- Panthenol
- Quercetin
- Rutin
- Salbutamol
- ....

- Tinidazole
- Urea
- Vitamins
- Xylometazoline
- Yeast
- Zinc sulphate
- ....

L = 135 cm
B = 75 cm

Leg rest

1 1-48
2 49-96
3
4 145-192
5 193-240
6 241-288

A

B

- Each bottle is labelled with the name of the substance and is assigned number such as 1-48, 49-96, 97-144 ... depending on the number of holes in a drawer.
- Record pertaining to issue of standards can be maintained on the lines of issue of books in a library.
- Amber-coloured bottles may preferably be used for storing standards.
- Table may preferably be placed in central instruments room which is normally air-conditioned.
- This storage system is excellent for substances to be stored in normal laboratory conditions.
- Complete inventory of the standards with assigned number can be placed on the table top under glass cover as shown in the diagram.

Fig. 5.8. A. Standard office table with three drawers on each side. Each drawer fitted with removable aluminium rack having circular holes to hold bottles containing reference/working standards. **B.** Diagrammatic sketch of the aluminium tray fitted in each drawer.

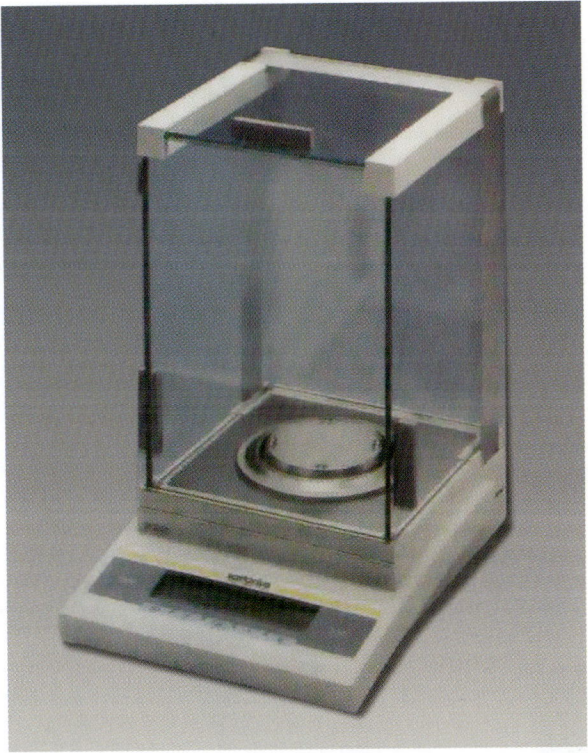

Fig. 5.9. Sartorius analytical balance, Model BP 210S having capacity of 210 g with reproducibility of ± 0.1 mg with built-in calibration weights & RS232 data interface. (*Courtesy:* Sartorius AG, Germany through SICO Ltd., New Delhi, India)

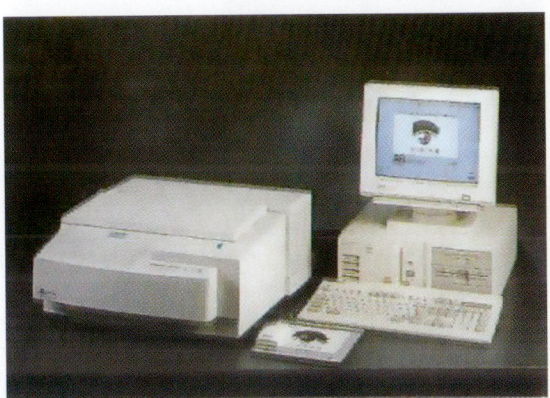

Fig. 5.10. Unicam double beam recording UV-Vis spectrophotometer. (*Courtesy:* Unicam, UK, through SICO Ltd., New Delhi, India)

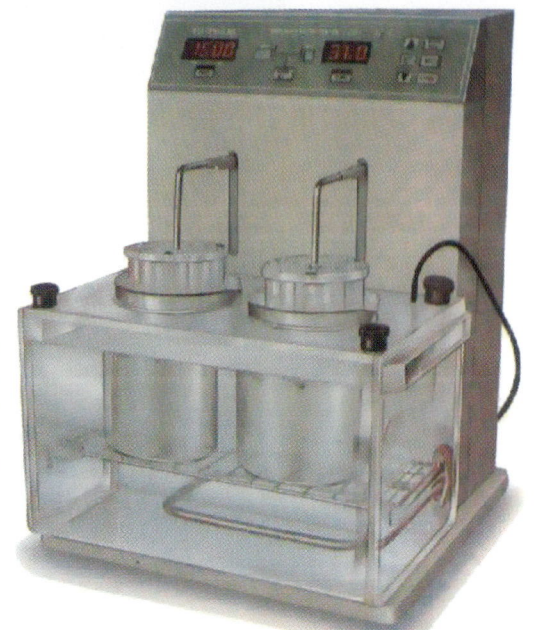

Fig. 5.11. Microprocessor based tablet disintegration tester for tablets, capsules and other dosage forms as per IP, BP, USP, fitted with programmable timer, swivel-free movements through snap-click loading mechanism, water-bath to ensure uniform temperature. (*Courtesy:* Electrolab, Mumbai, India)

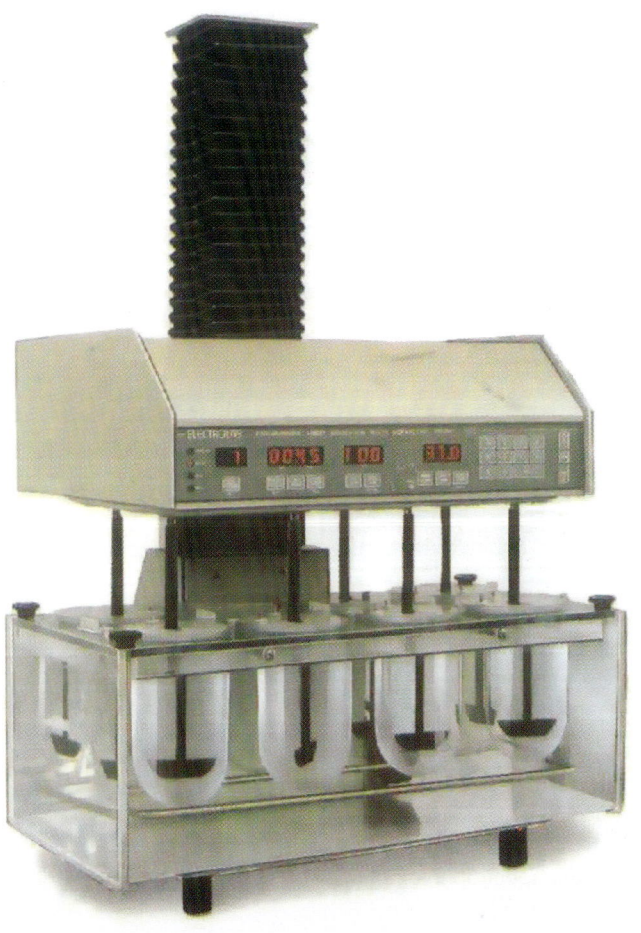

Fig. 5.12. Microprocessor programmable tablet dissolution tester as per IP, BP, USP and DAB specifications, for solid dosage forms as well as sustained and controlled release dosage forms, programmable temperature and speed and 12 sampling intervals, available with fraction collector and interface for attachment to UV-visible spectrophotometer. (*Courtesy:* Electrolab, Mumbai, India)

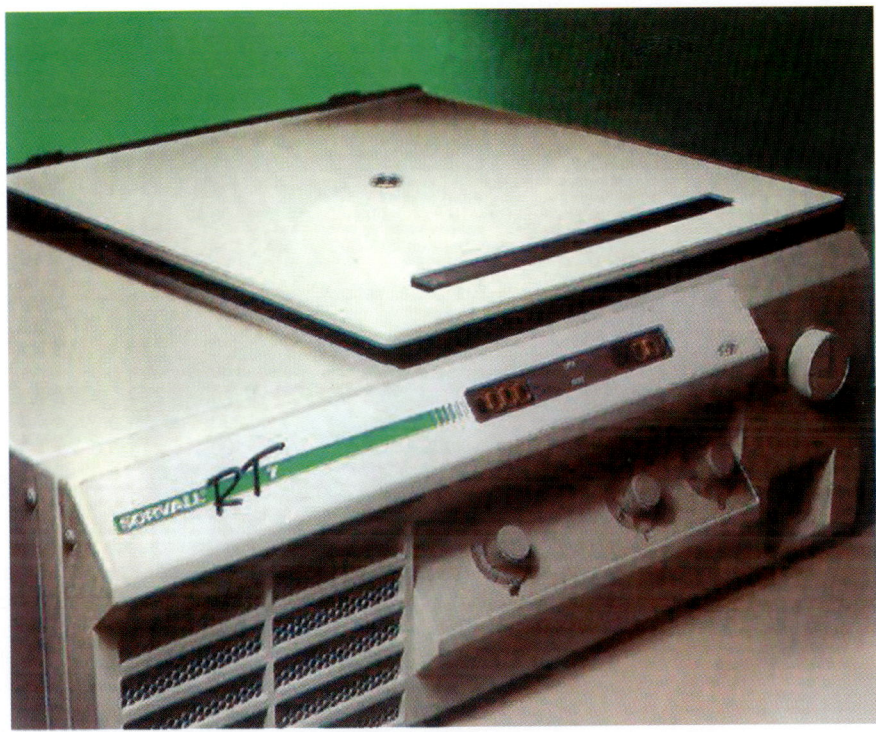

Fig. 5.13A. Sorvall benchtop refrigerated centrifuge, Model RT-7.

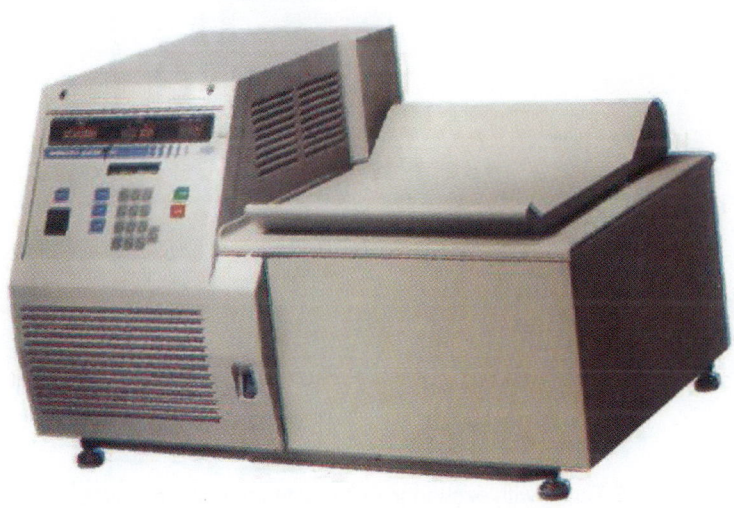

Fig. 5.13B. Sorvall superspeed benchtop centrifuge, Model Super T-21. (*Courtesy:* Sorvall Inc., USA; & 31B, Pocket A, Sidharth Ext., New Delhi through SICO Ltd., New Delhi)

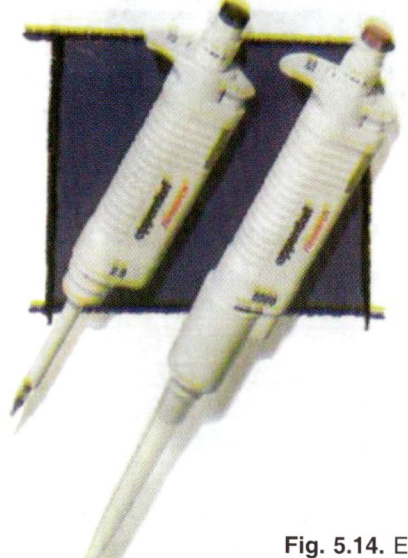

Technical data				
Range (µl)	Control button	Volume (µl)	Inaccuracy (%)	Imprecision (%)
0.1–2.5	Anthracite	0.2	± 12.0	≤ 6.0
		1.0	± 2.5	≤ 1.5
		2.5	± 1.4	≤ 0.7
0.5–10	Gray	0.5	± 5.0	≤ 2.8
		1	± 2.5	≤ 1.8
		10	± 1.0	≤ 0.4
2–20	Yellow	2	± 5.0	≤ 1.5
		20	± 1.0	≤ 0.3
10–100	Yellow	10	± 3.0	≤ 1.0
		100	± 0.8	≤ 0.2
20–200	Yellow	20	± 2.5	≤ 0.7
		200	± 0.6	≤ 0.2
100–1000	Blue	100	± 3.0	≤ 0.6
		1000	± 0.6	≤ 0.2
500–5000	Violet	500	± 2.4	≤ 0.6
		5000	± 0.6	≤ 0.15

Fig. 5.14. Eppendorf's fixed volume pipettes with ceramic piston, suitable for working with aggressive liquids, reduced risk of contamination or carry over, volume display during pipetting; four digit display and easy volume adjustability, autoclavable for microbiological work. (*Courtesy:* Eppendorf Research; Germany through M/s Micro-Devices & Computers, Chennai, India)

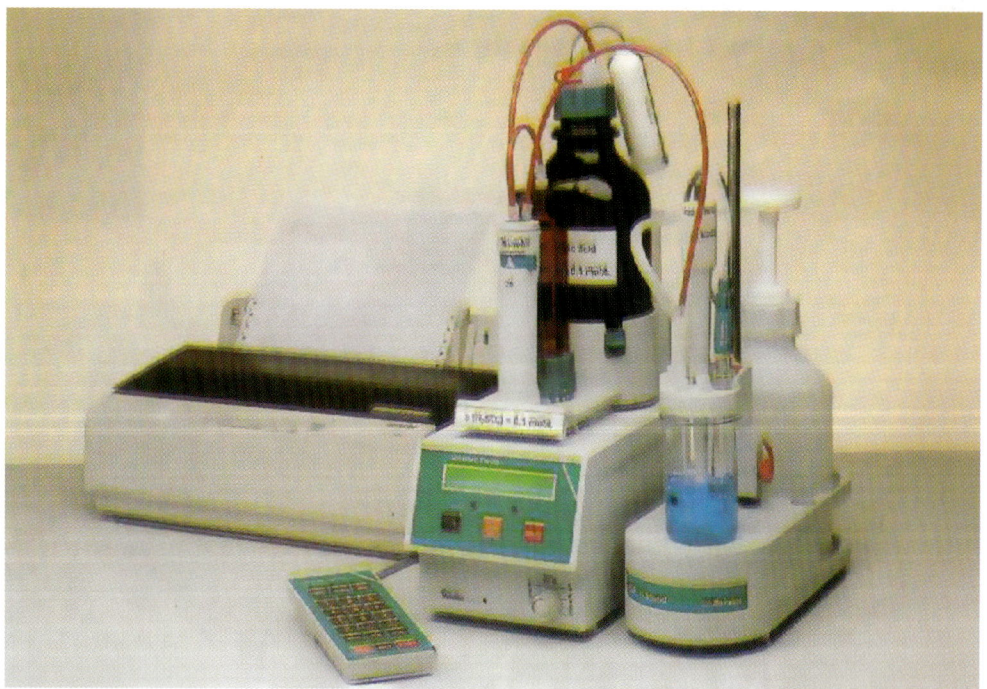

Fig. 5.15. Metrohm 716 DMS Titrino with exchange unit and titration stand, suitable for end-point titrations, Karl-Fischer titration, measurement of pH, U/mV (potentiometrically or with polarised electrodes) and temperature (°C), pH calibration with up to nine buffers and calculation of regression line. (*Courtesy:* Metrohm, Switzerland through M/s Micro-Devices & Computers, Chennai, India)

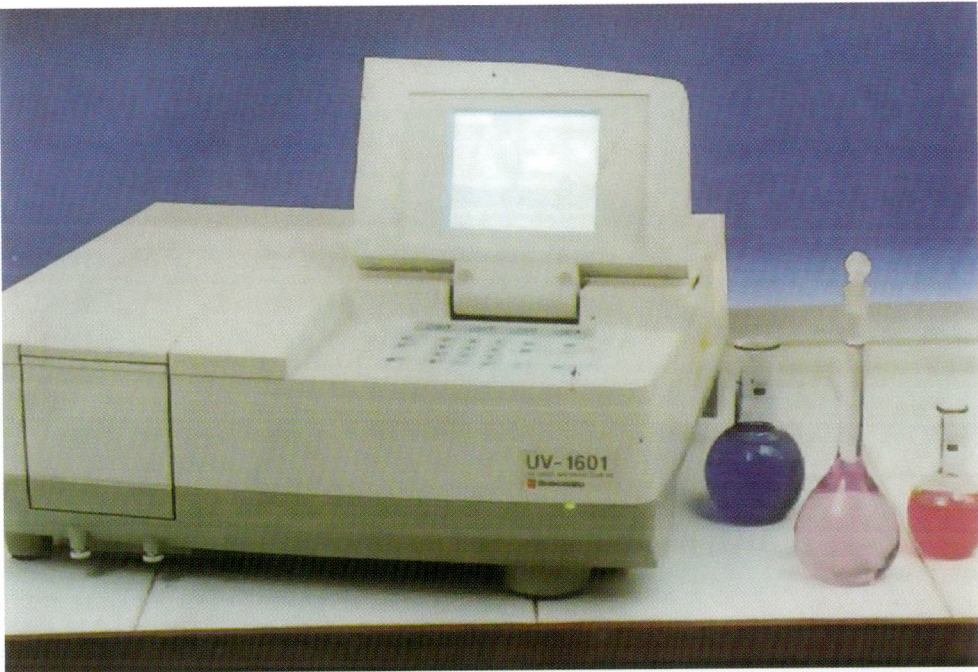

Fig. 5.16. Shimadzu double beam UV-Vis recording spectrophotometer, Model UV1601 (Standalone) with spectral range of 190-1100 nm, suitable for kinetic studies, quantitation, multi-component analysis and derivative (1st ~ 4th) methods. (*Courtesy:* Shimadzu Corp., Japan through Toshbro Ltd., 198 Jamshedji Tata Road, Mumbai, India)

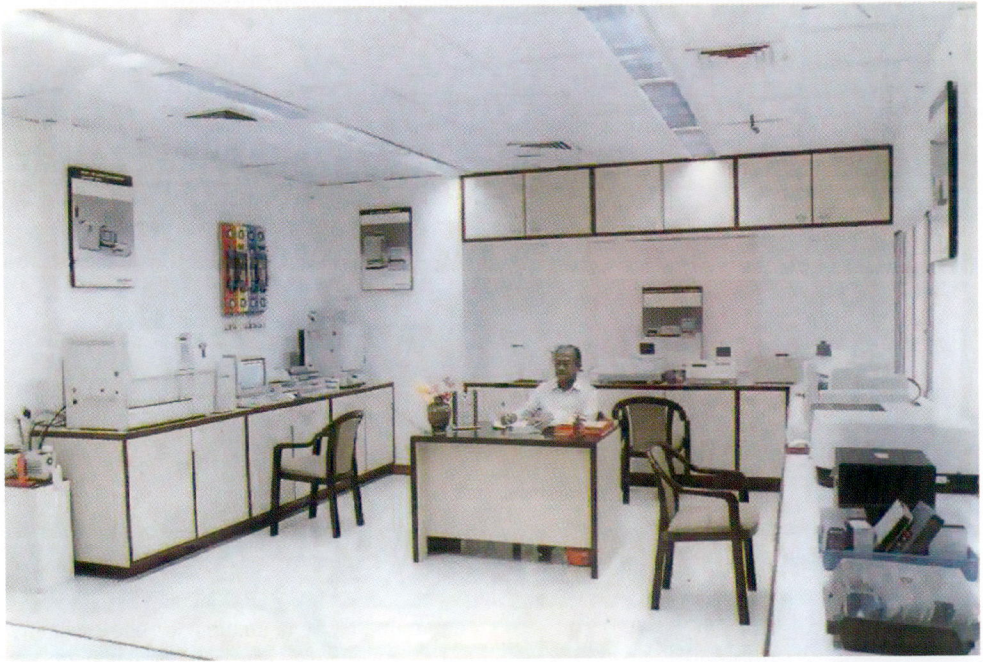

Fig. 5.17. Toshbro application/demonstration laboratory equipped with Shimadzu's GC/MS, GC, FTIR, UV1601, UV1601 PC, analytical balance and CZ microscope. (*Courtesy:* Toshbro Ltd., Mumbai, India)

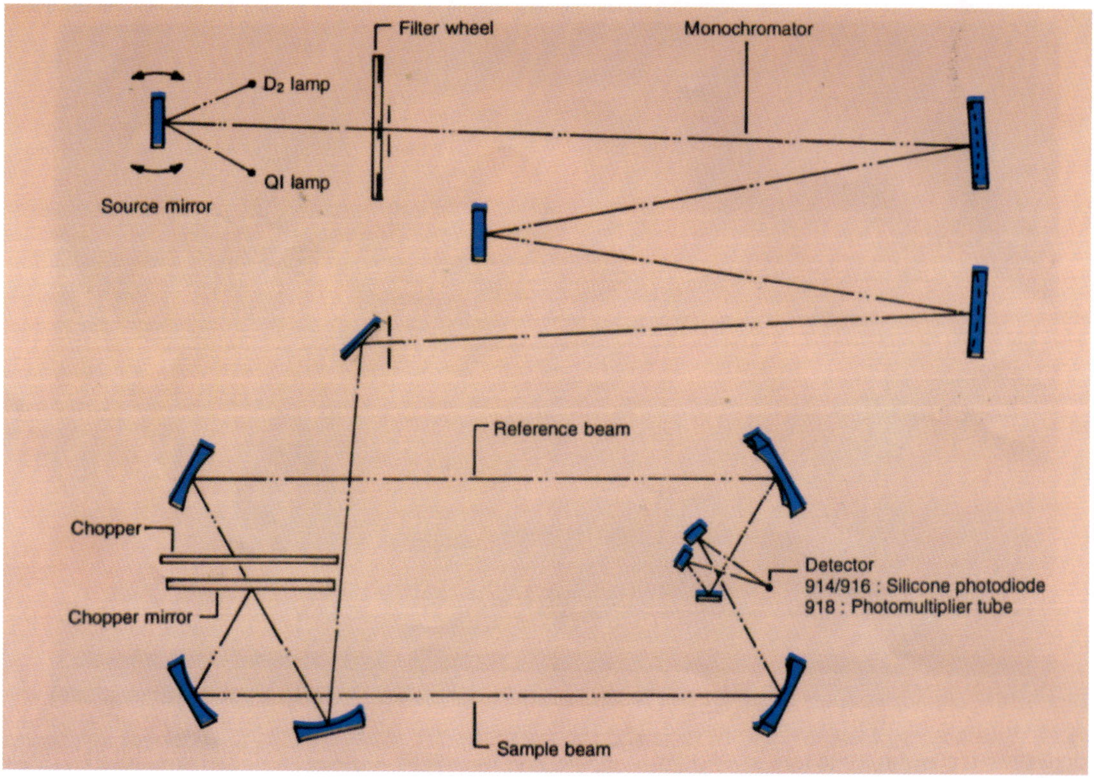

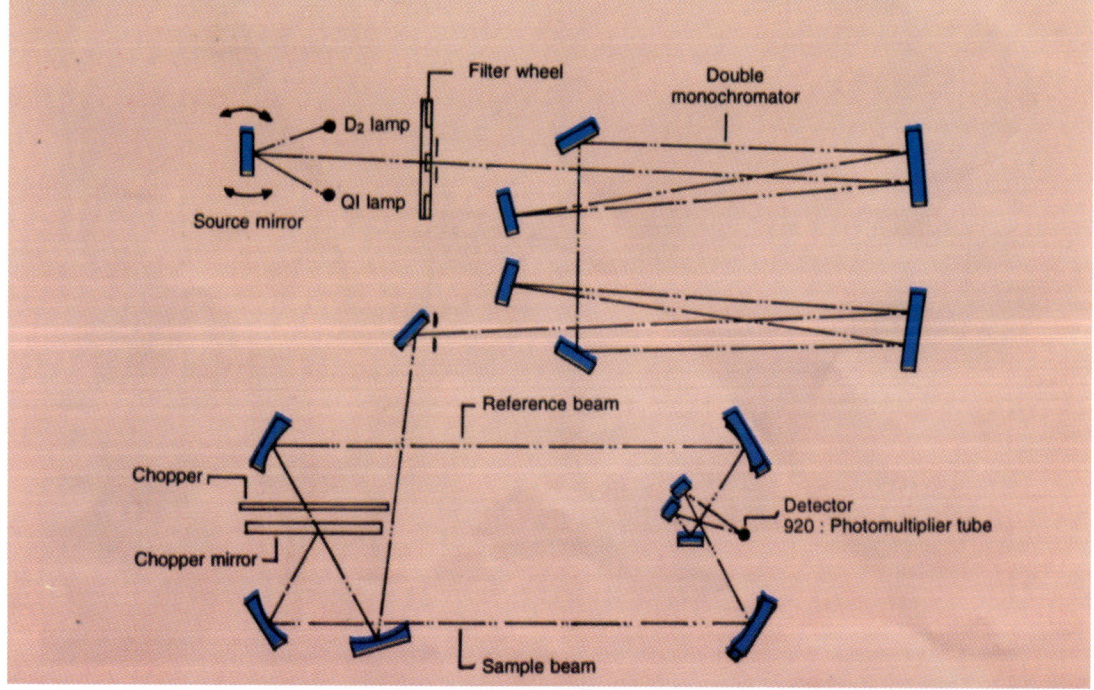

Fig. 5.18A. Optical system of a double beam UV-visible spectrophotometer.

Fig. 5.18B. Optical system of a double beam, double chromator UV-visible spectrophotometer.

Determine the dry weight fast and reliably

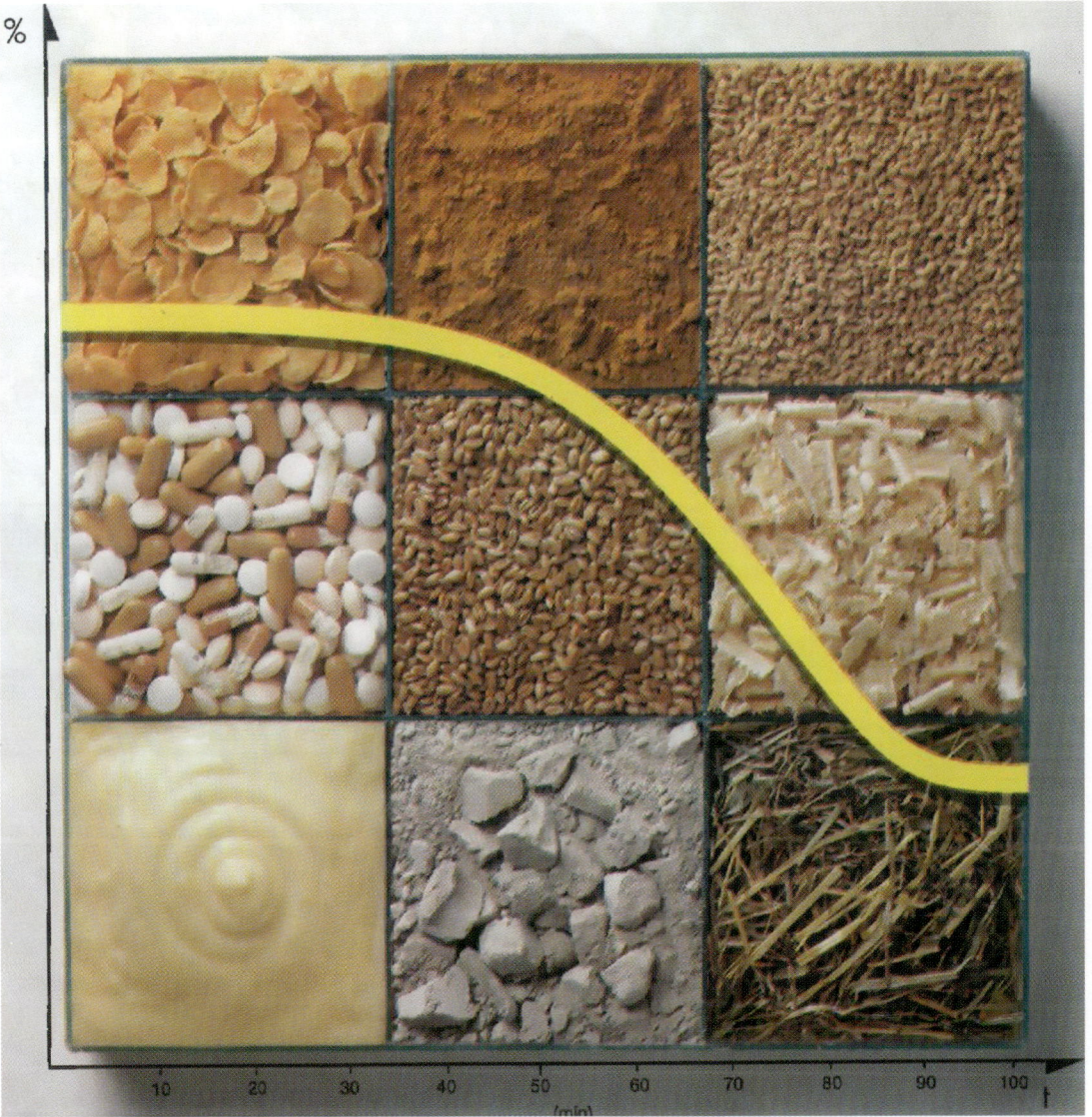

Fig. 5.19. To determine moisture (dry weight) incredibly faster, accurate and reliably, use Sartorius moisture analyser.

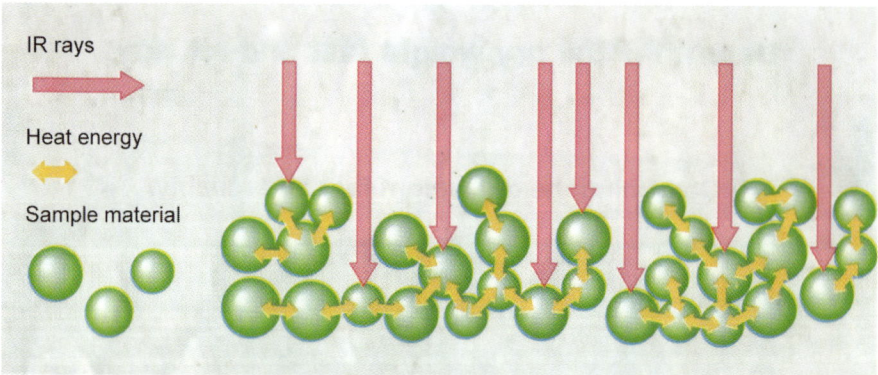

Fig. 5.20A. Principle of infrared drying; infrared rays penetrate the sample without being impeded, reach interior of the sample, get converted leading to heat energy to evaporation and subsequent drying. Infrared drying is faster and more reliable than conventional oven drying.

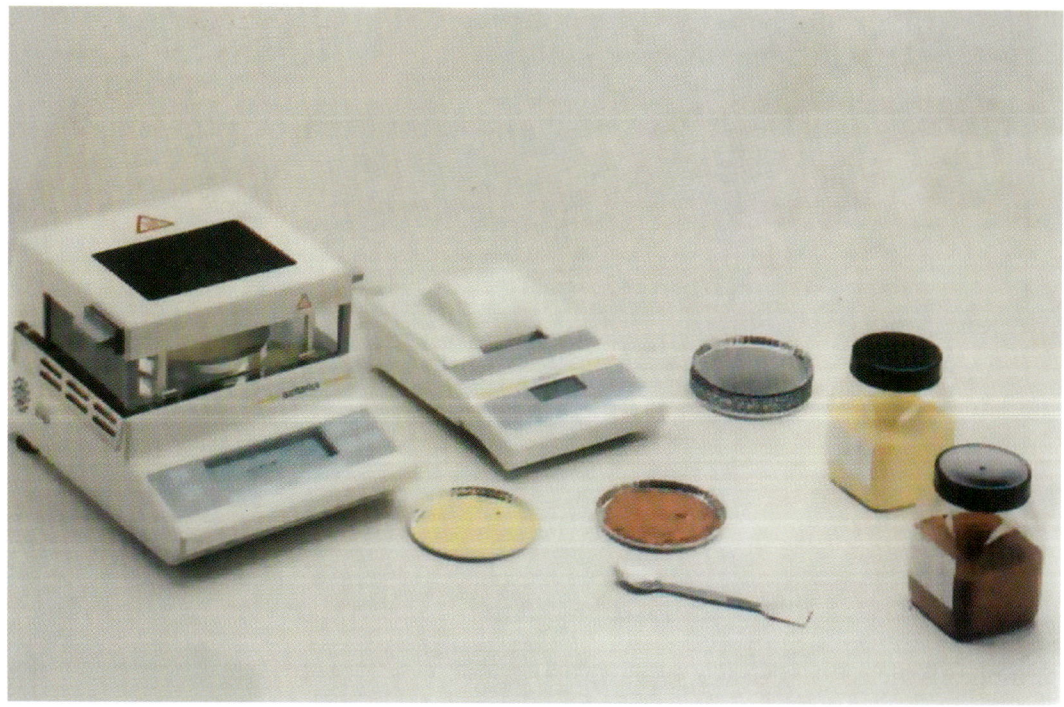

Fig. 5.20B. Sartorius automatic moisture balance MA30, fully microprocessed for thermogravimetric moisture determination with modes for moisture (%), dry weight (%), or % ratio, sample requirement 1 to 5 g. (*Courtesy:* Sartorius AG, Germany through SICO Ltd., New Delhi, India)

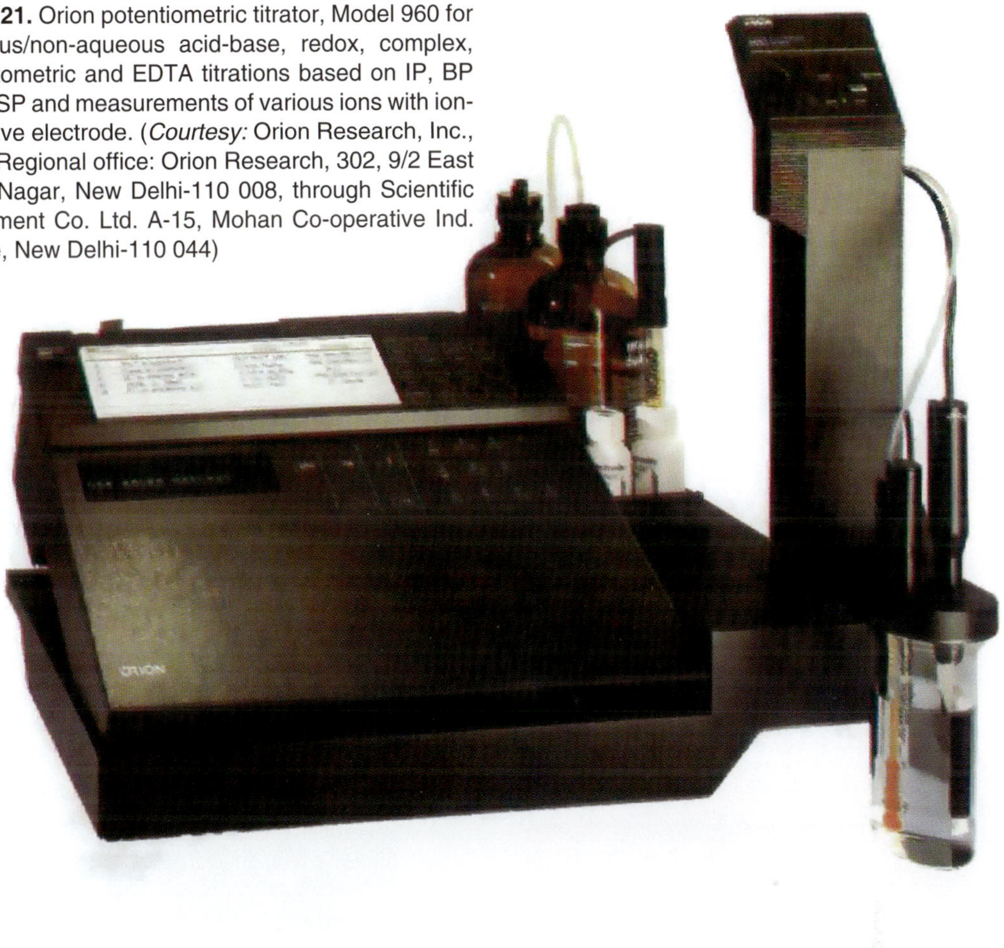

Fig. 5.21. Orion potentiometric titrator, Model 960 for aqueous/non-aqueous acid-base, redox, complex, argentometric and EDTA titrations based on IP, BP and USP and measurements of various ions with ion-selective electrode. (*Courtesy:* Orion Research, Inc., USA; Regional office: Orion Research, 302, 9/2 East Patel Nagar, New Delhi-110 008, through Scientific Instrument Co. Ltd. A-15, Mohan Co-operative Ind. Estate, New Delhi-110 044)

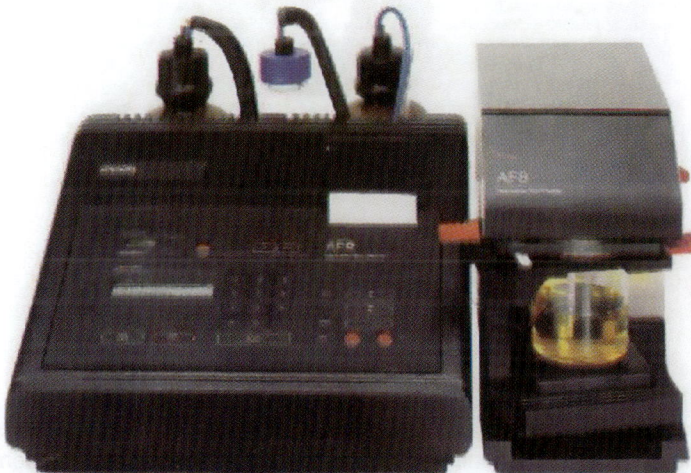

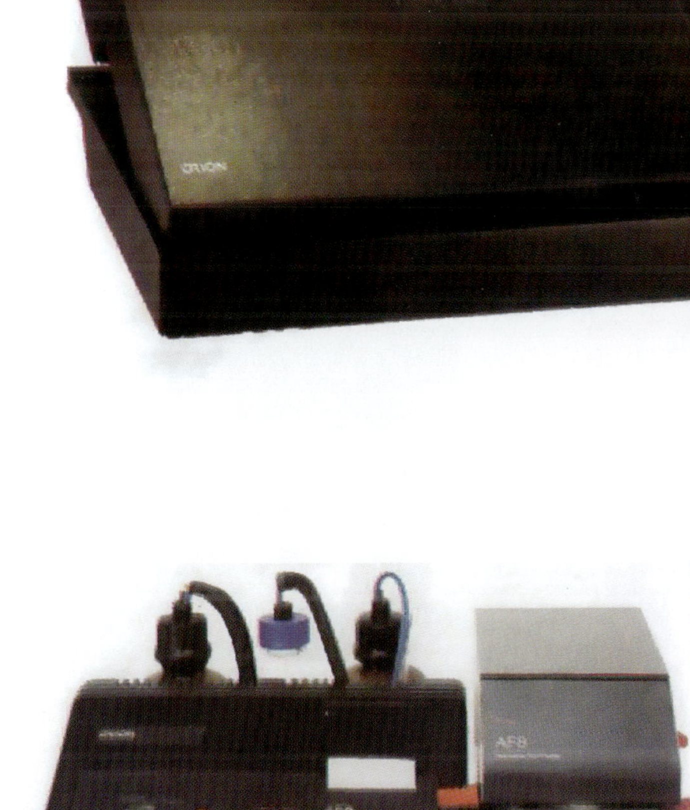

Salient features:
- Broad operating range 10 ppm to 100% H_2O
- System fully sealed for chemical handling
- Auto-fill/drain minimises any handling error
- Self-diagnosis to pass or fail calibration GLP-Cal
- Built-in printer, qualifies GLP-Doc
- Interfaces for connection with balances and computers

Fig. 5.22. Orion's Model AF8 volumetric Karl-Fischer titrator for moisture determination. (*Courtesy:* Orion Research, Inc., USA; Regional office: Orion Research, 302, 9/2 East Patel Nagar, New Delhi-110 008, through Scientific Instrument Co. Ltd., A-15, Mohan Co-operative Ind. Estate, New Delhi-110 044)

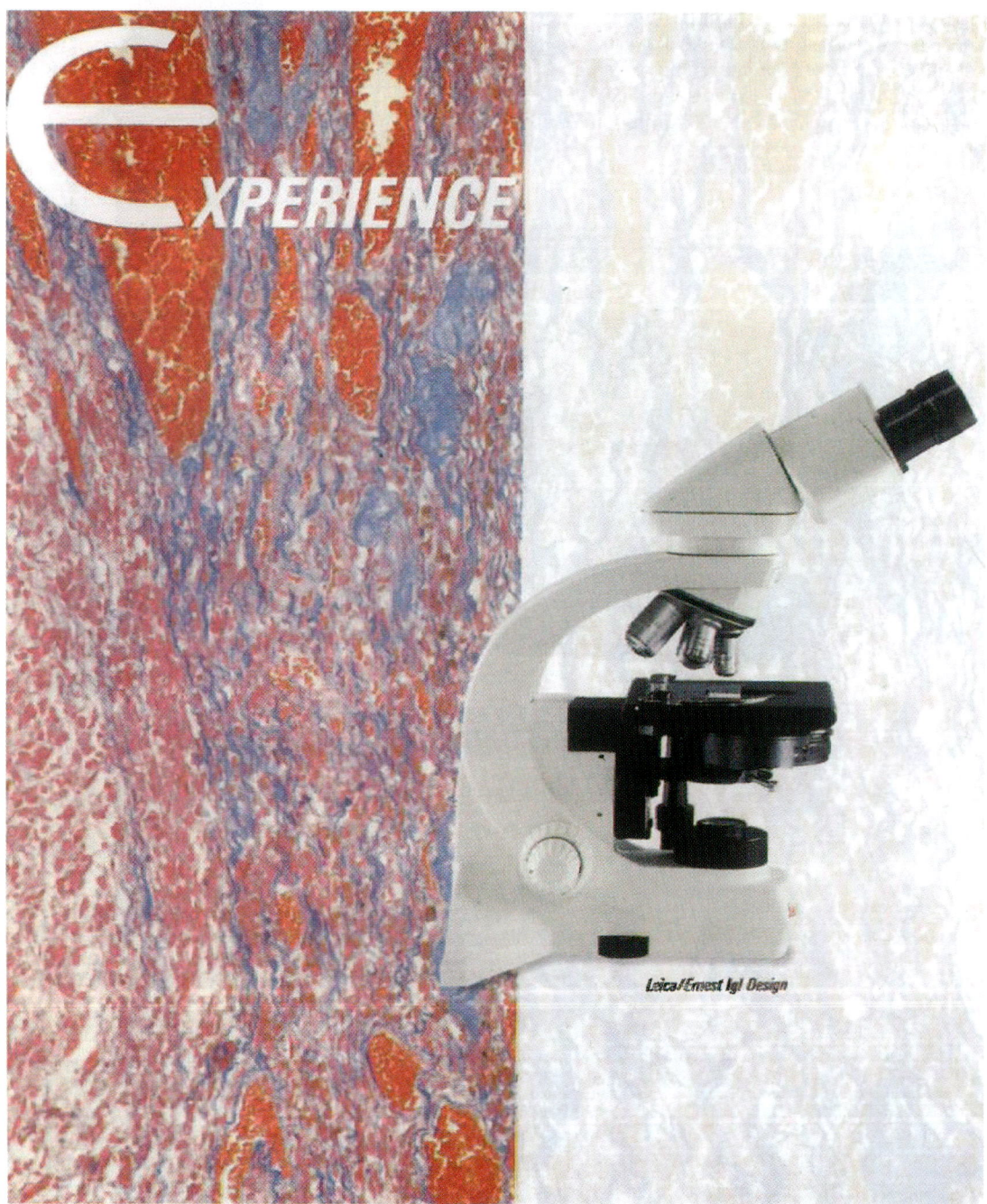

Fig. 5.23. Leica laboratory microscope, Model DMLS for medical practice and quality control laboratories; suitable for all contrast techniques (dark field, phase, differential interference, fluorescence) in transmitted and incident light. (*Courtesy:* Leica Microscopy and Scientific Instruments Group, Switzerland through SICO Ltd., New Delhi, India)

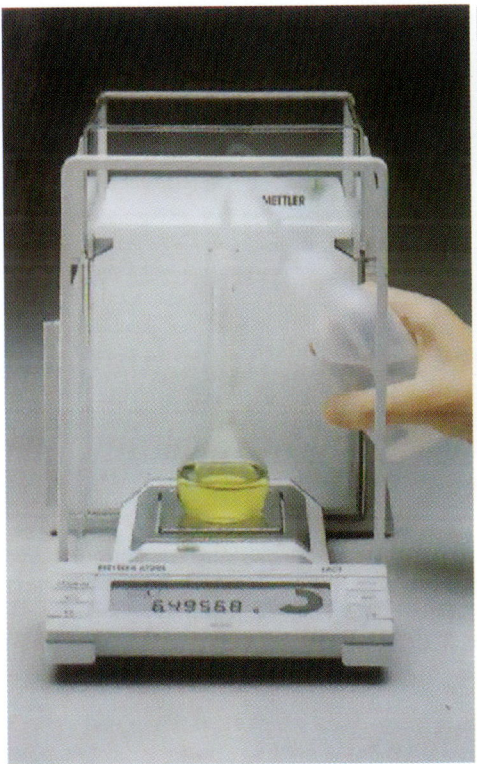

AT Micro, Analytical and Comparator Balances			
Model	**Max. capacity**		**Readability**
AT20	22 g		2 µg
AT201		205 g	0.01 mg
AT261 DeltaRange	◄62 g/0.01 mg►	205 g	0.1 mg
AT200		205 g	0.1 mg
AT400		405 g	0.1 mg
AT460 DeltaRange	◄ 62 g/0,1 mg ►	405 g	1 mg
AT21 Comparator	22 g		1 µg
AT106 Comparator		111 g	1 µg
AT1005 Comparator		1109 g	0.01 mg
AT1004 Comparator		1109 g	0.1 mg

Fig. 5.24. Mettler AT series analytical balance with auto-calibration system and auto-shut off, facilities of taring, piece counting, % weighing, density determination (solids, liquids). (*Courtesy:* Mettler-Toledo AG, Switzerland through Nulab Equipment Co. (P) Ltd., Mumbai, India)

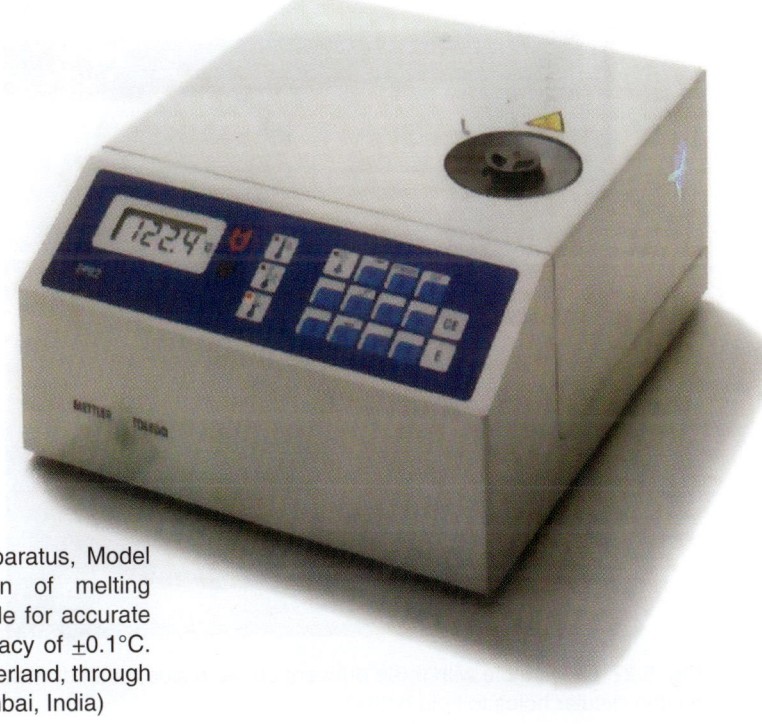

Fig. 5.25. Mettler melting point apparatus, Model FP62 for automatic determination of melting point, requires 2–3 mg of the sample for accurate determination of m.p. with an accuracy of ±0.1°C. (*Courtesy:* Mettler-Toledo AG, Switzerland, through Nulab Equipment Co. Pvt. Ltd., Mumbai, India)

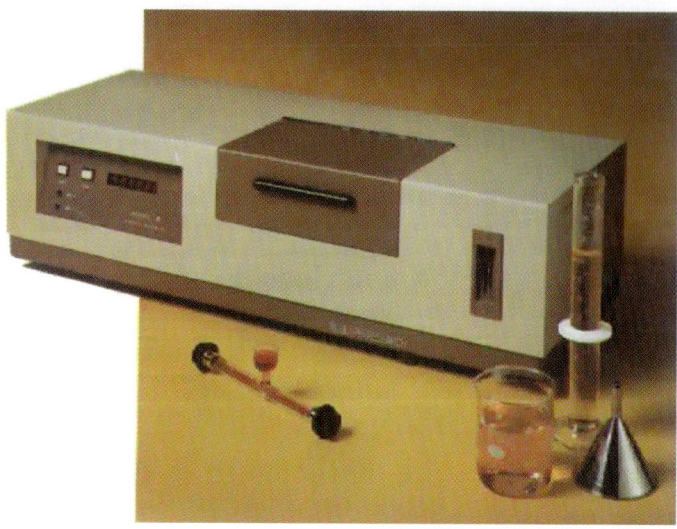

Fig. 5.26. Rudolph Autopol-III, multi-wavelengths (365, 405, 435, 546, 589, 633 nm), digital automatic polarimeter, sample chamber to accept tubes of 50, 100 and 200 mm with reproducibility of 0.002° arc, Autopol-IV is microprocessed suitable for measuring optical rotation, specific rotation and concentration, RS232 interface for printer. (*Courtesy:* Rudolph Research, Flanders, NJ, USA, through M/s Agaram Industries, Chennai, India)

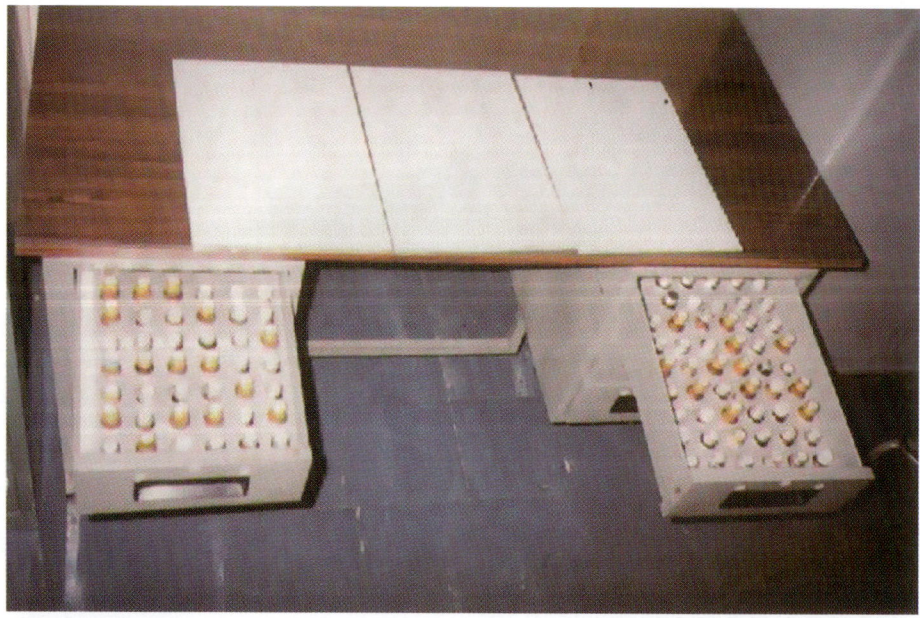

Fig. 5.27. Office table with three drawers on each side, each drawer fitted with removable aluminium rack having circular holes to hold bottles.

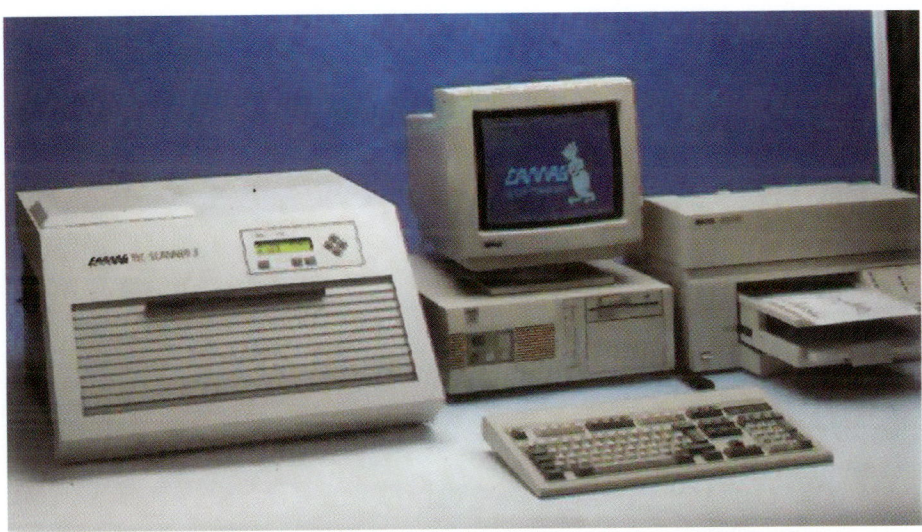

Fig. 5.28. Densitometric evaluation system with CAT software for scanning of thin layer chromatogram or electrophoresis objects in reflectance or transmission mode by absorbance or by fluorescence, spectral recording from 190-800 nm, facilities for single-level/multi-level calibration with linear or non-linear regression; content uniformity; quantification of sub-components (impurities) and statistical calculations (RSD & COV). [*Courtesy:* Camag, Switzerland through Anchrom Enterprises (I) Pvt., Mumbai, India]

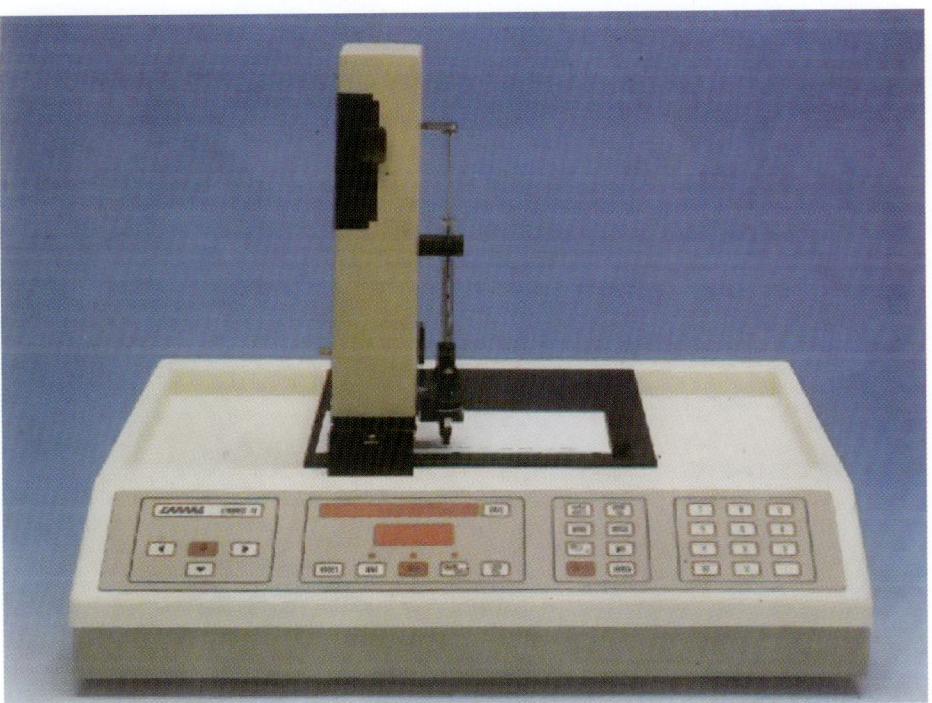

Fig. 5.29. Linomat IV sample application device; can handle volumes 1-99 μl with the spray-on technique for quantitative scanning and 5-490 μl for preparative separation. [*Courtesy:* Camag, Switzerland through Anchrom Enterprises (I) Pvt. Ltd., Mumbai, India]

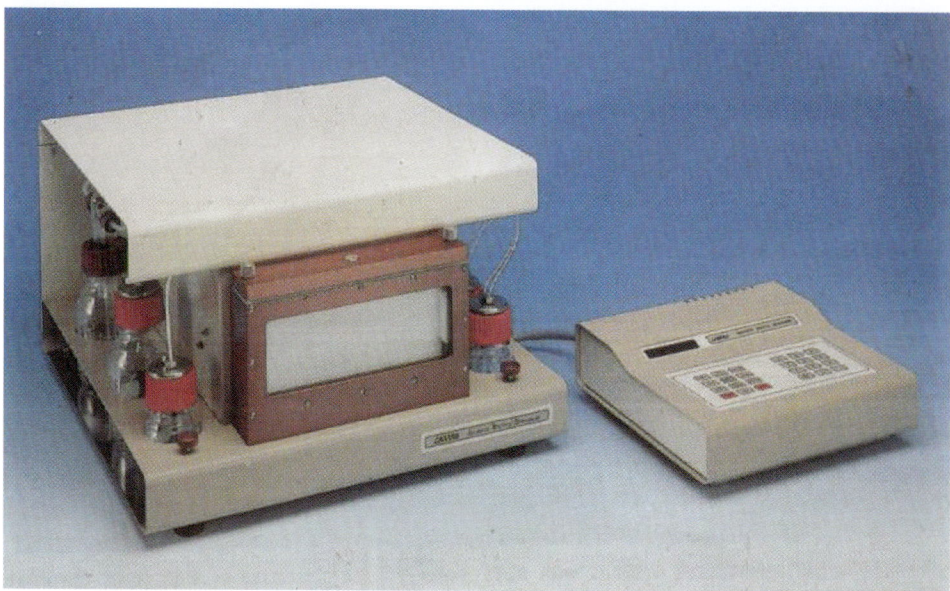

Fig. 5.30. Camag automated multiple development (AMD) system. Programmable for gradient elution of substances of widely differing polarities on one chromatogram. [*Courtesy:* Camag, Switzerland through Anchrom Enterprises (I) Pvt. Ltd., Mumbai, India]

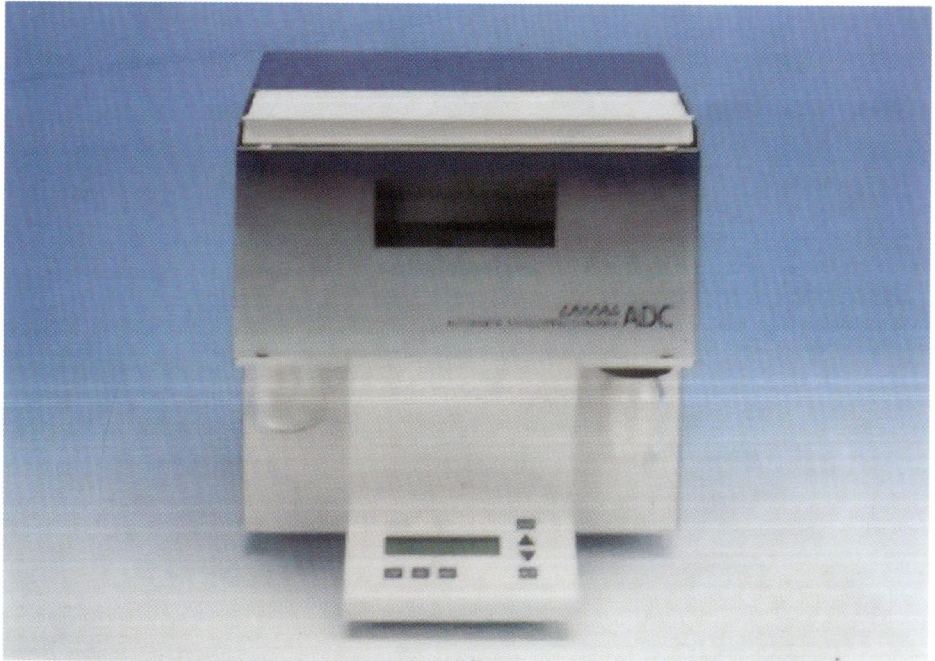

Fig. 5.31. Camag automatic developing chamber (ADC). Programmable for various chromatographic parameters; pre-conditioning, configuration (tank or sandwich), solvent migration distance and drying (cold or hot air) offers reproducible chromatogram development and avoids constant monitoring. [*Courtesy:* Camag, Switzerland through Anchrom Enterprises (I) Pvt. Ltd., Mumbai, India]

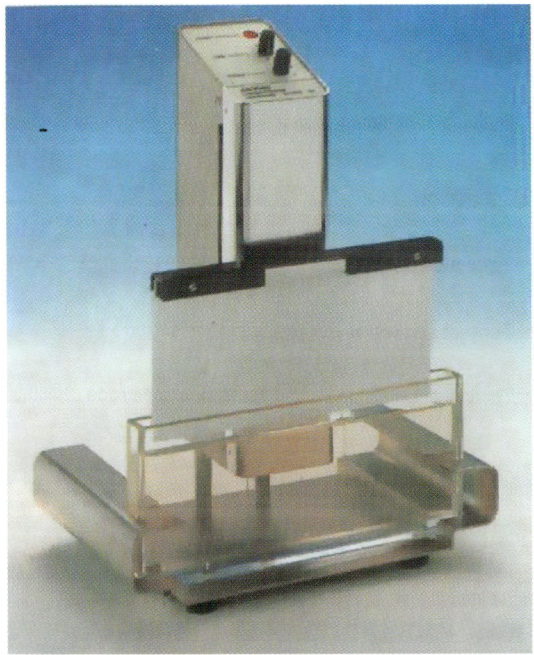

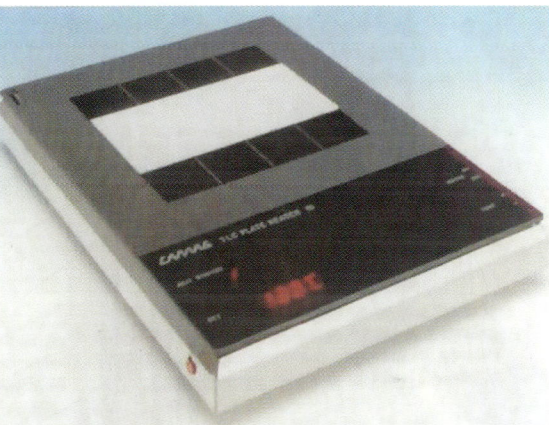

Fig. 5.32A. Camag chromatographic immersion device (battery-operated) for TLC/HPTLC plates with continually selectable vertical speed, immersion and withdrawal time, useful for pre-washing by dipping, impregnating and post-derivatisation.

Fig. 5.32B. Camag TLC plate heater with ceramic heating surface, resistant to common reagents and selectable temperature range between 25 and 200°C uniformly maintained over entire surface, programmable and digitally displayed.

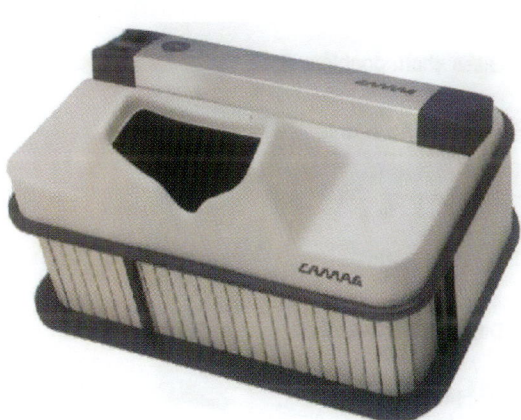

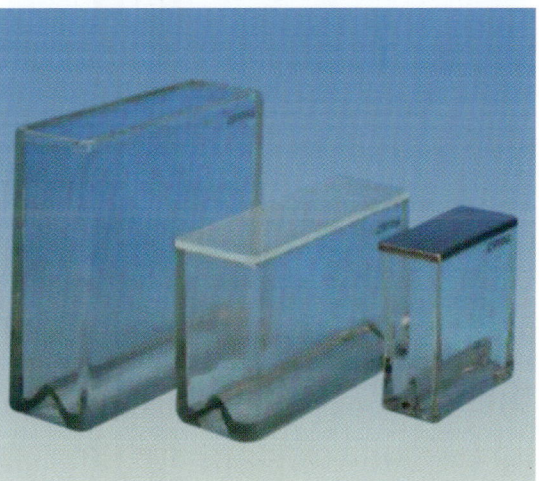

Fig. 5.32C. Camag dual wavelength (254/366 nm) viewing cabinet with automatic cutoff (2 min) device.

Fig. 5.32D. Camag twin-trough glass chamber for TLC plates (20 × 20, 20 × 10, 10 × 10 cm) with glass or SS lid, ensures low solvent consumption and reproducing pre-equilibrium.

[*Courtesy:* Camag, Switzerland, through Anchrom Enterprises (I) Pvt. Ltd., Mumbai, India]

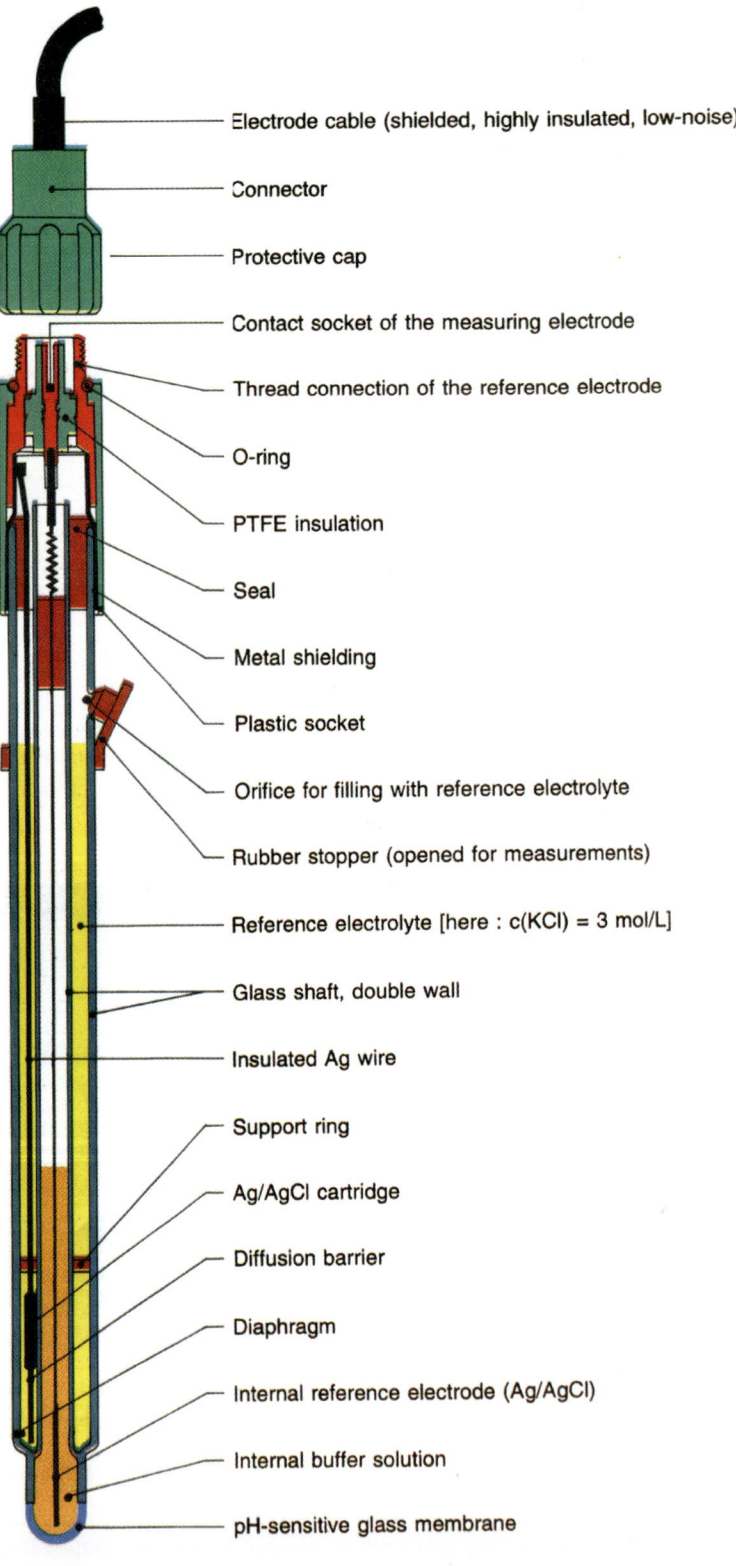

- Electrode cable (shielded, highly insulated, low-noise)
- Connector
- Protective cap
- Contact socket of the measuring electrode
- Thread connection of the reference electrode
- O-ring
- PTFE insulation
- Seal
- Metal shielding
- Plastic socket
- Orifice for filling with reference electrolyte
- Rubber stopper (opened for measurements)
- Reference electrolyte [here : c(KCl) = 3 mol/L]
- Glass shaft, double wall
- Insulated Ag wire
- Support ring
- Ag/AgCl cartridge
- Diffusion barrier
- Diaphragm
- Internal reference electrode (Ag/AgCl)
- Internal buffer solution
- pH-sensitive glass membrane

Fig. 5.33. Metrosensor long life (LL) combined pH electrode with Ag/AgCl cartridge; quicker response to temperature and more reliable pH measurements. (*Courtesy:* Metrohm, Switzerland through M/s Micro-devices & Computers, Chennai, India)

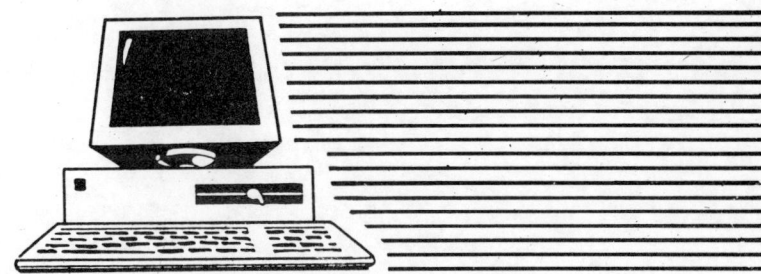

OASIS

LABORATORY INFORMATION MANAGEMENT SYSTEM (LIMS)

LABMASTER

Salient feature of the software package is test methods

- Acetyl, acid, ester, peroxide, iodine, hydroxyl and saponification values
- Titrations (direct, back and iodometric)
- Average weight and uniformity of weight (tablet, capsule, other solid dosage forms)
- Disintegration and dissolution (IP/BP/USP) including release pattern of sustained release formulations
- Uniformity of contents (IP/BP/USP)
- General tests : Specific optical rotation, pH, specific gravity, viscosity, thickness, diameter, hardness, friability, loss on drying/ignition, moisture contents, extractable volume, soluble extracts, m.p./b.p. range, sterility, particulate matter
- Spectrophotometric assay (single and multi-component)
- GLC/HPLC : internal standard technique
- Microbiological assay (test tubes—antibiotics, vitamins)
- Calculations of fiducial limits
- Computation of complete data for release pattern of sustained, controlled and modified release dosage forms
- On-line switch-over from one method to another in case of breakdown of instruments, non-availability of reagents, chemicals
- Record of vendor rating, trend analysis, stability scheduling, equipment calibration, recent reference standard details (source, assay)
- Protocols : raw material and finished product

Note : Software can be modified or developed to meet the needs of individual laboratory.

Fig. 5.34. Labmaster, complete solution for evaluating all the laboratory analytical data. (*Courtesy :* Oasis Infotech, Jaipur, India)

Chapter 6

Analgesics & Antipyretics

Aspirin, Caffeine citrate, Phenylephrine hydrochloride, Terpine hydrate, Ascorbic acid

ESTIMATION

Aspirin

Standard solution

15 mcg/ml of aspirin in 0.1 N sodium hydroxide.

Sample solution

Transfer accurately weighed portion of the powdered tablets equivalent to 150 mg of aspirin to a 100 ml volumetric flask. Add about 70 ml of 0.1 N sodium hydroxide and heat in a water bath for 30 min, cool and adjust the volume with 0.1 N sodium hydroxide. Filter and collect the filtrate after rejecting first 20-25 ml of filtrate. The filtrate is appropriately diluted with 0.1 N sodium hydroxide to get a concentration of 15 mcg/ml in respect of aspirin.

Procedure

Measure the extinction of both the solutions at maximum at about 292 nm using 0.1 N sodium hydroxide as blank and calculate the results by comparison.

Note : The extinction value of standard solution at 292 nm is quite constant on the same instrument and can be used for future estimations, so it is not necessary to run a standard every time i.e. A 1%, 1 cm value at 292 nm may be used for calculations.

Caffeine citrate

METHOD 1

Weigh accurately a quantity of powdered tablets equivalent to 10 mg of caffeine and transfer to a separating funnel. Add 10 ml of water and 10 ml of 1 N sodium hydroxide, shake well, and extract with four successive quantities, each of 20 ml of chloroform. Wash each chloroform extract with the same 10 ml of water contained in another separating funnel. Collect in a dry 100 ml volumetric flask after passing through a cotton plug and make up the volume with chloroform. Dilute 10 ml of the aliquot to 100 ml with chloroform. Measure the extinction of this solution at the maximum at about 276 nm using chloroform as blank. Calculate the contents of caffeine per tablet from the extinction of a standard caffeine solution (10 mcg/ml) in chloroform run simultaneously with the sample.

METHOD 2

Reagents

1. 0.1 N iodine.
2. 0.1 N sodium thiosulphate.
3. Dilute sulphuric acid.

Procedure

Follow the extraction procedure as described above under method 1 taking sample equivalent to 50 mg of caffeine citrate. Evaporate chloroform layer and dissolve the residue in 30 ml of dilute sulphuric acid. Add 50 ml of 0.1 N iodine and dilute to 100 ml with water, allow it to stand for 60 min. Filter, discarding the first 20 ml of the filtrate and titrate 25 ml of filtrate with 0.1 N sodium thiosulphate using starch solution as indicator. Each ml of 0.1 N iodine consumed is equivalent to 0.00485 g of caffeine.

METHOD 3

Reagents

1. 5% w/v silicotungstic acid solution in water.
2. A solvent mixture of ethyl alcohol and anhydrous ether (1 : 5) v/v.

Standard solution

500 mcg/ml of caffeine citrate in alcohol-ether mixture.

Sample solution

Weigh powdered material accurately equivalent to 20 mg of caffeine citrate, add 20 ml of dilute sulphuric acid and 30 ml of water. Reflux for 1 hr, cool and extract with four 25 ml portions of chloroform. Evaporate chloroform layer and dissolve the residue in solvent mixture to produce 50 ml.

Procedure

To 50 ml each of the sample and standard solutions, add 10 ml of silicotungstic acid solution, stir and filter through glass sintered funnel G_4. Wash the precipitate with solvent mixture. Dissolve the residue in water and dilute further with water to get 15 mcg/ml solution. Measure the extinction of both the solutions at 265 nm. The method obeys Beer's law over the concentration range of 10-90 mcg/ml.

Note : 1. The solvent should be absolutely free from water, a serious limitation of the method.
2. Paracetamol, analgin, codeine, salicylamide, atropine, phenobarbitone, vitamin B_1 and niacin do not interfere.

Phenylephrine hydrochloride

METHOD 1

This method is based on alkaline oxidation and coupling with 4-aminoantipyrine.

Reagents

1. 0.5% w/v solution of 4-aminophenazone (4-aminoantipyrine) in water.
2. 2.0% w/v solution of potassium ferricyanide in water.
3. 8.4% w/v solution of sodium bicarbonate in water.

Standard solution

100 mcg/ml of phenylephrine hydrochloride in water.

Sample solution

Weigh accurately a quantity of the powdered tablets equivalent to 10 mg of phenylephrine hydrochloride, dissolve in water to produce 100 ml, filter, reject first 15-20 ml of the filtrate.

Procedure

To 10 ml each of sample and standard solutions, add 5 ml of the 4-aminophenazone solution, 5 ml of the potassium ferricyanide solution and 1 ml of the sodium bicarbonate solution, allow to stand for 30 minutes and make up the volume to 100 ml. Measure the absorption at about 500 nm taking blank similarly treated but replacing test solution by water. Correct this result by taking a sample blank obtained by diluting 10 ml of the sample filtrate to 100 ml and reading at 500 nm, taking water as blank.

Note : Although the absorption can be measured even after 15 minutes but 30 minutes gives more reproducible results.

METHOD 2

Reagents

1. 0.15% w/v solution of nitroso-naphthol in ethyl alcohol.
2. 20% v/v nitric acid.

Standard solution

100 mcg/ml of phenylephrine hydrochloride in water.

Sample solution

Weigh accurately a quantity of powdered tablets equivalent to 10 mg of phenylephrine hydrochloride, extract with 100 ml of water, shake and filter (100 mcg/ml).

Procedure

To 2 ml each of sample and standard solutions, add 1 ml of nitrosonaphthol reagent and 1 ml of the nitric acid. Heat on a water bath at 55°C for 30 min, cool and extract with 10 ml of ethylene dichloride. Reject organic layer and measure extinction of yellow colour of the aqueous layer at about 420 nm.

Note : Chlorpheniramine maleate, aspirin, caffeine which are usually present along with this compound do not interfere.

METHOD 3

This method is based on formation of nitroso-derivative which is coupled with copper (Cu^{++}) to give pink coloured complex.

Reagents

1. 5% w/v solution of sodium nitrite in water.
2. 2.5% w/v solution of copper acetate in water.
3. 0.2 N hydrochloric acid.
4. 1% w/v solution of urea in water.

Standard solution

500 mcg/ml of phenylephrine hydrochloride in water.

Sample solution

Extract the sample with water to get 500 mcg/ml of phenylephrine hydrochloride.

Procedure

To 1 ml each of sample and standard solutions, add 1 ml of sodium nitrite solution, 1 ml of copper acetate solution, 3 ml of 0.2 N hydrochloric acid and 0.5 ml of urea solution, shaking after each addition. Keep in a boiling water bath for 15 minutes. Cool in ice for 1 minute and add 1 ml of 0.2 N hydrochloric acid and dilute to 10 ml with water. Measure the absorbance of both the solutions at about 520 nm. The coloured complex is stable for several hours.

Terpine hydrate

Reagent

1. Phosphotungstic-phosphomolybdic acid : To 10 g pure sodium tungstate and 2 g phosphomolybdic acid (free from nitrates and ammonium salts), add 10 g phosphoric acid and 70 ml of water. Boil over free flame for 2 hrs, cool, filter, if necessary, and dilute to 100 ml with water.

Standard solution

Dissolve 50 mg of terpine hydrate in 500 ml of chloroform (100 mcg/ml).

Sample solution

Transfer a quantity of powdered tablets accurately weighed equivalent to 10 mg of terpine hydrate to a dry 100 ml volumetric flask. Add about 75 ml of chloroform, shake well, make up the volume with chloroform and filter.

Procedure

In a series of 100 ml conical flasks, transfer respectively 5 ml each of standard solution, test solution and chloroform (to serve as blank). To each flask, add 5 ml water, 2 ml of phosphotungstic-phosphomolybdic acid reagent and shake well for 10 minutes. Evaporate chloroform layer in a water bath at 65-70°C. Cool in the ice bath, add very slowly 2 ml of ice-cooled sulphuric acid and allow to stand in the ice bath for half an hour with very light mixing at interval of 10 minutes. Heat the mixture on water bath (90-95°C) for exactly 10 minutes, with occasional shaking. Cool to room temperature (a turbid solution may be obtained which will subsequently become clear on further dilution). Add about 10 ml of acetone, shake and transfer to a 25 ml volumetric flask with the help of acetone and make up the volume with acetone. Measure the extinction at 630 nm using blank in the reference cell. Deduce the results by comparison.

Ascorbic acid (Vitamin C)

METHOD 1

Reagents

1. 2,6-dichlorophenol-indophenol solution : The dye is dissolved in alcohol to get a concentration of 0.25 mg/ml. The solution is filtered and stored in refrigerator. It is brought to room temperature just before use.
2. Citrate-buffer solution : Dissolve 70 g of citric acid (monohydrate) in 420 ml of 1 N sodium hydroxide and dilute to 1000 ml with water. Adjust the pH to 3.5 and store in refrigerator.

Standardization of the dye solution

Weigh accurately 15 mg of ascorbic acid and transfer to a volumetric flask with the help of sufficient volume of buffer solution to produce 50 ml. To 2 ml of the resulting solution, add 10 ml of buffer solution and titrate rapidly with the dye solution with constant shaking till distinct rose pink colour persists for about 10 seconds. Carry out the blank titration using 12 ml of buffer solution. Express the concentration of the dye solution (per ml) in term of its equivalent (mg) of ascorbic acid.

Sample solution

An accurately weighed/measured quantity of the sample equivalent to about 100 mg of ascorbic acid is shaken with 50 ml of citrate buffer and diluted to 100 ml with the buffer. 2 ml of the resulting solution is titrated with the previously standardized dye solution to a rose pink end point and the contents of ascorbic acid in the sample are calculated with the help of pre-determined equivalent factor.

Note : 1. As ascorbic acid is unstable in citrate buffer, the experiment should be completed within 60 minutes.
2. The dye solution in ethyl alcohol is stable for more than 45 days.

METHOD 2

Transfer accurately weighed portion of the powdered tablets equivalent to 250 mg of ascorbic acid to 100 ml volumetric flask, add 25 ml of sulphuric acid (10% v/v) and dilute to volume with water. Filter and titrate 20 ml of the filtrate with 0.1 N ceric ammonium sulphate using phenanthroline ferrous complex as indicator. Each ml of 0.1 N ceric ammonium sulphate is equivalent to 0.0088 g of ascorbic acid.

Salicylamide, Paracetamol

ESTIMATION

Salicylamide and Paracetamol
METHOD 1

(Simultaneous estimation of salicylamide and paracetamol without prior separation)

Standard solution of paracetamol

To 250 mg of paracetamol accurately weighed, add 10 ml of methyl alcohol and dilute to 250 ml with water (1 mg/ml).

Standard solution of salicylamide

To 250 mg of salicylamide accurately weighed, add 10 ml of methyl alcohol and dilute to 250 ml with water (1 mg/ml).

Solution A : Dilute 3 ml of standard solution of both salicylamide and paracetamol separately to 250 ml with 0.01 N sodium hydroxide (12 mcg/ml).

Solution B : Dilute 3 ml of standard solutions of both salicylamide and paracetamol separately to 250 ml with water (12 mcg/ml).

Sample solution

Weigh accurately a quantity of powdered tablets equivalent to 250 mg of paracetamol, add 10 ml of methyl alcohol, shake and dilute to 250 ml with water. Filter and carry out further dilutions as under standard solution A and B above.

Procedure

Measure the extinction of respective standard solution A at 262.5 nm and 329 nm using respective standard solution B as blank. Use the extinction value at 262.5 nm for calculation of paracetamol and that at 329 nm for calculation of salicylamide.

METHOD 2

Paracetamol

This method involves the formation of nitroso-derivative which shows absorption maxima at about 430 nm.

Reagents

1. 3% w/v solution of sodium nitrite in water.
2. 1 N hydrochloric acid.
3. 0.1 N hydrochloric acid.

4. 1 N sodium hydroxide.
5. 0.12% w/v solution of cobalt (11) bromide or chloride in water.
6. 3% w/v solution of ammonium sulphamate in water.

Standard solution

100 mcg/ml of paracetamol in 0.1 N hydrochloric acid.

Sample solution

Weigh accurately powdered tablets equivalent to 50 mg of paracetamol, add 70-80 ml of 0.1 N hydrochloric acid. Shake to dissolve paracetamol as completely as possible and dilute to 100 ml with 0.1 N hydrochloric acid. Filter and dilute the resulting solution with 0.1 N hydrochloric acid to get 100 mcg/ml.

Procedure

(a) To 5 ml each of sample and standard solutions, add 1 ml of 1 N hydrochloric acid and 2 ml of sodium nitrite solution. Mix and allow to stand for 5 minutes. Add 3 ml of 1 N sodium hydroxide, mix and allow to stand for further 5 minutes. Dilute to 50 ml with water and measure the absorbance of both standard and sample solutions at maximum at about 430 nm. Excess nitrous acid may also be neutralized by addition of 2 ml of ammonium sulphamate solution after addition of sodium nitrite. The method obeys Beer's law in the range of 4-36 mcg/ml.

(b) Carry out the above procedure till addition of 2 ml of sodium nitrite solution and keeping for 5 minutes. Add 5 ml of cobalt bromide/chloride solution and extract with three 5 ml portions of chloroform. Dilute the chloroform layer to 25 ml and measure the absorbance of chloroform extract of both the solutions at about 390 nm against reagent blank. Calculate the results by comparison. The method obeys Beer's law in the range of 4-36 mcg/ml.

Note : Salicylamide does not interfere as it does not yield cobalt derivative.

Paracetamol, Salicylamide, Caffeine citrate, Chlorpheniramine maleate

ESTIMATION

Paracetamol

Paracetamol is hydrolysed to p-aminophenol, diazotised and coupled with 'NED' to get pink dye which shows absorption maxima at about 550 nm.

Reagents

1. 0.1% w/v solution of sodium nitrite in water.
2. 0.5% w/v solution of ammonium sulphamate in water.
3. 0.1% w/v solution of N-1-naphthyl-ethylene diamine dihydrochloride (NED) in water.
4. 4 N hydrochloric acid.

Standard solution

Weigh accurately 250 mg of paracetamol, add 20 ml of hydrochloric acid and 30 ml of water. Reflux on water bath for 30 minutes, cool and dilute to 100 ml with water. 5 ml of the resultant solution is further diluted to 100 ml with water (125 mcg/ml).

Sample solution

Weigh accurately a quantity of powdered tablets equivalent to 250 mg of paracetamol and proceed with hydrolysis as described above under standard solution.

Procedure

To 10 ml of the sample and standard solutions, add 0.5 ml of 4 N hydrochloric acid and 1 ml of sodium nitrite solution. Shake vigorously and allow to stand for 3 minutes. Then, add 1 ml of ammonium sulphamate solution and keep at room temperature for 2 minutes. (This step ensures complete neutralization of nitrous acid.) Then, add 1 ml of 'NED' reagent, shake and keep in water bath (50°C) for 1 hr. Measure the extinction of both the solutions at about 550 nm against reagent blank and calculate the results by comparison.

Note : 1. Method described in formulation 4 of this chapter involving use of vanillin reagent can also be used.

2. On hydrolysis, free amino group is liberated, which can be titrated with sodium nitrite like any free aromatic amino group. Titrate appropriate aliquot of the hydrolysed sample solution as obtained above with 0.1 M sodium nitrite potentiometrically or using starch iodide paste as external indicator. Each ml of 0.1 N sodium nitrite is equivalent to 0.09512 g paracetamol.

Salicylamide

Reagents

1. 50% w/v solution of sodium hydroxide in water.
2. 4% w/v solution of boric acid in water.
3. 0.1 N sulphuric acid.

Procedure

Weigh accurately a quantity of powdered tablets equivalent to 200 mg of salicylamide and transfer to a distillation flask with the aid of 200 ml of water. Add 50 ml of sodium hydroxide solution and distil. The distillate is absorbed in boric acid solution. Titrate the distillate with 0.1 N sulphuric acid. Each ml of 0.1 N sulphuric acid is equivalent to 0.0137 g of salicylamide.

Caffeine citrate

Weigh accurately powdered sample equivalent to 20 mg of caffeine, suspend in water, basify, extract with chloroform. For details, refer to the method 1 described for estimation of caffeine citrate under formulation 1 of this chapter.

Chlorpheniramine maleate

Follow the cyanogen bromide method as described in formulation 1 of the chapter on rubefacients.

Formulation 4

Paracetamol, Caffeine citrate, Chlorpheniramine maleate, Phenylephrine hydrochloride, Ascorbic acid

ESTIMATION

Paracetamol

METHOD 1

Reagents

1. 1 N hydrochloric acid.
2. 5% w/v solution of vanillin in isopropyl alcohol.

Standard solution

Weigh accurately about 100 mg of pure paracetamol, add 50 ml of 1 N hydrochloric acid. Keep for 20 minutes and adjust to 100 ml with 1 N hydrochloric acid (1 mg/ml).

Sample solution

Weigh accurately a quantity of powdered tablets equivalent to 100 mg of paracetamol, add 50 ml of 1 N hydrochloric acid and process as per standard solution to get 1 mg/ml solution.

Procedure

To 2 ml each of standard and sample solutions, add 5 ml of 1 N hydrochloric acid and heat on boiling water bath for 5 minutes. Cool, add 10 ml of vanillin reagent and dilute to 50 ml with water. After 10 minutes, measure the absorbance of standard and sample solutions at maximum at about 395 nm and calculate the results by comparison.

METHOD 2

Reagents

1. 1% w/v solution of 2,4-dinitrobenzeldehyde (DNB) in 5% v/v sulphuric acid.
2. 0.1 N and 1 N hydrochloric acid.

Standard solution

Prepare the standard solution of paracetamol according to the method described under sample solution.

Sample solution

Weigh sample accurately equivalent to 150 mg of paracetamol, add 10 ml of methyl alcohol and dilute to 200 ml with 0.1 N hydrochloric acid.

Procedure

To 2 ml each of sample and standard solutions, add 5 ml of 1 N hydrochloric acid, heat on water bath for 30 min, cool, add 10 ml of 'DNB' reagent and after 10 minutes, measure the extinction of both the solutions at 430 nm against reagent blank. Calculate the results by comparison.

Caffeine citrate

METHOD 1

Weigh accurately a quantity of powdered tablets equivalent to 10 mg of caffeine and follow the method for estimation of caffeine involving measurement of extinction at 276 nm as described in formulation 1 of this chapter.

METHOD 2

Transfer accurately weighed quantity of the sample and carry out dry extraction with 70 ml of chloroform. Wash the chloroform layer with two 30 ml portions of saturated solution of sodium bicarbonate. Evaporate the organic layer and dissolve the residue in 100 ml of 0.01 N tartaric acid. Carry out further dilution with 0.01 N tartaric acid to get a concentration of 7.5 mcg/ml. Measure the extinction of the resulting solution at 271 nm and compare the results with standard solution of caffeine, 7.5 mcg/ml in 0.01 N tartaric acid.

Chlorpheniramine maleate

Follow the cyanogen bromide method as described in formulation 1 of the chapter on rubefacients.

Phenylephrine hydrochloride

METHOD 1

Follow the alkaline oxidation with potassium ferricyanide followed by coupling with 4-amino-phenazone as described in formulation 1 of this chapter.

METHOD 2

Suspend accurately weighed quantity of the sample equivalent to 20 mg of phenylephrine hydrochloride in 20 ml of water, basify with ammonia solution and extract with three 20 ml portions of chloroform. Wash the combined chloroform layer with water till free from alkali. Evaporate chloroform layer and dissolve the residue in glacial acetic acid and titrate with 0.01 N perchloric acid. Each ml of 0.01 N perchloric acid is equivalent to 0.0032037 g of phenylephrine hydrochloride.

METHOD 3

Reagents

1. 0.1% w/v solution of borax in water.
2. Dioxane.
3. 1 N hydrochloric acid.
4. Dinitrofluorobenzene (DNFB) reagent : Dilute 2.5 ml to 25 ml with acetone (store in refrigerator). Just before use, dilute 1 ml to 100 ml with borax solution.

Standard solution

100 mcg/ml of the substance in water.

Sample solution

(a) Eye/ear drops/liquid oral (syrups) : Directly dilute with water to get 100 mcg/ml.

(b) Ointments : Extract with 10% w/v sodium chloride solution by slight heating for 10 min to get solution of 100 mcg/ml.

(c) Tablets/capsules : Extract with water by heating in boiling water for 5 min, cool and dilute with water to get solution of 100 mcg/ml.

Procedure

To 2 ml each of sample and standard solutions, add 2 ml of DNFB reagent. Heat in boiling water bath for 10 min. Cool, add 1 ml of 1 N hydrochloric acid and 10 ml of dioxane (to dissolve the chromophore) and adjust the volume to 25 ml with water. Measure the absorbance of the sample and standard at about 385 nm against reagent blank. The method obeys Beer's law in the range of 2-10 mcg/ml.

Note : Betamethasone, lignocaine, diphenylpyraline, antipyrine, parabens did not interfere.

Ascorbic acid

Reagents

1. 85% v/v sulphuric acid in water.
2. 2% w/v solution of 2,4-dinitrophenylhydrazine in 9 N sulphuric acid.
3. 9 N sulphuric acid.
4. 50% w/v solution of oxalic acid in water.
5. Bromine water; saturated aqueous solution.
6. 1% w/v solution of thiourea in oxalic acid solution.

Standard solution

2.5 mg/ml of ascorbic acid in oxalic acid solution. To 1 ml of this solution, add 50 ml of oxalic acid solution and 10-12 drops of bromine water till faint yellow colour. Bubble air till colourless and dilute to 100 ml with oxalic acid solution (25 mcg/ml).

Sample solution

Weigh accurately a quantity of the sample equivalent to 100 mg of ascorbic acid, add 50 ml of water, shake for 15 minutes and dilute to 100 ml with same solvent. Filter, take 2.5 ml (2.5 mg), add 50 ml of oxalic acid solution and treat as per standard solution.

Procedure

To 5 ml each of sample and standard solutions, add 4 ml of thiourea solution and 2 ml of dinitro-phenylhydrazine solution. Prepare sample and standard blanks separately, using 5 ml of water instead of sample or standard. Allow all the tubes to stand at 37°C for 3 hrs. Cool in ice bath and then add 3 ml of 85% sulphuric acid drop by drop in each tube with continuous cooling. Then, add 1 ml of phenylhydrazine reagent to blanks and let all the tubes stand at room temperature for 20-30 minutes. Measure the absorbance at about 550 nm against respective blanks and calculate the results by comparison.

Aspirin, Salicylamide, Caffeine citrate, Codeine phosphate, Paracetamol

ESTIMATION

Codeine phosphate

METHOD 1

Reagents

1. Phosphate buffer, pH 5.0 or phthalate buffer, pH 5.0.
2. 0.1 N sulphuric acid, saturated with ether.
3. 0.2% w/v solution of methyl orange in water.
4. Acidified methanol : 3% v/v sulphuric acid in methanol.

Standard solution

80 mcg/ml of codeine phosphate in ether saturated 0.1 N sulphuric acid.

Sample solution

Weigh accurately a quantity of powdered tablets equivalent to 2 mg of codeine phosphate, add 20 ml of 0.1 N sulphuric acid (ether saturated) and extract with four 20 ml portions of chloroform. Collect acid layer and dilute to 25 ml with 0.1 N sulphuric acid. This step removes other ingredients present in the formulation.

Procedure

To 5 ml each of sample and standard solutions, add 5 ml of either buffer solution and 2 ml of methyl orange solution. Shake and extract with two 10 ml portions of chloroform. Separate chloroform layer and adjust with chloroform to 25 ml. Measure the absorbance of both the solutions at about 410 nm using chloroform as blank. Calculate the results by comparison.

Note : Sample directly extracted with buffer solution also gives satisfactory results.

METHOD 2

Proceed with formation of dye complex and extraction with chloroform as per method 1 above. To 10 ml of the resultant chloroform extract, add 1 ml of acidified methanol and measure the absorbance of both the solutions at about 510 nm. This method is more sensitive.

Note : Usually a buffer of pH 3.5 is employed for formation of ion-pair complex but due to presence of aspirin, pH of the extract is slightly lower, hence buffer of pH 5.0 is employed. Centrifuge chloroform layer before addition of acidified methanol for consistent results.

Salicylamide

Weigh accurately, a quantity of powdered tablets equivalent to 15 mg of salicylamide, shake with 25 ml of chloroform and adjust to 100 ml. Carry out further dilution with chloroform to get 10 mcg/ml solution and measure the extinction at maxima at about 308 nm. Calculate the results taking 350 as value of A 1%, 1 cm at 308 nm.

Note : Analgin, phenobarbitone, ascorbic acid and chloroquine do not interfere.

Alternatively, follow the method described in formulation 2 of this chapter, based on ammonia distillation.

Aspirin

Weigh accurately, a quantity of the sample equivalent to 150 mg of aspirin. Suspend in 25 ml of ether, shake vigorously for 5 minutes and filter through cotton plug, wash cotton plug with ether. Combine ether extracts and extract with 25 ml portions of 6% w/v sodium bicarbonate solution. Acidify the alkaline extract with dilute hydrochloric acid, cool and extract with four 20 ml portions of ether. Combine ether layer, wash each layer with the same 10 ml of water. Evaporate ether layer at room temperature under current of air. Dissolve the residue in neutralized methanol and titrate with 0.1 N sodium hydroxide using phenolphthalein as indicator. Each ml of 0.1 N sodium hydroxide is equivalent to 0.018016 g of aspirin.

Paracetamol

Follow the nitroso-derivative method or cobalt derivative method as described in formulation 2 of this chapter.

Note : Salicylamide yields nitroso-derivative only on boiling whereas paracetamol gives nitroso-derivative in cold.

As in salicylamide, ortho-position of phenolic function is occupied, formation of nitroso-derivative does not take place at room temperature due to hindrance of amide group at ortho-position. Further due to substitution at ortho-position, salicylamide does not form cobalt derivative.

Caffeine citrate

Reagents

1. 15% v/v phosphoric acid in water.
2. Phosphoric acid (1 : 1 v/v) in water.

Standard solution

10 mcg/ml of caffeine in 15% v/v phosphoric acid.

Sample solution

Weight accurately a quantity of sample equivalent to 5 mg of caffeine and dissolve in water to produce 25 ml. To 5 ml of this solution, add 20 ml of chloroform and extract with 30 ml of phosphoric acid (1 : 1). Collect acid layer, wash it with 20 ml of chloroform. Discard chloroform layer, dilute acid layer to 100 ml with water (10 mcg/ml). Concentration of phosphoric acid in final solution is 15% v/v.

Procedure

Measure the extinction of both standard and sample solutions at maximum at about 269 nm using 15% v/v phosphoric acid as blank and calculate the results by comparison.

Free salicylic acid (FSA)

This special procedure is described as salicylamide if present along with aspirin will interfere in the estimation of free salicylic acid by usual pharmacopoeal method.

Reagents

1. Petroleum ether (40-60°C).
2. Ferric nitrate solution : Dissolve 2.5 g of ferric nitrate monohydrate in about 200 ml of water. Add 1 ml of concentrated nitric acid and make volume to 250 ml with water. Dilute further 5 ml of the above solution to 100 ml with water.

Standard stock solution of salicylic acid

Weigh accurately 500 mg of salicylic acid and transfer to a dry 50 ml volumetric flask, make up the volume with methanol.

Working standard

Dilute 5 ml of the standard stock of salicylic acid to 100 ml with water. Each ml represents 500 mcg of salicylic acid. Take 1 ml in a 50 ml volumetric flask (A) and proceed for colour development.

Sample preparation

Weigh accurately a suitable quantity of the powdered sample and transfer to a dry 100 ml volumetric flask and make volume to 100 ml with petroleum ether (40-60°C). Shake vigorously for 2 minutes and allow it to stand for 5 minutes. Pipette 25 ml of the filtrate immediately into a 100 ml dry beaker, evaporate off the solvent to dryness at room temperature. Dissolve the residue in 5 ml of methanol and transfer to a 50 ml volumetric flask (B), rinse the beaker twice with 5 ml of water and proceed further for colour development.

Colour development

Add 5 ml of the diluted ferric nitrate solution to each 50 ml standard and sample flasks (A and B) and make volume with water and mix well. Measure the absorption of the colour at about 540 nm against water as blank and calculate the contents of salicylic acid in the tablets.

Paracetamol, Codeine phosphate, Caffeine citrate, Doxylamine succinate

ESTIMATION

Paracetamol

Follow the nitroso-derivative method as described in formulation 2 of this chapter.

Codeine phosphate

Follow the ion-pair complex method with methyl orange as described in formulation 5 of this chapter.

Caffeine citrate

Follow the method as described in formulation 5 of this chapter.

Doxylamine succinate

Reagents

1. Buffered solution of sulphanilic acid : Dissolve 2.5 g of sulphanilic acid and 10 g of anhydrous sodium acetate in 100 ml of methanol and dilute to 200 ml with methanol.
2. Cyanogen bromide solution : Prepare saturated solution of cyanogen bromide in water (to be freshly prepared).
3. 15% w/v solution of phosphoric acid in water.

Standard solution

40 mcg/ml of doxylamine succinate in 0.1 N hydrochloric acid.

Sample solution

Accurately weighed quantity of the powdered sample equivalent to 10 mg of the substance was suspended in 15% phosphoric acid and extracted with four 25 ml portions of chloroform. Organic layer was evaporated and residue taken up in 100 ml of 0.1 N hydrochloric acid.

Procedure

To 5 ml of sample and standard solutions, add 5 ml of buffered sulphanilic acid solution and 2 ml of cyanogen bromide solution. Allow it to stand for 10 min and measure the absorbance of both the sample and standard at 480 nm against respective blank and calculate the results by comparison.

Formulation 7

Paracetamol, Caffeine citrate, Codeine phosphate, Diphenhydramine hydrochloride

ESTIMATION

Paracetamol

Follow the method described in formulation 2 of this chapter.

Caffeine citrate

Follow the method described in formulation 5 of this chapter.

Codeine phosphate

Follow the method described in formulation 5 of this chapter or the method described in formulation 5 of the chapter on expectorants and cough suppressants.

Diphenhydramine hydrochloride

Follow the ammonium reineckate method or cobalt thiocyanate method described in formulation 5 or 6 of the chapter on expectorants and cough suppressants.

Paracetamol, Dicyclomine hydrochloride, Clidinium bromide

ESTIMATION

Clidinium bromide

Follow the method 1 or 2 described under formulation 1 of the chapter on sedatives and tranquilizers.

Paracetamol

Follow the method 1 or 2 described under formulation 2 of this chapter.

Dicyclomine hydrochloride

Follow the method described under formulation 20 of this chapter.

Ibuprofen, Colchicine

ESTIMATION

Ibuprofen

Accurately weighed quantity of the powdered sample equivalent to 400 mg of the substance was suspended in 25 ml of 1 N hydrochloric acid and extracted with three 20 ml portions of chloroform (reserve the acid layer for estimation of colchicine). Evaporate combined chloroform layer, take up the residue in neutral (phenol red) methanol and titrate with 0.1 N sodium hydroxide. Each ml of 0.1 N sodium hydroxide is equivalent to 20.63 mg of ibuprofen.

Colchicine

The acidic extract retained during estimation of ibuprofen was diluted to 50 ml with methanol and extinction measured at absorption maxima at about 243 nm. Calculate the results by comparing with the standard (5 mcg/ml) or by taking 730 as value of A 1%, 1 cm at 243 nm.

Paracetamol, Promethazine hydrochloride

ESTIMATION

METHOD 1

Standard solution

1. Paracetamol : 10 mcg/ml in 0.1 N hydrochloric acid.
2. Promethazine hydrochloride : 40 mcg/ml in 1% v/v sulphuric acid.

Promethazine hydrochloride

Take a measured volume of suspension equivalent to 100 mg (10 ml) of promethazine hydrochloride in a 250 ml separator. Add 5 ml of 1 N sodium hydroxide, mix thoroughly. Immediately extract the promethazine base with four 25 ml portions of chloroform. Collect the total chloroform in a second separator. The aqueous layer is acidified with 1 N hydrochloric acid and preserved for paracetamol estimation. The chloroform extract is washed with 2×10 ml of 1 in 9 hydrochloric acid and collect the chloroform extract in a 250 ml conical flask. Wash the acid portion with 25 ml chloroform and add this 25 ml chloroform to total chloroform layer. Evaporate the chloroform on a boiling water bath to dryness. Add 5-10 ml of methanol and evaporate. Dissolve the residue in 1 in 100 sulphuric acid and dilute to get a final concentration of 40 mcg/ml. Measure the absorbance at 298 nm and calculate the result by comparing with standard. Carry out the entire procedure under low actinic light.

Paracetamol

The above preserved solution is taken and warmed slightly on water bath till it is free from smell of chloroform. Dilute with 0.1 N hydrochloric acid to get a final concentration of 10 mcg/ml. Measure the extinction at 244 nm and calculate the results by comparing with standard solution (10 mcg/ml) (final concentration of 7.5 mcg/ml is preferable).

Typical laboratory analysis

1. Promethazine hydrochloride

Weight of standard promethazine hydrochloride = 0.0630 g

$$0.063 \text{ g of standard promethazine hydrochloride} \xrightarrow{\text{1 in 100 } H_2SO_4} 50 \text{ ml}$$

$$1.6 \text{ ml} \xrightarrow{\text{1 in 100 } H_2SO_4} 50 \text{ ml (40 mcg/ml)}$$

Sample :

$$\begin{array}{c} \text{10 ml of suspension} \\ \text{equivalent to 0.010 g} \\ \text{of promethazine} \end{array} \longrightarrow \begin{array}{c} \text{Extraction,} \\ \text{evaporation} \\ \text{and residue} \end{array} \xrightarrow{\text{1 in 100 } H_2SO_4} 250 \text{ ml (40 mcg/ml)}$$

Absorbance at 298 nm :
Standard reading : 0.398
Sample reading : 0.391

$$\text{Promethazine hydrochloride mg/5 ml} = \frac{0.391}{0.398} \times \frac{0.063}{50} \times \frac{1.6}{50} \times \frac{250 \times 5}{10}$$

$$= 4.95 \text{ mg}$$

$$\text{Claim} = 5 \text{ mg}$$

2. Paracetamol

$$0.0249 \text{ g of standard paracetamol} \xrightarrow{\text{0.1 N HCl}} 50 \text{ ml}$$

$$1 \text{ ml} \xrightarrow{\text{0.1 N HCl}} 50 \text{ ml (10 mcg/ml)}$$

10 ml of suspension $\xrightarrow{\text{1 N NaOH}}$ basified, extracted, acidic extract $\xrightarrow{\text{0.1 N HCl}}$ 100 ml
equivalent to 0.5 g
of paracetamol

$$1 \text{ ml} \xrightarrow{\text{0.1 N HCl}} 50 \text{ ml}$$

$$5 \text{ ml} \xrightarrow{\text{0.1 N HCl}} 50 \text{ ml (10 mcg/ml)}$$

Absorbance at 245 nm :
Standard reading : 0.760
Sample reading : 0.780

$$\text{Paracetamol mg/5 ml} = \frac{0.780}{0.760} \times \frac{0.0249}{50} \times \frac{1}{50} \times \frac{100}{0.50} \times \frac{50}{1} \times \frac{50}{5} \times \frac{5}{10}$$

$$= 255 \text{ mg}$$

$$\text{Claim} = 250 \text{ mg}$$

METHOD 2

Paracetamol

Reagents

1. 1 N hydrochloric acid
2. 1 N sodium hydroxide
3. 10% w/v solution of sodium nitrite in water.
4. 10% w/v solution of sulphamic acid in water.

Standard solution

Dissolve 100 mg of the substance in 50 ml of 1 N hydrochloric acid and dilute to 500 ml with water.

Sample solution

Accurately measured quantity of the sample equivalent to 100 mg of the substance is suspended in 50 ml of 1 N hydrochloric acid and diluted to 500 ml with water.

Procedure

To 5 ml each of sample and standard solutions add 5 ml of sodium nitrite solution, shake and allow to stand for 5 min. Add 5 ml of sulphamic acid solution drop by drop with constant shaking till the effervescence clears. Allow to stand for 5 min and dilute to 50 ml with 1 N sodium hydroxide. Measure the absorbance of both sample and standard solutions at about 430 nm against reagent blank and calculate the results by comparison.

Promethazine hydrochloride

Reagents

1. Buffer solution pH 2.7 : 6 g of citric acid and 3.9 g of disodium dihydrogen phosphate dissolved in about 900 ml of water, pH adjusted to 2.7-2.8 with citric acid and diluted to 1000 ml.
2. Bromocresol green solution : 69.8 mg of dye was dissolved in 2 ml of 0.1 N sodium hydroxide and made to 1000 ml with buffer solution.

Standard solution

1 mg/ml of promethazine hydrochloride in water.

Sample solution

The sample (suspension) containing 5 mg/5 ml of the substance was used as such.

Procedure

To 2 ml each of sample and standard solutions, add 50 ml of water, 25 ml dye solution. Mix and extract with three 30 ml portions of chloroform. Pass the chloroform layer through anhydrous sodium sulphate (already moistened with chloroform), make up to 100 ml. Measure the absorbance of both sample and standard solutions at about 415 nm using chloroform as blank and calculate the results by comparison.

Paracetamol, Pseudoephedrine hydrochloride, Chlorpheniramine maleate. Caffeine citrate

ESTIMATION

Paracetamol

Follow the method described in formulation 2 or 33 of this chapter.

Pseudoephedrine hydrochloride

As ephedrine/pseudoephedrine are volatile bases, this property has been used for quantitative estimation by steam distillation of the base. For details, refer to formulation 8 of the chapter on bronchospasm relaxants. Each ml of 0.1 N hydrochloric acid is equivalent to 20.17 mg of pseudoephedrine hydrochloride.

Alternatively, follow the method described in formulation 19 of the chapter on expectorants.

Chlorpheniramine maleate

Follow the method described in formulation 1 of the chapter on rubefacients.

Caffeine citrate

Standard solution

10 mcg/ml of caffeine in chloroform.

Sample solution

Accurately weighed quantity of the powdered sample was extracted with chloroform to get final concentration of 10 mcg/ml of caffeine.

Measure the absorption of both sample and standard solutions at maxima at about 276 nm using chloroform as blank and calculate the results by comparison.

Aspirin, Dipyridamole

ESTIMATION

Aspirin

METHOD 1

Follow the method described in formulation 5 of this chapter.

METHOD 2

Standard solution

20 mcg/ml of aspirin in 0.1 N sulphuric acid, solution is prepared by heating in boiling water bath.

Sample solution

Weigh accurately, powdered sample equivalent to 100 mg of aspirin, suspend in 60-70 ml of 0.1 N sulphuric acid. Heat in a boiling water bath, cool and make the volume to 100 ml with 0.1 N sulphuric acid. Dilute further to get solution of 20 mcg/ml.

Measure the absorbance of both sample and standard solution at about 229 nm using 0.1 N sulphuric acid as blank and calculate the results by comparison.

Dipyridamole

Standard solution

15 mcg/ml of dipyridamole in 0.1 N sulphuric acid.

Sample solution

Weigh accurately equivalent to 75 mg of dipyridamole, suspend in about 150 ml of 0.1 N sulphuric acid. Shake for 10 min and make up the volume to 250 ml with 0.1 N sulphuric acid. Further dilutions are appropriately done with 0.1 N sulphuric acid to get final dilution of 15 mcg/ml.

Measure the absorbance of both sample and standard solution at about 285 nm using 0.1 N sulphuric acid as blank and calculate the results by comparison.

Ibuprofen, Dextropropoxyphene hydrochloride, Paracetamol

ESTIMATION

Ibuprofen

Follow the method described in formulation 9 of this chapter which involves extraction with chloroform, followed by evaporation of organic layer, residue taken up in neutral methanol and titrated with 0.1 N sodium hydroxide. Each ml of 0.1 N sodium hydroxide is equivalent to 20.63 mg of ibuprofen.

Dextropropoxyphene hydrochloride

Follow the method based on formation of ion-pair complex with bromocresol green. For details, refer to formulation 25 of this chapter.

Paracetamol

Paracetamol is hydrolysed to p-aminophenol, diazotised and coupled with 'NED' to get pink dye having absorption maxima at about 530 nm. For details refer to formulation 3 of this chapter.

Phenylephrine hydrochloride, Caffeine citrate, Diphenhydramine hydrochloride

ESTIMATION

Phenylephrine hydrochloride

Follow the method described in formulation 1 of this chapter. The method is based on alkaline oxidation and coupling with 4-aminoantipyrine.

Caffeine citrate

Follow the method described in formulation 24 of this chapter.

Diphenhydramine hydrochloride

Reagents

1. Phthalate buffer, pH 3.00. Dissolve 2.042 g of potassium hydrogen phthalate in 100 ml of water. Add 40.6 ml of 0.1 N hydrochloric acid, make up to 200 ml with water. Check final pH.
2. Bromocresol green (BCG) solution : 34.9 mg of the dye is dissolved in 100 ml of 0.1 N sodium hydroxide and diluted to 500 ml with water.

Standard solution

20 mcg/ml of the substance in water.

Sample solution

Accurately weighed quantity of the sample extracted with water to get a concentration of 20 mcg/ml.

Procedure

To 15 ml each of sample and standard solutions, add 60 ml of the dye solution, add 1-2 drops of 1 N hydrochloric acid till yellow colour is obtained. Add 10 ml of buffer solution. Extract the complex with three 15 ml portions of chloroform. Combine the chloroform layer, dilute to 50 ml. Add few crystals of anhydrous sodium sulphate and shake. Measure the absorbance of each sample and standard solutions at 415 nm using chloroform as blank. Calculate the results by comparison.

Formulation 15

Paracetamol, Diclofenac sodium, Chlormezanone

ESTIMATION

Paracetamol

Follow the nitroso-derivative method described in formulation 2 of this chapter.

Diclofenac sodium

Follow the method based on colour development with methylene blue. For details refer to method 2 described under formulation 51 of this chapter.

Chlormezanone

Follow the method described in formulation 46 of this chapter. Chloroform extract can either be directly used for spectrophotometric measurements or it can be evaporated and residue taken up in 0.1 N sulphuric acid and appropriately diluted for subsequent spectrophotometric analysis at 227 nm.

Alternatively, combine the alkaline layer (formulation 46) and washings, make it acidic with 1 N HCl and extract with three 25 ml portions of chloroform. The combined extract is evaporated and residue taken up in 0.1 N NaOH to get final solution of 10 mcg/ml in respect of diclofenac sodium. Measure the absorbance at 276 nm (see formulation 51 of this chapter). The acidic layer is appropriately diluted to get solution of 10 mcg/ml in respect of paracetamol (see formulation 51 of this chapter).

Typical laboratory analysis

Paracetamol

Weight of standard paracetamol taken = 100.9 mg (W_s)

Weight of sample taken = 242.6 mg (W_u)

Average weight of the tablet = 1200 mg

$$\text{Paracetamol (mg)/tablet} = \frac{A_u}{A_s} \times \frac{W_s}{W_u} \times \text{dilution factor} \times 1200$$

$$= \frac{0.544}{0.540} \times \frac{100.9}{242.6} \times \text{dilution factor} \times 1200$$

$$= 499.62 \text{ mg}$$

$$\text{Claim} = 500 \text{ mg}$$

Diclofenac sodium

Weight of standard diclofenac sodium taken = 50.4 mg

Weight of sample taken = 1205.1 mg

$$\text{Diclofenac sodium (mg)/tablet} = \frac{A_u}{A_s} \times \frac{W_s}{W_u} \times \text{dilution factor} \times 1200$$

$$= \frac{0.496}{0.511} \times \frac{50.4}{1205.1} \times \text{dilution factor} \times 1200$$

$$= 48.62 \text{ mg}$$

$$\text{Claim} = 50 \text{ mg}$$

Chlormezanone

Weight of standard chlormezanone taken = 51.70 mg

Weight of sample taken = 609.40 mg

$$\text{Chlormezanone (mg)/tablet} = \frac{A_u}{A_s} \times \frac{W_s}{W_u} \times \text{dilution factor} \times 1200$$

$$= \frac{0.607}{0.644} \times \frac{51.7}{609.4} \times \text{dilution factor} \times 1200$$

$$= 94.79 \text{ mg}$$

$$\text{Claim} = 100 \text{ mg}$$

Formulation 16

Ibuprofen, Paracetamol, Chlorzoxazone

ESTIMATION

Paracetamol

Follow the method described in formulation 35 of this chapter.

Ibuprofen

Follow the method described in formulation 47 of this chapter.

Chlorzoxazone

Standard solution

20 mcg/ml of chlorzoxazone in methanol.

Sample solution

Suspend accurately weighed quantity of powdered sample equivalent to 50 mg of the substance in slightly warm water. Cool and extract with diethyl ether (4 × 20 ml). Combined ethereal layer is washed twice with water (2 × 20 ml) and passed through a bed of anhydrous sodium sulphate. Organic layer is evaporated to dryness and residue taken up in methanol to produce a working solution of 20 mcg/ml for analysis.

Measure the absorbance of both the solutions at about 282 nm and calculate the results by comparison.

Ibuprofen, Paracetamol, Magnesium trisilicate

ESTIMATION

Paracetamol

Follow the method described in formulation 57 of this chapter.

Ibuprofen

Follow the method described in formulation 19 of this chapter. Alternatively, the residue is taken up in 20 ml of neutralized methanol and titrated with 0.1 N sodium hydroxide using phenolphthalein as indicator. Each ml of 0.1 N sodium hydroxide is equivalent to 0.02063 g of ibuprofen.

Magnesium trisilicate

Follow the method described in formulation 1 of the chapter on anti-inflammatory drugs. Cooling the solution in ice-bath before titration gives better results.

Paracetamol, Orphenadrine citrate

ESTIMATION

Paracetamol

Follow the method described in formulation 53 of this chapter.

Orphenadrine citrate

Procedure

Accurately weighed quantity of the powdered sample equivalent to 70 mg of the substance was suspended in about 30 ml of 1 N sodium hydroxide and extracted with three 50 ml portions of chloroform. Combined chloroform layers are passed through anhydrous sodium sulphate and evaporated to dryness at 105°C. Dissolve the residue in 50 ml of neutralized glacial acetic acid and titrate with 0.02 N perchloric acid using crystal violet as indicator. Each ml of 0.1 N perchloric acid is equivalent to 9.23 mg of orphenadrine citrate.

Ibuprofen, Pseudoephedrine hydrochloride or Codeine phosphate

ESTIMATION

Pseudoephedrine hydrochloride

Standard solution

300 mcg of pseudoephedrine hydrochloride in water.

Procedure

An accurately weighed quantity of powdered sample (tablets) equivalent to 200 mg of ibuprofen is suspended in 20 ml of water, sonicated for 5 min and filtered through G_3 sintered glass funnel. The filtrate was diluted appropriately with water to get a concentration of 300 mcg/ml in respect of pseudoephedrine hydrochloride (the residue was retained for estimation of ibuprofen).

Measure absorbance of both sample and standard solutions at 257 nm and calculate the results by comparison.

Ibuprofen

Standard solution

400 mcg/ml of ibuprofen in chloroform.

Procedure

The residue retained in the crucible during extraction and estimation of pseudoephedrine was extracted with chloroform (2 × 25 ml) and filtered. The filtrate was further diluted to get final concentration of 400 mcg/ml. Absorption of both sample and standard solutions was measured at 264 nm and results calculated by comparison.

Note :   For estimating codeine phosphate, filtrate was diluted with water to get concentration of 100 mcg/ml and absorbance measured at 284 nm for calculating the results.

In case of suspension, accurately measured quantity of sample equivalent to 100-150 mg of ibuprofen was suspended in 4-5 ml of water and extracted with chloroform (4 × 25 ml). The combined chloroform extract was evaporated, residue taken up in 50 ml of neutral methanol (phenol red) and titrated with 0.1 N sodium hydroxide. Each ml of 0.1 N sodium hydroxide is equivalent to 0.02063 g of ibuprofen.

Another portion of sample equivalent to about 100-150 mg of pseudoephedrine hydrochloride was suspended in 5 ml of water and extracted with ether (4 × 25 ml) filtering each portion through cotton-plug. The combined ether layer was evaporated on water-bath and residue taken up in 40 ml of glacial acetic acid for non-aqueous titration with 0.1 N perchloric acid (crystal violet). Each ml of 0.1 N perchloric acid is equivalent to 0.02017 g of pseudoephedrine hydrochloride.

Paracetamol, Dicyclomine hydrochloride, Activated Dimethicone

ESTIMATION

Paracetamol

Follow the method described in formulation 53 of this chapter.

Dicyclomine hydrochloride

Reagent

1. Picric acid solution : 20 mg of picric acid and 2.90 g of sodium acetate anhydrous are dissolved in 70-80 ml of water, add 4 ml of glacial acetic acid and dilute to 100 ml with water.

Standard solution

20 mcg/ml of dicyclomine hydrochloride in 0.1 N hydrochloric acid.

Sample solution

Accurately weighed quantity of powdered sample is extracted with 0.1 N hydrochloric acid to get a final concentration of 20 mcg/ml in respect of dicyclomine hydrochloride.

Procedure

To 20 ml each of sample and standard solutions, add 5 ml of picric acid solution, shake and extract with chloroform (2 × 10 ml) passing each extract through bed of anhydrous sodium sulphate. Make up the volume to 25 ml and measure the absorbance of both the solutions at 405 nm against reagent blank and calculate the results by comparison. Alternatively, follow the method described in formulation 21 of this chapter.

Activated Dimethicone (Dimethylpolysiloxane) (DMP)

Weigh sample equivalent to 40 mg of the DMP, add 15 ml of concentrated hydrochloric acid. Digest on water-bath for 15 min till all the foam has disintegrated and emulsifying action has been destroyed. Extract the contents with four 40 ml portions of chloroform-ether (2 : 6) mixture. Wash the pooled organic layer with three 15 ml portions of 1 N sodium hydroxide followed by 3 × 15 ml of water. Pass the organic layer through cotton-plug and evaporate to dryness at 150°C for 45 min. Cool and weigh. The weight of the residue obtained represents the amount of DMP present in the sample initially taken for analysis.

Note : Washing with sodium hydroxide removes parabens, this step can be omitted if parabens are absent.

Mefenamic acid, Dicyclomine hydrochloride

ESTIMATION

Mefenamic acid

Weigh accurately powdered sample equivalent to 250 mg of mefenamic acid, suspend in 50-60 ml water and shake for 5 min and filter through G$_3$ glass sintered funnel, discard the filtrate. Wash the residue with water, rejecting the filtrate. Dissolve the residue in neutralized methanol (phenol red) and titrate with 0.1 N sodium hydroxide. Each ml of 0.1 N sodium hydroxide is equivalent to 0.02413 g of mefenamic acid.

Dicyclomine hydrochloride

Suspend accurately weighed quantity of finely powdered sample equivalent to about 10 mg of dicyclomine hydrochloride in 40-50 ml of water. Shake for 5-10 min, add 10 ml of 1 N sulphuric acid and 1 ml of potassium permanganate solution (0.1%). Allow the mixture to stand for 2 min, add 0.1 ml of dimethyl yellow solution (indicator) and 25 ml of chloroform. Shake and titrate with 0.004 M sodium lauryl sulphate to permanent pink colour in chloroform layer. Each ml of 0.004 M sodium lauryl sulphate is equivalent to 0.001384 g of dicyclomine hydrochloride.

Aspirin, Chlorpheniramine maleate, Salicylamide

ESTIMATION

Aspirin

Extract accurately weighed quantity of the powdered sample equivalent to 500 mg of aspirin with neutral acetone and titrate with 0.1 N sodium hydroxide using phenolphthalein solution as indicator. Each ml of 0.1 N sodium hydroxide is equivalent to 0.018016 g of aspirin. For estimation of free salicylic acid in the formulation, follow the method given in formulation 5 of this chapter.

Chlorpheniramine maleate

Follow the cyanogen bromide method as described in formulation 1 of the chapter on rubefacients.

Salicylamide

Reagents

1. 0.1% w/v solution 2,6-dichloroquinone chlorimide in isopropyl alcohol.
2. Buffer solution, pH 9.2.
3. Isopropyl alcohol : water (1 : 1) v/v mixture.

Standard solution

50 mcg/ml of salicylamide in alcohol-water solvent mixture.

Sample solution

Weigh accurately powdered tablets equivalent to 50 mg of salicylamide and extract with isopropyl alcohol-water mixture to make 100 ml. Dilute appropriately with the same solvent to get 50 mcg/ml solution.

Procedure

To 2 ml each of standard and sample solutions, add 2 ml of buffer solution, pH 9.2, 5 ml of isopropyl alcohol and 1 ml of chlorimide reagent. Shake for 1 minute and allow to stand for 30 minutes. Measure the absorbance of both the solutions at about 650 nm and calculate the results by comparison.

Paracetamol, Salicylamide, Chlorpheniramine maleate, Phenylephrine hydrochloride

ESTIMATION

Chlorpheniramine maleate

Follow the cyanogen bromide method as described in formulation 1 of chapter on rubefacients.

Phenylephrine hydrochloride

METHOD 1

Reagents

1. Amberlite IRC-50-sodium (a weak cationic exchanger).
2. 0.5 N sodium hydroxide.
3. 0.5 N hydrochloric acid.
4. 2 N sulphuric acid.
5. 5% w/v solution of sodium bicarbonate in water.

Treatment of resin (amberlite IRC-50 - Na$^+$)

Wash 25 g of the resin with water, repeat washing twice. Then suspend the resin in 2 N sulphuric acid. Allow the resin to remain in contact with the acid for 2 hours, discard the acid. Wash the resin with water till washings are free from sulphate. Suspend the resin in 500 ml of sodium bicarbonate solution and stir for 1 hour. Filter the resin through buchner funnel. Wash the resin with water till washings are free from carbonate. Suspend the resin in water, the pH of the suspension should be about 8.2-8.6. If the pH is less than 8.2, repeat the treatment with sodium bicarbonate. The resin is now ready for use. Store the resin always in water and it should not go dry and should have no fungus growth.

Preparation of the column : Glass column having a height of 125 mm and diameter of 15 mm with glass stop cock is used. Put a plug of glass wool at the bottom of the column to support the resin. Fill the column with suspended resin to a height of about 100 mm. Wash the column with water. Then put a thin plug of glass wool on the top so as the resin layer is not disturbed during elution. The column is ready for use.

Standard solution

1 mg/ml of phenylephrine hydrochloride in water. Use 2.5 ml of the solution for column chromatography.

Sample solution

Weight accurately a quantity of the sample equivalent to 2.5 mg of phenylephrine hydrochloride, suspend in water and dilute to 100 ml with water.

Procedure

Put standard solution and sample solution equivalent to 2.5 mg of the compound on two different columns. Run blank column as well. Wash the columns with 250 ml of distilled water and then elute phenylephrine hydrochloride with 0.5 N hydrochloric acid. Dilute the eluent to 100 ml. Dilute 2.5 ml of this solution to 10 ml with 0.5 N sodium hydroxide and measure the extinction at 238 nm against eluate obtained from blank column.

METHOD 2

Reagents

1. 1% w/v solution of copper sulphate in water.
2. 1% w/v solution of hydroxylamine hydrochloride.
3. Strong ammonia-ammonium chloride buffer solution.
4. Dilute ammonia-ammonium chloride buffer solution : Prepared by diluting 20 ml of strong buffer to 50 ml with water.

Standard solution

200 mcg/ml of phenylephrine hydrochloride in 0.1 N sulphuric acid.

Sample solution

Extract accurately weighed amount of the powdered tablets with 0.1 N sulphuric acid to get 200 mcg/ml.

Procedure

To 5 ml each of sample and standard solutions, add 1 ml of copper sulphate solution, 1 ml of dilute buffer solution and 1 ml of hydroxylamine hydrochloride solution. Extract with four 5 ml portions of n-butanol. Collect butanol layer and dilute to 25 ml with alcohol. Measure the extinction of both the solutions at about 415 nm and calculate the results by comparison.

Note : If the sample is coloured, prepare blank as under :

To 5 ml of the test solution, add 1 ml of buffer solution and extract with two 5 ml portions of n-butanol. Collect butanol layer. Add 1 ml of copper sulphate solution, 1 ml of buffer solution and 1 ml of hydroxylamine solution to butanol layer. Shake, collect butanol layer and dilute to 25 ml with butanol and use as sample blank.

The colour is stable for 24 hrs and obeys Beer's law in concentration range of 8-40 mcg/ml. Ascorbic acid, naphazoline nitrate, caffeine do not interfere.

Paracetamol

Follow the methods as described in formulation 3 of this chapter.

Salicylamide

Standard solution

Weigh accurately 100 mg of pure compound, dissolve in 5 ml of methanol and dilute to 100 ml with water (1 mg/ml). Dilute 3 ml of the resulting solution to 250 ml with 0.01 N sodium hydroxide.

Sample solution

Weigh powdered material accurately equivalent to 100 mg of salicylamide and proceed as under standard solution.

Blank solution

Prepare respective blank by diluting 3 ml of initial solutions (1 mg/ml) of both standard and sample to 250 ml with water.

Procedure

Measure absorbance of both the solutions against respective blanks at 331 nm and calculate the results by comparison.

Analgin, Paracetamol, Caffeine citrate, Codeine phosphate

ESTIMATION

Analgin

Reagents

1. 0.2 M phthalate buffer, pH 4.0.
2. 0.5% w/v solution of 1,2-naphthoquinone-4-sulphonic acid (sodium salt) in water.

Standard solution

1 mg/ml of analgin in water.

Sample solution

Weigh accurately a quantity of powdered tablets equivalent to 250 mg of analgin and extract with water to produce 250 ml (1 mg/ml).

Procedure

To 2 ml each of sample and standard solutions, add 10 ml of buffer solution and 1 ml of naphthoquinone reagent. Heat in water bath at 50°C for 60 minutes. Cool and extract with three 20 ml portions of chloroform. Combine chloroform layer, pass through anhydrous sodium sulphate and adjust to 100 ml with chloroform. Measure the absorbance of both standard and sample solutions at about 475 nm. Deduce the results by comparison.

Caffeine citrate

METHOD 1

Reagents

1. 10% w/v solution of phosphomolybdic acid in water.
2. 1 N hydrochloric acid.

Standard solution

1 mg/ml of caffeine in water.

Sample solution

Weigh accurately sample equivalent to 100 mg of caffeine, add 50 ml of chloroform or dichloromethane and boil on water-bath for few minutes. Filter hot, evaporate organic layer and dissolve the residue in water to produce 100 ml.

Procedure

To 25 ml each of sample and standard solutions, add 15 ml of 1 N hydrochloric acid and 3 ml of phosphomolybdic acid solution. Boil for 3 minutes, chill for 30 minutes. Filter the precipitates through dry glass sintered funnel G_4. Wash the residue with dilute hydrochloric acid till filtrate is colourless. Allow the acid layer to drain off completely. Dissolve the residue in acetone to produce 25 ml. Measure the absorbance of both standard and sample solutions at 440 nm, and calculate the results. The method obeys Beer's law in the range of 1-5 mg/ml.

METHOD 2

Reagents

1. 5% w/v solution of silicotungstic acid in alcohol-ether solvent mixture.
2. A solvent mixture of ethyl alcohol and anhydrous ether (1 : 5) v/v.

Procedure

Weigh accurately, a quantity of powdered tablets equivalent to 30 mg of caffeine, extract with 100 ml of alcohol-ether solvent mixture. Filter and add 10 ml of silicotungstic acid reagent. Allow to stand for 10 minutes, filter through G_4 sintered glass funnel, wash the precipitates with the solvent mixture and dry at 105°C to a constant weight.

Weight of caffeine (g) = Weight of the precipitates (g) × 0.1701

The precipitates obtained above can be dissolved in water to get a concentration of 10 mcg/ml in respect of caffeine which exhibits maxima at above 265 nm. For details, refer to the method for estimation of caffeine described under formulation 1 of this chapter.

Codeine phosphate

METHOD 1

This is based on estimation of phosphate moiety of the compound.

Reagents

1. 10 N sulphuric acid.
2. Stannous chloride solution : To 1 g stannous chloride, add 5 ml of concentrated hydrochloric acid. Heat on boiling water bath till clear solution is obtained. Just before use, dilute 1 ml of this solution to 100 ml with water.
3. Ammonium molybdate solution : To 6.4 g of ammonium molybdate, add 40 ml of water and 50 ml of 10 N sulphuric acid. Make up to 100 ml with water.

Standard solution

100 mcg/ml of codeine phosphate in water.

Sample solution

Weigh accurately powdered material equivalent to 10 mg of codeine phosphate and extract with water to produce 100 ml.

Procedure

To 10 ml each of sample and standard solutions, add 50 ml of water, 10 ml of 10 N sulphuric acid and 10 ml of ammonium molybdate solution. Then, add 5 ml of stannous chloride solution with care and shake. Keep at room temperature for 60 minutes and dilute with water to 100 ml. Measure the absorbance of both the solutions at 675 nm and calculate the results by comparison.

METHOD 2

Follow the ion-pair-complex method with methyl orange as described in formulation 5 of this chapter.

Paracetamol

METHOD 1

Follow the nitroso-derivative method followed by chelation with cobalt as described in formulation 2 of this chapter.

METHOD 2

Reagents

1. Hydrochloric acid solution : Dilute 50 ml of concentrated hydrochloric acid to 100 ml with water.
2. 10% w/v solution of sodium nitrite in water.
3. 5% w/v solution of sodium carbonate in water.

Standard solution

100 mcg/ml of paracetamol in water.

Sample solution

Accurately weighed quantity of the powdered sample is extracted with water by intermittent heating in water-bath for 60 min to get final solution of 100 mcg/ml.

Procedure

To 1 ml each of sample and standard solutions add 0.5 ml of hydrochloric acid solution and 1 ml of sodium nitrite solution. Shake well and allow to stand at room temperature for 10 min. Add 5 ml of sodium carbonate solution to each, shake and allow to stand at room temperature for 15 min. Measure the absorbance of both sample and standard solution at 430 nm against reagent blank and calculate the results by comparison.

Dextropropoxyphene napsylate, Paracetamol, Diazepam

ESTIMATION

Dextropropoxyphene napsylate

METHOD 1

Weigh accurately, a quantity of powdered tablets equivalent to about 500 mg of dextropropoxyphene napsylate, add 10 ml of water and 3 ml of solution of sodium hydroxide (10% w/v). Extract with four 30 ml portions of chloroform. Wash combined chloroform extract with water till washings are free from alkali. Pass organic layer through anhydrous sodium sulphate and titrate with 0.1 N perchloric acid using crystal violet solution as indicator (change of colour from violet to blue). Each ml of 0.1 N perchloric acid is equivalent to 0.05658 g of dextropropoxyphene napsylate. Alternatively, follow the method described in formulation 26 of this chapter which is based on optical rotation property of the compound.

METHOD 2

Reagents

1. Buffer solution, pH, 4. To 50 ml of 0.2 M potassium hydrogen phthalate, add 0.1 ml of 0.2 N hydrochloric acid and dilute to 200 ml with water. Check and adjust the pH to 4.0.
2. Bromocresol green solution, 0.01% w/v solution of the dye in water. Glasswares should be thoroughly washed with water before preparing the dye solution.

Standard solution

20 mcg/ml of dextropropoxyphene napsylate in water.

Sample solution

Extract accurately weighed quantity of the sample equivalent to 20 mg of dextropropoxyphene with water to make 100 ml. Dilute further with water to get 20 mcg/ml solution.

Procedure

To 10 ml each of sample and standard solutions, add 5 ml of pH 4.0 buffer solution and 2.5 ml of the dye solution. Mix and extract with two 10 ml portions of chloroform and dilute organic layer to 25 ml with chloroform. Measure the absorbance of both the solutions at about 420 nm using chloroform as blank. Deduce the results by comparison.

Paracetamol

METHOD 1

Add an accurately weighed quantity of the powdered sample equivalent to about 150 mg of paracetamol to 50 ml of 0.1 N sodium hydroxide taken in a 200 ml volumetric flask. Add 100 ml of water, shake for 15 minutes and add sufficient water to produce 200 ml. Mix, filter and dilute 10 ml of the filtrate to 100 ml with water. To 10 ml of the resulting solution, add 10 ml of 0.1 N sodium hydroxide and dilute to 100 ml with water. Measure the extinction of the resulting solution at maxima at about 257 nm and calculate the results taking 715 as value of A 1%, 1 cm at 257 nm.

METHOD 2

This method is based on bathochromic shift from 249 nm to about 460 nm as a result of alkaline hydrolysis.

Standard solution

100 mg of paracetamol is dissolved in methanol to produce 100 ml (1 mg/ml).

Sample solution

Extract the sample with methyl alcohol to get a concentration of 1 mg/ml in respect of the substance.

Procedure

To 1 ml each of sample and standard solutions, add 1 ml of 2 N sodium hydroxide solution and keep in water bath for 15 minutes. Remove and add immediately 1.5 ml of water and mix. Allow to stand for 60 minutes and dilute to 5 ml with water. Measure the absorbance at about 460 nm using reagent blank.

Note : Aspirin, oxyphenbutazone and phenobarbitone, if present, do not interfere.

Alternatively, to 10 ml of sample and standard solution, add 5 ml of hydrochloric acid (10%) and 2 ml of sodium nitrite solution (5% w/v). The absorbance of yellow colour so developed is measured at 440 nm and results calculated by comparison with standard.

Diazepam

Reagents

1. Acidified methanol : 3% v/v sulphuric acid in methanol.
2. Phosphate buffer, pH 7.0.

Standard solution

50 mg of diazepam is dissolved in acidified methanol to get 40 mcg/ml solution.

Sample solution

Weigh accurately, a quantity of powdered tablets equivalent to 2 mg of diazepam, add 20 ml of buffer solution, pH 7.0, extract with four 30 ml portions of ether (peroxide free). The combined ether layer is washed with 10 ml of 2 N sodium hydroxide solution and then with water to get free of alkali. Pass through sodium sulphate, anhydrous. Evaporate ether layer and dry at 105°C. Cool and take up the residue in acidified methanol to get 50 ml (40 mcg/ml).

Measure the extinction of standard and sample solutions at maximum at about 368 nm and calculate the results by comparison.

Paracetamol, Diazepam, Dextropropoxyphene hydrochloride, Dicyclomine hydrochloride

ESTIMATION

Paracetamol

The compound is hydrolysed and estimated by the method involving reaction with vanillin. For details, refer to method 1 for paracetamol described under formulation 4 of this chapter. Alternatively, carry out nitroso-derivative method as described in formulation 2 of this chapter.

Diazepam

An accurately weighed quantity of the sample equivalent to 2 mg of diazepam is suspended in pH 7 phosphate buffer, and extracted with ether. For further details, refer to formulation 25 of this chapter.

Dextropropoxyphene hydrochloride

The compound is dextro-rotatory. The other compounds present in the formulation being optically inactive do not interfere. An accurately weighed quantity of the sample equivalent to 650 mg of dextropropoxyphene hydrochloride is extracted with four 25 ml portions of chloroform. Combined chloroform layer is evaporated almost to dryness at low temperature to get final volume of 10 ml. Optical rotation of the resultant solution is used to determine the contents of the substance in the sample. Standard solution of the substance (65 mg/ml) is prepared in chloroform for comparison and calculation.

Note : The optical rotation of the substance is usually measured in water. Since paracetamol is the major component in this formulation, it is not feasible to extract 650 mg of dextropropoxyphene in 10 ml of water, hence extraction with chloroform followed by concentration has been used. Further paracetamol is insoluble in chloroform.

Dicyclomine hydrochloride

METHOD 1

Reagents

1. 0.004 M sodium lauryl sulphate solution : While preparing the solution in water, add 2 ml of sulphuric acid for each 1000 ml of the solution to prevent formation of precipitates. If precipitate is formed on storage, discard the solution. Standardise the solution against standard dicyclomine hydrochloride and dilute to get exact 0.004 M solution.
2. Dimethyl yellow solution, indicator.
3. 10% w/v solution of sodium hydroxide in water.

Procedure

Weigh accurately, a quantity of the sample equivalent to 10 mg of the dicyclomine hydrochloride.

Suspend in 10 ml of 0.1 N hydrochloric acid. Add 5 ml of sodium hydroxide solution and extract with five 25 ml portions of chloroform or petroleum ether (40-60°), the latter being preferred as emulsion is usually not formed. Wash the combined organic layer with water to get free of alkali. Dry over anhydrous sodium sulphate. Wash the sodium sulphate layer with the solvent and mix with the main extract. Evaporate on water-bath. Transfer the residue to a separating funnel with the aid of 5 ml of methanol. Add 25 ml water, 10 ml dilute sulphuric acid, 1 ml of indicator solution and 40 ml of chloroform. Shake and titrate with 0.004 sodium lauryl sulphate, shaking vigorously after each addition and allowing the layers to separate, until the colour begins to change from yellow to orange pink in lower layer. Record the volume of titrant consumed in the titration. From this, subtract the volume of titrant equivalent to the contents of dextropropoxyphene hydrochloride present in the weight of the sample initially taken for analysis of dicyclomine hydrochloride. Each ml of 0.004 M sodium lauryl sulphate is equivalent to 0.0015036 g of dextropropoxyphene hydrochloride. From remaining volume of the titrant, calculate the contents of dicyclomine hydrochloride in the sample. Each ml of 0.004 M sodium lauryl sulphate or 0.004 M sodium lauryl sulphate is equivalent to 0.001384 g of dicyclomine hydrochloride.

METHOD 2

Reagents

1. 0.004 M sodium lauryl sulphate.
2. 0.25% w/v solution of methylene blue in water.
3. Colour reagent : It is prepared by mixing 10 ml of 0.004 M sodium lauryl sulphate, 30 ml of chloroform and 1 ml of dye solution. Mix, gently shake, allow to separate and use the chloroform layer which is blue in colour.

Standard solution

2 mg/ml of dicyclomine hydrochloride in chloroform.

Sample solution

Weigh accurately powdered sample equivalent to 20 mg of dicyclomine hydrochloride, add 20 ml of water and 1 ml of concentrated hydrochloric acid. Extract with chloroform (4 × 25 ml), passing each extract through anhydrous sodium sulphate. Evaporate combined chloroform layer to 10 ml.

Procedure

To 1 ml each of sample and standard solutions, add 2 ml of colour reagent and 25 ml of water, shake vigorously. Collect the aqueous layer and measure the absorbance of both the solutions at 590 nm using water as blank and calculate the results by comparison.

Note : If the solution is turbid, extract blue colour with isobutyl alcohol.

METHOD 3

Reagents

1. 0.01 N hydrochloric acid.
2. Picric acid solution : Dissolve 20 mg of picric acid and 2.9 g of sodium acetate (anhydrous) in about 80 ml of water, add 4.0 ml of glacial acetic acid and dilute to 100 ml with water.

Standard solution

20 mcg/ml of dicyclomine hydrochloride in 0.01 N hydrochloric acid.

Sample solution

Accurately weighed quantity of powdered sample is extracted with 0.01 N hydrochloric acid to get final solution of 20 mcg/ml.

Procedure

To 20 ml each of sample and standard solutions, add 5 ml of picric acid solution. Mix and extract with 2 × 10 ml portions of chloroform. Combine chloroform layer, make up to 25 ml and add few crystals of sodium sulphate, anhydrous. Shake and allow to stand for 10 min. Concomitantly measure the absorbance of sample and standard solution at 450 nm using chloroform as blank and calculate the results by comparison.

Paracetamol, Pseudoephedrine hydrochloride, Azatadine maleate

ESTIMATION

Azatadine maleate

Weigh accurately powdered sample equivalent to 1 mg of the substance and suspend in 15-20 ml of water. Basify with 0.1 N sodium hydroxide and extract with four 25 ml portions of chloroform. Pass chloroform layer through anhydrous sodium sulphate and evaporate combined chloroform extract till no perceptible smell of chloroform (reserve alkaline aqueous layer for estimation of paracetamol). Take up the entire residue in 0.1 N hydrochloric acid to produce 100 ml (10 mcg/ml) and measure the absorbance at 285 nm. Calculate the contents of azatadine maleate in the sample by comparing with the standard solution (10 mcg/ml).

Note :   Pseudoephedrine hydrochloride has insignificant absorption at 285 nm.

Paracetamol

The alkaline aqueous layer reserved during extraction of azatadine maleate is appropriately diluted with 0.1 N sodium hydroxide to produce final concentration of 10 mcg/ml in respect of paracetamol. Measure the absorption at 257 nm and calculate the results by taking 715 as value of A 1%, 1 cm at 257 nm.

Pseudoephedrine hydrochloride

Follow the copper sulphate method described in formulation 19 of the chapter on expectorants and cough suppressants.

Dicyclomine hydrochloride, Paracetamol, Isopropylantipyrin, Chlordiazepoxide

ESTIMATION

Chlordiazepoxide

Reagents

1. Dilute hydrochloric acid.
2. 0.5% hydrochloric acid.
3. 2% w/v solution of p-dimethylaminobenzaldehyde (PDAB) in alcohol.

Standard solution

Weigh accurately 50 mg of chlordiazepoxide, add 25 ml of dilute hydrochloric acid and heat on water bath for 30 minutes; cool, dilute to 50 ml with water. 5 ml of the resulting solution is further diluted to 100 ml with water (50 mcg/ml).

Sample solution

Weigh accurately a quantity of the sample equivalent to 50 mg of the substance and proceed as for standard solution.

Procedure

To 1 ml each of sample and standard solutions, add 1.5 ml each of dilute hydrochloric acid and 'PDAB' reagent. Shake and dilute to 10 ml with water. Measure the absorbance of both the solutions at about 450 nm against reagent blank.

Isopropylantipyrin (Propyphenazone)

Follow the method 2 described under formulation 9 of the chapter on anti-inflammatory drugs.

Paracetamol

Follow the method described in formulation 33 of this chapter. The method is based on conversion of paracetamol to p-aminophenol, followed by alkaline oxidation with sodium nitroprusside.

Dicyclomine hydrochloride

Follow the method described in formulation 21 of this chapter. Each ml of 0.004 M sodium lauryl sulphate is equivalent to 0.001384 g of dicyclomine hydrochloride.

Paracetamol, Dicyclomine hydrochloride, Phenylisopropyl pyrazolone, Ethylmorphine hydrochloride

ESTIMATION

Paracetamol

Carry out the nitroso-derivative method described in formulation 2 of this chapter or the method described in formulation 3 of this chapter.

Dicyclomine hydrochloride

Follow the method described in formulation 21 of this chapter.

Phenylisopropyl pyrazolone

Follow the method 2 described in formulation 9 of the chapter on anti-inflammatory drugs.

Ethylmorphine hydrochloride

Reagents

1. Dilute sulphuric acid (75% v/v).
2. 1 N sodium hydroxide.
3. 1.0% w/v solution of p-dimethylaminobenzaldehyde in 75% v/v sulphuric acid.

Standard solution

80 mcg/ml of ethylmorphine hydrochloride in dilute sulphuric acid.

Sample solution

Measure appropriate quantity of the sample equivalent to 5 mg of the compound. Saturate the solution with sodium chloride and make alkaline with 1 N sodium hydroxide. Extract the alkaline solution with five 40 ml portions of chloroform. Wash the combined chloroform layers with 10 ml of sodium chloride solution. Dry chloroform extract over anhydrous sodium sulphate and evaporate to 25 ml. To 10 ml of the above solution, add 5 ml of dilute sulphuric acid and evaporate on water bath till the smell of chloroform is not perceptible. Dilute to 25 ml with dilute sulphuric acid.

Procedure

To 0.5 ml each of sample and standard solutions, add 8 ml of the benzaldehyde reagent, mix and allow the flasks to stand at room temperature for one hour in the dark. Measure the absorption of both solutions at about 450 nm against reagent blank. Results are calculated by comparison.

Paracetamol, Salicylamide, Codeine phosphate

ESTIMATION

Paracetamol

Sample solution

Take a quantity of powdered tablets equivalent to 250 mg of paracetamol, extract with three 60 ml portions of hot water and dilute to 200 ml with water (solution A). Take two equal volumes of solution A, dilute one portion with water and the other with 0.1 N sodium hydroxide to get 10 mcg/ml solutions.

Procedure

Measure the extinction of the alkaline solution at 262 nm against aqueous solution as blank. Process standard solution of paracetamol (10 mcg/ml) similarly and calculate the results.

Salicylamide

Process as per paracetamol but dilute to get 15 mcg/ml solution. Measure the extinction of alkaline solution at 329 nm using aqueous solution as blank. Process the standard solution of salicylamide similarly and calculate the results.

The above methods are similar to the one described in formulation 2 of this chapter except instead of methanol, water is used for extraction.

Codeine phosphate

Follow the ion-pair formation method with methyl orange using acetate buffer pH 3.5. For details, refer to the method described in formulation 5 of this chapter.

Ascorbic acid, Methapyriline hydrochloride, Phenylephrine hydrochloride

ESTIMATION

Ascorbic acid

While estimating ascorbic acid by iodine titration method, the end point is not very sharp due to reaction of iodine with starch. However, the following method involving cold extraction and filtration overcomes this problem.

Procedure

Weigh accurately, a quantity of powdered tablets equivalent to 500 mg of ascorbic acid and suspend in water to make 250 ml. Mix, filter and reject first 20-30 ml of the filtrate. To 75 ml of filtrate, add 3 ml of dilute sulphuric acid and titrate with 0.1 N iodine solution to a light yellow end point. Each ml of 0.1 N iodine is equivalent to 0.008806 g of ascorbic acid.

Methapyriline hydrochloride

Methapyriline in 0.1 N hydrochloric acid exhibits maximum at about 313 nm and the other two active components of this formulation do not absorb at 313 nm.

Standard solution

20 mcg/ml of pure methapyriline hydrochloride in 0.1 N hydrochloric acid.

Sample solution

Suspend accurately weighed quantity of the powdered tablets equivalent to 25 mg of methapyriline hydrochloride in 250 ml of 0.1 N hydrochloric acid. Shake and filter, rejecting first 25-30 ml of the filtrate. Dilute 20 ml of the filtrate to 100 ml with 0.1 N hydrochloric acid. Measure the extinction of both the solutions at maximum at about 313 nm against 0.1 N hydrochloric acid as blank. Calculate the results by comparison.

Phenylephrine hydrochloride

Follow any one of the three methods for estimation of phenylephrine hydrochloride as described in formulation 1 of this chapter.

Note : Ascorbic acid being a strong reducing agent interferes in the estimation of phenylephrine by alkaline oxidation method. This difficulty is overcome by using stronger solution of potassium ferricyanide as oxidizing agent.

Ascorbic acid, Analgin

ESTIMATION

Analgin

Reagent

1. 1% w/v solution of p-dimethylaminobenzaldehyde in 5% v/v sulphuric acid.

Standard solution

1 mg/ml of analgin in water.

Sample solution

Appropriate weight of the powdered sample is extracted with water to get 1 mg/ml of analgin.

Procedure

To 5 ml each of sample and standard solutions, add 5 ml of p-dimethylaminobenzaldehyde reagent. Keep for 5 minutes and make up the volume to 25 ml with water. Measure the absorbance of both the standard and the sample solutions at about 430 nm and calculate the results by comparison.

Ascorbic acid

Carry out the method involving titration with standardized 2,6-dichlorophenol-indophenol solution. For preparation of indophenol solution, refer to formulation 1 of this chapter.

Note : Iodine titration method is not applicable in this formation as both analgin and ascorbic acid react with iodine.

Ergotamine tartrate, Caffeine citrate, Paracetamol, Prochlorperazine maleate

ESTIMATION

Ergotamine tartrate

METHOD 1

Reagents

1. 0.125% w/v solution of tetrazolium blue in alcohol:
2. Tetramethyl ammonium hydroxide, 0.25% v/v : Mix 0.5 ml of tetramethyl ammonium hydroxide (10%) with ethyl alcohol to produce 20 ml.
3. 20% w/v sodium hydroxide solution in water.

Standard solution

Accurately weigh and transfer 20 mg of ergotamine tartrate to 50 ml dry volumetric flask containing 40 ml ethyl alcohol. Dissolve and make up the volume with ethyl alcohol. Dilute 5 ml of the resulting solution to 50 ml with ethyl alcohol (40 mcg/ml).

Sample solution

Accurately weigh and transfer a quantity of tablet powder equivalent to 2 mg of ergotamine tartrate to 40 ml of water, shake for 5 minutes and dilute to 50 ml with water. Transfer 25 ml of the clear filtrate to 250 ml separatory funnel. Add 1 ml of sodium hydroxide solution and extract with four 30 ml portions of chloroform. Wash the combined chloroform extracts with 10 ml of water. Pass chloroform extracts through anhydrous sodium sulphate. Wash the sodium sulphate layer with 20 ml of chloroform. Evaporate the chloroform on water-bath. Dissolve the residue in sufficient ethyl alcohol to produce 25 ml. Use clear solution for colour development.

Procedure

Transfer 3 ml each of ethyl alcohol (blank), standard solution, sample solution to separate 10 ml dry volumetric flask. Add 2 ml of tetrazolium blue reagent and mix. Add 2 ml of tetramethyl ammonium hydroxide, mix and wait for 60 minutes. Make up the volumes with ethyl alcohol, mix and measure absorption of sample and standard solutions against reagent blank at about 525 nm. Calculate the content by comparison.

METHOD 2

Reagents

1. 0.125% w/v solution of p-dimethylaminobenzaldehyde (PDAB) in water.
2. 2% w/v tartaric acid in water.

Standard solution

60 mcg/ml of ergotamine tartrate in 2% tartaric acid.

Sample solution

Weigh accurately, a quantity of powdered tablets equivalent to 3 mg of ergotamine tartrate, add 25 ml of dilute ammonia solution and extract with three 25 ml portions of solvent ether. Wash the combined ether layer with 10 ml of dilute ammonia solution. Pass ether layer through anhydrous sodium sulphate. Evaporate the ether layer on water bath. Cool and dissolve the residue in 2% tartaric acid to make 50 ml (60 mcg/ml).

Procedure

To 2 ml each of standard and sample solutions, add 4 ml of 'PDAB' solution and keep at room temperature for 30 minutes. Measure the absorbance of both the solutions at 650 nm against reagent blank. Calculate the results by comparison.

Caffeine citrate

Accurately weigh and transfer tablet powder equivalent to 100 mg of caffeine to 100 ml round bottom flask. Add 10 ml dilute sulphuric acid and reflux on low flame for one hour. Cool and transfer the contents to a 250 ml separatory funnel with the aid of 10 ml water. Extract with three 50 ml portions of chloroform. Wash the combined chloroform extracts with two 10 ml portions of water. Pass chloroform extracts through anhydrous sodium sulphate layer into 250 ml dry weighed conical flask. Wash the sodium sulphate layer and separatory funnel with 25 ml of chloroform and mix along with main chloroform extracts. Evaporate the chloroform extracts and dry the conical flask along with residue at 105°C for one hour or till constant weight. Cool the flask in dessicator and re-weigh. Weight of the residue represents amount of caffeine present in the weight of the sample taken for analysis or dissolve the residue in 0.01 N tartaric acid (7.5 mcg/ml) for spectrophotometric analysis. For further details refer to formulation 60 of this chapter.

Paracetamol

METHOD 1
Reagents

1. 4% w/v solution of sodium nitroprusside in water.
2. 4% w/v solution of sodium hydroxide in water.

Standard solution

To 100 mg of paracetamol, add 50 ml of concentrated hydrochloric acid and boil for 60 minutes in water bath. Cool, filter and adjust to 100 ml with water. Dilute 1 ml of the resultant solution to 100 ml with water (10 mcg/ml).

Sample solution

Weigh accurately sample equivalent to 100 mg of paracetamol and treat as under standard solution (conversion to p-aminophenol).

Procedure

To 5 ml each of the sample and standard solutions, add 0.5 ml of sodium nitroprusside solution and adjust to 10 ml with sodium hydroxide solution. Keep at room temperature for 10 minutes and measure the absorbance of both the solutions at about 725 nm. Calculate the results by comparison.

Note : 1. Aspirin, phenobarbitone, phenylbutazone, chlorpheniramine maleate, ephedrine hydro-chloride do not interfere.
2. Phenols with substitution as para-position except p-aminophenol do not interfere.

METHOD 2

Follow the method described in formulation 3 of this chapter. This method is based on acid hydrolysis to p-aminophenol, diazotization and coupling with 'NED'.

Prochlorperazine maleate

Reagent

1. 0.05% w/v solution of 1,2-naphthoquinone-4-sulphonate (Na$^+$) (NQS) in 62.5% v/v sulphuric acid. The reagent should be freshly prepared.

Standard solution

Weigh accurately 50 mg of prochlorperazine maleate and dissolve in water by heating to produce 100 ml. 10 ml of the resultant solution may be further diluted with water to produce 50 mcg/ml.

Sample solution

Weigh accurately powdered tablets equivalent to 10 mg of prochlorperazine maleate and dissolve in boiling water to produce 200 ml (50 mcg/ml).

Procedure

To 4 ml each of standard and sample solutions, add 8 ml of the 'NQS' reagent. Mix and allow to stand at room temperature for 30 minutes. Measure the absorbance of both the solutions at about 520 nm and calculate the results by comparison.

Ergotamine tartrate, Cyclizine hydrochloride, Caffeine citrate

Preparation of test solution

Transfer finely powdered quantity of sample equivalent to about 20 mg of ergotamine tartrate into a volumetric flask. Add 2.5 g of tartaric acid and 100 ml of water. Shake for 30 minutes and dilute to 250 ml with water. Filter, collect the filtrate rejecting first few ml of the filtrate.

ESTIMATION

Cyclizine hydrochloride

Transfer 10 ml of test solution into separating funnel, make alkaline with 5 N sodium hydroxide and extract with three 25 ml portions of cyclohexane. Wash the combined organic layer with two 10 ml portions of 0.1 N sodium hydroxide. Extract the organic layer with four 25 quantities of 0.05 N sulphuric acid. Dilute the combined acidic layer to 100 ml. Further dilution may be done with 0.05 N sulphuric acid to get a concentration of 10 mcg/ml. Measure the extinction at maximum at 225 nm using acid as blank. Calculate the results taking 390 as value of A 1%, 1 cm at 225 nm.

Caffeine citrate

Dilute the test solution with water to get concentration of 10 mcg/ml. Measure the absorbance of final solution at maximum at about 272 nm and calculate the results using 500 as value of A 1%, 1 cm. Each g of caffeine anhydrous is equivalent to 1.092 g of caffeine monohydrate.

Ergotamine tartrate

Standard solution

40 mcg/ml of ergotamine tartrate in 1% v/v acetic acid in methanol.

Sample solution

To accurately weighed quantity of the sample equivalent to about 4 mg of the substance add 1 ml of glacial acetic acid and about 80 ml of methanol, place in ultrasonic bath for 10 min and dilute to 100 ml with methanol.

Concomitantly measure the extinction of both the solutions at maximum at about 320 nm using 1% v/v solution of glacial acetic acid in methanol as blank and calculate the results by comparison. Use amber coloured glass apparatus.

Paracetamol, Pentazocine hydrochloride

ESTIMATION

Pentazocine hydrochloride

METHOD 1

Weigh accurately powdered tablets equivalent to 60 mg of pentazocine, add 20 ml of 1 N sodium hydroxide and extract with four 25 ml portions of chloroform. Pass chloroform layer through anhydrous sodium sulphate. Evaporate chloroform layer and take the residue (A) in 25 ml glacial acetic acid and titrate with 0.02 N perchloric acid using crystal violet as indicator. Each ml of 0.02 N perchloric acid is equivalent to 0.005708 g of pentazocine hydrochloride.

METHOD 2

Dissolve the residue (A) obtained after evaporation of chloroform in 0.1 N hydrochloric acid or 0.1 N sodium hydroxide to get 50 mcg/ml solution. Measure the extinction at 278 nm (acidic solution) or at 298 nm (alkaline solution). Calculate the contents of pentazocine using value of 69 as value of E 1%, 1 cm for acidic solution and 108 for the alkaline solution. The method obeys Beer's law in the concentration range of 10-200 mcg/ml.

METHOD 3

Reagents

1. 0.1 N and 1 N hydrochloric acid.
2. 1 N sodium hydroxide.
3. 3% w/v freshly prepared solution of sodium nitrite in water.

Standard solution

200 mcg/ml of pentazocine in 0.1 N hydrochloric acid.

Sample solution

(a) **Tablets and injections :** An accurately weighed or measured aliquot of the preparation is extracted and suitably diluted with 0.1 N hydrochloric acid to give a concentration of about 200 mcg/ml of pentazocine. Filter, if necessary.

(b) **Pentazocine in presence of paracetamol :** An accurately weighed amount of the sample equivalent to 20 mg of pentazocine is extracted with chloroform as described under method 1. The chloroform layer is evaporated and the residue is taken in 0.1 N hydrochloric acid to produce 100 ml.

Procedure

To 5 ml each of sample and standard solutions, add 2 ml of sodium nitrite solution and 1 ml of 1 N hydrochloric acid. Heat the mixture on water bath for 30 minutes, cool and add 3 ml of 1 N sodium hydroxide. Allow to stand at room temperature for five minutes and dilute to 25 ml with water. Measure the extinction of both the solutions at about 430 nm against reagent blank. Pentazocine may be converted into its hydrochloride salt by multiplying with a factor of 1.1278. The method follows Beer's law in the concentration range of 50-500 mcg/ml.

Paracetamol

Standard solution

10 mcg/ml of paracetamol in 0.1 N hydrochloric acid.

Sample solution

Extract powdered tablets equivalent to 10 mg of paracetamol with 0.1 N hydrochloric acid to produce 100 ml. Filter and dilute 10 ml of the filtrate to 100 ml with same solvent.

Procedure

Measure the extinction of both sample and standard solutions at absorption maximum at about 244 nm using 0.1 N acid as blank. Pentazocine does not interfere at this wavelength.

Aspirin, Caffeine citrate

ESTIMATION

Caffeine citrate

Standard solution

10 mcg/ml of caffeine citrate in water.

Sample solution

Dissolve powder equivalent to 30 mg of caffeine in 2 ml of water by gentle shaking and filter through a sintered glass funnel G_4 (retain the residue for estimation of aspirin). Dilute 0.5 ml of the filtrate with water suitably to produce a final concentration of about 10 mcg/ml of caffeine citrate.

Measure the extinction at maximum at about 272 nm taking water as blank. Calculate the results by comparison.

Note : The total filtrate so obtained should be presumed to be 2 ml and contains 30 mg of caffeine and further dilutions are done accordingly.

Aspirin

Standard solution

10 mcg/ml of aspirin in 7% v/v ammonia.

Sample solution

Dissolve entire insoluble residue obtained above under caffeine in 6 ml of 7% ammonia solution and filter. Dilute the filtrate suitably with 7% ammonia solution to produce concentration of about 10 mcg/ml.

Measure the extinction of sample and standard solutions at maximum at about 240 nm taking 7% ammonia solution as blank. Calculate the results by comparison.

Note : 1. The above method has been extensively used with excellent results. In the opinion of the author, the method can be adopted for regular use by manufacturers of above combination.
2. The methods based on differential solubilities have been extensively used in the text for separation and quantitative estimation of individual component in several formulations. These methods are suitable for routine quality control.

Aspirin, Caffeine citrate, Dextropropoxyphene hydrochloride

ESTIMATION

Aspirin

Follow the method described in formulation 5 of this chapter.

Caffeine citrate

Follow the method described in formulation 5 of this chapter.

Dextropropoxyphene hydrochloride

Follow the method described in formulation 26 of this chapter.

Formulation 38

Aspirin, Caffeine citrate, Diphenhydramine hydrochloride

ESTIMATION

Aspirin

Follow the method described in formulation 5 of this chapter.

Caffeine citrate

Follow the method described in formulation 5 of this chapter.

Diphenhydramine hydrochloride

Follow the ammonium reineckate precipitation method as described in formulation 5 or colour development method with cobalt thiocyanate as described in formulation 6 of the chapter on expectorants and cough suppressants.

Aspirin, Caffeine citrate, Noscapine, Chlorpheniramine maleate

ESTIMATION

Caffeine citrate

Triturate accurately weighed quantity of powdered material equivalent to 100 mg of caffeine with 30-40 ml of 0.1·N hydrochloric acid. Extract the aqueous suspension with four 20 ml portions of chloroform, washing each extract with the same 10 ml of 0.1 N hydrochloric acid. Combine the acid washing with main acidic extract and reserve for estimation of chlorpheniramine maleate. Extract the chloroform layer with four 20 ml portions of 1 N sodium hydroxide and reserve alkaline layer for estimation of aspirin. Filter chloroform layer and evaporate on water-bath to dryness and then dry to a constant weight in an oven at 80°C. Weigh the material which represents caffeine only. Alternatively dissolve the residue in 0.01 N tartaric acid to get a concentration of 7.5 mcg/ml. For details refer to formulation 60 of this chapter.

Chlorpheniramine maleate

The acidic extract reserved during estimation of caffeine above is diluted appropriately and contents of chlorpheniramine are estimated by cyanogen bromide method as described in formulation 3 of the chapter on expectorants and cough suppressants or formulation 1 of the chapter on rubefacients.

Aspirin

Acidify the alkaline extract reserved during estimation of caffeine with dilute hydrochloric acid. Extract with ether, dry ethereal layer by passing over anhydrous sodium sulphate and evaporate at low temperature. Final drying is done under current of air. Dry the residue in a dessicator and weigh salicylic acid (salicylic acid tends to sublime).

Each g of salicylic acid is equal to 1.305 g of aspirin.

Noscapine

Take powdered material, accurately weighed, equivalent to 25 mg of noscapine. Add 5 ml of 1 N hydrochloric acid and extract with three 20 ml portions of ether. The combined ether extract is shaken with 10 ml of 0.02 N hydrochloric acid. The acidic extracts are combined, made alkaline and extracted with five 20 ml portions of ether. The combined ethereal layer is extracted with 0.02 N hydrochloric acid to produce 50 mcg/ml solution. Measure the extinction of the sample solution at 312 nm and calculate the results by comparing with the standard (50 mcg/ml) solution of noscapine in 0.02 N hydrochloric acid.

Aspirin, Paracetamol, Caffeine citrate

ESTIMATION

Aspirin

Follow the method as described in formulation 5 of this chapter.

Caffeine citrate

Carry out chloroform extraction, followed by spectrophotometric measurement at 276 nm as described in formulation 1 of this chapter.

Paracetamol

Follow the nitroso-derivative method as described in formulation 2 of this chapter.

Typical laboratory analysis

Each tablet contains :
Paracetamol	250 mg
Aspirin	250 mg
Caffeine	30 mg

Average weight = 0.599 g

Aspirin

(Method followed : See formulation 5 of this chapter.)

Weight of sample taken for analysis = 0.486 g

Volume of 0.1 N sodium hydroxide consumed = 11.2 ml

$$\text{Aspirin, mg/tablet} = \frac{11.2 \times 0.018016 \times 0.599}{0.486}$$

$$= 249 \text{ mg}$$

$$\text{Claim} = 250 \text{ mg}$$

Caffeine citrate

(Method followed : Basification, followed by chloroform extraction, see formulation 1 of this chapter.)

Dilutions to be done with chloroform.

Standard 0.0133 g → 100 ml; 10 ml → 100 ml

Sample 0.602 g → 250 ml; 10 ml → 100 ml

Extinction values at 276 nm Sample 0.56 Standard 0.66

$$\text{Caffeine, mg/tablet} = \frac{0.56}{0.66}\left(\frac{0.0133}{100} \times \frac{10}{100} \times \frac{250}{0.602} \times \frac{100}{10}\right)0.599$$

$$= 28 \text{ mg}$$

$$\text{Claim} = 30 \text{ mg}$$

Paracetamol

(Method followed : Nitroso-derivative, followed by coupling with cobalt—see formulation 2 of this chapter.)

Dilutions to be done with water.

Sample 0.293 g → 50 ml; 1 ml → 100 ml

Standard 0.059 g → 25 ml; 1 ml → 100 ml

Extinction values at 390 nm : Sample 0.420, Standard 0.400

$$\text{Paracetamol, mg/tablet} = \frac{0.420}{0.400}\left(\frac{0.059}{25} \times \frac{1}{100}\right)\left(\frac{50}{0.293} \times \frac{100}{1}\right)0.599$$

$$= 253.2 \text{ mg}$$

$$\text{Claim} = 250 \text{ mg}$$

Formulation 41

Aspirin, Caffeine citrate, Phenylephrine hydrochloride, Pseudoephedrine hydrochloride

ESTIMATION

Aspirin

Reagents

1. 1% w/v solution of ferric chloride in 0.01 N hydrochloric acid.
2. 0.01 N and 1 N hydrochloric acid.

Standard solution

To about 100 mg of aspirin accurately weighed, add 10 ml of 1 N hydrochloric acid and 70 ml of water. Heat in water-bath for 30 minutes, cool and dilute to 100 ml with water.

Sample solution

Weigh sample accurately equivalent to 100 mg of the compound and treat as under standard solution.

Procedure

To 2 ml each of the sample and standard solutions, add 2 ml of ferric chloride reagent and dilute to 25 ml with water. After 5 minutes, measure absorption of both the solutions at about 530 nm using 0.01 N hydrochloric acid as blank and calculate the results by comparison.

Pseudoephedrine hydrochloride

Follow the method 1 for pseudoephedrine as described in formulation 19 of the chapter on expectorants and cough suppressants.

Caffeine citrate

Follow the method as described in formulation 1 of this chapter, which involves basification, extraction with chloroform, followed by spectrophotometric measurements at 276 nm.

Phenylephrine hydrochloride

METHOD 1

Follow the method as described in formulation 1 of this chapter.

METHOD 2

Reagents

1. Borate buffer, pH 9.2.
2. 0.04% w/v solution of 2,6-dichloroquinone chlorimide in isopropyl alcohol.

Standard solution

50 mcg/ml of pure substance in water.

Sample solution

Extract accurately weighed amount of the sample with water to produce 50 mcg/ml.

Procedure

To 2 ml each of sample and standard solutions, add 5 ml of isopropyl alcohol and 1 ml of borate buffer (if the solution is cloudy, add 2 ml of water to clear the solution). Finally, add 1 ml of chlorimide reagent and keep for 10 minutes at room temperature. Measure the absorbance of both the solutions at 625 nm against reagent blank. Calculate the results by comparison.

Aspirin, Noscapine, Caffeine, Pseudoephedrine hydrochloride, Chlorpheniramine maleate

ESTIMATION

Aspirin

Extract the powdered sample with 100 ml of 1 N sodium hydroxide and dilute to 500 ml with water. Take 10 ml of the solution in iodine flask, add 20 ml of 0.1 N bromine solution and 5 ml of concentrated hydrochloric acid. Immediately stopper the flask to avoid any loss of bromine. Keep for 30 min, shake from time to time, add 10 ml of potassium iodide solution (10%) and titrate with 0.1 N sodium thiosulphate using starch mucilage as indicator. Perform the blank. Each ml of 0.1 N bromine is equivalent to 0.006 g of aspirin.

Chlorpheniramine maleate (CPM)

Standard solution

20 mcg/ml of CPM in water.

Sample solution

Accurately weighed quantity of the sample equivalent to 10 mg of the substance is suspended in 20 ml of water and 5 ml of 0.1 N hydrochloric acid. Extract with five 40 ml portions of chloroform, washing each chloroform layer with 10 ml of 0.1 N hydrochloric acid. Collect the acidic extract and acidic washing and dilute to 500 ml with water (use for estimation of CPM).

(Wash the chloroform layer with 1 N sodium hydroxide to remove aspirin and dilute to 250 ml with chloroform. The solution is used for estimation of noscapine and caffeine.)

Follow the cyanogen bromide method as described in formulation 1 of the chapter on rubefacients.

Noscapine

Standard solution

40 mcg/ml of noscapine in chloroform.

Sample solution

Dilute the chloroform solution obtained during estimation of CPM after washing with sodium hydroxide to get solution of 40 mcg/ml.

Measure the absorbance of each sample and standard solutions at 312 nm using chloroform as blank and calculate the results by comparison.

Standard solution

10 mcg/ml of caffeine in 0.1 N hydrochloric acid.

Sample solution

Appropriate volume of chloroform solution obtained during estimation of CPM after washing with 1 N sodium hydroxide is evaporated and residue taken up in 0.1 N hydrochloric acid to get final concentration of 10 mcg/ml of caffeine.

Measure the absorbance of both sample and standard solutions at 271 nm and calculate the results by comparison.

Pseudoephedrine hydrochloride

Follow the method described in formulation 19 of the chapter on expectorants and cough suppressants.

Analgin, Salicylamide

ESTIMATION

Analgin

Weigh a quantity of powdered tablets equivalent to 200 mg of analgin and dissolve in water to produce 200 ml (1 mg/ml). Prepare standard solution of analgin of same concentration (1 mg/ml) and follow the colorimetric method involving the use of p-dimethylaminobenzaldehyde. The coloured complex exhibited absorption maxima at 430 nm. For details, refer to formulation 32 of this chapter.

Salicylamide

Standard solution

10 mcg/ml of salicylamide in 1 N sodium hydroxide.

Sample solution

Weigh a quantity of powdered tablets equivalent to 100 mg of salicylamide, extract with 1 N hydroxide and dilute appropriately with the same solvent to get a concentration of 10 mcg/ml.

Standard and sample solutions exhibit maximum at 328 nm. The results are calculated by comparing with the standard. A solution containing 10 mcg/ml of salicylamide shows absorption value of about 0.42.

Analgin, Paracetamol, Diazepam, Chlorpheniramine maleate

ESTIMATION

Analgin

Follow the method as described in formulation 32 of this chapter.

Paracetamol

Follow the nitroso-derivative method as described in formulation 2 of this chapter.

Diazepam

Follow the method as described in formulation 25 of this chapter.

Chlorpheniramine maleate

Follow the cyanogen bromide method as described in formulation 1 of the chapter on rubefacients.

Analgin, Paracetamol, Caffeine citrate

ESTIMATION

Analgin

Reagent

1% w/v solution of p-dimethylaminobenzaldehyde (PDAB) in 5% v/v sulphuric acid.

Standard solution

1 mg/ml of analgin in water.

Sample solution

Weigh accurately powdered sample equivalent to 250 mg of analgin, add 200 ml of water, shake for 5 minutes to dissolve and make up the volume to 250 ml with water.

Procedure

To 5 ml each of sample and standard solutions, add 5 ml of **PDAB** reagent. Allow to stand for 5 minutes at room temperature and make up the volume to 25 ml with water. Measure the absorption of both the solutions at maximum at about 430 nm against reagent blank. Calculate the results by comparison.

Note :   PDAB reagent should preferably be prepared freshly, as it tends to darken. The reagent is stable if stored in refrigerator using amber coloured bottle.

Paracetamol

Reagents

1. 1 N hydrochloric acid.
2. 10% w/v solution of sodium nitrite in water—freshly prepared.
3. 10% w/v solution of ammonium sulphamate in water.
4. 20% w/v solution of sodium hydroxide in water.

Standard solution

100 mcg/ml in 1 N hydrochloric acid.

Sample solution

Take sample accurately weighed equivalent to 25 mg of paracetamol in 250 ml volumetric flask. Add about 200 ml of 1 N hydrochloric acid, shake vigorously for 15 minutes to dissolve the substance and make up the volume (100 mcg/ml).

Procedure

Take 5 ml each of sample and standard solutions in different 50 ml volumetric flasks. To each, add 5 ml of 1 N hydrochloric acid and 5 ml of sodium nitrite solution. Allow to stand for 5 minutes with intermittent shaking. To neutralize excess of nitrous acid, add 5 ml of freshly prepared ammonium sulphamate solution to each flask. Shake vigorously and further allow to stand for 5 minutes, followed by addition of 5 ml of sodium hydroxide solution. Make up the volume and measure the absorption of both the solutions at 430 nm against reagent blank. Deduce the results by comparison.

Caffeine citrate

Reagents

1. 0.15% w/v solution of tartaric acid in water.
2. 1 N sodium hydroxide.
3. Dilute sulphuric acid.
4. Chloroform.

Standard solution

7.5 mcg/ml of caffeine in tartaric acid solution.

Sample solution

Weigh powdered sample accurately equivalent to 30 mg of caffeine. Add 40 ml of dilute sulphuric acid and reflux on a burner for 10 minutes, cool, transfer to a separating funnel. Basify with 1 N sodium hydroxide and extract with four 50 ml portions of chloroform, washing each organic layer with the same 20 ml of water. Pass combined chloroform layer through anhydrous sodium sulphate pre-moistened with chloroform. Evaporate chloroform layer and dry at low temperature at last stage to get the residue of caffeine. Dissolve the residue in tartaric acid solution to get final concentration of 7.5 mcg/ml.

Measure the extinction of both sample and standard solutions at maximum at about 271 nm and calculate the results by comparison.

Paracetamol, Chlormezanone

ESTIMATION

Chlormezanone

Standard solution

10 mcg/ml of chlormezanone in chloroform.

Sample solution

Suspend a quantity of the powdered sample equivalent to 10 mg of chlormezanone in 10 ml of water in a separating funnel. Basify with dilute ammonia and extract with four 20 ml portions of chloroform. Wash the combined chloroform extract with four 15 ml portions of ammonia solution and then with two 10 ml portions of water. Combine the washings with main aqueous ammoniacal layer and retain for estimation of paracetamol. Dry the chloroform layer by passing through anhydrous sodium sulphate, collect in a 100 ml volumetric flask, make up the volume with chloroform. Carry out further dilution with chloroform to get a final concentration of 10 mcg/ml.

Measure the extinctions of both standard and sample solutions at the maximum at about 239 nm using chloroform as the blank. Deduce the results by comparison. Alternatively, chloroform may be evaporated and residue taken up in methanol-water (3 + 1) and extinction measured at 227 nm.

Paracetamol

Standard solution

10 mcg/ml of paracetamol in dilute ammonia solution.

Sample solution

Wash the aqueous ammoniacal layer, obtained in the estimation of chlormezanone, with 10 ml of chloroform. Make up the aqueous layer with dilute ammonia to 100 ml. Dilute appropriately with dilute ammonia to get a final concentration of 10 mcg/ml.

Measure the extinction of standard and sample solutions at the maximum at about 257 nm using ammonia as the blank. Deduce the results by comparison.

Ibuprofen, Paracetamol, Chlormezanone

ESTIMATION

Ibuprofen/Ketoprofen

Weigh accurately a quantity of the powdered sample equivalent to about 200 mg of ibuprofen. Extract with four 25 ml portions of ether. Evaporate the combined ether layer and dry with the aid of current of air. Dissolve the entire residue in methanol previously neutralized to phenol red and titrate with 0.1 N sodium hydroxide using phenol red solution as indicator. Each ml of 0.1 N sodium hydroxide is equivalent to 0.02063 g of ibuprofen or 0.02543 g of ketoprofen.

Note : Chloroform can be used instead of ether for extraction.

Paracetamol

METHOD 1

Follow the nitroso-derivative described in formulation 2 of this chapter.

METHOD 2

Reagents

1. 0.1 N cerric ammonium sulphate.
2. 2 N sulphuric acid.
3. Ferroin sulphate solution (indicator).

Procedure

Weigh accurately quantity of the sample equivalent to about 50 mg of paracetamol, dissolve in mixture of 10 ml of water and 30 ml of 2 N sulphuric acid. Reflux for 60 minutes, cool, add about 50 ml of water, cool in ice bath and add 15 ml of 2 N hydrochloric acid and titrate with cerric ammonium sulphate using ferroin sulphate solution as indicator. Each ml of 0.1 N cerric ammonium sulphate solution is equivalent to 0.00756 g of paracetamol.

Method based on diazotization and coupling with 'NED' as described in formulation 3 of this chapter is also suitable.

Chlormezanone

Follow the method described in formulation 46 of this chapter. By basification, both paracetamol and ibuprofen will remain in the alkaline phase, whereas chlormezanone can be extracted into chloroform. Basification with 0.1 N sodium hydroxide instead of dilute ammonia solution gives better results. Chloroform layer is evaporated till no perceptible smell of chloroform. The residue is taken up with methanol and water (3 : 1) or in 0.1 N sulphuric acid and absorbance measured at 227 nm.

Paracetamol, Oxyphencyclimine hydrochloride

ESTIMATION

Paracetamol

Reagents

1. 1 N sodium hydroxide.
2. 0.2% w/v solution of sodium nitroprusside in water.

Standard solution

Weigh 100 mg of standard paracetamol, add 50 ml of dilute hydrochloric acid.

Sample solution

Powdered sample equivalent to 100 mg of paracetamol is transferred to 100 ml volumetric flask, add 50 ml of dilute hydrochloric acid.

Procedure

Keep both sample and standard solutions in boiling water bath for one hour. Cool and dilute to 100 ml with water. Filter and dilute 1 ml of the filtrate to 100 ml with water.

To 5 ml each of sample and standard solutions, add 0.5 ml of sodium nitroprusside solution and 4.5 ml of sodium hydroxide solution. Measure the absorbance of both the solutions at 730 nm after 10 minutes and calculate the results by comparison.

Oxyphencyclimine hydrochloride

Procedure

Transfer accurately weighed quantity of the powdered tablets equivalent to about 25 mg of oxyphencyclimine hydrochloride to a separator. Basify with sodium hydroxide solution (5% w/v). Extract with five 25 ml portions of chloroform. Pass chloroform extract through anhydrous sodium sulphate and evaporate the combined chloroform extract on water bath till the volume is reduced to about 2 ml. Cool, add 5 ml of acetic anhydride and 10 ml of glacial acetic acid. Carry out non-aqueous titration with 0.02 N perchloric acid using crystal violet solution as indicator. Each ml of 0.02 N perchloric acid is equivalent to 0.0076189 g of oxyphencyclimine hydrochloride.

Paracetamol, Triprolidine hydrochloride

ESTIMATION

Paracetamol

Follow the nitroso-derivative method described under formulation 2 of this chapter.

Triprolidine hydrochloride

Weigh sample accurately equivalent to about 1.5 mg of triprolidine hydrochloride, suspend in 2 ml of dilute sulphuric acid. Extract with two 40 ml portions of ether. Wash the ether layer with 2 ml of dilute sulphuric acid and 20 ml of water before rejecting it. Combine the main acid layer and washings. Make alkaline with sodium hydroxide solution (20% w/v) and extract with three 30 ml portions of ether. Combine the ether layers and wash with water till the water washing is neutral to litmus. Extract the ether extract with four 40 ml portions of 0.1 N hydrochloric acid. Mix the acidic layer and dilute to 200 ml with acid. Measure the extinction of resulting solution at maxima at about 290 nm and calculate the contents of triprolidine in the sample taking 290 as value of A 1%, 1 cm at 290 nm.

Paracetamol, Dichloralphenazone

ESTIMATION

Paracetamol

Follow the nitroso-derivative method described under formulation 2 of this chapter.

Dichloralphenazone

Reagents

1. 10% w/v solution of sodium hydroxide.
2. 10% w/v solution of sodium acetate.
3. 0.1 N iodine solution.
4. 0.1 N sodium thiosulphate solution.
5. Chloroform.

Procedure

Transfer accurately weighed quantity of the sample equivalent to about 250 mg of dichloralphenazone to a separating funnel. Make it distinctly alkaline with sodium hydroxide solution and extract with four 25 ml portions of chloroform. Wash the combined chloroform layer with water till washings are neutral to litmus. Evaporate the chloroform layer and take up the residue in sodium acetate solution. Add to this 25 ml of 0.1 N iodine and allow to stand in stoppered flask for 20 minutes with occasional shaking. Add 10 ml of chloroform and shake well to dissolve any precipitates formed. Titrate excess of iodine with sodium thiosulphate solution. Each ml of 0.1 N iodine consumed is equivalent to 0.02595 g of dichloralphenazone.

Paracetamol, Diclofenac sodium

ESTIMATION

Paracetamol

Standard solution

10 mcg/ml of paracetamol in 0.1 N hydrochloric acid.

Sample solution

Weigh accurately powdered sample equivalent to about 100 mg of paracetamol. Carry out the dry extraction with three 25 ml portions of 0.1 N hydrochloric acid, filtering through G_4 sintered glass funnel. Dilute the combined filtrate to 100 ml with acid. Dilute further appropriately with the acid to get final concentration of 10 mcg/ml.

Measure the extinction of both sample and standard solutions at maxima at about 244 nm and deduce the results by comparison. Alternatively, follow the method described in formulation 3 of this chapter.

Diclofenac sodium

METHOD 1

Standard solution

The entire residue left after the extraction of paracetamol as described above is used for estimation of diclofenac sodium. Transfer the residue left in the conical flask and on the top of sintered funnel quantitatively to 100 ml volumetric flask with the help of 0.1 N sodium hydroxide. Make up the volume and carry out the further dilutions appropriately with sodium hydroxide to get final concentration of 10 mcg/ml.

Measure the extinction of standard and sample solutions at maxima at about 276 nm using 0.1 N sodium hydroxide solution as blank. Deduce the results by comparison.

METHOD 2 (a & b)

Reagents

1. 0.2% w/v solution of ferric chloride in methanol.
2. 2,2'-bipyridine solution : 0.5% w/v solution in methanol.
3. Mixed phosphate buffer pH 6.8 (0.1 M). To 500 ml of 0.1 M potassium dihydrogen phosphate, add sufficient quantity of 0.2 M sodium phosphate to adjust pH to 6.8, dilute to 1000 ml with water.
4. Methylene blue solution : 0.025% w/v solution in phosphate buffer, pH 6.8 (extract with chloroform and discard organic layer).

Standard solution

(a) 25 mcg/ml of diclofenac sodium in water.
(b) 50 mcg/ml of diclofenac sodium in phosphate buffer, pH 6.8.

Sample solution

Accurately weighed quantity of the powdered sample equivalent to 500 mg of diclofenac sodium was shaken for 5 min with 30 ml of water, made up to 50 ml and filtered.

  (a) Dilute 5 mg of the filtrate to 200 ml with water.
  (b) Dilute 5 ml of the filtrate to 100 ml with phosphate buffer.

Procedure

  (a) To 5 ml each of sample and standard solutions, marked "a" above, add 1 ml each of ferric chloride and 2,2′-bipyridine solution, keep in water bath for 5 min, cool to room temperature and dilute to 10 ml with water. Measure absorbance of both sample and standard solution at 520 nm against reagent blank and calculate the results by comparison.
  (b) To 10 ml each of sample and standard solutions marked "b" above, add 5 ml of methylene blue solution and the complex extracted with chloroform (10 + 10 + 5 ml), passing each extract through anhydrous sodium sulphate, diluted to 25 ml with chloroform. Absorbance of the resulting solution was measured at 650 nm against reagent blank and results calculated by comparison.

Note : Both these methods were found to be suitable for gels also.

Alternatively, diclofenac sodium can be estimated by non-aqueous titration by dissolving the powdered sample equivalent to 250 mg of the substance in 50 ml of glacial acetic acid and titrating with 0.05 N perchloric acid (crystal violet).

Each ml of 0.05 N perchloric acid is equivalent to 15.905 mg of diclofenac sodium.

Paracetamol in the above combination can be directly estimated by UV method described in formulation 25 or 52 of this chapter.

Diclofenac sodium has insignificant absorption at 257 nm, the absorption maxima of paracetamol. However, if contents of diclofenac sodium are more than 10% of the paracetamol contents, it will interfere in the assay of paracetamol.

METHOD 3

To 1 ml each of sample and standard solutions (1 mg/ml in water) add 5 ml of methanol, 1 ml of orthophosphoric acid and 1 ml of 0.25% solution of sodium cobaltinitrite. Heat in a water bath at 45-50°C for 30 min, cool and dilute to 10 ml with methanol. Measure the absorbance of both sample and standard solutions at 368 nm against reagent blank and calculate the results by comparison.

METHOD 4

Reagents

  1. 2% w/v solution of ferric chloride in 0.1 N hydrochloric acid, filter if necessary.
  2. 0.1 N solution of 3-methyl-2-benzothiazolinone hydrazone hydrochloride.

Standard solution

25 mcg/ml solution of diclofenac sodium in 0.01 N sodium hydroxide.

Sample solution

Sample is extracted with 0.01 N sodium hydroxide, filtered and used for analysis.

Procedure

To 3 ml each of sample and standard solutions, add 1 ml of 1 N hydrochloric acid, 1 ml of ferric chloride solution, shake and add 1 ml of the hydrazone reagent. Heat in a water bath at 40°C for 15 min, cool and dilute to 250 ml with acetone. Measure the absorbance of sample and standard solutions at 590 nm against blank and calculate the results by comparison.

METHOD 5

Reagent

1. Copper chloride solution : Dissolve 3 g of copper (II) chloride in 250 ml of pyridine and dilute to 100 ml with water.

Standard solution

1 mg/ml of diclofenac sodium in water.

Sample solution

Extract accurately weighed quantity of the sample with warm water to get final concentration of 1 mg/ml.

Procedure

To 4 ml each of sample and standard solutions, add 6 ml of copper chloride solution, shake and extract the complex with 10 ml of chloroform, shaking intermittently for 10 min. Separate chloroform layer and measure its absorbance at about 730 nm against blank prepared by following above procedure except the sample. The method obeys Beer's law in the concentration range of 1-10 mg/ml of diclofenac sodium.

Paracetamol, Metoclopramide hydrochloride

ESTIMATION

Paracetamol

Standard solution

10 mcg/ml of paracetamol in 0.01 N sodium hydroxide.

Sample solution

Weigh accurately sample equivalent to about 50 mg of paracetamol. Add 25 ml of 0.1 N sodium hydroxide and shake for 10-15 min, dilute to 100 ml with water, mix and filter. Dilute further appropriately with 0.01 N sodium hydroxide solution to get final concentration of 10 mcg/ml.

Measure the extinction of both sample and standard solutions at 257 nm. Calculate the results by comparison or by using 715 as value of A 1%, 1 cm at 257 nm.

Metoclopramide hydrochloride

Reagents

1. Bromothymol blue solution : Dissolve 150 mg of bromothymol blue and 150 mg of anhydrous sodium carbonate in water to make 100 ml.
2. Citric acid-phosphate buffer, pH 5.7. Buffer is prepared by mixing appropriately 10% w/v solutions of citric acid and disodium phosphate.
3. 2% w/v solution of boric acid in methanol.

Standard solution

100 mcg/ml of metoclopramide hydrochloride in water.

Sample solution

Weigh accurately a quantity of the sample equivalent to about 10 mg of the substance. Add about 50 ml of water and warm in a warm-bath for 20-25 min to effect complete solution. Cool to room temperature and adjust the volume to 100 ml with water.

Procedure

To 5 ml each of sample and standard solutions, add 1 ml of dye solution and 20 ml of phosphate buffer solution. Mix and extract with three 25 ml portions of chloroform. Pass each chloroform layer through anhydrous sodium sulphate. Add 25 ml of boric acid solution and dilute to 100 ml with chloroform. Measure the absorbance of both the solutions at about 425 nm using chloroform as blank. Calculate the results by comparison.

Note : 1. Allow complete separation of layers after each extraction.
2. Extract the dye solution with chloroform till chloroform layer is colourless before using the dye for colour development, this will reduce the blank value.
3. Centrifuge the chloroform layer for consistent results.

Paracetamol, Mefenamic acid

ESTIMATION

Paracetamol

METHOD 1

Standard solution

10 mcg/ml of paracetamol in 0.1 N hydrochloric acid.

Sample solution

Weigh accurately powdered sample equivalent to about 100 mg of paracetamol. Dry extract with three 25 ml portions of 1 N hydrochloric acid filtering through G_4 sintered glass funnel (reserve the residue left on the funnel for estimation of mefenamic acid). Collect the filtrate and dilute to 100 ml with the acid. Further dilutions are done appropriately with the acid to get a concentration of 10 mcg/ml.

Measure the extinction of sample and standard solutions at 244 nm and deduce the results by comparison.

Note :   As the mefenamic acid is insoluble in acid, it does not interfere in estimation of paracetamol.

METHOD 2

Follow the nitroso-derivative method as described in formulation 2 of this chapter.

Mefenamic acid

METHOD 1

Standard solution

10 mcg/ml of mefenamic acid in 0.1 N sodium hydroxide.

Sample solution

Dissolve the entire residue obtained on the sintered funnel during the estimation of paracetamol in 1 N sodium hydroxide by slowly adding the alkali on the top of funnel and filtering by slow suction, dilute to 100 ml. Dilute 10 ml of the resultant solution to 100 ml with water. Further dilutions are done with 0.1 N sodium hydroxide to get 10 mcg/ml concentration.

Measure the extinction of both sample and standard solutions at 284 nm using 0.1 N sodium hydroxide as blank. The results may be deduced by comparison.

METHOD 2

Standard solution

10 mcg/ml of mefenamic acid in 0.1 N methanolic hydrochloric acid.

Sample solution

Dissolve accurately weighed quantity of the sample equivalent to about 100 mg of mefenamic acid in 100 ml of 0.1 N methanolic hydrochloric acid. Filter, rejecting first few ml of the filtrate. Dilute the filtrate suitably with 0.1 N methanolic hydrochloric acid to get concentration of 10 mcg/ml.

Measure the extinction of both sample and standard solutions at maxima at about 350 nm using methanolic hydrochloric acid as blank. Deduce the results by comparison.

Note : Paracetamol has no absorption at 350 nm, hence no interference.

METHOD 3

Weigh accurately powdered sample equivalent to about 500 mg of mefenamic acid, dissolve in neutralized (phenol red) methanol by slight warming. Titrate with 0.1 N sodium hydroxide using phenol red as indicator. Each ml of 0.1 N sodium hydroxide is equivalent to 0.02413 g of mefenamic acid. Paracetamol does not interfere.

METHOD 4

Reagents

1. 1% w/v solution of potassium ferricyanide in water.
2. 0.1% solution of aminophenazone in water (freshly prepared).

Standard solution

50 mcg/ml of mefenamic acid in methanol.

Sample solution

Accurately weighed quantity of the powdered tablets equivalent to 100 mg of mefenamic acid was extracted with methanol and finally diluted to get a solution of 50 mcg/ml.

Procedure

To 1 ml each of sample and standard solutions, add 2 ml of phenazone reagent and 5 ml of potassium ferricyanide. The contents were mixed and allowed to stand for 15 min and diluted to 25 ml with water. The absorbance was measured at 590 nm against reagent blank and results calculated by comparison. The chromogen was stable for 45 min. The method obeyed Beer's law in concentration range of 0.5-4 mcg/ml.

Methocarbamol, Paracetamol, Diclofenac sodium

ESTIMATION

Methocarbamol

Follow the method 1 or 2 described under formulation 55 of this chapter.

Diclofenac sodium

Standard solution

15 mcg/ml of diclofenac sodium in methanol.

Sample solution

To alkaline aqueous extract obtained during estimation of methocarbamol, add dilute hydrochloride to make it distinctly acidic and extract with four 20 ml portions of chloroform, washing each chloroform layer with the same 10 ml of water. Combine the aqueous layers and resume estimation of paracetamol. Dilute chloroform layer to 100 ml. Further dilution is done with methanol to get final solution of 15 mcg/ml. Measure extinction of both the sample and standard at 282 nm against solvent blank.

Typical laboratory analysis

$$\text{Diclofenac sodium (mg)/tablet} = \frac{A_v}{A_s} \times \frac{W_s}{W_t} \times \text{dilution factor} \times \frac{\text{Av. wt.}}{1} \times 1000$$

$$= \frac{0.530}{0.540} \times \frac{0.0747}{0.2678} \times \frac{0.9366}{5} \times 1000$$

$$= 51.09$$

$$\text{Claim} = 50 \text{ mg/tab}$$

Note : Sometimes higher results are obtained due to interference by excipients. Under these circumstances chloroform layer is evaporated. Residue is taken up in neutralized methanol (phenol red) and diluted with 0.1 N sodium hydroxide for estimation.

Paracetamol

Follow the procedure (a) described under formulation 2 of this chapter.

Methocarbamol, Paracetamol

ESTIMATION

Methocarbamol

METHOD 1

Transfer accurately weighed quantity of the powdered sample equivalent to 400 mg of methocarbamol to a separating funnel with the aid of 5-10 ml of water. Basify with 2-3 ml of 1 N sodium hydroxide solution. Extract with 4 × 25 ml of chloroform. Shake the combined chloroform layer with 20 ml of water, add washing to the alkaline layer (reserve for estimation of paracetamol). Pass the combined chloroform layer through anhydrous sodium sulphate placed over cotton plug and pre-moistened. Evaporate the chloroform on a steam bath, finally drying in an oven at 50°C to a constant weight. From the weight initially taken for analysis, calculate the contents of methocarbamol (mg) in each tablet.

METHOD 2

Standard solution

100 mg of the substance accurately weighed and dissolved in chloroform to make 100 ml. 5 ml of the resultant solution is diluted to 50 ml with methanol (100 mcg/ml).

Sample solution

Extract the powdered sample equipment to 100 mg of the substance with chloroform after basifying with 1 N sodium hydroxide. The chloroform layer is made up to 100 ml. 5 ml of the solution is further diluted to 50 ml with methanol (100 mcg/ml).

Measure the extinction of both the sample and standard solutions at 274 nm against solvent blank and calculate the results by comparison.

Paracetamol

To the combined alkaline aqueous layer obtained during estimation of methocarbamol (method 1), add 2.5 ml of 1 N sodium hydroxide solution and dilute to 250 ml with water. Further dilutions are made appropriately with 0.1 N sodium hydroxide to obtain a solution of 10 mcg/ml. Measure extinction of the resulting solution at 257 nm against reagent blank. Calculate the results by using 715 as value of A 1%, 1 cm at 257 nm.

Paracetamol, Methionine

ESTIMATION

Paracetamol

Follow the nitroso-derivative method as described in formulation 2 of this chapter.

Methionine

Weigh accurately powdered sample equivalent to 150 mg of methionine and transfer to iodine flask containing 50 ml of water. Add 2.5 g of potassium dihydrogen phosphate and 1 g of potassium iodide. Shake to dissolve the contents. Add 25 ml of 0.1 N iodine, seal the flask tightly with glass stopper and allow to stand for 30 min. Immerse in ice water and titrate excess of iodine with 0.1 N sodium thiosulphate using starch as indicator. Run the blank. Each ml of 0.1 N iodine consumed is equivalent to 7.461 mg of methionine.

Methionine could also be assayed by formol titration using phenolphthalein or thymol blue as indicator.

Note : The method involving oxidation with sodium nitroprusside as described in the chapter on vitamins is not applicable as paracetamol will interfere.

Paracetamol, Ibuprofen, Dextropropoxyphene hydrochloride

ESTIMATION

Paracetamol

METHOD 1

(a) Follow the nitroso-derivative method described under formulation 2 of this chapter.

(b) Dilute the aqueous layer obtained in estimation of ibuprofen to 100 ml with water and take appropriate portion for estimation by nitroso-derivative method as described in formulation 2 of this chapter, or follow method 1 or 2 described under the estimation of paracetamol in formulation 4 of this chapter.

METHOD 2

Standard solution

10 mcg/ml of paracetamol in 0.1 N hydrochloric acid.

Sample solution

Weigh accurately a quantity of the sample equivalent to 100 mg of paracetamol. Extract the dry powder with three 25 ml portions of 1 N hydrochloric acid, filtering each portion through the same G_4 sintered glass funnel (reserve the residue for estimation of ibuprofen). Adjust the filtrate to 100 ml with 1 N hydrochloric acid. Dilute further appropriately and stepwise with 0.1 N hydrochloric acid to get a final concentration of 10 mcg/ml in respect of paracetamol.

Measure the extinction of both the solutions at maxima at about 244 nm using 0.1 N hydrochloric acid as blank. Calculate the results by comparison.

Ibuprofen

METHOD 1

Weigh accurately quantity of the sample equivalent to 200 mg of the substance, suspend in 20 ml of water and extract with four 25 ml portions of chloroform (retain aqueous layer for estimation of paracetamol as above). Pass combined chloroform layer through anhydrous sodium sulphate placed on cotton plug (pre-moistened with chloroform). Evaporate chloroform on water bath and take up the residue in 25 ml of neutralized (phenol red) methyl alcohol. Add 20 ml of water and titrate with 0.1 N sodium hydroxide. Each ml of 0.1 N sodium hydroxide is equivalent to 0.02063 g of ibuprofen.

Note : 1. Do not use filter paper for filtration as it may result in loss of the substance, filtration through sintered glass funnel (G_2) is preferred.

2. The powdered sample can also be directly extracted with ether, ether layer evaporated and residue taken up in neutral methanol for titration with 0.1 N sodium hydroxide.

METHOD 2

Standard solution

50 mcg/ml of ibuprofen in methanol.

Sample solution

Dissolve the entire residue obtained in the estimation of paracetamol above in methanol to make 100 ml. Further dilutions are done appropriately and stepwise with methanol to get a final concentration of 50 mcg/ml.

Measure the extinction of both sample and standard solutions at maxima at about 267 nm using methanol as blank. Calculate the results by comparison.

METHOD 3

As ibuprofen being propionic acid derivative contains free carboxyl (COOH) group, it can be directly titrated with sodium carbonate, paracetamol containing hydroxyl (OH^-) group will not interfere.

Reagents

1. 1 N sodium carbonate.
2. Solution of phenol red (indicator).

Procedure

Accurately weighed quantity of the powdered sample equivalent to 500 mg of the substance was dissolved in methanol (neutralized) and titrated with sodium carbonate using phenol red as indicator. Each ml of 1 N sodium carbonate is equivalent to 0.02063 g of ibuprofen.

Dextropropoxyphene hydrochloride

Follow the method 2 described in formulation 25 of this chapter.

Methocarbamol, Ibuprofen

ESTIMATION

Methocarbamol

Follow the method described under formulation 55 of this chapter.

Ibuprofen

Standard solution

50 mcg/ml of ibuprofen in 0.1 N methanolic sodium hydroxide.

Sample solution

Combined alkaline aqueous extract obtained during estimation of methocarbamol under formulation 55 is appropriately diluted with methanol to get concentration of 50 mcg/ml.

Measure the extinction of both the standard and sample solutions at maxima at about 267 nm against solvent blank. Deduce the results by comparison with the standard.

Alternatively, appropriate quantity of the sample can be extracted with water. Ibuprofen being insoluble is retained on the sintered funnel, whereas the filtrate containing only methocarbamol can be further diluted with water to get a concentration of 40 mcg/ml having absorption maxima at 272 nm. The residue can be taken in 0.1 N sodium hydroxide for spectrophotometric analysis (λ_{max} 264 nm) or residue dissolved in neutralized methanol (phenol red) and titrated with 0.1 N sodium hydroxide. Each ml of 0.1 N sodium hydroxide is equivalent to 20.63 mg of ibuprofen.

Isopropylantipyrin, Ketoprofen/Ibuprofen

ESTIMATION

Ketoprofen/Ibuprofen

Follow the method described in formulation 47 of this chapter. Each ml of 0.1 N sodium hydroxide is equivalent to 0.02543 g of ketoprofen or 0.02063 g of ibuprofen.

Isopropylantipyrin (Propyphenazone)

Follow the method described under formulation 9 of the chapter on anti-inflammatory drugs. Each ml of 0.1 N perchloric acid is equivalent to 0.02303 g of propyphenazone.

Formulation 60

Paracetamol, Caffeine citrate, Phenyl-Dimethyl-Isopropylpyrazolone, Diethyl-Dioxo-Tetrahydropyridine

ESTIMATION

Paracetamol

Follow the nitroso-derivative method described under formulation 2 of this chapter.

Phenyl-dimethyl-isopropylpyrazolone (Propyphenazone/Isopropylantipyrin/Isopropylphenazone)

Follow the method described under formulation 10 of the chapter on anti-inflammatory drugs.

Caffeine citrate

METHOD 1

Reagents

1. Saturated solution of sodium bicarbonate in water.
2. 0.01 N tartaric acid.
3. Chloroform.

Standard solution

7.5 mcg/ml caffeine citrate in 0.01 N tartaric acid.

Sample solution

Weigh powdered sample accurately equivalent to about 20 mg of caffeine citrate, carry out dry extraction of the sample with four 25 ml portions of chloroform. Wash the combined chloroform layer with 25 ml of sodium bicarbonate solution. Discard the aqueous layer, the chloroform layer is evaporated and the residue is taken up in 0.01 N tartaric acid and further diluted with the acid to get final concentration of 7.5 mcg/ml.

Measure the extinction of both sample and standard solutions at maxima at about 271 nm against solvent blank. Calculate the results by comparison.

METHOD 2

Extract accurately weighed quantity of the sample equivalent to about 1 g of total weight of all the four active ingredients present in the formulation with methanol. Filter and evaporate the filtrate to constant weight. This gives total weight of all the four ingredients. Subtract the total weight of other three ingredients estimated individually by various methods described in the formulation to obtain the net contents of caffeine citrate present in the sample under analysis.

Diethyl-dioxo-tetrahydropyridine

METHOD 1

Standard solution

10 mcg/ml of substance in methanol.

Sample solution

Accurately weighed quantity of the sample equivalent to 20 mg of the substance is extracted with methanol and made up to 100 ml. The resultant solution is further diluted appropriately to get final concentration of 10 mcg/ml.

The extinction of both the solutions is measured at 310 nm using methanol as blank. The results are calculated by comparison.

Note : Although maxima of the compound in methanol is observed at 305 nm, but at this wavelength, there is slight interference from paracetamol and propyphenazone. However, at 310 nm, the interference due to above ingredients is almost nil, hence, the latter wavelength is preferred for estimation.

METHOD 2

Follow the above method using 0.1 N sodium hydroxide instead of methanol. Measure the extinction of both sample and standard solutions at about 366 nm and calculate the results by comparison.

Paracetamol, Phenylpropanolamine hydrochloride, Caffeine citrate, Chlorpheniramine maleate

ESTIMATION

Paracetamol

Follow the nitroso-derivative method described under formulation 2 of this chapter.

Caffeine citrate

Transfer accurately weighed quantity of powdered tablets equivalent to 20 mg of caffeine citrate to a separating funnel. Add 20 ml of saturated solution of sodium chloride, shake to disperse. Extract with three 25 ml portions of chloroform, washing each extract with same 10 ml of saturated solution of sodium bicarbonate (reserve aqueous layer for estimation of phenylpropanolamine hydrochloride). Filter the combined chloroform layer through moistened cotton plug and make up to 100 ml with chloroform. Take 5 ml of chloroform extract into volumetric flask, evaporate, take up the residue in 0.01 N tartaric acid and follow the method described in formulation 60 of this chapter.

Phenylpropanolamine hydrochloride

METHOD 1

Reagents

1. 2% w/v solution of sodium carbonate in water.
2. 2% w/v solution of sodium metaperiodate in water.
3. 6 N hydrochloric acid.

Standard solution

1.5 mg/ml of the substance in water. To 10 ml of this solution, add 40 ml of saturated solution of sodium bicarbonate, 30 ml of 6 N hydrochloric acid, stir to remove carbon dioxide and dilute to 200 ml with water.

Sample solution

To the aqueous extract reserved during estimation of caffeine, add 30 ml of 6 N hydrochloric acid and dilute to 200 ml with water.

Sample solution

To the aqueous extract reserved during estimation of caffeine, add 30 ml of 6 N hydrochloric acid and dilute to 200 ml with water.

Procedure

To 10 ml each of sample and standard solutions, add 10 ml each of sodium carbonate and sodium metaperiodate solutions, mix, allow to stand. Make slightly acidic with hydrochloric acid. Extract with three 30 ml portions of dichloromethane, passing each extract through same layer of anhydrous sodium sulphate. Dilute to 100 ml with dichloromethane. Concomitantly measure the absorbance of both standard and sample solutions at about 242 nm against solvent blank and calculate the results by comparison.

METHOD 2

Reagents

1. 1.5% w/v solution of ninhydrin in pyridine : methanol mixture (1 : 1).
2. 0.05% w/v solution of ascorbic acid in water.

Standard solution

50 mcg/ml of phenylpropanolamine hydrochloride in water.

Sample solution

Weigh the powdered sample equivalent to 25 mg of the substance, dissolve in 200-300 ml of water by mechanical stirring, dilute to 500 ml with water.

Procedure

To 2 ml each of sample and standard solutions, add 1.0 ml of ascorbic acid solution, 2 ml of ninhydrin solution. Place the test tubes in boiling water bath for 25 minutes, cool in ice bath and dilute to 25 ml with water. After 10 minute, measure at about 570 nm against reagent blank and deduce the results by comparison.

Chlorpheniramine maleate

Standard solution

Weigh accurately 20 mg of the substance, add 10 ml of water, 2.5 ml of 1 N hydrochloric acid and dilute to 50 ml with water.

Sample solution

Transfer accurately weighed quantity of the powdered sample equivalent to 20 mg of chlorpheniramine maleate to 100 ml volumetric flask. Add 10 ml of water, 2.5 ml of 1 N hydrochloric acid and dilute to 50 ml with water.

Follow the cyanogen bromide method described under formulation 1 of the chapter of rubefacients.

Chlorpheniramine maleate, Trithioparamethoxyphenylpropene

ESTIMATION

Chlorpheniramine maleate

Standard solution

30 mcg/ml of chlorpheniramine maleate in water.

Sample solution

Transfer accurately weighed quantity of the powdered sample equivalent to 10 mg of chlorpheniramine maleate to 100 ml volumetric flask. Add about 50 ml of water, shake vigorously and make up the volume. Further dilutions are done appropriately with water to get a concentration of 30 mcg/ml.

Measure the extinction of both the solutions at maxima at about 262 nm and deduce the results by comparison. Alternatively, follow the cyanogen bromide method.

Trithioparamethoxyphenylpropene

Standard solution

10 mcg/ml of trithioparamethoxyphenylpropene in methanol.

Sample solution

Remove the sugar coating (if coated) of the tablets with wet cotton. Dry the core and determine average weight of the core. Transfer accurately weighed quantity of the powdered sample equivalent to 10 mg of the substance to a dry 100 ml volumetric flask. Add about 50 ml of methanol and dissolve by slight warming in water-bath. Make up the volume and filter. The filtrate is appropriately diluted with methanol to get a final concentration of 10 mcg/ml.

Measure the absorption of both the sample and standard solutions at about 435 nm using methanol as blank and calculate the results by comparison.

Chapter 7

Alimentary Drugs
(Antidiarrhoeals, Antacids, Oral Rehydration Salts)

Formulation 1

Di-iodohydroxyquinoline, Metronidazole, Chloroquine phosphate, Belladonna dry extract

ESTIMATION

Di-iodohydroxyquinoline

METHOD 1

Standard solution

2.5 mcg/ml of di-iodohydroxyquinoline in methanol.

Sample solution

Weigh sample accurately equivalent to 50 mg of di-iodohydroxyquinoline in a 200 ml volumetric flask, add absolute alcohol to make up the volume. Dilute appropriately with absolute alcohol to get 2.5 mcg/ml. Measure the absorbance of both standard and sample solutions at 253 nm using methanol as blank and calculate the results by comparison.

METHOD 2

Reagents

1. 0.1% v/v acetone in dimethylformamide (DMF).
2. 25% v/v benzyl trimethylammonium hydroxide (BTAH) in distilled water.

Standard solution

10 mcg/ml of the substance in dimethylformamide (DMF).

Sample solution

Weigh accurately powdered sample equivalent to 100 mg of the compound and add 'DMF' to produce 100 ml, shake and filter. The filtrate is suitably diluted with 'DMF' to get concentration of 10 mcg/ml.

Procedure

To 0.5 ml each of standard and sample solutions, add 0.2 ml of acetone solution and 0.1 ml of 'BTAH' reagent and make up the volume to 5 ml with 'DMF'. Measure the absorbance after 10 minutes at 360 nm against reagent blank. The method obeys Beer's law in the range of 2-14 mcg/ml. The yellow complex is stable for 20 minutes.

METHOD 3

Reagents

1. 0.02% w/v vanadyl sulphate in ethyl alcohol.
2. Hydrochloric acid, dilute.
3. Cyclohexane.

Standard solution

200 mcg/ml of di-iodohydroxyquinoline in dilute hydrochloric acid.

Sample solution

Weigh accurately powdered sample equivalent to about 20 mg of the compound, add 75 ml of dilute hydrochloric acid, shake and make up to 100 ml with the acid (200 mcg/ml).

Procedure

To 2.5 ml each of standard and sample solutions, add 7 ml of vanadyl reagent and 10 ml of cyclohexane. Shake for 2 minutes, allow to separate the cyclohexane layer. Measure absorbance of the organic layer at 415 nm against reagent blank. The method obeys Beer's law in the range of 10-100 mcg/ml. The yellow colour is stable for 45 minutes.

METHOD 4

Reagents

1. 0.1% w/v p-aminophenol solution in 0.2 N hydrochloric acid (freshly prepared).
2. 0.5 N sodium carbonate.
3. 1,4-dioxane.

Standard solution

100 mg of the compound is dissolved in 1,4-dioxane to produce 100 ml (1 mg/ml).

Sample solution

Powdered sample accurately weighed equivalent to 25 mg of the compound is shaken with 20 ml of dioxane and filtered. The final volume is adjusted to 25 ml with dioxane (1 mg/ml).

Procedure

To 0.4 ml each of the sample and standard solutions, add 3 ml of sodium carbonate solution and 0.4 ml of p-aminophenol reagent. Keep at room temperature for 5 minutes and then dilute to 10 ml with water. The absorbance of the resultant solution is measured at 570 nm after 15 minutes against reagent blank. The contents of di-iodohydroxyquinoline are calculated by comparison with the standard. The method obeys Beer's law in the concentration range of 15-500 mcg/ml.

Note : 1. The colour attains maximum intensity after 15 minutes and is stable for 50 minutes.
2. Metronidazole, chloramphenicol, chloroquine, brobenzoxalidine, hyoscine and hyoscyamine do not interfere.

Metronidazole

METHOD 1

Transfer a quantity of the sample accurately weighed equivalent to 200 mg of metronidazole in a 125 ml separating funnel. Extract with six 30 ml portions of warm acetone. Collect the acetone extracts, cool and pass through a pledget of cotton and collect in a beaker. Add to the beaker, 50 ml of acetic anhydride and 2 drops of 1% w/v solution of brilliant green in glacial acetic acid. Titrate this solution with 0.1 N perchloric acid to a yellowish green end point. Repeat the operation without the sample (blank) and subtract the blank reading from the main reading. Each ml of 0.1 N perchloric acid consumed is equivalent to 0.01712 g of metronidazole.

METHOD 2

Weigh accurately a quantity of the sample equivalent to about 50 mg of metronidazole, add 80-90 ml 0.1 N hydrochloric acid, shake for 15 minutes, add sufficient 0.1 N hydrochloric acid to produce 200 ml. Filter and dilute 5 ml of the filtrate to 100 ml with 0.1 N hydrochloric acid. Measure the extinction of the resulting solution at the maximum at about 277 nm and calculate the content of metronidazole taking 380 as the value of A 1%, 1 cm at 277 nm.

METHOD 3

Standard solution

1 mg/ml of metronidazole in water.

Sample solution

(a) Tablets : Weigh accurately powdered sample equivalent to about 100 mg of metronidazole, and 60-70 ml of water, shake and make up the volume to 100 ml with water. Filter and use for colour development.

(b) Syrups/suspensions : Measure sample equivalent to about 100 mg of substance, extract with three 30 ml portions of chloroform. Combine chloroform layer and evaporate on water-bath. Dissolve the residue in water to produce 100 ml and use appropriate volume for colour development.

Procedure

To 2 ml each of the standard and sample solutions, add 3 ml of 20% w/v sodium hydroxide solution and keep at room temperature for 8 minutes (this is the optimum time for completion of the reaction). Adjust to 10 ml with water and read at 500 nm within 12 minutes against reagent blank. The method obeys Beer's law in the concentration range of (100-150 mcg/ml).

Note : The colour is stable for 13 minutes and starts fading after that.

METHOD 4

Reagents

1. Hydrochloric acid.
2. Zinc dust.
3. 1% w/v solution of vanillin in water.

Standard solution

Weigh accurately about 100 mg of metronidazole and dissolve in 25 ml of water. Add 10 ml of hydrochloric acid and 3 g of zinc dust. Keep in water-bath for 15 minutes for completion of the reaction. Cool, filter and wash the residue with water till filtrate is free of acidity. Washings and main filtrate are combined and adjusted to 100 ml. 10 ml is further diluted to 100 ml with water.

Sample solution

Prepare the initial sample (tablets, syrups and suspensions) solutions as per procedure described under method 3 under sample solution. These solutions are further treated and diluted as described under standard solution in this method.

Procedure

To 2.5 ml each of the standard and sample solutions, 1 ml of vanillin solution is added and heated on water-bath for 20 minutes. Cool to room temperature, adjust the volume to 10 ml with water and read at about 410 nm. The yellow complex thus produced is quite stable. The method obeys Beer's law in the concentration range of 10-50 mcg/ml.

METHOD 5

The final standard and sample solutions obtained after zinc and acid treatment as described under method 4 above are used in this method.

Reagents

1. 1% w/v solution of sodium nitrite in water.
2. 0.5% w/v solution of ammonium sulphamate in water.
3. 0.1% w/v solution of N-1-naphthyl-ethylenediamine dihydrochloride in water.

Procedure

To 2.5 ml each of sample and standard solutions as indicated above, 0.5 ml of sodium nitrite solution is added. Keep for 3 minutes, neutralize excess of nitrous acid by adding 0.5 ml of ammonium sulphamate solution. Again leave the solution for 3 minutes and finally add 0.5 ml of naphthyl-ethylenediamine dihydrochloride solution. Determine the absorption of resulting solutions at about 550 nm against reagent blank and calculate the results by comparison.

Chloroquine phosphate

Standard solution

10 mcg/ml of chloroquine phosphate in water.

Sample solution

Weigh accurately a portion of the sample equivalent to about 200 mg of chloroquine phosphate and dissolve in 20 ml of water. Filter the solution to 250 ml separator, wash any undissolved residue with several small portions of water, add 5 ml of ammonia, agitate, and extract the liberated base with five 25 ml portions of chloroform. Wash the combined chloroform extract with 10 ml of water, then extract the water washing with 10 ml of chloroform. Evaporate the combined chloroform extracts on a steam-bath to about 10 ml, add 50 ml of dilute hydrochloric acid and continue heating in the steam-bath until the odour of chloroform is no longer perceptible. Transfer the aqueous acidic solutions to a 200 ml volumetric flask, wash the evaporating dish with portion of dilute acid, adding the washings to the volumetric flask and dilute to volume. Dilute the solution further quantitatively and step-wise with dilute acid to give a concentration of about 10 mcg per ml.

Determine the absorbance of both the solutions at maximum at about 343 nm in a suitable spectro-photometer. Calculate the contents of chloroquine phosphate by comparison or use A 1%, 1 cm value of 360 for calculations.

Total belladonna alkaloids calculated as atropine

Reagents

1. Chloroform.
2. Acetone (water contents not more than 0.02% v/v).
3. Anhydrous sodium sulphate, granular.
4. Phosphoric acid (88% w/w).
5. Solvent (6% v/v of acetic acid in 5% v/v alcohol) : Take 6 ml of the glacial acetic acid and 5 ml of dehydrated alcohol in a 250 ml conical flask. Add 89 ml of distilled water and shake well.
6. Dehydrated alcohol.
7. Fuming nitric acid (it is highly corrosive; handle with care).
8. Potassium hydroxide (pellets).
9. Methyl alcohol.
10. 50% v/v alcohol.

Standard stock solution

Take about 80 mg of atropine sulphate accurately weighed in 100 ml volumetric flask and dissolve in solvent. Make up the volume to 100 ml with the solvent. Prepare this solution once every month and store in a refrigerator to serve as stock solution.

Dilute standard solution

Dilute 10 ml of the standard stock solution to 100 ml with the solvent (80 mcg/ml). Prepare this solution freshly before use.

Calculate the contents of atropine (base) in mg/ml in the diluted standard solution as follows :

$$\text{Weight of atropine sulphate taken} = \frac{578.76 \times 10}{694.86 \times 100 \times 100}$$

Sample solution

Take sample accurately weighed in a 250 ml stoppered conical flask. Extract the alkaloids by shaking the sample twice, each with 50 ml of a mixture of 2 ml of phosphoric acid and 48 ml of 50% v/v alcohol in a mechanical shaker. Filter both the extracts through the same Whatman filter paper No. 4 into 500 ml beaker and wash the residue with a further 50 ml of mixture of 0.5 ml of phosphoric acid and 49.5 ml of ethyl alcohol. Add the washings to the filtrate and reduce the volume of the combined filtrate and the washings on a water-bath to about 50 ml. Transfer to a separator with the aid of little alcohol. Wash the container with chloroform and add the washings to the separator. Make distinctly alkaline with dilute solution of ammonia and extract with four 30 ml portions of chloroform. Wash each chloroform layer with same 10 ml of water. Filter organic layer through anhydrous sodium sulphate and evaporate just to dryness. Add 2 ml of ethyl alcohol and finally dry at 105°C for 3 h. Dissolve the residue in 9 ml of chloroform and transfer into stoppered 25 ml cylinder. Wash the flask with 15 ml of solvent and add to the cylinder. Shake vigorously for 2 minutes and allow to settle till the aqueous portion is distinctly clear. Transfer 5 ml of the aqueous layer into a porcelain dish and completely evaporate off the liquid to dryness. Add 5 drops of fuming nitric acid, keep on water-bath for 3 minutes and transfer quickly to a 10 ml volumetric flask with the aid of acetone. Make up the volume with acetone and mark the flask as 'sample'.

Take 1 ml of standard solution and 1 ml of water in two 25 ml porcelain dishes and proceed according to preceding para beginning with "completely evaporate off the liquid to dryness". Mark these flasks as 'standard' and 'blank' respectively.

Procedure

Dissolve one pellet of sodium hydroxide in 5 ml of methyl alcohol and add 0.1 ml of this solution to each of three 10 ml volumetric flasks marked as 'standard', 'sample' and 'blank'. Shake and allow to stand for 3 minutes. Measure immediately the optical densities of the standard and sample at 550 nm in a spectrophotometer against the blank. Calculate the total belladonna alkaloids as hyoscyamine by comparison.

Note : If morphine is also present, it should be oxidized with ferric chloride as described below and then tropane alkaloids extracted as usual.

Take sample equivalent to 1 mg of the alkaloids, add 0.5 ml of ferric chloride solution (5%), allow to stand for 2 minutes, add 2 g of sodium citrate and shake until dissolved. Make alkaline with ammonium hydroxide and then follow general extraction procedure and colour development for belladonna alkaloids.

Di-iodohydroxyquinoline, Phthalylsulphathiazole

ESTIMATION

Di-iodohydroxyquinoline

METHOD 1

Reagents

1. Dilute hydrochloric acid.
2. Dimethylformamide (DMF).

Standard solution

Weigh accurately 100 mg of pure compound, add 10 ml of 'DMF' and shake vigorously for 5 minutes. Further make appropriate dilution with dilute hydrochloric acid to obtain a concentration of 50 mcg/ml.

Sample solution

Weigh accurately a quantity of powdered sample equivalent to 100 mg of the compound, add 10 ml of 'DMF' and treat as per standard solution.

Concomitantly determine the extinctions of both the standard and sample solutions at absorption maximum at about 390 nm and calculate the results by comparison.

METHOD 2

Follow the method 4 described for estimation of di-iodohydroxyquinoline under formulation 1 of this chapter.

METHOD 3

Reagents

1. 0.4% w/v solution of 2,6-dichloroquinone chlorimide in isopropyl alcohol.
2. Buffer solution : 3.3% w/v solution of dipotassium hydrogen phosphate in water.
3. 1,4-dioxane.

Standard solution

100 mcg/ml of the compound in 1,4-dioxane.

Sample solution

Weigh accurately powdered sample or measure aliquot equivalent to 25 mg of the compound and extract with 1,4-dioxane to get 100 mcg/ml solution.

Procedure

To 1 ml each of the sample and standard solutions, add 2 ml buffer and 5 ml chlorimide reagent and dilute to 10 ml with water. After 5 minutes, measure the absorbance of both the solutions at 650 nm against reagent as blank. The method obeys Beer's law in the range of 1-16 mcg/ml.

Metronidazole, metronidazole benzoate and tetracycline hydrochloride do not interfere.

Phthalylsulphathiazole

METHOD 1

Weigh accurately a quantity of sample equivalent to about 0.25 g of phthalylsulphathiazole. Add 100 ml of 25% w/v sodium hydroxide solution and reflux for four hours. Cool, filter through cotton, wash with water and acidify with hydrochloric acid. Cool below 15°C and titrate against 0.1 M sodium nitrite with constant shaking using starch iodide paste as an external indicator. Each ml of 0.1 M sodium nitrite is equivalent to 0.04034 g of phthalylsulphathiazole.

METHOD 2

Transfer a quantity of powder equivalent to about 400 mg of phthalylsulphathiazole in a dry beaker. Add 30-40 ml of ethyl acetate, boil on water-bath, stir and decant the solution through filter paper. Repeat the extraction 4-5 times with boiling ethyl acetate and filter while hot. Iodochlorhydroxy-quinoline, soluble in hot ethyl acetate gets removed by above extraction procedure. Collect the residue, dry and reflux for 30 minutes with water and 20 ml of hydrochloric acid. Cool to 15°C and proceed for estimation as under method 1 above.

Chloroquine phosphate, Di-iodohydroxyquinoline, Phthalylsulphathiazole

ESTIMATION

Chloroquine phosphate

METHOD 1

Follow the method 2 for estimation of chloroquine phosphate described under formulation 1 of this chapter.

METHOD 2

Reagents

1. 0.4% w/v solution of bromothymol blue in water.
2. Chloroform.
3. Buffer solution, pH 5.6 : Weigh 41.5 g of disodium hydrogen phosphate and 8.72 g of citric acid and dissolve in water to produce 1000 ml.

Standard solution

Weigh chloroquine phosphate or sulphate equivalent to 40 mg of the chloroquine base and dissolve in water to produce a solution of 10 mcg/ml (base).

Sample solution

Weigh accurately powdered sample equivalent to 40 mg of chloroquine base, shake with water and adjust the volume to 100 ml with water. Filter and dilute the filtrate appropriately to get a sample solution of 10 mcg/ml (base).

Procedure

To 5 ml each of the sample and standard solutions, add 5 ml of the buffer solution, pH 5.6 and 5 ml of the dye solution. Shake and add 10 ml of chloroform. Shake vigorously for 1 minute, and allow the chloroform layer to separate. Measure absorption of chloroform layer of both the solutions at about 410 nm and calculate the contents of chloroquine phosphate by comparison.

Phthalylsulphathiazole

METHOD 1

Reagents

1. 10% w/v solution of sodium bicarbonate in water.
2. 0.1 M sodium nitrite solution.

Procedure

To accurately weighed quantity of the sample equivalent to 500 mg of the substance, add 50 ml of sodium bicarbonate solution and allow the mixture to stand for 30 minutes with occasional stirring. After the suspended matter has settled down, the supernatant liquid is filtered through G_4 sintered crucible. Extract the residue with further three successive 25, 15, 10 ml portions of bicarbonate solution, filtering each through the same crucible. Neutralize the combined filtrate with hydrochloric acid and add 10 ml of the acid in excess. Reflux for 1 hour, cool to 15°C and slowly titrate with 0.1 M sodium nitrite. Each ml of 0.1 M sodium nitrite is equivalent to 0.04034 g of phthalylsulphathiazole.

METHOD 2

Follow the method described under formulation 2 of this chapter.

Di-iodohydroxyquinoline

Follow the method 4 described under formulation 1 of this chapter.

Broxyquinoline, Brobenzoxalidine, Hyoscyamine, Hyoscine

ESTIMATION

Broxyquinoline and Brobenzoxalidine as Broxyquinoline

METHOD 1

Reagents

1. Glacial acetic acid.
2. Acetic anhydride.
3. Methylene chloride.
4. 0.1 N perchloric acid in glacial acetic acid.
5. Crystal violet solution, indicator.

Procedure

Weigh accurately quantity of the sample equivalent to 250 mg of both the ingredients. Transfer to sintered glass funnel (G_4) and percolate ten times 10 ml portions of methylene chloride. Evaporate the organic layer under reduced pressure to dryness below 40°C. Dissolve the residue thus obtained in 100 ml of mixture of glacial acetic acid and acetic anhydride (1 : 1) and titrate with 0.1 N perchloric acid using crystal violet as indicator. Each 1 ml of 0.1 N perchloric acid is equivalent to 0.0303 g of broxyquinoline.

METHOD 2

This method is specific for broxyquinoline.

Reagents

1. 0.5 N sodium carbonate.
2. 0.1% w/v solution of p-aminophenol in 0.2 N hydrochloric acid (freshly prepared).
3. 1,4-Dioxane.

Standard solution

500 mcg/ml of the substance in dioxane.

Sample solution

Weigh accurately quantity of the sample equivalent to about 25 mg of substance. Shake with 30 ml of dioxane, filter, adjust the final volume to 50 ml with dioxane (500 mcg/ml).

Procedure

To 0.5 ml each of the sample and standard solutions, add 4 ml of sodium carbonate solution and 0.5

ml of p-aminophenol reagent. Keep at room temperature for 10 minutes and then dilute to 10 ml with water and shake to mix. The absorbance of solutions is measured after 20 minutes at 570 nm against reagent blank. The method obeys Beer's law in the concentration range of 5-40 mcg/ml. The colour attains maximum intensity after 20 minutes and is stable for 45 minutes. Calculate the contents of broxyquinoline per tablets/capsule by comparison.

From the weight of broxyquinoline thus found, calculate equivalent volume of 0.1 N perchloric acid. Each ml of 0.1 N perchloric acid is equivalent to 0.0303 g of broxyquinoline.

Subtract the volume of 0.1 N perchloric acid thus calculated from the total volume of 0.1 N perchloric acid used in the titration for determination of both broxyquinoline and Brobenzoxalidine (see method 1). This will give the net volume of 0.1 N perchloric acid required for brobenzoxalidine.

Note : While estimating broxyquinoline and brobenzoxalidine in suspension, add 10 g of silica gel (column chromatography grade) to the accurately weighed quantity of the suspension, mix to get homogeneous free flowing powder. Extract the powder with methylene chloride for further determination as per details discussed above under method 1 and 2. To calculate the contents in each 5 ml, specific gravity of the sample is required to be determined.

Hyoscyamine and Hyoscine (total alkaloids)

METHOD 1

Follow the method described in formulation 1 of this chapter.

METHOD 2

Reagents

1. 0.1 M citric acid.
2. 0.2 M disodium hydrogen phosphate, dihydrate.
3. Citric acid-phosphate buffer, pH 7.5 : Dilute 7.5 ml each of 0.1 M citric acid and 0.2 M disodium hydrogen phosphate to 100 ml with water.
4. Bromothymol blue solution : Dissolve 0.15 g bromothymol blue and 0.15 g of anhydrous sodium carbonate in 100 ml of water.
5. Alcoholic solution of boric acid : Dissolve 20 g of boric acid in 800 ml of ethanol and 80 ml of water and then make up to 1000 ml with ethanol.

Standard solution

100 mcg/ml of the substance in water.

Sample solution

Quantity of the sample equivalent to 5 mg of the substance is accurately weighed and dissolved in water to produce 50 ml (100 mcg/ml).

Procedure

Pipette 5 ml each of the sample and standard solutions and 0.5 ml of 0.1 N sodium hydroxide into separate 100 ml separating funnels. To each separating funnel, add 2 ml of bromothymol blue solution and 20 ml of buffer solution. Extract by shaking for about one minute with exactly 30 ml of chloroform. Separate chloroform layer and make up to 50 ml with alcoholic boric acid solution to clear the chloroform phase. Determine the extinctions of the sample and standard solutions at about 420 nm against chloroform as a blank. Compute the results by comparison.

METHOD 3

Reagents

Solution 1 : Phosphate buffer solution of pH 2.5. To 55 ml of 7.8% w/v solution of potassium phosphate dibasic, add 20 ml of 9.6% w/v solution of citric acid and dilute to 100 ml with water.

Solution 2 : Bromocresol purple : To 400 mg of bromocresol purple, add 6.5 ml of 0.1 N sodium hydroxide and make up to 500 ml with water.

Dye solution : Mix equal volumes of solution 1 and solution 2, extract with chloroform and reject chloroform layer. This step reduces the blank value.

Standard solution

50 mcg/ml of L-hyoscyamine in 0.1 N hydrochloric acid.

Sample solution

Weigh accurately a quantity of the sample equivalent to 5 mg of substance and shake with 0.1 N hydrochloric acid to produce 100 ml.

Procedure

To 10 ml each of the sample and standard solutions, add 10 ml of dye solution and exactly 25 ml chloroform. Shake for 2 minutes, and allow the layers to separate out. Filter the chloroform layer through cotton plug. Read extinction of sample and standard solutions at about 440 nm against chloroform as blank and calculate the results by comparison.

Chloramphenicol, Broxyquinoline, Brobenzoxalidine

ESTIMATION

Chloramphenicol

Standard solution

150 mg of chloramphenicol is shaken with water to dissolve and adjusted to 100 ml. 5 ml is further diluted to 50 ml with methanol.

Sample solution

Weigh accurately a quantity of powdered tablets or capsule material equivalent to about 150 mg chloramphenicol. Add 50 ml of distilled water, shake for 15-20 minutes and make up the volume to 100 ml with water. Filter and dilute 5 ml of the filtrate to 50 ml with methyl alcohol.

Procedure

Measure the extinction of both the solutions at maxima at about 275 nm using 90% methyl alcohol as blank and deduce the results by comparison.

Broxyquinoline and Brobenzoxalidine

Follow the method 1 and 2 as described under formulation 4 of this chapter.

Streptomycin sulphate, Chloramphenicol, Diloxanide furoate

ESTIMATION

Diloxanide furoate

METHOD 1

Standard solution

10 mcg/ml of diloxanide furoate in chloroform.

Sample solution

Transfer an accurately weighed quantity of the mixed contents of capsules equivalent to 0.2 g of diloxanide furoate to a separating funnel containing 25 ml of water. Shake well and acidify with 1 N sulphuric acid. Shake well and extract with three quantities each of 40 ml of chloroform. Wash each chloroform extract in succession with same 15 ml of 0.1 N sulphuric acid and 15 ml of water, contained in two different separators. Collect the washed chloroform extracts into a dry, 200 ml volumetric flask after passing through anhydrous sodium sulphate held over a plug of cotton wool. Dilute the combined extracts to volume with chloroform and mix. Dilute further appropriately with chloroform to get a concentration of 10 mcg/ml.

Procedure

Concomitantly determine the extinctions of the standard and sample solutions at the absorption maximum at about 260 nm using chloroform as blank. Calculate average net content per capsule using a value of 690 for A 1%, 1 cm at 260 nm.

METHOD 2

Diloxanide furoate on acid hydrolysis gives blue colour with sodium nitroprusside in alkaline medium.

Reagents

1. 4 N hydrochloric acid.
2. Ethyl alcohol.
3. 0.2% w/v solution of sodium nitroprusside in water.
4. 1 N sodium hydroxide.

Standard solution

100 mg of pure diloxanide furoate is dissolved in ethyl alcohol to get 1 mg/ml solution. To 10 ml of this solution, add 10 ml of 4 N hydrochloric acid, boil on water-bath for 60 minutes, cool and dilute to 100 ml with water. 10 ml of the resultant solution is further diluted with water to 100 ml.

Sample solution

Accurately weigh sample equivalent to 100 mg of diloxanide furoate, add 50 ml of ethyl alcohol, warm

Streptomycin sulphate

and sample at about 490 nm using blank similarly prepared but replacing sample solution/standard solution by water. Calculate the results by comparison.

METHOD 2

Reagents

1. 0.25% ferric chloride solution : Dissolve 5 g of ferric chloride in 50 ml of 0.1 N hydrochloric acid. Dilute 2.5 ml of the solution to 100 ml with 0.01 N hydrochloric acid.
2. 1 N sodium hydroxide.
3. 1 N hydrochloric acid.

Standard solution

1 mg/ml of streptomycin (base) as streptomycin sulphate in water.

Sample solution

Weigh accurately, a quantity of the sample equivalent to about 100 mg of streptomycin (base) and prepare the sample solution (1 mg/ml base) as described under method 1 above.

Procedure

To 10 ml each of sample and standard solutions, add 2 ml of sodium hydroxide solution. Heat in boiling water-bath for 10 minutes and cool in ice water for 3 minutes. Acidify with 2.5 ml of 1 N hydrochloric acid. Add 5 ml of iron reagent and dilute to 25 ml with water. Measure the absorbance of sample and standard solutions at about 530 nm against reagent blank and calculate the results by comparison.

Chloramphenicol

Reagents

1. 5% w/v solution of sodium nitrite in water.
2. 5% w/v solution of sulphamic acid in water.
3. 0.5% w/v solution of N-1-naphthyl-ethylenediamine dihydrochloride in water.

Standard solution

Accurately weigh 250 mg of pure chloramphenicol and transfer quantitatively into a 100 ml volumetric flask with the aid of alcohol. Dissolve and make up the volume with alcohol.

Sample solution

Transfer an accurately weighed quantity of the mixed contents of 20 capsules equivalent to 25 mg of chloramphenicol to a 100 ml round bottom flask, add 10 ml of alcohol. To another round bottom flask, transfer 10 ml of standard solution. To each flask, add 30 ml of 1 N hydrochloric acid and 1.5 g of small pieces of metallic aluminium wire. Reflux on a water-bath the contents of each flask for one hour. Cool and with the help of water, transfer quantitatively the contents of each flask into separate 100 ml volumetric flasks, make up the volume with water and filter.

Procedure

To 1 ml each of reduced standard and sample solutions and water (to serve as blank) add 1 ml of solution of sodium nitrite and 5 to 10 drops of hydrochloric acid. Shake and leave for 2 minutes. Add 5 ml of solution of sulphamic acid, shake well and remove any nitrous acid fumes present in the flask under mild suction. Add 1 ml of n-naphthyl ethylenediamine solution. Dilute the solutions to 50 ml with water and read the extinction of both the solutions at about 558 nm using blank in the reference cuvette. Calculate the results by comparison.

Diloxanide furoate, Chloroquine phosphate, Streptomycin sulphate

ESTIMATION

Diloxanide furoate

Follow any one of the methods described for estimation of diloxanide furoate under formulation **6** of this chapter.

Streptomycin sulphate

Follow the method 1 for estimation of streptomycin as described under formulation 6 of this chapter.

Chloroquine phosphate

Standard solution

25 mcg/ml of chloroquine phosphate in water.

Sample solution

Weigh accurately a quantity of powdered tablets equivalent to about 100 mg of chloroquine phosphate, add 150 ml of water and shake for 30 minutes. Adjust the volume to 200 ml and filter. Reject the first 25 ml and dilute 5 ml of the filtrate to 100 ml with water.

Concomitantly measure the extinction of standard and sample solutions at the absorption maxima at about 343 nm or use 360 as value of A 1%, 1 cm at 343 nm for calculation of the results.

Diloxanide furoate

Metronidazole

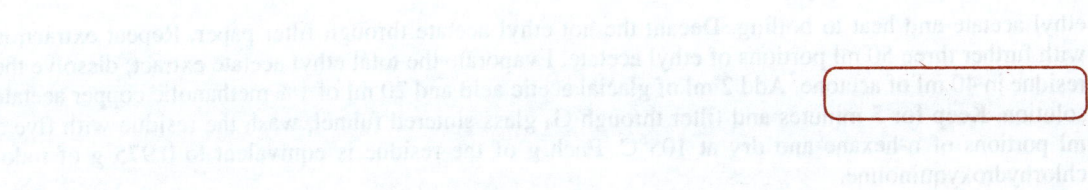

Metronidazole

Iodo-chlorhydroxyquinoline

ethyl acetate and heat to boiling. Decant the hot ethyl acetate through filter paper. Repeat extraction with further three 50 ml portions of ethyl acetate. Evaporate the total ethyl acetate extract, dissolve the residue in 40 ml of acetone. Add 2 ml of glacial acetic acid and 20 ml of 1% methanolic copper acetate solution. Keep for 5 minutes and filter through G$_4$ glass sintered funnel, wash the residue with five 5 ml portions of n-hexane and dry at 105°C. Each g of the residue is equivalent to 0.975 g of iodo-chlorhydroxyquinoline.

Di-iodohydroxyquinoline, Metronidazole

ESTIMATION

Di-iodohydroxyquinoline

Standard solution

5 mcg/ml of di-iodohydroxyquinoline (DIHQ) in absolute alcohol.

Sample solution

Weigh sample accurately equivalent to 50 mg of substance, add sufficient absolute alcohol to produce 200 ml. Dilute appropriately with absolute alcohol to get 5 mcg/ml.

Measure the extinction of both sample and standard solutions at 253 nm using alcohol as blank and calculate the results by comparison.

Metronidazole

METHOD 1

Weigh accurately a quantity of the sample equivalent to 50 mg of the substance, add 80-90 ml of 0.1 N hydrochloric acid, shake for 15 min and add sufficient 0.1 N hydrochloric acid to produce 200 ml. Filter and dilute 5 ml to 100 ml with 0.1 N hydrochloric acid. Measure the extinction of the resultant solution at maxima at about 277 nm and calculate the results taking 380 as value of A 1%, 1 cm at the maxima.

Note : The residue obtained during estimation of metronidazole is dissolved in alcohol and used for estimation of 'DIHQ' as described.

Alternatively, methods described in formulation 1 and 9 of this chapter may be used. Extraction with ethyl acetate will separate both the compounds.

METHOD 2

Reagents

1. 0.2% w/v solution of benzocaine in methanol.
2. 0.1% w/v solution of sodium nitrite in water.
3. Acid mixture : To 85 ml of trichloroacetic acid (15%) add 20 ml of 2 M sulphuric acid and dilute to 200 ml with water.

Standard solution

1 mg/ml in 1,4-dioxan.

Sample solution

Extract the powdered sample with dioxan by slight warming, cool, dilute to get solution of 1 mg/ml.

Metronidazole

Furazolidone

Metronidazole benzoyloxylate

sample equivalent to 200 mg of the substance. Transfer into 25 ml separating funnel and extract with four 20 ml portions of chloroform-acetone mixture. Collect the clear chloroform-acetone layer and pass through anhydrous sodium sulphate. Add 2-3 glass beads and evaporate carefully on warm water-bath to about 10 to 15 ml. To it, add 25 ml glacial acetic acid and again evaporate further for 10 minutes on warm water-bath to remove chloroform/acetone. Cool it to room temperature, add 1 ml indicator and titrate it against 0.1 N perchloric acid.

Each ml of 0.1 N perchloric acid is equivalent to 0.01712 g of metronidazole or 0.02753 g of metronidazole benzoate. Calculate the contents in each 5 ml, taking into consideration weigh per ml of the sample preparation.

Note : 1. Since metronidazole is only slightly soluble in chloroform, alcohol and ether, several successive extractions are required for complete extraction of the compound into organic layer.

2. As metronidazole is more soluble in water than organic solvent, further addition of water is to be avoided.

3. Extraction procedure is necessary to eliminate water for non-aqueous titration.

4. 1 g of metronidazole is equivalent to 1.61 g of benzoylmetronidazole.

METHOD 2

Metronidazole

Reagent

1 N hydrochloric acid.

Procedure

Shake the preparation mechanically for 10 minutes for uniform making and pipette out quantity of the sample equivalent to 100 mg of the substance into 100 ml volumetric flask containing 70 ml 1 N hydrochloric acid. Rinse the pipette with the acid. Shake it mechanically for 15 minutes and make the volume to 100 ml with 1 N acid. Shake well and filter through No. 1 filter paper, discard first 10-15 ml of the filtrate. Reserve insoluble material for estimation of furazolidone. Dilute 10 ml of the clear filtrate to 100 ml with 1 N acid. Further dilution is done with water to get a concentration of 10 mcg/ml of metronidazole. Measure the extinction of the solution at 277 nm against 0.1 N acid as blank. A value of 390 as A 1%, 1 cm at 277 nm can be used for calculations of the contents.

Furazolidone

Dissolve the insoluble material as obtained above in 1% v/v DMF (aqueous) to produce 10 mcg/ml. Measure the extinction at about 367 nm against 1% DMF and calculate the results by comparison with the standard. Alternatively follow the colour development procedure as described under method 1 above.

METHOD 3

This method has been found to give excellent results in solid dosage forms (capsules and tablets).

Furazolidone

Standard solution

0.5 mg/ml of furazolidone in dimethylformamide (DMF). Dilute 2 ml of the solution to 100 ml with water (100 mcg/ml).

Sample solution

Weigh accurately a quantity of powdered material equivalent to 50 mg of furazolidone. Add 50 ml of water and warm on a water-bath. Shake vigorously and filter through G_4 glass sintered funnel. Repeat the above process thrice. Combine the filtrate and adjust to 250 ml with water and reserve for estimation of metronidazole. Dissolve the residue obtained above in 'DMF' to get a concentration of 1 mg/ml. 2 ml of the resultant solution is further diluted to 100 ml with water (10 mcg/ml).

Measure the extinction of both the solutions at maxima at about 367 nm using 2% v/v DMF solution in water as blank and calculate the results by comparison. Alternatively, colorimetric method involving reaction with alcoholic potassium hydroxide may be used.

Metronidazole

Standard solution

10 mcg/ml of metronidazole in water.

Sample solution

Dilute the filtrate obtained in the estimation of furazolidone appropriately to get a concentration of 10 mcg/ml with water.

Measure the absorbance of both the solutions at maxima at about 320 nm against water as blank. Calculate the contents by comparing with the standard.

Alternatively, the filtrate obtained in the estimation of furazolidone under method 3 above is suitably diluted with water to get 500 mcg/ml.

To 2 ml each of sample and standard solutions, add 3 ml of sodium hydroxide solution (20% w/v). Keep at room temperature for 8 min and dilute to 10 ml with water. Measure the absorption of both the solutions at about 500 nm within 12 min against reagent blank. Calculate the results by comparison.

Note : The colour starts fading after 13 min.

Iodochlorhydroxyquinoline (Chinoform)

Berberine hydrochloride

Tinidazole

ESTIMATION

METHOD 1

Accurately weigh a quantity of the sample equivalent to 450 mg of tinidazole and transfer to 500 ml volumetric flask. Make up the volume with methanol and stir for 30 minutes. Filter the resulting solution through a Whatman No. 1 filter paper, rejecting the first 20 ml and dilute 5 ml of the filtrate to 500 ml with methanol. Measure the absorbance of this final solution on a suitable spectrophotometer at 310 nm against methanol and calculate the result by using 355 as value of E 1%, 1 cm at 310 nm. The method obeys Beer's law in the range of 5-25 mcg/ml.

Note : 1. Tinidazole is light sensitive. Therefore, all solutions must be protected from light either by using amber glassware or by covering the glassware with opaque material like carbon paper.

2. Several other solvents can be used for extraction and spectrophotometric determination. The absorption maxima and values of E 1%, 1 cm in different solvents are given as under :

Solvent	λ_{max} (nm)	E 1%, 1 cm	range of Beer's law
Chloroform	315	400	
Ethyl alcohol	310	355	
Methyl alcohol	310	355	5-25 mcg/ml
Benzene	322	380	
0.1 N hydrochloric acid	277	244	0.5-4 mcg/ml

METHOD 2

Standard solution

100 mcg/ml of tinidazole in methyl alcohol.

Sample solution

Weigh accurately powdered sample equivalent to 10 mg of tinidazole. Add 70-80 ml methyl alcohol, shake, filter, wash the residue with methyl alcohol and adjust the filtrate to 100 ml with methanol (100 mcg/ml).

Procedure

2 ml each of sample and standard solutions are evaporated to dryness on boiling water-bath. Cool and add 2.5 ml of 20% w/v aqueous sodium hydroxide solution and dilute to 10 ml with water. Measure the absorbance of standard and sample solutions at maximum at about 268 nm and calculate the result. The method obeys Beer's law in the range of 5-25 mcg/ml.

METHOD 3

Reagents

1. 0.1 N hydrochloric acid.

2. Hydrochloric acid.
3. Zinc dust.
4. 1.0% w/v solution of vanillin in 0.1 N hydrochloric acid.

Standard solution

1 mg/ml of tinidazole in 0.1 N hydrochloric acid.

Sample solution

Weigh accurately sample equivalent to 100 mg of tinidazole, add 50 ml of 0.1 N hydrochloric acid, shake and filter through G₄ glass sintered funnel. Wash the residue with 0.1 N acid and adjust to 100 ml with the acid.

Procedure

To 25 ml each of the standard and sample solutions, add 2.5 ml of 0.1 N hydrochloric acid, 5 g zinc dust and 4 ml of hydrochloric acid. Keep aside for 30 minutes to ensure complete reaction (reduction). Dilute both sample and standard reduced solutions to get 100 mcg/ml. To 2.5 ml each of standard and sample reduced solutions, add 1 ml of vanillin reagent and heat on water-bath for 20 minutes, cool and dilute to 10 ml with water. Measure the extinction of solutions at about 410 nm against reagent blank and calculate the results. The method obeys Beer's law in the range of 10-50 mcg/ml. The coloured complex is stable for 6 hours.

METHOD 4
Reagents

1. 0.1% w/v solution of potassium ferricyanide in water.
2. 0.1% w/v solution of sodium nitroprusside in water.
3. 0.1% w/v solution of sodium hydroxide in water.
4. Methyl alcohol.

Standard solution

Weigh accurately 100 mg of pure tinidazole, add 50 ml of methyl alcohol, shake to dissolve and dilute to 100 ml with methanol. Suitable quantity of above methanolic solution (1 mg/ml) is diluted with water to produce solution of 40 mcg/ml.

Sample solution

Weigh accurately a quantity of the sample equivalent to 100 mg of tinidazole and extract with methanol as described under method 1 above. 5 ml of the resultant solution (1 mg/ml) is diluted with water to produce 25 ml.

Procedure

To 5 ml each of the standard and sample solutions, add 3 ml each of sodium hydroxide, sodium nitroprusside and potassium ferricyanide solution. Keep aside for 30 minutes for colour to develop. Adjust the volume to 25 ml with distilled water. Measure the absorption of standard and sample solutions at about 460 nm against reagent blank and calculate the contents of tinidazole in the formulation. The method obeys Beer's law in the range of 8-80 mcg/ml.

Diloxanide furoate, Tinidazole, Methylpolysiloxane

ESTIMATION

Diloxanide furoate

Weigh accurately a quantity of powdered tablets equivalent to 200 mg of diloxanide furoate. Add 25 ml of 0.1 N hydrochloric acid, shake well and extract with four 25 ml portions of chloroform, washing each chloroform layer with the same 10 ml of 0.1 N hydrochloric acid. Preserve acidic layer for determination of tinidazole. Evaporate chloroform layer, dry at 105°C and weigh which represents the amount of diloxanide furoate present in the sample taken for analysis.

Alternatively, the combined chloroform extract may be diluted quantitatively with chloroform and subjected to spectrophotometric analysis. For details, refer to method 1 for estimation of diloxanide furoate under formulation 6 or 8 of this chapter.

Tinidazole

METHOD 1

Dilute acidic layer obtained above appropriately with 0.1 N hydrochloric acid to get a concentration of 500 mcg/ml in respect of tinidazole. Dilute 5 ml of resultant solution with 0.1 N hydrochloric acid to 200 ml and measure the extinction at absorption maximum at 277 nm. Calculate the results using 244 as value of A 1%, 1 cm at 277 nm. Alternatively, other methods described in formulation 13 of this chapter may be employed.

METHOD 2

Standard solution

10 mcg/ml of tinidazole in methanol.

Sample solution

An accurately weighed quantity of the powdered sample equivalent to 25 mg of tinidazole was shaken with about 60 ml of methanol, filtered through G_4 sintered funnel. The residue was washed with methanol, filtrate adjusted to 100 ml. 2 ml of the filtrate was further diluted to 50 ml with methanol.

The absorbance of both sample and standard solutions was measured at about 311 nm and results calculated by comparison. Diloxanide furoate showing zero absorbance at 311 nm, the absorption maximum for tinidazole. The method obeys Beer's law in the concentration range of 5-15 mcg/ml.

METHOD 3

Transfer accurately weighed powdered sample equivalent to 300 mg of tinidazole, add 50 ml of glacial acetic acid, shake well and add 2-3 ml of acetic anhydride and titrate against 0.1 N perchloric acid (crystal violet). Each ml of 0.1 N perchloric acid is equivalent to 0.02473 g of tinidazole.

Estimation of Tinidazole and Diloxanide furoate

Standard solution

Prepare mixed standard by dissolving 40 mg of tinidazole and 50 mg of diloxanide furoate in 50 ml of

DMF, keep aside for 15 min and dilute to 100 ml with water. 1 ml of resultant solution is diluted to 50 ml with water.

Sample solution

To accurately weighed quantity of the sample equivalent to 40 mg of tinidazole, add 50 ml of DMF, stir to dissolve and dilute to 100 ml with water. Filter and dilute 1 ml to 50 ml with water.

Measure the absorption of both the sample and standard solutions at 262 nm (diloxanide furoate) and 318 nm (tinidazole) and calculate the results by comparison.

Activated methylpolysiloxane (MPS)

METHOD 1

Suspend a quantity of powdered tablets equivalent to 50 mg of activated methylpolysiloxane in 25 ml of dilute hydrochloric acid. Extract with four 40 ml of petroleum ether (40 to 60°C), wash the organic layer with two 10 ml portions of water, filter the organic layer through anhydrous sodium sulphate, collect the filtrate in a pre-dried, weighed beaker and dry it on a water-bath and then in air oven at 105°C for one hour.

The difference in weight is the amount of activated methylpolysiloxane present in the weighed quantity of the sample taken for analysis.

METHOD 2

Silicates give yellow colour with ammonium molybdate in acidic medium.

Reagent

1. Ammonium molybdate solution : Dissolve 8.0 g of ammonium molybdate monohydrate in 9 ml of concentrated sulphuric acid, dilute to 100 ml with water.

Standard solution

Weigh accurately 50 mg of MPS, add 20 ml of carbon tetrachloride and 15 ml of dilute hydrochloric acid. Heat to boiling, cool and separate organic layer. Pass the organic layer through anhydrous sodium sulphate placed over a plug of cotton.

Sample solution

Weigh accurately the sample equivalent to 50 mg of MPS and proceed as under standard solution.

Procedure

Evaporate 5 ml each of sample and standard solutions in platinum dish. Add 1 g of sodium carbonate, anhydrous, ignite, cool and dissolve the residue in 20 ml of water.

Wash the crucible with 10 ml of water, mix with main aqueous extract. Adjust the pH to 5.0 (± 0.5) with dilute sulphuric acid and dilute to 50 ml with water (use for estimation).

To 5 ml each of the above solutions, add 2 ml of ammonium molybdate solution. Set aside for 10 min. Measure the absorption of both the solutions at about 400 nm using water instead of sample solution for blank. Calculate the results by comparison.

Loperamide hydrochloride, Furazolidone

ESTIMATION

Loperamide hydrochloride

Reagents

1. Tropeolin reagents : Weigh accurately 50 mg of tropeolin-00 (acid orange) in a 50 ml volumetric flask, dissolve and make up the volume with water.
2. Acidified methanol : Dilute 1 ml of concentrated sulphuric acid to 100 ml with methanol.
3. Buffer, pH 3.0 : Dissolve 11 g of dibasic sodium phosphate and 18.3 g of citric acid mono-hydrate in 800 ml of distilled water. Adjust the pH to 3.0 with citric acid or dibasic sodium phosphate and make up the volume to 1000 ml with water.

Standard solution

20 mcg per ml of loperamide hydrochloride in chloroform.

Sample solution

Extract the powdered sample equivalent to 2 mg of loperamide hydrochloride with 100 ml of chloroform.

Procedure

Pipette out 20 ml each of standard and sample solutions in separate stoppered centrifuge tube. Add 10 ml of buffer pH 3.0 and 3 ml of tropeolin reagent to each tube. Shake the tubes for five minutes and centrifuge. Pipette out 10 ml of chloroform, add 3 ml of acidified methanol. Measure the extinctions of both standard and sample solutions at about 540 nm using chloroform as the blank and deduce the results by comparison.

Furazolidone

Sample solution

Dissolve the powdered sample equivalent to 20 mg of furazolidone in 25 ml of dimethylformamide in a 100 ml volumetric flask. Shake well and make up the volume with water. Dilute 25 ml with distilled water.

Procedure

Measure the extinction of sample solution at the maximum at about 367 nm against blank prepared by diluting 1.5 ml of dimethyl formamide to 25 ml with water. Calculate the contents of furazolidone using 750 as value of the A 1%, 1 cm at 367 nm.

Loperamide hydrochloride, Streptomycin sulphate

ESTIMATION

Loperamide hydrochloride

Follow the colour reaction with tropeolin-00 (acid orange) as described in formulation 15 of this chapter.

Streptomycin sulphate

Follow the method 1 (reaction with oxidised sodium nitroprusside) for estimation of streptomycin sulphate described in formulation 6 of this chapter.

Furazolidone, Diphenoxylate hydrochloride, Atropine sulphate

ESTIMATION

Furazolidone

Follow the method described under formulation 11 of this chapter.

Diphenoxylate hydrochloride

Transfer accurately weighed quantity of the sample equivalent to 100 mg of the substance to a separating funnel. Add 25 ml of water and 2 ml of 10 N sodium hydroxide solution. Extract with five 25 ml portions of chloroform. Wash the combined chloroform layer with water and pass through anhydrous sodium sulphate placed over cotton plug (pre-moistened). Evaporate chloroform layer to dryness and take up the residue in 50 ml of glacial acetic acid. Titrate with 0.05 N perchloric acid using crystal violet solution as indicator. Each ml of 0.05 N perchloric acid is equivalent to 0.02445 g of diphenoxylate hydrochloride.

Atropine sulphate

Reagents

1. 88% sulphuric acid (44 ml of concentrated sulphuric acid and 6 ml of water).
2. Acetic anhydride.
3. 16.0% w/v solution of p-dimethylaminobenzaldehyde (PDAB) in 88% sulphuric acid.

Standard solution

50 mcg/ml of atropine sulphate in methanol.

Sample solution

Accurately weigh the sample equivalent to 1 mg of atropine sulphate. Add about 100 ml of water, boil on water-bath for 15 min, cool and make up to 200 ml with water. Acidify 100 ml of the resultant solution with 0.1 N sulphuric acid and extract with four 25 ml portions of chloroform. Discard the chloroform layer. Basify the acidic layer with 5 N ammonium hydroxide and extract with five 25 ml portions of chloroform, washing each separated layer with the same 20 ml water. Shake the combined chloroform layer with 25 ml of 0.1 N sulphuric acid, discard the organic layer. Repeat the process of basification and extraction into chloroform as descibed above. The final chloroform extract is passed through anhydrous sodium sulphate and evaporated to dryness. The residue is taken in methanol to get a concentration of 50 mcg/ml.

Procedure

Evaporate 2 ml each of sample and standard solutions on water-bath. Add 0.5 ml of 'PDAB' solution and allow to stand for 2 minutes. Heat on water-bath exactly for 5 minutes, cool, add 5 ml of acetic anhydride, mix and allow to stand for 30 minutes. Measure the absorption of both the solutions at about 515 nm against reagent blank. Calculate the results by comparison.

Furazolidone, Iodochlorhydroxyquinoline, Homatropine methyl bromide

ESTIMATION

Furazolidone

Standard solution

Transfer accurately weighed 25 mg of furazolidone to a 50 ml volumetric flask, add 25 ml of dimethylformamide, heat to dissolve and make up the volume with dimethyl formamide. Dilute 2 ml of the resultant solution to 200 ml with water (5 mcg/ml).

Sample solution

Transfer accurately weighed quantity of the sample equivalent to 25 mg of furazolidone to a 50 ml volumetric flask, add 25 ml of dimethylformamide, heat to dissolve and make up the volume. Filter and dilute 2 ml of the filtrate to 200 ml with water (5 mcg/ml).

Measure the absorption of both the solutions at 367 nm using dimethylformamide as blank. Deduce the results by comparison or by using 750 as value of A 1%, 1 cm at 367 nm.

Iodochlorhydroxyquinoline

Reagents

1. 1% w/v solution of ferric chloride in water.
2. Acetone.

Standard solution

Dissolve accurately weighed quantity of iodochlorhydroxyquinoline in acetone with slight warming to get a concentration of 500 mcg/ml.

Sample solution

Extract accurately weighed quantity of sample with acetone by slight warming to produce 500 mcg/ml of iodochlorhydroxyquinoline.

Procedure

To 2 ml each of sample and standard solutions, add 1 ml of ferric chloride solution and make up the volume to 25 ml with acetone. Measure the absorption of both the solutions at about 650 nm against reagent blank. Calculate the results by comparison.

Homatropine methyl bromine

Reagents

1. 0.2 M cerric ammonium sulphate.

2. 1 N sodium hydroxide.

3. Anion-exchange resin-1R-400 (Cl⁻).

4. Glass column 50 cm × 1.5 cm (ID) fitted with G_2 sintered disc.

Column preparation

Place a small quantity of fine glass wool on the base of the column. Suspend the resin in water and pour over the column to an height of 25 cm. Cover the tip of the column with a glass wool plug. Wash the column with 150-200 ml of water. The column is ready for use.

Sample solution

Transfer accurately weighed quantity of the sample equivalent to 5 mg of the substance to a 100 ml volumetric flask, add 40-50 ml of water. Shake well and make up the volume with water. Filter and add the entire filtrate to the prepared column. Wash the column first with 30 ml of water and discard the eluate. Collect subsequent eluates and make up to 100 ml with water.

Standard solution

Equivalent to 5 mg of the substance is treated as sample solution.

Procedure

Transfer 10 ml each of sample and standard solutions to a stoppered flask. To each add 20 ml of sodium hydroxide solution and heat in a water-bath at 80°C for 15 min. Cool, add 8 ml of 0.2 M cerric ammonium sulphate and mix, add 25 ml of n-hexane and shake for 15 min. Decant the organic layer and concomitantly determine the absorbance of both the solutions at about 242 nm using n-hexane as blank. Calculate the results by comparison.

Note : Separation through column is not often required. Directly basify the sample, standard solutions and follow the procedure as described above.

Norfloxacin/Ciprofloxacin, Tinidazole

ESTIMATION

Norfloxacin/Ciprofloxacin

METHOD 1

Reagents

1. 0.1 N hydrochloric acid.
2. 1% w/v solution of ferric chloride in water (freshly prepared).

Standard solution

100 mcg/ml of norfloxacin in 0.1 N hydrochloric acid.

Sample solution

Weigh accurately powdered sample equivalent to 100 mg of the substance, add 60-70 ml of 0.1 N hydrochloric acid, shake for 10 min and make up to 100 ml with the acid. Further dilution is done with the acid to get final concentration of 100 mcg/ml.

Procedure

To 5 ml each of sample and standard solutions, add 1 ml of freshly prepared ferric chloride solution and make up to 50 ml with 0.1 N hydrochloric acid. Measure the absorption of both the solutions at a maximum at about 438 nm against reagent blank (1 ml of ferric chloride solution diluted to 50 ml with the acid) and calculate the contents of norfloxacin by comparison.

METHOD 2

Reagents

1. 0.005 M solution of p-chloranil (Cl) in acetonitrile.
2. 0.005 M solution of chloranilic acid (CLA) in acetonitrile.

Standard solution

500 mcg/ml of norfloxacin in acetonitrite.

Sample solution

An accurately weighed quantity of the sample equivalent to 50 mg of the substance was extracted with acetonitrite to produce 100 ml (500 mcg/ml).

Procedure

To 2 ml each of the sample and standard solutions, add 2.5 ml of either of the reagents and heat on water-bath at 60°C for 10 min, cool and make up to 25 ml with acetonitrile. Measure the absorption of the sample and standard solutions against reagent blank at 550 nm (Cl) and 531 nm (CLA). The method obeys Beer's law in the concentration range of 10-230 mcg/ml (Cl) and 20-250 mcg/ml (CLA) and the colour is stable for about 2 hrs. The reaction is based on exchange of π electrons, norfloxacin being the donor and p-chloranil/chloranilic acid being the π electron acceptors.

Tinidazole

Reagents

1. Dimethyl formamide (DMF).
2. 1% v/v tetramethyl ammonium hydroxide (TMAH) in methanol.

Standard solution

100 mg of the substance accurately weighed and dissolved in 20 ml of DMF and diluted to 100 ml with water. Further dilutions are done with water to get final concentration of 100 mcg/ml.

Sample solution

To accurately weighed quantity of powdered sample, add 20 ml of DMF and 20 ml of water. Shake for 15 min to effect solution and dilute to 100 ml with water. Filter and further dilute appropriately with water to get final concentration of 100 mcg/ml.

Procedure

To 5 ml each of sample and standard solutions, add 5 ml of TMAH solution. Allow it to stand for 60 min at room temperature and dilute to 50 ml with water.

Measure extinction of both sample and standard solutions at about 370 nm against reagent blank and calculate the contents of tinidazole by comparison.

Typical laboratory analysis

Each tablet contains 400 mg of norfloxacin and 600 mg of tinidazole.

Average weight of tablet = 1201 mg

Norfloxacin

Weight of standard (S) = 99.6 mg

Weight of sample (U) = 300.8 mg

$$\text{Norfloxacin (mg)/tablet} = \frac{A_u}{A_s} \times \frac{S}{U} \times \text{dilution factor} \times 1201$$

$$= \frac{0.587}{0.584} \times \frac{99.6}{300.8} \times \text{dilution factor} \times 1201$$

$$= 389.38 \text{ mg}$$

$$\% \text{ claim} = 97.35$$

Tinidazole

Weight of standard (S) = 101.4 mg

Weight of sample (U) = 200.7 mg

$$\text{Tinidazole (mg)/tablet} = \frac{A_u}{A_s} \times \frac{S}{U} \times \text{dilution factor} \times 1201$$

$$= \frac{0.884}{0.892} \times \frac{101.4}{200.7} \times \text{dilution factor} \times 1201$$

$$= 601.34 \text{ mg}$$

$$\% \text{ claim} = 100.20$$

Formulation 20

Furazolidone, Berberine hydrochloride

ESTIMATION

Furazolidone

Standard solution

40 mcg/ml of furazolidone in DMF.

Sample solution

Weigh accurately finely powdered sample equivalent to 100 mg of furazolidone, add 60-70 ml of dimethyl formamide (DMF) and warm on water-bath for 15-20 min, cool and dilute to 100 ml with DMF. Filter through G₄ sintered funnel rejecting 15-20 ml of the filtrate. Dilute 2 ml of the filtrate to 50 ml with DMF—40 mcg/ml. All the apparatus should be absolutely dry.

Procedure

To 2 ml each of sample and standard solutions, add 2 ml of 0.1 N tetrabutyl ammonium hydroxide and dilute to 25 ml with DMF. Measure the absorption of both sample and standard solutions at 570 nm against reagent blank and calculate the results by comparison.

Berberine hydrochloride

Follow the method described in formulation 12 of this chapter.

Tinidazole, Diloxanide furoate, Dicyclomine hydrochloride

ESTIMATION

Tinidazole and Diloxanide furoate

Follow the method described in formulation 14 of this chapter.

Dicyclomine hydrochloride

Reagents

1. Sulphuric acid : Add 3 ml of concentrated sulphuric acid to 100 ml of water.
2. Methyl orange solution : Dissolve 300 mg of methyl orange in 800 ml of water, add 30 ml of sulphuric acid. Stir and filter to get clear solution.
3. Sodium acetate solution : Dissolve 2 g of sodium acetate in 400 ml of methanol, filter to get clear filtrate.
4. Hydrochloric acid : 1 ml of concentrated hydrochloric acid is diluted to 100 ml with water.

Standard solution

(a) 250 mcg/ml in hydrochloric acid.
(b) 10 ml of (a) diluted to 100 ml with methanol—25 mcg/ml.

Sample solution

Accurately weighed quantity of the sample equivalent to 2.5 mg of the substance is suspended in 10 ml of hydrochloric acid and heated at 80°C with stirring for dissolving the substance. Dilute to 100 ml with methanol and filter.

Procedure

To 10 ml of sample and standard solutions, add 50 ml of methyl orange solution. Mix and extract with 3 × 15 ml portions of chloroform. Combine the organic layers and dilute to 100 ml with sodium acetate solution. Measure the absorption of both the solutions at 420 nm against blank. Repeat the experiment without the substance and calculate the results by comparison.

Dried aluminium hydroxide gel, Magnesium hydroxide, Deglycyrrhizinated liquorice, Dimethyl polysiloxane

ESTIMATION

Aluminium hydroxide

Reagents

1. Concentrated hydrochloric acid.
2. 0.05 M EDTA solution.
3. 0.05 M zinc sulphate solution.
4. Acetic acid-ammonium acetate buffer. Dissolve 7.71 g of ammonium acetate in water, add 5.7 ml of glacial acetic acid and dilute to 100 ml with water.
5. Dithizone solution : Dissolve 25.6 mg of dithizone in 100 ml of methanol. Stable for 2 months if stored in cold place.

Sample preparation

Weigh powdered sample equivalent to 500 mg of aluminium hydroxide, add 20 ml of concentrated hydrochloric acid and boil for 5 min, cool and make up to 250 ml with water. Filter and use this solution for assay. To 25 ml of the sample solution, add 25 ml of 0.05 M EDTA solution, 25 ml of buffer solution with constant stirring. Add 20 ml of methanol and 1 ml of dithizone solution and titrate with 0.05 M zinc sulphate solution to a bright rose pink colour. Perform blank. Each ml of 0.05 M EDTA is equivalent to 2.549 mg of aluminium oxide (Al_2O_3).

Magnesium hydroxide

Reagents

1. Triethanolamine.
2. Ammonia-ammonium chloride buffer.
3. 0.05 M EDTA.

Procedure

To 25 ml of sample solution as prepared under estimation of aluminium hydroxide, add 25 ml of triethanolamine and 10 ml of ammonia-ammonium chloride buffer solution and titrate with 0.05 M EDTA using eriochrome black T as indicator. Each ml of 0.05 M EDTA is equivalent to 2.916 mg magnesium hydroxide $Mg(OH)_2$.

Glycyrrhizic acid

Follow the method described in formulation 1 of the chapter on urinary anti-infectives. Deglycyrrhizinated liquorice usually contains not more than 3% of the acid.

Estimation of Dimethicone in creams such as Triamcinolone acetonide

Mix the cream with 5 g of anhydrous sodium sulphate in a beaker till uniform mixture is obtained. Extract with warm toluene (6 × 15 ml), filtering each extract through G_3 sintered funnel, make up to 50 ml with toluene. Record the IR in 4% liquid paraffin in toluene and compare with standard.

Note : Anhydrous sodium sulphate abstracts water from cream as decahydrate, leaving readily filtered organic layer.

Dimethylpolysiloxane (DMP)

METHOD 1

This method is based on defoaming activity of the compound. The foam is generated by dissolving 200 mg of sodium lauryl sulphate or ordinary detergent in 100 ml of purified water at 37°C in a 250 ml graduated cylinder. Adjust pH of the foam solution to 1.2 with 0.1 N hydrochloric acid.

Sample solution

Transfer powdered tablets corresponding to 200 mg of the compound in 150 ml dried conical flask. Extract 4 times with 30 ml portions of boiling benzene. Concentrate total benzene extract to exactly 10 ml in a 10 ml volumetric flask.

Procedure

Transfer 1 ml of the sample solution to 250 ml graduated cylinder containing 100 ml of foam solution. The cylinder is then stoppered and shaken till slightly more than 150 ml of foam is generated. When foam level comes to 150 ml, the reading in the cylinder will be 250 ml. Counting of time is started and at every 15 second interval, the volume of remaining foam is noted. Not less than 80% of the foam should disappear within 5 minutes. Alternatively, the time required for complete disappearance of the foam is noted and co-related with the standard solution of polysiloxane in benzene.

METHOD 2

This method is based on the estimation of silicone dioxide contents of the compound. To the sample equivalent to 100 mg of the compound, add 10 ml of 1 N sulphuric acid and heat on water-bath for ninety minutes. Filter through an ashless filter paper. The residue is washed with hot water and transferred to a platinum crucible. Heat to dryness, incinerate and ignite at 1000°C, cool and weigh (a). The residue is moistened with water and then add 5 ml of hydrofluoric acid and few drops of sulphuric acid. Evaporate to dryness and ignite at 1000°C, cool and weigh (b). The difference between weights (a) and (b) represents the weight of silicone dioxide.

Note : Silicone dioxide forms volatile complex (silicone tetrafluoride) with hydrofluoric acid.

METHOD 3

Measure 10 ml of suspension or weigh powdered tablets equivalent to 200 mg of the compound and transfer to a separating funnel. Add 50 ml of 5 N hydrochloric acid and 50 ml of saturated solution of sodium chloride. Shake well and extract with four 50 ml portions of ether. Wash the combined ethereal extract with 20 ml of saturated solution of sodium chloride. In turn, wash the saline layer with 20 ml of ether, combine the latter ether extract with the main ether extract. Filter through anhydrous sodium sulphate placed over cotton plug. Rinse the sodium sulphate with two 10 ml portions of ether. Evaporate combined ether layer on steam-bath to about 2-3 ml. Transfer to a tared 30 ml Kjeldahl flask. Wash the flask 3-4 times each with 4 ml of ether. Evaporate the oily liquid to dryness on steam-bath using nitrogen gas to prevent bumping. Add 2 ml of concentrated sulphuric acid and 0.5 ml concentrated nitric acid. Place the Kjeldahl flask on a sand-bath equipped with a thermometer (0-360°C). Heat slowly to 140°C and maintain at this temperature for 30 minutes. Draw back the flash and place on direct flame slowly at the beginning to prevent bumping, then strongly heat to constant weight which represents silicone dioxide present in the sample.

METHOD 4

Take sample accurately weighed equivalent to 50 mg of the compound, add 50 ml water and extract with four 50 ml portions of chloroform. Pool chloroform layer, evaporate on rotary evaporator and proceed as per method 1 or 2 above.

Note : Use ground glass joint apparatus and separating funnel free of silicone. Alternatively the sample is neutralized with 1 N hydrochloric acid (amount of acid required can be calculated from acid consuming capacity) and neutralized sample solution is used directly for defoaming actively. Aqueous sample solution gives more satisfactory results.

METHOD 5

Silicates give yellow colour with ammonium molybdate in acidic medium. For details refer to method described in formulation 14 of this chapter.

Aluminium hydroxide, Magnesium trisilicate, Sodium bicarbonate, Alginic acid

ESTIMATION

Aluminium hydroxide and Magnesium trisilicate

Sample preparation

Weigh accurately, powdered sample equivalent to 200 mg of aluminium hydroxide, add 10 ml of water, mix, allow to stand and then add 30 ml of 6 N hydrochloric acid, allow to stand at room temperature for 45 min. Add 30 ml of water and heat on a water-bath for 40-45 min with continuous stirring to prevent charring. Cool and filter, wash filter paper with water and adjust the volume of filtrate to 250 ml with water. Use this solution for estimation of aluminium hydroxide and magnesium trisilicate (if the solution is coloured, treat with acid-washed charcoal and filter).

Aluminium hydroxide

Neutralise 20 ml of the sample solution with dilute ammonia solution (Congo red paper) and proceed as per method described in formulation 22 of this chapter.

Magnesium trisilicate

50 ml of the sample solution is made alkaline with ammonia (litmus paper) and then follow the method described in formulation 22 of this chapter.

Alginic acid

Accurately weighed quantity of sample equivalent to 250 mg of alginic acid is transferred to a stoppered flask. Add 60 ml of acetone and 40 ml of dilute hydrochloric acid (10% w/v). Stopper the flask and shake occasionally for 30 min. Filter through Whatman No. 4 filter paper transferring as much of the precipitate as possible to a filter paper. Transfer precipitates and filter paper to a flask. Ensure that all the precipitates/residue sticking to the funnel are also removed to the flask. Add 25 ml of 0.1 N sodium hydroxide and shake for 15 min. Titrate excess of the alkali with 0.1 N hydrochloric acid using phenolphthalein as indicator. Treat 250 mg of working standard of alginic acid simultaneously. Carry out the blank determination and calculate by comparison.

Isopropamide iodide, Trifluoperazine

ESTIMATION

Isopropamide iodide

Reagents

1. Buffer solution, pH 10.2 : Dissolve 43.5 g of potassium phosphate, dibasic and 21 g of sodium bicarbonate anhydrous in 1000 ml of water. Adjust the pH to 10.2 with phosphoric acid.
2. Methyl orange solution : Add 0.2 g of methyl orange to about 190 ml of pH 10.2 buffer in a 500 ml conical flask and stir on a steam-bath for 30 min. Dilute to 200 ml with pH 10.2 buffer while hot. Stir mechanically until cold and then continue to stir overnight. Filter through a Whatman filter paper (No. 1) and extract the filtrate with successive 20 ml of chloroform until the chloroform extracts are colourless and do not yield a red colour on shaking with 2% hydrochloric acid (extraction with chloroform results in lower blank values).
3. 1% w/v solution of sodium sulphite in water.

Standard solution

Accurately weigh about 200 mg of isopropamide iodide in a 100 ml volumetric flask. Add 0.1 N sulphuric acid to dissolve and to make up to 100 ml. Pipette 10 ml into a 250 ml volumetric flask, add 0.1 N sulphuric acid to about 200 ml. Add 2 ml of sodium sulphite solution and shake for 20 minutes. Dilute to 250 ml with 0.1 N sulphuric acid and mix well.

Sample solution

Powder tablets finely and weigh accurately powder, equivalent to 15 mg of isopropamide into a 250 ml volumetric flask, add about 200 ml of 0.1 N sulphuric acid, 2 ml of sodium sulphite solution and shake for 20 minutes. Dilute to 250 ml with 0.1 N sulphuric acid and mix well. Filter through Whatman paper (No. 1), discarding the first few ml of the filtrate.

Procedure

Place 50 ml of chloroform and 30 ml of methyl orange solution each in two separators. Pipette 5 ml each of the standard and sample solutions into the separators, shake well and allow to stand for 3 to 4 minutes or until the layers are completely separated. Slowly run the chloroform layer into another separator through a pledget of cotton pre-moistened with chloroform. Repeat the extraction with two more 50 ml portions of chloroform and wash the cotton pledget with 25 ml of chloroform. Extract the combined chloroform layer with 20 ml of dilute hydrochloric acid and 30 ml of water. Discard the chloroform layer and run the acid phase into a 100 ml volumetric flask. Rinse the separator, dilute to 100 ml with water. Measure the absorbance of the final solutions at about 510 nm using 1% v/v hydrochloric acid as blank. Calculate the results by comparison.

Trifluoperazine

Powder tablets finely and transfer accurately weighed quantity of the powder equivalent to 5 mg of trifluoperazine into 500 ml volumetric flask. Shake for 15 min with 400 ml of a mixture of one volume of hydrochloric acid and 19 volumes of water. Dilute to 500 ml with the same solvent mixture, mix and filter. Measure the extinction of the filtrate at maxima at about 256 nm and calculate the results by taking 743 as value of A 1%, 1 cm at 256 nm.

Hyoscyamine-N-butyl bromide, Analgin

ESTIMATION

Hyoscyamine-N-butyl bromide

METHOD 1

Reagents

1. 0.1 M citric acid.
2. 0.2 M disodium hydrogen phosphate dihydrate.
3. Citric acid-phosphate buffer, pH 7.5 : Dilute 7.5 ml each of 0.1 M citric acid and 0.2 M disodium hydrogen phosphate to 100 ml with water.
4. Bromothymol blue solution : Dissolve 0.15 g of bromothymol blue and 0.15 g of anhydrous sodium carbonate in 100 ml of water.
5. Alcoholic solution of boric acid : Dissolve 20 g of boric acid in 800 ml of methanol and 80 ml of water and then make up to 1000 ml with methanol.

Standard solution

100 mcg/ml of the substance in water.

Sample solution

Quantity of the sample equivalent to 5 mg of the substance is accurately weighed and dissolved in water to produce 50 ml (100 mcg/ml).

Procedure

Pipette 5 ml each of the sample and standard solutions and 0.5 ml of 0.1 N sodium hydroxide into separate 100 ml separating funnels. To each separating funnel, add 2 ml of bromothymol blue solution and 20 ml of buffer solution. Extract by shaking for about one minute with exactly 30 ml of chloroform. Separate chloroform layer and make up to 50 ml with alcoholic boric acid solution to clear the chloroform phase. Determine the extinctions of the sample and standard solutions at about 420 nm against chloroform as a blank. Compute the results by comparison.

METHOD 2

Reagents

1. Iodine solution : 0.250 mg/ml in ethylene dichloride.
2. Phosphate buffer, pH 9.0.

Standard solution

Dissolve the pure compound in water to get concentration of 500 mcg/ml. To 1 ml of standard solution, add 5 ml of buffer solution and 10 ml of ethylene dichloride. Shake vigorously for 5 minutes and allow the layers to separate. Pass organic layer through anhydrous sodium sulphate and dilute to 10 ml with ethylene dichloride (50 mcg/ml).

Sample solution

Weigh accurately sample equivalent to 0.5 mg of hyoscyamine-N-butyl bromide. Add 5 ml of buffer solution, 10 ml of ethylene dichloride and proceed as described under standard solution.

Procedure

To 1 ml each of standard and sample solutions, add 1 ml of iodine solution and 10 ml of ethylene dichloride. Shake and measure the extinction at maxima at about 280 nm (atropine, homatropine and scopolamine exhibit maxima at about 295 nm).

Analgin (Dipyrone)

METHOD 1

Standard solution

20 mcg/ml of analgin in 0.01 N hydrochloric acid.

Sample solution

In a 100 ml volumetric flask, shake up powdered tablets, accurately weighed equivalent to 200 mg of analgin with about 80 ml of 0.01 N hydrochloric acid for 15 minutes and then make up to volume with 0.01 N hydrochloric acid. Pipette 5 ml of the filtrate into a 500 ml volumetric flask and make up the volume with 0.01 N hydrochloric acid.

Determine the extinctions of the sample and standard solutions at the maximum at about 257 nm against 0.01 N acid as blank. Deduce results by comparison.

METHOD 2

Weigh accurately, powdered sample equivalent to 0.5 g of analgin, add 10 ml of water and shake for one minute. Immediately add 25 ml of methyl alcohol, shake and make up the volume to 50 ml with methyl alcohol. Filter immediately and to 25 ml of the filtrate, add 5 ml of 0.01 N hydrochloric acid and titrate with 0.1 N iodine till pale yellow colour persists for 30 seconds. Each ml of 0.1 N iodine is equivalent to 0.01757 g of analgin.

Diazepam, L-Hyoscyamine

ESTIMATION

Diazepam

Standard solution

50 mcg/ml of diazepam in alcoholic sulphuric acid.

Sample solution

Weigh accurately powdered sample equivalent to 10 mg of diazepam, add 10 ml of water, 20 ml of borate buffer, pH 9.0 or phosphate buffer, pH 7.0 and extract with four 25 ml portions of solvent ether. For further details, refer to formulation 25 of the chapter on analgesics and antipyretics.

Note : Diazepam usually contains a hydrolytic decomposition product, 2-methylamino-5-chloro-benzophenone which interferes in the above assay as its absorbance overlaps at 368 nm and 285 nm. To eliminate the interference due to decomposition product, the following procedure is usually recommended :

    (a) Process the sample as above.

    (b) Follow the ether extraction procedure as above, however, reconstitute the residue with alcohol instead of acidified alcohol and read the resultant solution at 405 nm. This absorbance is multiplied by 19.314 to get amount (mg) of the diazepam present as decomposition product in the sample. This amount is subtracted from the amount of diazepam determined by the main method.

L-Hyoscyamine

Reagents

1. Solution 1 : Phosphate buffer solution, pH 2.5 : To 55 ml of 7.8% w/v solution of potassium phosphate dibasic, add 20 ml of 9.6% w/v solution of citric acid and dilute to 100 ml with water.
2. Solution 2 : Bromocresol purple : To 400 mg of bromocresol purple, add 6.5 ml of 0.1 N sodium hydroxide and make up to 500 ml with water.
3. Dye solution : Mix equal volumes of solution 1 and solution 2, extract with chloroform and reject chloroform layer. This step reduces the blank value.

Standard solution

50 mcg/ml of L-hyoscyamine in 0.1 N hydrochloric acid.

Sample solution

Weigh accurately a quantity of the sample equivalent to 5 mg of substance and shake with 0.1 N hydrochloric acid to produce 100 ml (50 mcg/ml).

Procedure

To 10 ml each of the sample and standard solutions, add 10 ml of dye solution and exactly 25 ml chloroform. Shake for two minutes, and allow the layers to separate out. Filter the chloroform layer through cotton plug. Read extinction of sample and standard solution at about 440 nm against chloroform as blank and calculate the results by comparison.

Formulation 27

Propantheline bromide, Meprobamate, Dried aluminium hydroxide gel

ESTIMATION

Propantheline bromide

Weigh accurately quantity of the powdered tablets equivalent to 50 mg of the substance and transfer to a 250 ml conical flask. Add 20 ml of water and 5 ml of dilute nitric acid. Boil, cool and add 25 ml of 0.01 N silver nitrate solution. Shake and titrate excess silver nitrate with 0.01 N ammonium thiocyanate using ferric alum as indicator. Run a blank with 25 ml of 0.01 N silver nitrate, 5 ml of dilute nitric acid and 20 ml of water. Difference in titration values gives the amount of 0.01 N silver nitrate consumed by the sample. Each ml of 0.01 silver nitrate is equivalent to 0.00448 g of propantheline bromide.

Meprobamate

This method is based on formol titration.

Extract the powdered tablets equivalent to 100 mg of meprobamate accurately weighed with three 50 ml portions of acetone and filter. Evaporate the solvent on a water-bath. To the residue, add 40 ml of hydrochloric acid (1 : 1) and reflux on a burner for 90 minutes. Remove the condenser and boil until the volume is reduced to about 8 ml. Cool the flask in ice, add 50 ml of water, 1 drop of methyl red indicator and neutralise with 10 N sodium hydroxide, until the colour is just changed. If necessary, add 1 N hydrochloric acid to restore the pink colour. Then carefully neutralise with 0.1 N sodium hydroxide. Add a mixture of 15 ml of formaldehyde solution and 15 ml of water previously neutralised to phenolphthalein with 0.1 N sodium hydroxide. Titrate with 0.1 N sodium hydroxide until the solution becomes yellow. Add 0.2 ml of phenolphthalein and continue to titrate with 0.1 N sodium hydroxide to a distinct pink colour. Each ml of 0.1 N sodium hydroxide is equivalent to 0.01091 g of meprobamate.

Total aluminium calculated as aluminium oxide

Transfer an accurately weighed powder of the sample equivalent to 100 mg of the gel. Add 30 ml of dilute hydrochloric acid and warm on a water-bath for 30 minutes and cool. Add 40 ml of 0.05 N disodium edetate and neutralise with sodium hydroxide solution (10% w/v) using methyl red as indicator and keep on water-bath for 30 minutes. Cool, add 6 g of hexamine and titration with 0.05 M lead nitrate solution using xylenol orange as indicator. Run a blank omitting the sample. Each ml of 0.05 M disodium edetate consumed is equivalent to 0.002549 g aluminium oxide.

Meprobamate, Ethoheptazine citrate, Aspirin

ESTIMATION

Meprobamate

Weigh accurately powdered tablets equivalent to 100 mg of meprobamate and follow the method described for meprobamate under formulation 27 of this chapter.

Ethoheptazine citrate

Reagents

1. 0.1 N perchloric acid in glacial acetic acid.
2. 1% w/v crystal violet solution.
3. Carbon tetrachloride.
4. Alkaline salt solution : 100 ml of saturated ammonium chloride solution in water containing 2 g of sodium hydroxide.

Procedure

Weigh sample equivalent to about 200 mg of ethoheptazine. Add 20 ml of alkaline salt solution, shake vigorously for 5 minutes and extract with four 30 ml portions of carbon tetrachloride. Pass organic layer through anhydrous sodium sulphate, add 20 ml of glacial acetic acid, 2 drops of crystal violet solution and titrate with 0.1 N perchloric acid to blue colour. Each ml of 0.1 N perchloric acid is equivalent to 0.04535 g of ethoheptazine citrate. From the total volume of the acid consumed in the above titration, calculate the amount of ethoheptazine citrate present in the sample.

Aspirin

Weigh accurately quantity of powdered tablets equivalent to 500 mg of aspirin, add 25 ml of 0.5 N sodium hydroxide, boil gently for ten minutes and titrate excess of alkali with 0.5 N hydrochloric acid using phenol red as indicator. Each ml of 0.5 N sodium hydroxide is equivalent to 0.04507 g of aspirin.

Analgin, Diazepam, Papaverine hydrochloride, Homatropine sulphate

ESTIMATION

Analgin

Follow the colorimetric method using p-dimethylaminobenzaldehyde reagent as described in formulation 32 of the chapter on analgesics and antipyretics.

Diazepam

Suspend accurately weighed quantity of the sample equivalent to 2 mg of the compound in phosphate buffer, pH 7. Extract into ether (peroxide free) and follow the method as described in formulation 25 of the chapter on analgesics and antipyretics.

Homatropine sulphate

Reagents

1. 1 N sodium hydroxide.
2. 0.2 M cerric ammonium sulphate in 6 N sulphuric acid.

Standard preparation

Weigh accurately 50 mg of homatropine sulphate into a 100 ml volumetric flask, dissolve and make up to 100 ml with water. 10 ml of this solution is further diluted to 100 ml with water (50 mcg/ml).

Sample preparation

Weigh accurately the sample equivalent to 5 mg of homatropine into a 100 ml volumetric flask and add 50 ml of water. Shake well and make up with water (50 mcg/ml).

Procedure

Transfer 10 ml each of the standard and sample preparations to separate glass-stoppered 100 ml flasks. To each flask, add 20 ml of 1 N sodium hydroxide and heat in a water-bath at 80°C for 15 minutes. Cool to room temperature, wash the solution with two 25 ml portions of chloroform before addition of cerric reagent. Add 8 ml of 0.2 M cerric ammonium sulphate and mix. To each flask add 25 ml of iso-octane and shake for 15 minutes. Decant the organic layer and concomitantly determine the absorbance of both the solutions, at the maximum at about 242 nm, on a suitable spectrophotometer using iso-octane as the blank.

Papaverine hydrochloride

Reagents

1. 1% w/v ammonium molybdate solution in water.

2. 10% w/v solution of catechol in water.
3. 0.1 N hydrochloric acid.

Standard solution

To 50 mg of pure papaverine, add 10 ml of 1 N hydrochloric acid and 50 ml of water. Boil on water-bath for 10 min, cool and dilute to 100 ml with water (0.5 mg/ml)

Sample solution

Weigh accurately a quantity of the powdered tablets equivalent to 50 mg of papaverine and proceed as per standard (0.5 mg/ml) solution.

Procedure

To 2 ml each of standard and sample solutions, add 1 ml of ammonium molybdate solution and 3 ml of catechol solution. Mix and extract with three 15 ml portions of chloroform. Pass chloroform layer through dry filter paper (do not use anhydrous sodium sulphate) and adjust to 50 ml with chloroform. Measure the absorbance of both the solutions at about 635 nm and calculate the results by comparison.

Analgin, Baralgan ketone (Pitofenone hydrochloride), Baralgan amide (Diphenyl-piperidinoethyl acetamide methobromide)

Preparation of test solution

Powdered sample accurately weighed equivalent to 25 mg of baralgan ketone is extracted with four 10 ml portions of 0.1 N hydrochloric acid, diluted to 50 ml with acid.

ESTIMATION

Analgin

Standard solution

20 mcg/ml of analgin in 0.01 N hydrochloric acid.

Sample solution

2 ml of the test solution is diluted to 100 ml with water. Further dilutions are done with 0.01 N hydrochloric acid to get a solution of 20 mcg/ml.

Measure the extinction of standard and sample solutions at maxima at about 257 nm using 0.01 N hydrochloric acid as blank. Calculate the results by comparison.

Baralgan ketone (p-piperidionethoxy-o-carbomethoxy benzophenone hydrochloride)

Reagents

1. 30% w/v solution of sodium hydroxide in water.
2. 0.1 N hydrochloric acid.
3. 0.2% w/v solution of sodium hydroxide in water.
4. n-hexane.

Standard solution

10 mcg/ml of baralgan ketone in water.

Sample solution

To 10 ml of test solution prepared above, add 5 ml of sodium hydroxide solution. Extract with three 20 ml portions of n-hexane (reserve the alkaline extract for estimation of baralgan amide). Combine the organic layer and shake vigorously with 40 ml of dilute sodium hydroxide solution and allow complete separation of layers. Reject the alkaline layer. The organic layer is extracted with three 20 ml portions of 0.1 N hydrochloric acid, the acidic extract is combined and diluted to 500 ml with water (10 mcg/ml).

The extinction of both sample and standard solutions is measured at maximum at about 290 nm and results calculated by comparison.

Baralgan amide

Reagents

1. 5% w/v solution of EDTA (disodium) in water.
2. 0.12% w/v solution of dithizone in chloroform.
3. 1 N hydrochloric acid.
4. Dithizone reagent : To 5 g of potassium cyanide and 11 g of sodium hydroxide, add 30 ml water, shake to dissolve and dilute to 100 ml with water. Add 8 ml each of EDTA solution and dithizone solution. Wash the above solution twice with 25 ml of chloroform, rejecting organic layer. The alkaline aqueous solution is the dithizone reagent. (The reagent is to be freshly prepared).
5. Saturated solution of sodium sulphate in water.

Standard solution

100 mcg/ml of baralgan amide in water.

Sample solution

The entire alkaline solution reserved during estimation of baralgan ketone is used for estimation of amide contents in the sample.

Procedure

Transfer 10 ml of standard solution and the entire sample solution to separating funnel containing 10 ml of freshly prepared ice cold dithizone reagent and 10 ml of sodium sulphate solution. Add 20 ml of chloroform and shake vigorously for about 2 minutes. Allow the layers to separate. The chloroform layer is shaken with 5 ml of 1 N hydrochloric acid. The separated chloroform layer is passed through a layer of anhydrous sodium sulphate placed over the plug of non-absorbent cotton.

The absorption of sample and standard solutions is measured at about 605 nm and results calculated by comparison.

Ibuprofen/Ketoprofen, Baralgan ketone, Baralgan amide

ESTIMATION

Ibuprofen/Ketoprofen

Weigh accurately quantity of powdered sample equivalent to about 500 mg of ibuprofen/ketoprofen and dry extract with 20 ml of chloroform. Filter chloroform extract through cotton plug and wash the powder and cotton plug with three more 10 ml portions of chloroform. Evaporate the combined filtrate to dryness by gentle heating with the aid of current of air. Dissolve the residue in 100 ml of methanol previously neutralized to phenol red and titrate with 0.1 N sodium hydroxide solution using phenol red solution as indicator. Each ml of 0.1 N sodium hydroxide solution is equivalent to 0.02063 g of ibuprofen or 0.02543 g of ketoprofen.

Note :   Do not employ filter paper for filtration as lower assay values are often obtained. Instead of dry extraction, suspend in 0.1 N hydrochloric acid and extract with chloroform. This procedure will give more consistent results.

Baralgan ketone and amide

Preparation of test solution

Weigh accurately powdered sample equivalent to 2.5 mg of baralgan ketone and extract with four 10 ml portions of 0.1 N hydrochloric acid, dilute to 50 ml with acid.

Estimate both baralgan ketone and amide by the methods described in formulation 30 of this chapter.

Alternatively, sample equivalent to 500 mg of ibuprofen is suspended in 20 ml of 0.1 N hydrochloric acid and extracted with chloroform as described above under ibuprofen. The acidic extract may be used for estimation of baralgan amide and ketone as per methods described in formulation 30 of this chapter.

Propyphenazone, Pitofenone hydrochloride, Baralgan amide

ESTIMATION

Propyphenazone

Weigh accurately powdered sample equivalent to 300 mg of the substance and dry extract with four 30 ml portions of dry ether. Evaporate the combined ether layer to remove water completely, adding few drops of methanol during last stages of evaporation to ensure complete removal of moisture. Add 40 ml of glacial acetic acid and 10 ml of acetic anhydride and titrate with 0.1 N perchloric acid using crystal violet as indicator. Each ml of 0.1 N perchloric acid is equivalent to 0.023031 g of propyphenazone.

Pitofenone hydrochloride (baralgan ketone)

Accurately weighed quantity of the sample equivalent to 50 mg of the substance is extracted thrice (3 × 50 ml) with boiling water. The combined aqueous extract is cooled. Add 10 ml of 0.05 N hydrochloric acid and back titrate with 0.05 N sodium hydroxide (phenolphthalein). Carry out blank titration. Each ml of 0.05 N hydrochloric acid is equivalent to 20.175 mg of ketone.

Baralgan amide

Standard solution

5 mcg/ml of baralgan amide in water.

Sample solution

Dry extract the powdered sample equivalent to 0.2 mg of the substance with chloroform (3 × 25 ml), filter through G₄ sintered funnel. Evaporate the combined organic layer and take up the residue in 40 ml of water.

Procedure

To 40 ml of the standard solution and entire sample solution, add 5 ml of 1 N sodium hydroxide and 5 ml of tropeolin OO solution (0.1%). Extract with chloroform (3 × 40 ml), and extract combined organic layer with dilute hydrochloric acid (3 × 30 ml). Make up the volume to 100 ml and measure the absorbance of both sample and standard solutions at about 535 nm against blank prepared by using 40 ml of water. Calculate the results by comparison.

Sodium chloride, Potassium chloride, Sodium citrate, Dextrose

ESTIMATION

Dextrose

Weigh accurately powder equivalent to 10 g of dextrose, add 80 ml of water and 0.2 ml of ammonia solution. Shake and dilute to 100 ml with water. Determine the angular rotation in a 0.2 metre tube at 25°C and calculate the result as under :

$$x \text{ (g \% of glucose)} = \frac{a \times 100}{1 \times 53}$$

where a = angle of rotation observed;

l = length of tube in metres;

x = % w/v of glucose present in the solution under test;

53 = claimed optical rotation of 10% w/v solution of glucose.

Note : If the powder contains colouring material and flavouring agents (flavouring agents produce opalescence on dilution), they will interfere in the assay of glucose by the above method. It is, therefore, desirable to add 0.5 g of activated charcoal to the glucose solution. Shake for 5 minutes and filter. This treatment will yield a clear solution. Alternatively method described under formulation 2 of this chapter may be used.

Total chlorides

METHOD 1

Weigh powder accurately equivalent to 10 mg of total chlorides, add 25 ml of distilled water and 3 ml of nitric acid. While agitating, add 50 ml of 0.1 N silver nitrate and 5 ml of nitrobenzene. Shake vigorously for 1 minute and add 2 ml of ferric ammonium sulphate solution (indicator) and titrate excess of silver nitrate with 0.1 N ammonium thiocyanate. Each ml of 0.1 N silver nitrate is equivalent to 0.003545 g of chloride.

METHOD 2

Weigh accurately powder equivalent to 100 mg of total chloride. Add 20 ml of water, 10 ml of dilute nitric acid, 50 ml of water and boil the solution. Add 50 ml of 0.1 N silver nitrite solution to the boiling liquid. Digest the precipitate for 30 minutes on a water-bath. Filter, wash the precipitate with water for 4-5 times and titrate the combined washing with 0.1 N ammonium thiocyanate, using ferric alum solution as indicator. Each ml of 0.1 N silver nitrate equivalent to 0.003545 g of chloride. Carry out a blank titration side by side.

Potassium chloride

Take powder equivalent to 5 mg of potassium chloride, add 5 ml of water and 1.5 ml alcohol. Then, add drop-wise and with continuous shaking, 2 ml of solution of sodium cobaltinitrite (30% w/v in water). Allow to stand at room temperature for 1 hr, centrifuge till precipitates are firmly packed at the bottom. Decant and drain for 5 min. Wash the precipitates with 5 ml of 70% alcohol. Centrifuge for 5 minutes and again drain. Dry at 80°C for 1 hr. Add 25 ml of 0.02 N cerric sulphate and 1 ml of sulphuric acid (50% v/v) and heat in water-bath till precipitates disappear. Cool to room temperature and add a drop of orthophenanthroline-ferrous complex and titrate excess cerric sulphate with 0.02 N ferrous ammonium sulphate. Each ml of 0.02 N cerric sulphate is equivalent to 0.2485 mg of potassium chloride.

Sodium chloride

From the total chlorides determined above, subtract the amount of chloride corresponding to the amount of potassium chloride determined above (1 g of potassium chloride contains 478 mg of chloride (Cl^-). The remaining amount of chloride corresponds to the amount of sodium chloride present in the sample. Convert this to sodium chloride (1 g of sodium chloride contains 607 mg of chloride Cl^-).

Calcium chloride, Potassium chloride, Sodium lactate, Dextrose

All the electrolytes can be estimated without separation by flame photometric method.

Reagents

1. **Calcium carbonate** : Dry at 285°C for 2 hrs, cool in desiccator and use for preparation of standard solutions.
2. **Potassium chloride** : Dry at 500-600°C for 2 hrs, cool in desiccator and use.
3. **Sodium chloride** : Dry at 500-600°C for 2 hrs, cool in desiccator and use.

Note : All solutions are prepared in glass distilled water.

(a) **Standard solution of calcium carbonate (10 mg/ml)** : Take 24.975 g of dried calcium carbonate accurately weighed, add 150 ml of distilled water, acidify gradually with 45 ml of hydrochloric acid. Cool to room temperature and dilute to 100 ml with distilled water. Dilute 10 ml further to 200 ml with distilled water.

(b) **Standard solution of potassium chloride (1 mg/ml)** : Transfer 1.907 g accurately weighed of dried potassium chloride and dilute to 1000 ml with distilled water.

(c) **Standard solution of sodium chloride** : Dissolve 25.240 g of dried sodium chloride accurately weighed in distilled water and adjust the volume to 1000 ml with distilled water.

Mixed cationic standard solution : Take 10 ml of solution (a), 10 ml of solution (b) and 20 ml of solution (c), and dilute to 200 ml with distilled water.

Note : 1. Store the mixed standard solution in a clear polyethylene bottle. This is stable for more than 1 month.
2. The readings on the instrument with the standard solutions should be adjusted between 20% and 95% of the scale.
3. Prepare median range of standards for different cations from standard solution of mixed cations.

The sample should be appropriately diluted with distilled water to give ionic concentrations close to the standard solution for better comparison. For calcium (Ca^{++}), read at 422.7 nm; for potassium (K^+) at 766.5 nm and for sodium (Na^+) at 589.0 nm.

Dextrose

Weigh sample accurately equivalent to about 100 mg of dextrose, dissolve in 5 ml of distilled water, add 25 ml of buffer solution (containing 14.3% w/w of sodium carbonate and 4% w/v of potassium iodide and 25 ml of 0.1 N iodine). Stopper and allow to stand exactly for 30 minutes at 20°C. Add 30 ml of dilute hydrochloric acid and titrate immediately the excess iodine with 0.1 N sodium thiosulphate. Repeat the entire procedure with 5 ml of distilled water. The difference between the titrations represent the amount of iodine required to oxidize dextrose. Each ml of 0.1 N iodine is equivalent to 0.00901 g of dextrose. Alternatively, follow the method described in formulation 33 of this chapter.

Calcium lactate, Potassium chloride, Sodium chloride, Magnesium sulphate, Sodium acid phosphate, Dextrose, Sodium citrate

ESTIMATION

Dextrose

Follow the methods described for determination of glucose under formulation 33 or 34 of this chapter.

Electrolytes

Weigh accurately appropriate quantity of the sample powder and dissolve in water. Use this solution (A) for determination of various electrolytes present in the formulation as under :

Magnesium sulphate

Magnesium sulphate is estimated gravimetrically by precipitating with barium chloride as barium sulphate. Take 100 ml of aliquot (A) in a 250 ml beaker and add 50 ml of dilute hydrochloric acid. Boil the solution and add 5 ml of 10% w/v aqueous solution of barium chloride. Keep it overnight after digestion. Filter through a weighed G_4 sintered glass crucible under vacuum. Give washings with water until free from chloride. Dry the precipitate to a constant weight at 105°C and calculate the percentage of magnesium sulphate as follows :

$$\frac{\text{Weight of barium sulphate precipitate} \times 1.056 \times 250 \times 100}{100 \times \text{Weight of the powder taken for analysis}}$$

Calcium lactate

Take 100 ml of aliquot (A) in a 250 ml beaker, add 5 ml of hydrochloric acid and boil. To the hot solution, add 15 ml of saturated solution of ammonium oxalate. Add with constant stirring, dilute ammonia solution until the solution is alkaline to litmus paper. Acidify with glacial acetic acid and digest on a water-bath for 30 minutes. Filter, wash the precipitate with water until free from oxalate. Puncture the filter paper and transfer the precipitates along with the filter paper to 500 ml conical flask. Dissolve the precipitates in about 5 ml of hydrochloric acid, add 5 ml of 0.02 M magnesium sulphate and 10 ml of strong ammonia-ammonium chloride buffer and titrate with 0.02 M disodium edetate using solochrome black as indicator. From the volume of 0.02 M disodium edetate required, subtract the volume 0.02 M magnesium sulphate equivalent to disodium edetate. Each ml 0.02 M disodium edetate is equivalent to 0.006168 g of calcium lactate.

Note : Conventional methods of combined estimation of calcium and magnesium using solochrome black as indicator by EDTA titration is not possible because in presence of phosphates, both calcium and magnesium get precipitated out with ammonia.

Sodium acid phosphate

This is based on estimation of phosphate moiety of the salt.

Reagents

1. Molybdate reagent : 5 g of ammonium molybdate is dissolved in about 80 ml of water. Add slowly 10 ml of sulphuric acid to dissolve the powder, cool, make up the volume to 100 ml with water.
2. Metol reagent : Dissolve 100 mg of p-N-methyl aminophenol sulphate in about 50 ml of distilled water in a 100 ml volumetric flask. Add 20 g of sodium metabisulphite and 1 g of sodium sulphite. Dissolve adding more water and make up to 100 ml.

Stock standard solution of sodium acid phosphate

Dissolve 20 mg of sodium acid phosphate in 50 ml water and dilute to make up 100 ml with water.

Working standard solution

Dilute 10 ml of stock solution to 100 with water (200 mcg/ml).

Sample solution

10 ml aliquot of solution (A) is diluted appropriately with water to get a concentration of 200 mcg/ml.

Procedure

Transfer 5 ml each of the sample and standard solutions to 50 ml volumetric flasks. To each of the flasks, add 1 ml of dilute sulphuric acid and about 20 ml of distilled water. Then, add 5 ml of molybdate reagent, mix and add 2 ml of the metol reagent, mix and allow to stand for 10 minutes. Make up the volume to 50 ml with distilled water and shake well. Measure the absorption of both the solutions at about 650 nm against blank and calculate the results by comparison.

Total chlorides

Follow the method described for total chlorides under formulation 33 of this chapter.

Calcium lactate, Sodium chloride and Potassium chloride

Follow the flame photometric method described for calcium lactate, sodium chloride and potassium chloride under formulation 33 of this chapter.

Sodium citrate

Follow the method 4, based on colour reaction with ferric chloride, as described for estimation of sodium citrate under formulation 6 of the chapter on expectorants and cough suppressants.

Typical calculations for various ions and ingredients (mEq/L, mmol/L, total osmolarity) in ORS-A (I.P.)

I.P. formula (ORS-A) g/L

Sodium chloride	1.25 g	Sodium citrate	2.9 g
Potassium chloride	1.5 g	Dextrose anhydrous	27.0 g

Calculations :

1 g of sodium chloride = 0.3934 g of Na^+; 0.6066 g of Cl^-
1 g of sodium citrate = 0.2345 g of Na^+; 0.6430 g of citrate ion
1 g of potassium chloride = 0.5245 g of K^+; 0.4756 g of Cl^-

$$mEq/L = \frac{mg/L}{Equivalent\ wt.} \qquad mmol = \frac{mEq/L}{Valency}$$

1250 mg of sodium chloride contains 491.75 mg of Na^+ = 21.38 mEq/L or mmol/L $\left(\dfrac{491.75}{23}\right)$

Sodium in sodium citrate

100 mg of sodium citrate contains 234.5 mg of Na^+

2900 mg of sodium citrate will contain $\dfrac{234.5 \times 2900}{1000}$ = 680.05 mg of Na^+

$$\text{or } \frac{680.05}{23} = 29.5 \text{ mEq/L or mmol/L}$$

Total sodium in ORS-A = 21.38 + 29.5 = 50.88 or 51 mEq/L (mmol/L)

Chloride in sodium chloride

1000 mg of sodium chloride contains 606.6 mg of Cl^-

1250 mg of sodium chloride will contain $\dfrac{606.6 \times 1250}{1000}$ = 758.25 mg of Cl^-

$$\text{or } \frac{758.25}{35.453} = 21.39 \text{ mEq/L (mmol/L)}$$

Chloride in potassium chloride

1000 mg of KCl contains 475.6 mg of Cl^-

1500 mg of KCl will contain $\dfrac{475.6 \times 1500}{1000}$ = 713.4 mg of Cl^-

$$\text{or } \frac{713.4}{35.453} = 20.12 \text{ mEq/L (mmol/L)}$$

Total chloride in ORS-A = 21.39 + 20.12 = 41.50 mEq/L or 41.00 mEq/L

Potassium in potassium chloride

1000 mg of potassium chloride contains 524.5 mg of K^+

1500 mg of potassium chloride will contain $\dfrac{524.5 \times 1500}{1000}$ = 786.75 mg of K^+

$$\text{or } \frac{786.75}{39} = 20.12 \text{ mEq/L (mmol/L)}$$

Citrate in sodium citrate

1000 mg of sodium citrate contains 643 mg of citrate

2900 mg of sodium citrate will contain

$$\frac{643 \times 2900}{1000} = 1864.7 \text{ mg of citrate}$$

$$= 29.60 \text{ mEq/L or 30 mEq/L or 10 mmol/L of citrate}$$

(valency of citrate ion = 3)

mEq of glucose/L

Amount of glucose per litre = 27.0 g or 27000 mg

Mol. wt./Eq. wt. of glucose = 180

$$\text{mEq of glucose/L} = \frac{27000}{180} = 150$$

Total osmolarity of ORS-A (total ions or ingredients in mmol/L)

Na^+	51	$Citrate^{3-}$	10
K^+	20	Glucose	150
Cl^-	41	Total osmolarity	272

Chapter 8

Antibiotics
(Anti-tubercular, Penicillins, Cephalosporins, Anthelmintics, Antimalarials)

Isoniazid, Calcium gluconate, Pyridoxine hydrochloride

ESTIMATION

Isoniazid

METHOD 1

To sample accurately measured or weighed equivalent to 50 mg of isoniazid, add 50 ml of distilled water and 1.5 of sodium bicarbonate. Add 50 ml of 0.1 N iodine solution, stopper and allow to stand for 90 minutes. Cautiously add 20 ml of dilute hydrochloric acid and titrate excess iodine with 0.1 N sodium thiosulphate. Each ml of 0.1 N iodine is equivalent to 0.003429 g of isoniazid.

METHOD 2

Reagents

1. Ammonia-ammonium chloride buffer, pH 10.8.
2. 0.33% w/v solution of 2,3-dichloro-1,4-naphthoquinone in absolute alcohol.

Standard solution

100 mcg/ml of isoniazid in water.

Sample solution

Sample equivalent to 100 mg of the substance is extracted and diluted with water to produce 100 mcg/ml.

Procedure

To 2 ml each of sample and standard solutions, add 1 ml of buffer solution, 6 ml of naphthoquinone reagent and dilute to 25 ml with water. Cool the mixture in ice-bath for 40 min. Measure the absorbance of purple blue complex of both sample and standard solutions at 610 nm against reagent blank. The method obeys Beer's law in the concentration range of 2-14 mcg/ml. The colour is stable for more than 2 hours. Thiacetazone and PAS do not interfere.

Note : If isoniazid is present as calcium methane sulphonate, estimate on the basis of calcium contents by the method : Extract the powdered sample with warm water to produce 2 mg/ml. Take aliquot equivalent to 200 mg (100 ml) and titrate with 0.1 N sodium edetate using erochrome-T as indicator.

Each ml of 0.1 M sodium edetate is equivalent to 0.025 g of calcium methane sulphonate of isoniazid.

METHOD 3

Reagents

1. 2% w/v solution of p-dimethylaminobenzaldehyde (PDAB).
2. 1% oxalic acid in methanol.

Standard solution

100 mcg/ml of isoniazid in alcohol.

Sample solution

Extract the accurately weighed quantity of the sample equivalent to 50 mg of isoniazid with alcohol to get 1 mg/ml. Dilute further with alcohol to get 100 mcg/ml.

Procedure

To 1 ml each of sample and standard solutions, add 2 ml of 'PDAB' solution. Allow to stand at room temperature for 10 min, add 15 ml of methanol, 10 ml of oxalic acid and dilute to 50 ml with methanol. After 10 min, measure absorbance of yellow complex at about 395 nm against reagent blank. The method obeys Beer's law in the concentration range of 2-8 mcg/ml.

Note : Thiacetazone does not interfere.

METHOD 4

Reagents

1. Buffer solution, pH 6.0.
2. Modified Grote's reagent : 10 ml of solution of sodium nitroprusside and 5 ml of hydroxylamine hydrochloride solution are taken in 50 ml beaker, mixed and allowed to stand for 2 min. Then, add 10 ml of the sodium bicarbonate solution, 1 ml of bromine is slowly added and after 10 min, 5 ml of the phenol solution is added. The reagent is allowed to stand at room temperature for 5-12 h. Filter and store at 5°C. This stock solution is stable for 75 days. Dilute one part of the reagent with 19 parts of buffer solution, pH 6 just before use.
3. 5% w/v solution of sodium nitroprusside in water.
4. 10% w/v solution of sodium bicarbonate in water.
5. 2% w/v solution of phenol in water.
6. 10% w/v solution of hydroxylamine hydrochloride in water.

Standard solution

500 mcg/ml of isoniazid in pH 6.0 buffer.

Sample solution

Extract accurately weighed amount of the powdered tablets with pH 6.0 buffer to get concentration of 500 mcg/ml.

Procedure

To 0.5 ml each of sample and standard solutions, add 5 ml of diluted Grote's reagent and dilute to 10 ml with pH 6.0 buffer. Shake and after 5 min, measure the absorbance of both the solutions at about 440 nm against reagent blank.

Note : In addition to calcium gluconate and vitamin B_6, vitamin D_2, proteolysed liver, lysine and common colouring agents do not interfere.

Calcium gluconate

To sample equivalent to 200 mg of calcium gluconate, add 3 ml of hydrochloric acid. Bring to boiling and add hot ammonium oxalate solution, followed by dilute ammonia solutions. Heat on water-bath for 1 hr and cool. Transfer precipitates to G_4 sintered funnel with the aid of 0.1% w/v ammonium oxalate solution. Wash precipitates with water till free of chloride. Dissolve the precipitates in dilute sulphuric acid, heat to 70°C and titrate with 0.1 N potassium permanganate maintaining solution at 70°C throughout titration. Each ml of 0.1 N potassium permanganate is equivalent to 0.02242 g of calcium gluconate, pentahydrate.

Pyridoxine hydrochloride

Follow method 1 or 3 as described in general methods for estimation of pyridoxine hydrochloride.

Thiacetazone, Isoniazid

ESTIMATION

METHOD 1

This involves spectrophotometric method for estimation of both the components without prior separation.

Standard solution

25 mg each of thiacetazone and isoniazid were accurately weighed, separately dissolved in methanol and diluted to 250 ml with the solvent. 5 ml of each solution was further diluted to 100 ml with 0.1 N methanolic hydrochloric acid.

Sample solution

A quantity of sample equivalent to 50 mg of isoniazid was accurately weighed, dissolved in methanol and diluted to 100 ml with the solvent. 2 ml of the solution was further diluted to 100 ml with 0.1 N methanolic hydrochloric acid.

Procedure

The extinction of the sample and standard solutions was immediately measured at 268 nm and 328 nm, the absorption maxima of isoniazid and thiacetazone respectively. The concentration of thiacetazone in the sample was directly calculated by using predetermined absorptivity value with standard thiacetazone solution in methanolic hydrochloric acid at 328 nm. Isoniazid does not interfere at this wavelength. The concentration of isoniazid was calculated by applying the following equation :

$$C_1 = \frac{E_1 \times A_2 - E_2 \times A_1}{A_2 \times B_1}$$

where C_1 = concentration (g/L) of isoniazid in the final sample solution;
E_1 and E_2 = extinction values of the sample solution at 268 nm and 328 nm respectively;
A_1 and A_2 = absorptivity values of thiacetazone at 268 and 328 nm respectively;
B_1 = absorptivity value of isoniazid at 268 nm.
The values of A_1, A_2 and B_2 were found to be 18, 188 and 37 respectively.

Note : 1. The extinction value of thiacetazone in acidic methanol tends to decrease if the solution is stored at room temperature beyond 30 minutes. It is, therefore, desirable that the extinction should be measured immediately after the preparation of the solutions.
2. Vitamins commonly present in such formulations interfere in the estimation of isoniazid but no such interference is observed in the estimation of thiacetazone.

METHOD 2

This method is based on the fact that isoniazid is highly soluble in water, whereas thiacetazone is practically insoluble.

Isoniazid

Weigh accurately quantity of the sample equivalent to 100 mg of isoniazid. Extract with three 25 ml portions of 0.01 N hydrochloric acid filtering each portion through the same sintered glass funnel (G_4), the filtrate is diluted to 100 ml with 0.01 N hydrochloric acid. Further dilutions are done appropriately with 0.01 N hydrochloric acid to final concentration of 10 mcg/ml. Measure the extinction of resultant solution at maxima at about 266 nm and calculate the results taking 378 as value of A 1%, 1 cm at 266 nm.

Thiacetazone

The entire residue left after the extraction of isoniazid as described above is used for estimation. The residue is transferred to a volumetric flask with the aid of ethanol, used in small portions and diluted to 100 ml and filtered. The filtrate is appropriately diluted with ethanol to get final concentration of 10 mcg/ml. Measure the extinction of resulting solution at maxima at about 328 nm using ethanol as blank. Calculate the results taking 580 as value of A 1%, 1 cm at 328.

Ethambutol hydrochloride, Isoniazid

ESTIMATION

Ethambutol hydrochloride

METHOD 1

Reagent

1. 1.67×10^{-4} M iodine in anhydrous chloroform.

Standard solution

50 mcg/ml of ethambutol hydrochloride in chloroform is processed as per sample to get standard solution (50 mcg/ml).

Sample solution

Transfer sample equivalent to 50 mg of ethambutol accurately weighed to a separating funnel. Add 3 ml of 3 N sodium hydroxide and extract with five 15 ml portions of dry chloroform (shake for 5 minutes for each extraction). Dry total chloroform layer over anhydrous sodium sulphate previously washed with chloroform and dilute to 100 ml with the same solvent. 5 ml of the resultant solution is further diluted to 50 ml with chloroform (50 mcg/ml).

Procedure

To 1 ml each of the sample and standard solutions, add 5 ml of the iodine reagent and dilute to 10 ml with anhydrous chloroform. Allow to stand in dark for 1 h and measure the extinction of both sample and standard solutions at 293 nm. The method follows Beer's law in the final concentration range of 1.5-7.5 mcg/ml.

Note : Although the peaks are observed at 293 and 360 nm but the one at 293 nm is quite linear.

METHOD 2

This is based on iodometric estimation of the substance.

Reagents

1. 0.5 N periodic acid solution : Dissolve 5.5 g of pure periodic acid in water to produce 500 ml. Store in dark glass bottle and standardize before use.
2. 0.2 N sodium thiosulphate.
3. 20% w/v solution of potassium iodine in water.

Procedure

Weigh accurately, a quantity of powdered tablets equivalent to 200 mg of ethambutol. Dissolve in water, followed by 5 ml of 1 N sodium hydroxide. Add 25 ml of periodic acid solution and keep for

1 hr. Then, add 15 ml of potassium iodide solution and 20 ml of dilute sulphuric acid and titrate against 0.2 N sodium thiosulphate solution using starch as indicator. Each ml of 0.1 N sodium thiosulphate is equivalent to 0.00698 g of ethambutol hydrochloride.

Note : PAS, thiacetazone and rifampicin do not interfere in this procedure.

Comments on assay method official in IP, 1996

1. Filtration of chloroform extract through filter paper will give lower assay values because of absorption by filter paper; filtration through layer of anhydrous sodium sulphate is recommended.
2. Basification with 2 N sodium hydroxide requires more chloroform for complete extraction (71% is extracted with single extraction of 25 ml of chloroform); use 3 N sodium hydroxide for basification for better extraction (89.5% is extracted with single extraction of 25 ml of chloroform).

METHOD 3
Reagents

1. 3 N sodium hydroxide.
2. 0.1 N perchloric acid.

Sample solution

Weigh accurately a quantity of the sample equivalent to 200 mg of ethambutol hydrochloride. Add 10 ml of 3 N sodium hydroxide solution and extract with five 25 ml portions of chloroform. Pass the combined chloroform layer through anhydrous sodium sulphate and evaporate to dryness and take up the residue in 100 ml of glacial acetic acid and titrate with 0.1 N perchloric acid using α-naphthol-benzein or crystal violet as indicator. Each ml of 0.1 N perchloric acid is equivalent to 0.01386 g of ethambutol hydrochloride.

Note : For extraction and filtration, follow instructions described in formulation 3 of this chapter.

Isoniazid

Follow the methods described in formulation 1 of this chapter.

Pyrazinamide, Rifampicin, Isoniazid

ESTIMATION

Pyrazinamide

Weigh accurately quantity of the sample equivalent to about 300 mg of pyrazinamide, suspend in 25 ml of chloroform and extract with five 30 ml portions of 0.1 N hydrochloric acid. Discard the chloroform layer. Transfer the combined acidic layer to ammonia distillation flask, add 100 ml of water and 100 ml of sodium hydroxide solution (50% w/v). Carry out ammonia distillation, collecting the distillate in 0.1 N sulphuric acid. Titrate excess acid with 0.1 N sodium hydroxide using methyl red as indicator. Each ml of 0.1 N sulphuric acid is equivalent to 0.01231 g of pyrazinamide.

Rifampicin

METHOD 1

Reagents

1. 5.0% w/v solution of potassium dichromate in water.
2. Phosphate buffer, pH 7.4.
3. Methyl isobutyl ketone (solvent).

Standard solution

1 mg/ml of rifampicin in methanol.

Sample solution

Weigh accurately the sample equivalent to about 100 mg of the rifampicin, add 50 ml of methyl alcohol, shake and make up to 100 ml with methyl alcohol.

Procedure

Take 5 ml each of potassium dichromate solution and buffer solution in two separators. Add 2 ml each of sample and standard solutions. Stir well and after 1 minute, extract with two 10 ml portions of methyl isobutyl ketone. Make up the volume to 25 ml with the solvent. Measure the absorbance of resulting solutions at about 540 nm against reagent blank. Deduce the results by comparison.

METHOD 2

Prepare solution of sample in methanol (1 mg/ml). Further dilution is done with pH 7.4 buffer (prepared as per IP 1996) to get final concentration of 20 mcg/ml. Measure the extinction at about 475 nm and calculate the results taking 187 as the value of A 1%, 1 cm at 475 nm.

Isoniazid

Reagents

1. 10% w/v solution of potassium iodide in water.

2. 0.1 N sodium thiosulphate.
3. 0.1 N bromine solution.
4. 0.1 N hydrochloric acid.
5. Starch solution (indicator).

Procedure

Weigh accurately quantity of the sample equivalent to about 25 mg of isoniazid. Suspend in 20 ml of 0.1 N hydrochloric acid and extract with five 50 ml portions of dichloromethane, allowing the layers to separate completely after each extraction. Transfer the combined acidic layer to iodine flask, cool, add 10 ml of concentrated hydrochloric acid and 25 ml of bromine solution, allow to stand for 30 min. Add 20 ml of potassium iodide solution, allow it to stand for 10 min and titrate with sodium thiosulphate solution using starch solution as indicator. Each ml of 0.1 N bromine is equivalent to 0.003429 g of isoniazid. Run a blank to calculate volume of bromine consumed by the drug.

Note : Acidic solution can be directly titrated with 0.1 N bromine solution using methyl red as indicator or potentiometrically.

Isoniazid, Rifampicin, Pyridoxine hydrochloride

ESTIMATION

Isoniazid

Follow the method 3 described in formulation 1 of this chapter based on reaction with aldehyde reagent. Alternatively, suspend the sample in 0.01 N hydrochloric acid and extract with 2 × 40 ml portions of chloroform. Chloroform layer may be washed with 25 ml of 0.1 N hydrochloric acid. The acidic layers are combined and diluted appropriately to get solution of 10 mcg/ml. See method 2 under formulation 2 of this chapter.

Rifampicin

Follow the method 2 described in formulation 4 of this chapter. The extinction of the substance is measured at 475 nm in phosphate buffer.

Pyridoxine hydrochloride

Follow the method based on the reaction with chlorimide reagent as described for estimation of pyridoxine hydrochloride.

Ampicillin

ESTIMATION

METHOD 1

Reagents

1. 0.1 N hydrochloric acid.
2. 0.1% w/v solution of ninhydrin in 0.1 N hydrochloric acid.
3. Methyl alcohol.

Standard solution

1 mg/ml of ampicillin in 0.1 N hydrochloric acid.

Sample solution

(a) Capsule and tablets : Contents are accurately weighed and dissolved in 0.1 N hydrochloric acid to produce 1 mg/ml of ampicillin, and filter.

(b) Dry syrup : The granules are just diluted with water to the desired volume. Aliquot equivalent to 100 mg of the compound is taken and diluted to 100 ml with 0.1 N hydrochloric acid.

Procedure

To 0.3 ml each of sample and standard solutions (300 mcg), add 5 ml of 0.1 N hydrochloric acid and 5 ml of ninhydrin solution. Keep the flask in boiling water-bath for 30 minutes ensuring uniform heating of all the flasks. Take out and immediately add 10 ml of methyl alcohol, shake, cool to room temperature and dilute to 50 ml with 0.1 N hydrochloric acid. After 10 minutes, measure the absorption at about 490 nm. The method obeys Beer's law in the concentration range of 2-10 mcg/ml. The colour is stable for more than 1 h.

Note : 1. Addition of methyl alcohol immediately after the reaction is over is necessary to prevent formation of precipitates.

2. Other semisynthetic penicillins such as benzyl penicillin, oxacillin, cloxacillin do not give measurable colour with this reagent.

3. Ensure that all the flasks are uniformly heated, failing which unsatisfactory results are obtained. This is the major drawback with this method.

METHOD 2

Reagents

1. Fehling reagent : Prepared by mixing 2 ml of Fehling solution A and 2 ml of Fehling solution B and diluting to 50 ml with water.

Standard solution

Dissolve accurately weighed quantity of ampicillin (anhydrous) in water to produce 1 mg/ml.

Sample solution

(a) Raw material : 1 mg/ml in water.

(b) Accurately weigh powder from capsule equivalent to 100 mg of ampicillin, add 80 ml of water, shake and dilute to 100 ml.

(c) Dry syrup : Add sufficient water so as to represent the labelled volume. Shake and keep for 45 minutes. Transfer aliquot of the syrup equivalent to 100 mg of anhydrous ampicillin, adjust the pH to 6.8-7.0, dilute to 100 ml and shake to mix.

Procedure

To 2 ml each of sample and standard solutions, add 3.5 ml of water. To all the tubes, add 0.5 ml of Fehling reagent. After 1 minute, measure the absorbance of all the solutions at about 558 nm using 5.5 ml of water instead of drug solution as blank. The method obeys Beer's law over the concentration range of 50-350 mcg/ml.

This method is highly specific as 6-aminopenicillinic acid, penicillin G sodium, phenoxymethyl penicillin and degradation products of ampicillin do not react with this reagent. Amoxycillin and cloxacillin do not interfere.

Note : Nucleophilic species which will produce hydrobromic acid are likely to interfere in this method.

METHOD 3

This method has been found to give good results for capsules. The acidic hydrolysis of ampicillin with 1% formaldehyde in 0.3 N hydrochloric acid yields a degradation product identified as 2-hydroxy-3-phenyl-6-methyl pyrazine, which has a well-defined U.V. absorption at 380 nm (for details, refer to formation 2 of this chapter).

Note : 1. It is absolutely essential that the temperature is maintained within specified limits.

2. For dissolving ampicillin, slight warming is necessary.

Ampicillin/Amoxycillin, Cloxacillin sodium

ESTIMATION

Ampicillin/Amoxycillin

METHOD 1

Reagents

1. 0.1 N sodium hydroxide.
2. 0.1 N hydrochloric acid.
3. Phenolphthalein solution (indicator).

Procedure

Weigh accurately quantity of the sample equivalent to about 0.25 g of ampicillin and transfer to a conical flask. Add about 25 ml of freshly boiled, cooled and neutralized (phenolphthalein) water. Slightly warm in boiling water-bath and titrate immediately with 0.1 N sodium hydroxide using phenolphthalein solution as indicator till faint pink colour appears. Warm slightly and continue titration till distinct pink colour persists. The volume of 0.1 N sodium hydroxide used in the titration represents the amount of ampicillin present in the sample. Each ml of 0.1 N sodium hydroxide is equivalent to 0.03495 g of ampicillin (anhydrous) or 0.03654 g of amoxycillin.

METHOD 2

The method is based on formation of Schiff's base.

Reagents

1. 0.1% w/v solution of p-dimethyl aminocinnamaldehyde (PDAC) in methanol.
2. 50% w/v solution of trichloroacetic acid (TCA) in methanol.

Standard solution

50 mcg/ml of ampicillin in water.

Sample solution

Accurately weighed quantity of the sample was extracted with water to get a concentration of 50 mcg/ml.

Procedure

To 2 ml each of sample and standard solutions in 100 ml volumetric flasks, add 2 ml of PDAC reagent, followed by 10 ml of TCA, shake and allow to stand for 10 min and dilute to 100 ml with methanol. Keep the final diluted solution to stand at room temperature for 60 min and measure the absorbance of both sample and standard solutions at absorption maxima at about 500 nm and calculate the results by comparison.

Cloxacillin

To the solution obtained after completing the titration for ampicillin/amoxycillin (method 1), add exactly 50 ml of 0.1 N sodium hydroxide solution and heat in a boiling water-bath for not less than 30 min. Cool and titrate excess of alkali with 0.1 N hydrochloric acid till the pink colour disappears.

From the volume of sodium hydroxide consumed in the second titration, subtract the volume of alkali used in the first titration i.e. for ampicillin. The difference represents the volume of alkali consumed by cloxacillin present in the sample. Each ml of 0.1 N sodium hydroxide is equivalent to 0.04350 g of cloxacillin.

Note : 1. The method gives excellent results with solid dosage forms (capsules). However in case of dry syrups, colour present tends to interfere. Charcoal treatment can remove interference to great extent.

2. The method is not suitable if ampicillin is present as sodium salt.

METHOD 2

Reagents

1. 0.3 N hydrochloric acid.
2. 1% v/v solution of formaldehyde in 0.3 N hydrochloric acid.

Standard solution

500 mcg/ml of ampicillin, amoxycillin or cloxacillin in water.

Sample solution

Accurately weighed quantity of the sample (capsule, syrup) equivalent to 50 mg of the substance is suspended in 70-80 ml of water and sonicated for 5 min or slightly warm in boiling water-bath to ensure complete dissolution. Dilute with water to 100 ml, filter and use the filtrate for analysis.

Procedure

Dilute 2 ml each of the standard and sample solutions to 50 ml with formaldehyde reagent and proceed as under :

(a) Maintain part of both the solutions at room temperature and after 20 min measure the absorbance of sample and standard solutions at 346 nm against reagent blank and calculate the contents of cloxacillin in the sample by comparison.

(b) Heat other portion of both the sample and standard solutions at 90°C (± 0.5°C) in constant temperature water-bath for 60 min, cool to room temperature and measure the absorbance at 380 nm (ampicillin) and 397 nm (amoxycillin) against reagent blank and calculate the contents by comparison.

Note : 1. On treatment with acidic formaldehyde, β-lactam ring of penicillin present in cloxacillin opens up resulting in the formation of penicillinic acid, an intermediate compound having absorption maximum at 346 nm. Penicillinic acid being unstable undergoes further degradation to form D-penicillamine and penaldic acid, both of which have negligible absorbance. This explains the reason for decrease in absorbance after 20 min.

2. In case of ampicillin/amoxycillin, intra-molecular aminolysis occurs; as a result, α-amino-benzoyl group present in the side chain of both the drugs attack nucleophilically carbonyl group present in the β-lactam ring resulting in formation of pyrazine derivative.

3. Formaldehyde plays no role in the acid hydrolysis of cloxacillin.

4. Under acidic conditions, the free amino group is in its cationic form ($R-NH_3^+$) resulting in decrease in its nucleophilic ability and hence formation of pyrazine derivative. On addition of formaldehyde, the free amino group forms Schiff's base which being unstable in acidic medium releases unionised form of amino group which reacts with carbonyl group present in the β-lactam ring, resulting in enhanced formation of pyrazine derivative.

Amoxycillin

ESTIMATION

All the methods described below are based on phenolic function of the molecule, hence ampicillin does not interfere.

METHOD 1

Reagent

1. Dimethylaminobenzaldehyde (PDAB) reagent : Weigh 400 mg of p-dimethylamino-benzaldehyde, add 10 ml of ethyl alcohol, 2 ml of concentrated sulphuric acid and dilute to 50 ml with water.

Standard solution

1 mg/ml of amoxycillin in water.

Sample solution

Weigh material accurately equivalent to 25 mg of amoxycillin, add 15 ml of water and heat on water-bath to dissolve, adjust to 25 ml with water.

Procedure

To 2 ml of the standard and sample solutions, add 4 ml of 'PDAB' reagent and heat on water-bath at 65°C for 1 hr. Cool to room temperature and adjust to 10 ml with water. Measure the absorbance of both the solutions at about 410 nm. The method obeys Beer's law in the concentration range of 10-600 mcg/ml.

Note : 1. Penicillin G sodium and ampicillin do not give similar colour reaction.
2. 6-aminopenicillinic acid (6-APA), an impurity gives colour reaction at very high concentration, above 600 mcg/ml. For aged samples, it would be necessary to ascertain that 6-APA is not present in such samples in quantities greater than 600 mcg/ml.

METHOD 2

Reagents

1. 0.1% w/v solution of p-dimethylaminocinnamaldehyde (PDAC) in isopropyl alcohol.
2. Acetic acid-isopropanol mixture (2 : 3 v/v).

Standard solution

1 mg/ml of amoxycillin in acetic acid-isopropanol mixture.

Sample solution

Dissolve accurately measured or weighed quantity of the sample in acetic acid-isopropanol mixture to produce 1 mg/ml.

Procedure

Dilute 1 ml aliquot each of the standard and sample solutions as obtained above to 25 ml with isopropanol. To 1 ml of these solutions, add 1 ml of 'PDAC' reagent, followed by 1 ml of acetic acid. Immerse all the flasks in water-bath for 2 min, cool and dilute to 10 ml with isopropanol. Measure the absorbance at about 480 nm against a reagent blank. The colour is stable for 15 min.

Note : 1. This method has advantage over method 1 as more stable colour is obtained.
  2. This method requires only two minutes of heating while the method 1 requires longer heating period.

METHOD 3

Reagents

  1. 5% w/v solution of sodium cobaltinitrite in water.
  2. 20% w/v solution of sodium hydroxide in water.

Standard solution

0.5 mg/ml of anhydrous amoxycillin in water.

Sample solution

Weigh accurately, a quantity of sample equivalent to 250 mg of anhydrous compound and dissolve in water to produce 500 ml. Shake well and filter. Use the filtrate for estimation.

Procedure

  (a) To 2 ml each of the sample and standard solutions, add 5 ml of water, 2 ml of glacial acetic acid and 2 ml of sodium cobaltinitrite solution. Heat the solution in water-bath for 15 min, cool and dilute to 50 ml with water. Measure the absorbance of both the solutions at about 370 nm against reagent blank.
  (b) Proceed as under method (a) above. After heating for 15 minutes, cool and add 20 ml of sodium hydroxide solution. Filter, wash the precipitates with three 5 ml portions of water, collect the filtrate and dilute to 50 ml with water. Measure the absorption at about 430 nm against reagent blank.

Note : 1. 6-APA does not interfere.
  2. Procedure (b) is more sensitive.
  3. Procedure (b) is not applicable to dry syrups due to interference of excipients present.

METHOD 4

Reagents

  1. 0.04% w/v solution of 2,6-dichloroquinone chlorimide in isopropyl alcohol. The solution is stable for 7 days if stored in refrigerator.
  2. Borate buffer, pH 9.4.

Standard solution

100 mcg/ml of amoxycillin in water.

Sample solution

Accurately weighed quantity of the powdered material is extracted with water to produce 100 mcg/ml.

Procedure

To 2 ml each of standard and sample solutions, add 1.5 ml of buffer and 1.5 ml of the chlorimide reagent. Allow to stand for 5 minutes at room temperature and then dilute to 10 ml with water. Measure the absorption of blue indophenol derivative at about 620 nm against reagent blank. Calculate the results by comparison. Blue chromophore is stable for 24 h and the method obeys Beer's law in the range of 0.5-6 mcg/ml.

METHOD 5

This method is based on alkaline oxidation, followed by condensation with 4-aminophenazone. The complex has absorption maximum at about 505 nm.

Reagents

1. 1% w/v solution of sodium carbonate in water.
2. Methanol : water mixture (1 : 3 v/v)—solvent.
3. 0.5% w/v solution of 4-aminophenazone in the solvent.
4. 2% w/v solution of potassium ferricyanide in water.

Standard solution

200 mcg/ml of amoxycillin in water.

Sample solution

Accurately weighed or measured aliquot of the sample equivalent to 10 mg of amoxycillin is dissolved in water to get 50 ml (200 mcg/ml).

Procedure

To 1 ml each of sample and standard solutions, add 1 ml each of aminophenazone solution, potassium ferricyanide solution and sodium carbonate solution, dilute to 25 ml with water. The absorbance of the resulting solutions is measured at 505 nm against reagent blank. The colour reaches maximum intensity within 5 min and is stable for more than 2 h. Beer's law is obeyed in the concentration range of 4-24 mcg/ml. Other penicillins do not interfere in this method.

METHOD 6

Reagents

1. 0.05% w/v solution of N-chlorosuccinimide (NCS) or N-bromosuccinimide (NBS) in water (prepare fresh).
2. 0.1 N sodium hydroxide.

Standard solution

Dissolve 50 mg of the substance in 1 ml of methanol and dilute to 50 ml with water. Further dilutions are done with water to get solution of 50 mcg/ml.

Sample solution

Accurately weighed or measured amount of the sample equivalent to 100 mg of the substance is dissolved in 2 ml of methanol and final volume made up to 100 ml with water. Further dilutions are carried out with water to get solution of 50 mcg/ml.

Procedure

To 1 ml each of sample and standard solutions, add 1 ml of sodium hydroxide solution immediately followed by 1 ml of NCS or NBS reagent. Mix well and dilute to 10 ml with methanol. Measure the absorbance of both the solutions at 395 nm against reagent blank.

Note : 1. The intense yellow colour is stable for at least 30 min.
2. The method obeys Beer's law in the range of 1-20 mcg.
3. Amoxycillin and cefadroxil, the only phenolic compounds among the β-lactam antibiotics behave differently from the penicillins and cephalosporins on oxidation with NCS or NBS in alkaline medium.
4. The method is applicable to the estimation of cefadroxil, a phenolic compound.
5. Potassium clavulanate, cloxacillin, dicloxacillin, flucloxacillin and other related penicillins or structurally related degradation products such as penicillic acid, 6-aminopenicillinic acid and D-penicillamine do not interfere.
6. Amoxipenicilloic and amoxipenicillenic acid, alkaline and acid hydrolysis products interfere. Their interference can be eliminated by adding 0.4 ml of 0.025% methanolic solution of iodine and allowing the mixture to stand for 5 min before proceeding with the method involving oxidation with NCS or NBS.

Ampicillin, Probenecid

ESTIMATION

Probenecid

Reagents

1. Chloroform.
2. 0.1 N methanolic hydrochloric acid.

Standard solution

Prepare 100 mcg per ml solution of probenecid in chloroform. Evaporate 5 ml of it and dissolve the residue in 50 ml of 0.1 N methanolic hydrochloric acid (10 mcg/ml).

Sample solution

Weigh accurately the powdered sample equivalent to 100 mg of probenecid, extract the dry powder with three 25 ml portions of chloroform, filtering each through the same G₄ sintered glass funnel. Dilute the combined filtrate to 100 ml with chloroform. Evaporate 5 ml of the filtrate on a water-bath and take up the residue in 0.1 N methanolic hydrochloric acid to get a final concentration of 10 mcg per ml.

Measure the extinction of the sample and standard solutions at the maximum at about 248 nm using 0.1 N methanolic hydrochloric acid as blank and deduce the results by comparison.

Ampicillin

Reagents

1. 0.3 N hydrochloric acid.
2. 1% v/v formaldehyde in 0.3 N hydrochloric acid.

Standard solution

1 mg/ml of ampicillin in 0.3 N hydrochloric acid.

Sample solution

Use the entire residue left after the extraction of probenecid as described above. Dissolve the residue left in the G₄ sintered funnel in 100 ml of 0.3 N hydrochloric acid.

Procedure

Dilute 2 ml each of standard and sample solutions to 50 ml with 1% v/v formaldehyde in 0.3 N hydrochloric acid. Heat on a water-bath at 90 ± 0.5°C for 60 minutes. Cool to room temperature and measure the absorbance of both standard and sample solutions at the maximum at about 380 nm using 1% v/v formaldehyde in 0.3 N hydrochloric acid treated in the same manner as the blank and deduce the results by comparison.

Amoxycillin, Probenecid

ESTIMATION

Probenecid

Follow the method described under formulation 9 of this chapter. The method makes use of the fact that probenecid is soluble in chloroform whereas amoxycillin is totally insoluble in chloroform. The solution of the compound in 0.1 N methanolic hydrochloric acid exhibits maxima at about 248 nm. Sample equivalent to about 100 mg of probenecid is initially taken for analysis.

Amoxycillin

The residue obtained after extraction of probenecid is subjected to quantitative analysis for amoxycillin contents. For estimation, follow the method 6 described under formulation 8 of this chapter.

Cephalexin, Probenecid

ESTIMATION

Probenecid

Follow the method described under formulation 9 of this chapter. Probenecid is soluble in chloroform. Cephalexin, ampicillin and amoxycillin are insoluble in chloroform.

Cephalexin

METHOD 1

Standard solution

10 mcg/ml of cephalexin in 0.1 N methanolic hydrochloric acid.

Sample solution

The entire residue left after extraction of probenecid with chloroform is used for analysis of cephalexin. The residue left on sintered funnel is taken in 0.1 N methanolic hydrochloric acid and further diluted appropriately to get a concentration of 10 mcg/ml.

   Measure the extinction of both sample and standard solutions at maxima at about 258 nm using 0.1 N methanolic hydrochloric acid as blank and calculate the results by comparison.

METHOD 2

Reagents

  1. 50% v/v sulphuric acid.
  2. 0.1% w/v solution of ninhydrin in 50% sulphuric acid.

Standard solution

200 mcg/ml of cephalexin in water.

Sample solution

The residue left after extraction of probenecid was taken up in water.

Procedure

To 1 ml each of sample and standard solutions, add 2 ml of water, 1 ml of 50% sulphuric acid. Heat in steam-bath for 5 min, then add 2 ml of ninhydrin solution. Heat for another 10 min, cool and extract with chloroform (2 × 10 ml). Dilute the combined chloroform layer to 25 ml and measure the absorbance of both the sample and standard solutions at 520 nm within 10 min and calculate the results by comparison.

Piperazine and its salts

ESTIMATION

METHOD 1

Reagents

1. Phosphate buffer, pH 5.7.
2. Bromothymol blue solution : 0.0001 M solution of the dye in phosphate buffer of pH 5.7. The dye solution is shaken with chloroform and chloroform layer, which may be coloured, is rejected. (This step reduces the blank value).
3. Chloroform.

Standard solution

400 mcg/ml of piperazine hexahydrate in water.

Sample solution

The sample is appropriately diluted with water to get a concentration of 400 mcg/ml of piperazine hexahydrate.

Procedure

To 10 ml each of the sample and standard solutions, add 10 ml of the dye solution, mix and add 15 ml of chloroform and shake vigorously for one min. Separate chloroform layer and measure the extinction of chloroform layer at about 420 nm against reagent blank prepared by substituting water for piperazine solution. The method obeys Beer's law in the concentration range of 100 mcg/ml of piperazine hexahydrate.

METHOD 2

The method is based on spectrophotometric measurement of N-nitroso-derivative formed by interaction of piperazine with nitrous acid. This method is suitable for the complex calcium piperazine edetate (1 + 1 + 1).

Reagents

1. 1% w/v solution of sodium nitrite in water.
2. 5% w/v solution of ammonium sulphamate in water.
3. Ethyl alcohol.
4. Britton-Robinson buffer, pH 2.3 : 0.6 g of citric acid, 0.39 g of potassium dihydrogen phosphate, 0.18 g of boric acid and 0.53 g of diethyl barbituric acid in 100 ml of water.
5. 4 N hydrochloric acid.

Standard solution

100 mcg/ml of piperazine or its equivalent of citrate, adipate, phosphate or edetate salts.

Sample solution

Accurately weigh or measure composite sample (syrup, tablets, granules) equivalent to about 50 mg of piperazine (base), add 30 ml of water, shake thoroughly (in case of effervescent granules, wait until effervescence ceases; stir for 30 minutes in case of tablets) and dilute to 500 ml with water.

Procedure

To 2 ml each of the standard and sample solutions, add 1 ml of buffer solution and 0.5 ml of sodium nitrite solution. Heat at 80°C for 15 minutes on water-bath and cool. Add 1 ml of 4 N hydrochloric acid, 1 ml of ammonium sulphamate solution and 5 ml of ethyl alcohol. Shake and dilute to 100 ml with water and measure the extinction at about 249 nm against blank prepared by substituting water for the sample. The method obeys Beer's law in the concentration range of 1-15 mcg/ml of piperazine.

Note : It is a stability indicating method.

METHOD 3

Reagents

1. Saturated solution of ammonium reineckate in water, prepare fresh on day of use.
2. Wash solution : Dilute 2 ml of saturated solution of ammonium reineckate to 1000 ml with water.
3. Hydrochloric acid.
4. Acetone.

Standard solution

1 mg/ml of piperazine hexahydrate or its equivalent citrate, phosphate, edetate or adipate in water.

Sample solution

Accurately weigh or measure quantity of the sample equivalent to about 100 mg of the compound, add 50-60 ml water, shake, filter and make up the volume to 100 ml with water (1 mg/ml).

Procedure

To 20 ml each of the standard and sample solutions, add 3 ml of hydrochloric acid and 25 ml of saturated solution of ammonium reineckate. Mix and allow to stand for 15 min. Filter the precipitates through G_4 sintered glass funnel. Wash the precipitates with 4 ml of wash solution. Transfer the precipitates to 50 ml volumetric flask with the help of acetone and adjust the volume with acetone. Measure the absorbance at about 525 nm using acetone as blank. Calculate the results by comparison.

METHOD 4

Reagents

1. 4% w/v solution of 2,6-dichloroquinone chlorimide in isopropyl alcohol.
2. Isopropyl alcohol.
3. Hydrochloric acid.

Standard solution

7.5 mcg/ml of piperazine or its corresponding salt in water.

Sample solution

(a) Tablets or granules : Accurately weigh a quantity of powdered tablets equivalent to about 0.3 g of the piperazine. Add 20 ml of water and shake for 1 h. Filter, wash the residue with five

15 ml portions of water and dilute the combined filtrate to 100 ml. Further dilute the solution with water to get a concentration of 7.5 mcg/ml.

(b) Syrups : Dilute the sample with water to get a concentration of 7.5 mcg/ml.

Procedure

To 5 ml each of the sample and standard solutions, add 1 ml of chlorimide reagent. Heat gently on water-bath for 30 minutes, cool to room temperature and add 1 ml of hydrochloric acid. Adjust the volume to 25 ml with water and measure the extinction at about 525 nm against reagent blank. The method obeys Beer's law in the concentration range of 5-50 mcg/ml.

METHOD 5

Reagents

1. 1% w/v solution of trinitrophenol (picric acid) in water.
2. 10% w/v sulphuric acid : 5 ml of concentrated sulphuric acid is diluted to 100 ml with water.
3. Piperazine dipicrate, wash solution : To 200 mg of piperazine in a beaker, add 10 ml 1 N sulphuric acid, 20 ml of water, mix and add 100 ml of phenol solution. Allow to stand for two hours and filter through a medium porosity (G_2) sintered glass crucible. Wash the precipitates with water till the filtrate is free of sulphate. Transfer the residue to a two litre bottle, add water and shake for two hours. Filter this solution and use as wash solution as described in the procedure.

Procedure

Transfer 5 ml of homogeneous suspension of the sample to a 50 ml volumetric flask, rinsing the pipette with water into the flask, add water to volume, mix and filter. To 5 ml of the sample filtrate in a beaker, add 10 ml of 10% sulphuric acid, 15 ml water, mix and add 100 ml of trinitrophenol solution. Allow to stand for two hours and filter through a pre-tared medium porosity (G_2) sintered glass crucible, washing the beaker and crucible with five 20 ml portions of piperazine dipicrate wash solution. Dry the residue at 105°C for 2 hours, cool and weigh.

Anhydrous piperazine (mg) = mg of the residue × 0.1582 × dilution factor

Typical laboratory analysis

Each 5 ml of the sample is labelled to contain 750 mg of piperazine citrate

Quantity of the sample taken for analysis = 2 ml

Weight of the precipitates obtained (as dipicrate) = 0.659 g

Each g of the precipitate (dipicrate) is equal to 0.357 g of piperazine hexahydrate

Contents of piperazine hexahydrate/5 ml of the sample $= \dfrac{0.659 \times 0.357 \times 5}{2}$

$$= 0.5874 \text{ g}$$

0.5874 g of piperazine hexahydrate = 0.734 g of piperazine citrate

or 100 mg of piperazine hexahydrate = 125 mg of piperazine citrate

Contents of piperazine citrate $= \dfrac{0.659}{2} \times \dfrac{0.357}{1} \times \dfrac{5}{1} \times \dfrac{125}{100}$

$$= 734 \text{ mg}$$
$$\text{Claim} = 750 \text{ mg}$$

METHOD 6

Reagents

2. 10% w/v solution of sodium hydroxide in water.

Standard solution

250 mcg/ml of piperazine in chloroform.

Sample solution

Piperazine salts such as hexahydrate, phosphate, adipate or citrate, equivalent to 25 mg of piperazine (base) are quantitatively dissolved in 20-30 ml of water, add 10 ml of sodium hydroxide solution and extract with three 30 ml portions of chloroform. The combined organic extract is made up to 100 ml with chloroform.

Procedure

To 2 ml each of sample and standard solutions, add 1 ml of benzoquinone reagent. Mix and dilute to 10 ml with chloroform. After 3 minutes, measure the absorbance of both the solutions at about 590 nm using reagent blank. The method obeys Beer's law in the concentration range of 5-50 mcg/ml and the coloured complex is stable for 24 hrs.

METHOD 7

Two secondary amino groups of piperazine condense with acetaldehyde to form N,N-divinylpiperazine (a strong nucleophile) which displaces chloro group from DDQ to produce substituted coloured quinone.

Reagents

1. 10% w/v solution of acetaldehyde in dioxane or dichloromethane.
2. 0.5% w/v solution of dichlordicyanobenzoquinone (DDQ) in dioxane or dichloromethane.

Standard solution

100 mcg/ml of piperazine in dioxane or dichloromethane.

Sample solution

Dilute or extract appropriate aliquot of the sample with dioxane or dichloromethane to get 100 mcg/ml.

Procedure

To 1 ml each of sample and standard solutions, add 0.1 ml of acetaldehyde solution and 0.1 ml of benzoquinone reagent. Heat for 3 minutes in water-bath maintained at 70°C, cool to room temperature and dilute to 10 ml with dioxane or dichloromethane. Measure the absorbance of both the solutions at about 570 nm (dioxane) or 600 nm (dichloromethane) using reagent blank prepared with 1 ml of the solvent. The method obeys Beer's law in the concentration range of 1-12 mcg/ml.

Note : 1. The method is insensitive for primary and tertiary amines.
2. The coloured product exhibits two maxima; at 330 and 570 nm in dioxane and at 330 and 600 nm in dichloromethane.
3. The developed chromogen is stable at least for 1 hour.
4. Methanol, ethanol, acetone, n-butanol, benzene, dioxane, dichloromethane, isopropanol have been examined as solvents for dilution, but dioxane and dichloromethane have been found to be best as they yield highest absorption values and most stable coloured complex.
5. 2,3-dichloro-1,4-naphthoquinone reagent prepared in DMS can also be used instead of DDQ and colour developed at room temperature; Beer's law 0.5-3 mcg/ml, λ_{max} 580 nm.

Piperazine, Pyrvinium pamoate

ESTIMATION

Pyrvinium pamoate

Standard solution

Weigh accurately about 57 mg of pyrvinium pamoate and transfer quantitatively into 50 ml volumetric flask. Dissolve in and dilute to volume with dimethylformamide. Pipette 1 ml of this solution into 100 ml volumetric flask and dilute to volume with the same solvent. Use low actinic glassware in preparing solutions of pyrvinium pamoate.

Sample solution

Transfer a volume of homogeneous sample suspension equivalent to 57 mg of pyrvinium pamoate into a 100 ml volumetric flask. Wash the pipette with two 3 ml portions of water, followed by three 20 ml portions of dimethylformamide into the flask to ensure complete transfer of the contents. Mix the contents and heat on a water-bath until all of the pyrvinium pamoate is dissolved (it takes about 30 minutes). Cool to about 25°C, add dimethylformamide to volume and mix. Centrifuge a portion of this mixture and dilute 3 ml of the clear supernatant liquid to 100 ml with dimethylformamide, mix.

Concomitantly measure the absorbance of the sample and standard solutions against dimethyl-formamide as blank at about 508 nm.

Note : Complete the procedure without prolonged interruption.

Calculations

$$\text{Pyrvinium base (mg) per ml} = \frac{A_u}{A_s} \times \frac{0.6644}{1} \times \frac{S}{V} \times d_f.$$

where A_u = absorbance of the sample solution; A_s = absorbance of the standard solution; V = volume of the sample taken for analysis; S = weight of the standard taken for analysis; d_f = dilution factor.

0.6644 is the factor for the conversion of anhydrous pyrvinium pamoate (575.71) to the formula weight of pyrvinium base (382.53) ratio.

$$\frac{382.53}{575.71} = 0.6644$$

Piperazine

Follow method 5 as described under formulation 12 of this chapter.

Mebendazole

ESTIMATION

METHOD 1

This involves alkaline hydrolysis of the compound to 2-amino-5-benzyol benzimidazole and measurement of the resultant yellow colour at 420 nm.

Reagents

1. Formic acid (90%).
2. Formic acid-isopropyl alcohol mixture (1 : 9 v/v).
3. Methanol.
4. 30% w/v solution of potassium hydroxide in water.

Standard solution

To 25 mg of mebendazole, accurately weighed, add 2.5 ml of formic acid, shake to dissolve and make up the volume to 25 ml with isopropyl alcohol (1 mg/ml).

Sample solution

Weigh accurately a quantity of powdered tablets equivalent to 50 mg of the compound. Add 40 ml of formic acid-isopropanol mixture, shake for 5 minutes and filter. Wash the residue with two 5 ml portions of the mixture and adjust the volume to 50 ml with above mixture (1 mg/ml).

Procedure

To 2 ml each of standard and sample solutions, add 3 ml of methanol and 3 ml of potassium hydroxide solutions. Allow to stand for 30 minutes for maximum colour to develop. The absorbance of both the solutions is measured at about 420 nm against reagent blank. The method obeys Beer's law in the concentration range of 25-250 mcg/ml.

METHOD 2

Standard solution

To 50 mg of pure compound accurately weighed, add 10 ml of perchloric acid, shake and dilute to 50 ml with water (1 mg/ml). 1 ml of this solution is further diluted to 100 ml with water (10 mcg/ml).

Sample solution

Powdered tablets equivalent to 50 mg of the compound are accurately weighed and to this, 10 ml of perchloric acid (70%) is added. Shake for 10 minutes and dilute to 50 ml with water. 1 ml of this solution is further diluted with water to get 10 mcg/ml of mebendazole.

Measure the extinction of sample and standard solutions at 288 nm against blank prepared by mixing 0.2 ml of perchloric acid with 89.8 ml of water. The method obeys Beer's law in the range of 5-15 mcg/ml.

METHOD 3

When dissolved in appropriate solvent, mebendazole exhibits either basic or acidic properties.

(a) **Basic equivalent :** Accurately weigh a quantity of sample equivalent to about 250 mg of mebendazole and dissolve in 125 ml of glacial acetic acid. Warm, cool, filter, wash the residue in the flask with two 10 ml portions of glacial acetic acid and filter. Titrate the combined filtrate with 0.1 N perchloric acid using crystal violet solution as indicator. Each ml of 0.1 N perchloric acid is equivalent to 0.02953 g of mebendazole.

(b) **Acid equivalent.**

Reagents

1. 0.1% w/v solution of thymol blue in methanol (indicator).
2. Neutral dimethylformamide : Add 10 drops of thymol blue solution to 50 ml of dimethyl-formamide and neutralize to blue end point with 0.02 N sodium methoxide.
3. 0.02 N sodium methoxide.

Procedure

Accurately weigh powdered tablets equivalent to 50 mg of mebendazole, dissolve in neutralized (thymol blue) dimethylformamide and titrate with 0.02 N sodium methoxide to a green end point. Each ml of 0.02 N sodium methoxide corresponds to 0.005906 g of mebendazole.

Mebendazole, Levamisole hydrochloride

ESTIMATION

Mebendazole

METHOD 1

Standard solution

To an accurately weighed about 50 mg of the substance, add 10 ml of formic acid, keep in boiling water-bath for few minutes. Add 70 ml of isopropyl alcohol, cool to room temperature and make up the volume (100 ml). Dilute further appropriately with isopropyl alcohol to get 10 mcg/ml.

Sample solution

Weigh powdered sample accurately equivalent to 50 mg of the substance. Add 10 ml of formic acid and keep in boiling water-bath and make up to 100 ml with isopropyl alcohol. Shake well and centrifuge at moderate speed to get clear solution. The resultant clear solution is further diluted appropriately with isopropyl alcohol to get 10 mcg/ml.

Measure the extinction of both sample and standard solutions at maximum at about 310 nm using isopropyl alcohol as blank. Calculate the results by comparison.

METHOD 2

The residue obtained during dry extraction of levamisole under method 2, is taken up in glacial acetic acid for non-aqueous titration using crystal violet as indicator. Each ml of 0.1 N perchloric acid is equivalent to 0.02953 g of mebendazole.

Levamisole hydrochloride

METHOD 1

Reagents

1. 6% w/v solution of sodium hydroxide in water.
2. 5% w/v solution of sodium nitroprusside in water.
3. 2% w/v boric acid in water.

Standard solution

250 mcg/ml of levamisole hydrochloride in water.

Sample solution

Transfer accurately weighed powdered sample equivalent to 50 mg of levamisole to a 200 ml volumetric flask. Add about 150 ml of water, shake well and make up the volume. Centrifuge and use the clear supernatant solution for estimation (250 mcg/ml).

Procedure

To 1 ml each of sample and standard solutions, add 0.5 ml of sodium hydroxide solution and 1 ml of nitroprusside solution, followed by 5 ml of boric acid solution. Shake well and allow to stand for 2 minutes, dilute to 10 ml with water. The absorption of resultant purple coloured solution is measured at about 540 nm against reagent blank. Calculate the results by comparison. Each g of levamisole hydrochloride is equivalent to 0.8486 g of levamisole (base).

METHOD 2

Weigh accurately powdered sample equivalent to 100 mg of levamisole. Extract the dry powder with four 25 ml portions of chloroform (retain the residue for estimation of mebendazole). Pass the organic layer through anhydrous sodium sulphate. Evaporate to about 50 ml, add glacial acetic acid. Carry out non-aqueous titration using brilliant green solution as indicator. Each ml of 0.1 N perchloric acid is equivalent to 0.02408 g of levamisole.

Diethylcarbamazine citrate, Chlorpheniramine maleate

ESTIMATION

Diethylcarbamazine citrate

Reagent

1. 20% w/v sodium hydroxide solution in water.

Procedure

Take the powdered sample equivalent to about 30 mg of diethylcarbamazine citrate in a 250 ml separating funnel. Add 75 ml of water and 5 ml of sodium hydroxide solution and extract with three 25 ml portions of chloroform. Dry combined chloroform layer by passing through anhydrous sodium sulphate and titrate with 0.1 N perchloric acid using thymol blue as indicator. Each ml of 0.1 N perchloric acid is equivalent to 0.03914 g of diethylcarbamazine citrate.

Chlorpheniramine maleate

Procedure

Take the sample equivalent to about 10 mg of chlorpheniramine maleate, add solution of sodium hydroxide (50% w/v) to produce pH of about 11.0. Transfer the mixture to a 500 ml separator with the aid of three 10 ml portions of saturated solution of sodium chloride and extract with two 50 ml portions of n-hexane. Shake gently to avoid formation of emulsion. Wash the combined organic extract with 2 × 10 ml of water. Wash the aqueous layer with 2 × 20 ml of n-hexane and discard the aqueous layer. Pass the combined hexane layer through cotton and evaporate to dryness. To the residue, add 5 ml of acetic anhydride and 25 ml of glacial acetic acid and allow to stand for 15 minutes. Add 2 drops of crystal violet indicator and titrate with 0.01 N perchloric acid. Each ml of 0.01 N perchloric acid is equivalent to 0.001945 g of chlorpheniramine maleate.

Chapter 9

Anti-Inflammatory Drugs

Formulation 1

Analgin, Phenylbutazone/Calcium phenylbutazone, Dried aluminium hydroxide gel, Magnesium trisilicate, Diazepam

ESTIMATION

Analgin

METHOD 1

Weigh accurately a quantity of the sample equivalent to 500 mg of analgin and transfer to a 250 ml conical flask. Add 25 ml of alcohol and 5 ml of 0.01 N hydrochloric acid. Shake well to dissolve analgin and titrate immediately with 0.1 N iodine till yellow colour of iodine persists for about 30–60 seconds. Each ml of 0.1 N iodine is equivalent to 0.01757 g of analgin.

METHOD 2

This method involves the formation of formaldehyde which reacts with chromotropic acid to give pink coloured complex with maxima at 550 nm.

Reagents

1. Sulphuric acid.
2. 2.5% w/v solution of chromotropic acid (sodium salt) in water.

Standard solution

50 mcg/ml of analgin in water.

Sample solution

Weigh powdered material equivalent to 50 mg of analgin, add about 50 ml of water and allow to stand for 1 hr, shaking occasionally. Make up the volume to 1000 ml with water. Filter, collect the filtrate, rejecting first few millilitres.

Procedure

To 1 ml each of the sample and standard solutions, add drop by drop, 10 ml of sulphuric acid (previously cooled in ice) to each flask, keeping flask in ice-bath. Allow to stand in ice-bath for about 5 minutes. Add 1 ml of chromotropic acid solution and allow to stand in ice-bath for 45 minutes. Bring it to room temperature and measure the extinction of both the solutions at about 550 nm against blank, prepared by using 1 ml of water instead of chromotropic acid solution and calculate the results.

Note : 1. Above experiment conducted at room temperature has been found to give reproductive results. The maximum intensity of the colour is obtained within 5 minutes.
2. Paracetamol and caffeine do not interfere.

Aluminium hydroxide and Magnesium trisilicate

Preparation of sample solution

Weigh accurately a quantity of the powdered tablets equivalent to 500 mg of aluminium hydroxide in a silica crucible and ash it in a furnace till almost white. Cool and dissolve the ash in 10 ml of concentrated hydrochloric acid. Transfer it into a 100 ml volumetric flask quantitatively, warm if necessary, cool and make up the volume with water.

(a) **Estimation of aluminium :** 25 ml of above sample solution taken in 250 ml conical flask is neutralized with sodium hydroxide solution (Congo red paper). Follow the method 3 for estimation of aluminium described in formulation 1 of the chapter on antacids. Each ml of 0.05 M sodium edetate is equivalent to 0.001349 g of aluminium.

(b) **Estimation of magnesium trisilicate :** To 25 ml of the above sample solution, add 1 g of ammonium chloride and 10 ml or sufficient quantity of triethanolamine to dissolve precipitates. Add 150 ml of water and 5 ml ammonia-ammonium chloride buffer solution. Add few drops of mordant black-II solution as an indicator and titrate immediately with 0.05 M disodium edetate solution till full blue colour is obtained. Each ml of 0.05 M edetate is equivalent to 0.001215 g of magnesium.

Note : Phenylbutazone and oxyphenbutazone tablets are often coated with calcium carbonate which will interfere in the estimation of magnesium as it will consume considerable quantity of edetate solution. The following procedure is recommended in which calcium is first removed as oxalate.

To accurately weighed powder equivalent to 100 mg of magnesium trisilicate, add 2-3 ml of hydrochloric acid and few ml of water. Place on steam-bath for 5-10 minutes to dissolve as much as possible and adjust the volume to 100 ml. Shake well, set aside for 15 minutes and filter. To 15 ml of the filtrate, add 0.5 g of ammonium chloride, 0.5 g of ammonium oxalate and shake to dissolve. Neutralize the solution to litmus paper with dilute ammonia, and then add slight excess. Boil for few minutes and keep at room temperature for 2 h. Filter, wash precipitates 3-4 times with water. The combined filtrate is titrated with 0.02 M edetate for magnesium contents.

Diazepam

It is hydrolysed to 2-methylamino-5-chlorobenzophenone and yellow colour is measured at 410 nm.

Standard stock solution

Accurately weigh about 100 mg of diazepam standard and transfer to 100 ml volumetric flask, dissolve in alcohol and make volume with alcohol.

Working standard

20 ml of the standard stock solution is diluted to 100 ml with alcohol (200 mcg/ml).

Sample solution

Weigh accurately sample equivalent to 10 mg of diazepam and transfer to 50 ml volumetric flask. Add about 40 ml alcohol, carefully boil for one minute on steam-bath by shaking, cool and dilute to volume with alcohol. Filter solution through Whatman filter paper (No. 1), discard first 10 ml and collect the remaining filtrate.

Procedure

Place 5 ml each of sample and standard solutions in duplicate into separate 100 ml boiling tubes. Add 25 ml of 6 N hydrochloric acid, plug tubes loosely with cotton wool and heat for 1 h in boiling water-bath. Cool to room temperature by dipping in cold water. Extract solution with four 10 ml portions of chloroform. Combine chloroform extracts and make to 50 ml with chloroform in dry volumetric flask. Measure absorbance of both the solutions at about 410 nm against solvent blank. The method obeys Beer's law in the concentration range of 1-30 mcg/ml. Simultaneously take 5 ml aliquot of the sample and standard and treat as above except hydrolysis. Measure their absorbance and subtract the values from the respective hydrolysed values to get net extinction values which are used for calculations.

Note : 1. Vitamin B_6, common excipients and colouring agents do not interfere.
          2. The method can be applied to other 1,4-benzodiazepines such as chlordiazepoxide.

Phenylbutazone/Calcium phenylbutazone

Weigh a quantity of the sample accurately equivalent to 400 mg of phenylbutazone, add 50 ml of neutral acetone (bromothymol blue). Boil on water-bath and filter. Wash the residue with neutral acetone and titrate the combined acetone extract with 0.1 N sodium hydroxide. Each ml of 0.1 N sodium hydroxide is equivalent to 0.03084 g of phenyl-butazone or 0.03630 g of calcium phenylbutazone or 0.03302 g of sodium phenylbutazone or 0.03424 g of oxyphenbutazone.

Note : 1. It has been observed that in formulations containing phenylbutazone and oxyphenbutazone along with magnesium trisilicate, analgin, paracetamol, lower assay values are obtained in respect of phenylbutazone/oxyphenbutazone when determined by the usual method involving acetone extraction, followed by alkaline titration. This problem is more serious with the older sample. This is probably due to adsorption of phenylbutazone/oxyphenbutazone by magnesium trisilicate. The following method has been found to give satisfactory results :
"Take powder accurately weighed equivalent to 250-300 mg of the substance. Add 25-30 ml of dilute sulphuric acid and heat in boiling water-bath for 30 minutes under reflux condenser. Cool and extract with four 25 ml portions of chloroform or ether. Wash each organic layer with the same 10 ml of water. Evaporate organic layer, the last traces of organic layer should be removed under current of air, otherwise there are chances of decomposition in case of phenylbutazone. Dissolve the residue in neutral acetone and carry out the titration as above. This extraction procedure is also essential for injectible and liquid formulations."
          2. Diphenhydramine, salicylamide, thiamine hydrochloride and ascorbic acid do not interfere.

Oxyphenbutazone, Diazepam, Pyridoxine hydrochloride

ESTIMATION

Oxyphenbutazone

Weigh accurately a quantity of the sample equivalent to 400 mg of oxyphenbutazone, add 4 ml of hydrochloric acid, 1 g of sodium chloride and extract with ether or chloroform. Evaporate organic layer and take up the residue in neutral acetone (bromothymol blue) and titrate with 0.1 N sodium hydroxide. Each ml of 0.1 N sodium hydroxide is equivalent to 0.03424 g of oxyphenbutazone.

Note : If the sample is first suspended in appropriate quantity of 0.1 N sodium hydroxide, filtered and then acidified for extraction, it will ensure complete extraction of the substance from matrix (see formulation 2 of this chapter).

Diazepam

Weigh accurately quantity of the sample equivalent to 2 mg of diazepam and carry out the estimation as described in formulation 9 of the chapter on analgesics and antipyretics, involving extraction from buffer solution, pH 7.0 or 9.0, followed by extinction at 368 nm in acidified methanol.

Note : Diazepam solution in acidified methanol exhibits maxima at 284 and 368 nm. Pyridoxine hydrochloride having maxima at 291 nm will interfere at 284 nm, hence extinction should be taken at 368 nm.

Alternatively the compound can be subjected to acid hydrolysis and the coloured product measured at 410 nm. For details refer to formulation 1 of this chapter.

Pyridoxine hydrochloride

Follow the method 3 for estimation of pyridoxine hydrochloride as described under general analytical methods for vitamins.

Formulation 3

Aspirin, Oxyphenbutazone, Diazepam, Dried aluminium hydroxide gel

ESTIMATION

Oxyphenbutazone

METHOD 1

This is based on pH induced changes.

Standard solution

20 mg of the pure substance is dissolved in 25 ml of ethyl alcohol and diluted to 200 ml with water, 100 mcg/ml (A).

    (a) 5 ml of solution (A) is diluted to 50 ml with 0.01 N sodium hydroxide (10 mcg/ml).
    (b) 5 ml of solution (A) is diluted to 50 ml with 0.01 N sulphuric acid (10 mcg/ml).

Sample solution

Accurately weighed quantity of the sample equivalent to 20 mg of oxyphenbutazone is extracted with alcohol and diluted with water to get 100 mcg/ml. Further dilutions are carried out with acid alkali as described under standard solution to get solution (a) and (b).

Procedure

Record the extinction of solution (a) of both standard and sample solutions against solution (b) as blank. Both standard and sample solutions exhibit maximum at about 260 nm. The results are calculated by comparison.

METHOD 2

Reagents

    1. 1% w/v solution of vanillin in glacial acetic acid.
    2. 4% w/v solution of p-dimethylaminobenzaldehyde (PDAB) in glacial acetic acid.

Standard solution

1 mg/ml of oxyphenbutazone in glacial acetic acid.

Sample solution

Weigh accurately sample equivalent to 100 mg of oxyphenbutazone and extract with five 15 ml portions of glacial acetic acid. Filter through G$_4$ glass sintered funnel, wash the funnel with glacial acetic acid and dilute the filtrate to 100 ml with glacial acetic acid.

Procedure

To 1 ml each of the standard and sample solutions, add 2 ml of hydrochloric acid and keep on water-bath for 30 minutes, cool under running water. To each flask, add 2 ml of either vanillin or 'PDAB' reagent and dilute to 10 ml with glacial acetic acid. Keep for 10 minutes and measure the absorbance of both the solutions as about 424 nm (vanillin reagent) and at 406 nm (dimethylaminobenzaldehyde reagent) using respective reagent blank.

Aspirin

METHOD 1

Extract accurately weighed quantity of the sample equivalent to 10 mg of aspirin with 0.5 N sodium hydroxide by boiling for 10 minutes and dilute to 100 ml with 0.5 N sodium hydroxide. Dilute further with the same solvent to get 20 mcg/ml and measure the extinction at 300 nm. Calculate the results by using a value of 260 as A 1%, 1 cm for salicylic acid at 300 nm.

METHOD 2

Standard solution

10 mcg/ml of aspirin in 0.1 N sulphuric acid.

Sample solution

10 mcg/ml of aspirin in 0.1 N sulphuric acid.

Procedure

Measure the extinction of the solutions at maximum at about 230 nm using 0.1 N sulphuric acid as blank. Calculate the results by comparison.

Diazepam

Sample accurately weighed equivalent to 10 mg of diazepam is extracted with ethyl alcohol to get 10 ml. The volume of the sample solution equivalent to 1 mg of the substance is hydrolysed with 6 N hydrochloric acid to give 2-methylamino-5-chlorobenzophenone which is extracted into chloroform and absorbance of yellow colour measured at 410 nm. For details, refer to formulation 1 of this chapter or follow the method involving extraction with chloroform from phosphate buffer, pH 7.0 or 9.0 followed by extinction measurement at 368 nm in acidified methanol. For details, refer to formulation 25 of the chapter on analgesics and antipyretics.

Aluminium hydroxide

Follow the sodium edetate titration method described in formulation 1 of the chapter on antacids.

Phenylbutazone/Oxyphenbutazone, Salicylamide

ESTIMATION

Phenylbutazone and Salicylamide

This method is based on ultraviolet spectrophotometric measurements in 0.1 N sodium hydroxide at their respective maxima i.e. 264 and 328 nm. They do not interfere with each other at their respective maxima and can be estimated without prior separation.

Standard solution of phenylbutazone

10 mcg/ml of phenylbutazone in 0.1 N sodium hydroxide.

Standard solution of salicylamide

10 mcg/ml of salicylamide in 0.1 N sodium hydroxide.

Sample solution

Weigh accurately powdered tablets equivalent to 50 mg of salicylamide and extract with 0.1 N sodium hydroxide to get a concentration of 10 mcg/ml in respect of salicylamide.

Procedure

Measure the extinction of the sample and standard solutions at 264 nm and 328 nm and calculate the results from A 1%, 1 cm values at their respective maxima.

Phenylbutazone exhibits maxima at 264 nm (A 1%, 1 cm = 660) and salicylamide at 328 nm (A 1%, 1 cm = 435).

Oxyphenbutazone in 0.1 N sodium hydroxide exhibits maxima at 254 nm with A 1%, 1 cm value of 750.

Phenylbutazone, Paracetamol

ESTIMATION

Paracetamol

METHOD 1

Weigh accurately a quantity of the sample equivalent to 50 mg of paracetamol, add 50 ml of 0.1 N hydrochloric acid, shake and dilute to 100 ml with acid. Filter and collect the filtrate. To 10 ml of the filtrate, add 10 ml of 0.1 N sodium hydroxide and dilute to 100 ml with water. To 10 ml of the resultant solution, add 10 ml of 0.1 N sodium hydroxide and dilute to 100 ml with water. Mix well and measure absorbance of the above solution at 257 nm against blank prepared by mixing 10 ml of 0.1 N sodium hydroxide with 90 ml of water. Calculate the results taking 715 as value of E 1%, 1 cm of paracetamol at 257 nm.

METHOD 2

This method is based on the formulation of a complex (Schiff's base) with p-dimethylamino-benzaldehyde after hydrolysis, which has absorption maxima at about 440 nm.

Reagents

1. Dilute hydrochloric acid.
2. 3% w/v solution of p-dimethylaminobenzaldehyde (PDAB) in alcohol.

Standard solution

0.5 mg/ml of paracetamol in water, shake to dissolve.

Sample solution

Weigh accurately a quantity of the sample equivalent to 25 mg of paracetamol. Add about 40 ml of water and shake for 10-15 min. Dilute to 50 ml and filter.

Hydrolysis of sample and standard solutions

To 25 ml of the sample and standard solutions as prepared above, add 10 ml of dilute hydrochloric acid. Heat on water-bath for 60 min, cool and dilute to 100 ml with water.

Procedure

To 2 ml of hydrolysed solutions of sample and standard, add 2 ml of dilute hydrochloric acid and 5 ml of (PDAB) reagent. Mix and dilute to 50 ml with alcohol. Measure the extinction of golden yellow complex at about 440 nm against reagent blank, treated similarly.

Note : Analgin, caffeine, phenylbutazone, meprobamate, chloroquine phosphate, oxyphenbutazone, diazepam, dextropropoxyphene and noscapine do not interfere.

The colorimetric method for paracetamol described in formulation 25 of the chapter on analgesics and antipyretics can be used in such combination. This method involves bathochromic shift from 249 to 463 nm in alkaline medium. The method described in formulation 6 of this chapter can also be used.

Phenylbutazone

Weigh a quantity of the sample, equivalent to 200 mg of phenylbutazone. Extract with four 30 ml portions of chloroform. Combine and evaporate total chloroform extract (see instruction for evaporation under formulation 1 of this chapter). For further details, refer to formulation 1 of .this chapter.

Note : For complete extraction from matrix, refer to note under estimation of oxyphenbutazone in formulation 2 of this chapter.

Alternatively, the method based on the fact that paracetamol is soluble in 0.1 N hydrochloric acid, whereas both phenylbutazone and oxyphenbutazone are insoluble in acid. For details of the procedure, refer to formulation 7 of this chapter. Phenylbutazone thus separated can be taken up in 0.1 N sodium hydroxide and contents calculated by using 660 as value of A 1%, 1 cm at 264 nm.

Paracetamol, Oxyphenbutazone, Magnesium trisilicate

ESTIMATION

Paracetamol

Standard solution

10 mcg/ml of paracetamol in 0.1 N hydrochloric acid.

Sample solution

Extract an accurately weighed quantity of the sample equivalent to about 100 mg of paracetamol with three 25 ml portions of 1 N hydrochloric acid. Filter through G_4 sintered glass funnel. Collect the filtrate and dilute to 100 ml with acid. Dilute appropriately with 0.1 N hydrochloric acid to get a final concentration of 10 mcg/ml.

Concomitantly measure the extinction of both sample and standard solutions at maxima at about 242 nm using 0.1 N hydrochloric acid as blank. Deduce the results by comparison.

Oxyphenbutazone

Standard solution

10 mcg/ml of oxyphenbutazone in 0.01 N sodium hydroxide solution.

Sample solution

Use the entire residue left after extraction of paracetamol as described above. Transfer the powder left in the flask and on the top of sintered funnel to 100 ml volumetric flask with the aid of 0.01 N sodium hydroxide. Further dilute appropriately with 0.01 N sodium hydroxide to get a final concentration of 10 mcg/ml.

Simultaneously measure the extinction of both the solutions at maxima at about 254 nm and calculate the results by comparison. Alternatively dissolve the entire residue in neutral (phenolphthalein or bromothymol blue) acetone and titrate with 0.1 N sodium hydroxide. Each ml of 0.1 N sodium hydroxide solution is equivalent to 0.03424 g of oxyphenbutazone.

Magnesium trisilicate

Follow the method described in formulation 1 of this chapter.

Oxyphenbutazone, Paracetamol, Diazepam, Dextropropoxyphene hydrochloride, Dicyclomine hydrochloride

ESTIMATION

Oxyphenbutazone

Follow the method described in formulation 2 or 3 of this chapter.

Paracetamol

METHOD 1

In this method, advantage is taken of the fact that paracetamol is sparingly soluble in water and oxyphenbutazone is insoluble in water.

Standard solution

Dissolve 100 mg of paracetamol in 10 ml of alcohol and dilute with water to 100 ml. 1 ml of this solution is further diluted with water to 100 ml (10 mcg/ml).

Sample solution

Weigh accurately the sample equivalent to 250 mg of paracetamol. Add 50 ml of water, shake vigorously and dilute to 200 ml with water. Filter and dilute 1 ml of the filtrate to 100 ml with water.

Measure the absorbance of both the solutions at about 244 nm against blank and calculate the results by comparison.

Note : 1. By using 0.1 N hydrochloric acid instead of water, better separation is obtained.

2. Dextropropoxyphene hydrochloride being poor UV absorbing compound, does not interfere.

METHOD 2

Suspend accurately weighed amount of the sample equivalent to 50 mg of the compound in 20 ml of water and extract with three 30 ml portions of chloroform, washing each chloroform layer with the same 20 ml of water. Combine aqueous layers, add 50 ml of 0.1 N sodium hydroxide and dilute with water to 200 ml. 2 ml of the resulting solution is further diluted to 200 ml with 0.01 N sodium hydroxide. Measure extinction of the solution at 257 nm and calculate the results by comparing with the standard solution (10 mcg/ml in 0.01 N sodium hydroxide). Alternatively, calculate the amount of paracetamol taking 715 as value of A 1%, 1 cm at 257 nm (see method 1 for paracetamol under formulation 5 of this chapter).

Diazepam

This method is based on the fact that at 362 nm, paracetamol shows no absorption and oxyphenbutazone is insoluble in 0.1 N hydrochloric acid, the medium used for extraction of diazepam. Hence both the ingredients, oxyphenbutazone and paracetamol, do not interfere in the method described below.

Standard solution

20 mcg/ml of diazepam in 0.1 N hydrochloric acid.

Sample solution

Weigh accurately powdered material equivalent to 2 mg of the substance and dilute to 100 ml with acid and filter.

Measure the absorbance of both the solutions at 362 nm against 0.1 N hydrochloric acid as blank and calculate the results by comparison.

Note : Analgin and diphenhydramine do not interfere in this method.

Dextropropoxyphene hydrochloride

Weigh sample accurately equivalent to 350 mg of dextropropoxyphene hydrochloride and suspend in 15-20 ml of water. Add 1 g of sodium chloride and 3.5 ml of 2 N sodium hydroxide. Extract with four 25 ml portions of chloroform, washing each chloroform layer with the same 20 ml of water. Filter organic layer through anhydrous sodium sulphate and evaporate on a water-bath, removing last 5 ml of the extract under current of air. To the residue, add 30 ml of glacial acetic acid and warm on water-bath to dissolve. Carry out the non-aqueous titration using crystal violet solution or α-naphthol-benzein solution as indicator. From the total volume of 0.1 N perchloric acid consumed in the above titration, subtract the volume equivalent to diazepam contents as estimated above to get net volume of the acid equivalent to dextropropoxyphene contents. Each ml of 0.1 N perchloric acid is equivalent to 0.03759 g of dextropropoxyphene hydrochloride.

Note : On basification, both oxyphenbutazone and paracetamol remain in aqueous medium and do not get extracted into chloroform, hence no interference.

Alternatively, the combined chloroform extract after passing through anhydrous sodium sulphate is reduced to 10 ml and subjected to optical measurements for quantitation. For details, refer to formulation 26 of the chapter on analgesics and antipyretics.

Dicyclomine hydrochloride

Reagents

1. 0.04 M sodium lauryl sulphide (SLS). If precipitates appear, discard the solution.
2. Methylene blue 0.25% w/v in water.
3. Colour reagent : To 10 ml of 0.04 M SLS, add 30 ml of chloroform and 1 ml of methylene blue solution. Mix, separate chloroform layer which is blue in colour and is used as colour reagent.
4. Concentrated hydrochloric acid.

Standard solution

Take 20 ml of dicyclomine hydrochloride and transfer to a separatory funnel. Add 10 ml of chloroform.

Sample solution

Transfer finely powdered sample equivalent to 20 mg of dicyclomine hydrochloride to separatory funnel, add 25 ml of water and 1 ml of concentrated hydrochloric acid. Extract 4 × 25 ml portions of chloroform. Pass organic layer through anhydrous sodium sulphate. Evaporate chloroform layer to 10 ml and transfer to a separatory funnel.

Procedure

To each funnel containing sample and standard, add 10 ml of colour reagent and 10 ml of water. Shake and allow the layer to separate. Discard chloroform layer. Measure the absorbance of aqueous layer (blue) of both sample and standard solutions at 590 nm using water as blank and calculate the results.

Note : If the solution is turbid, extract the blue colour into isobutanol and use isobutanol as blank.

Phenylbutazone, Quercetin

ESTIMATION

METHOD 1

Phenylbutazone

Weigh accurately a quantity of the sample equivalent to 100 mg of phenylbutazone and extract dry with three 20 ml portions of toluene. Mix toluene extract with acetone, heat and titrate with 0.1 N sodium hydroxide using phenolphthalein solution as indicator. Each ml of 0.1 N sodium hydroxide is equivalent to 0.03084 g of phenylbutazone. For extraction, chloroform may be used instead of toluene.

Quercetin

The entire toluene insoluble residue obtained above is dissolved in dimethylformamide to get a concentration of 10 mcg/ml in respect of quercetin. Measure the absorbance of the solution at about 377 nm and calculate the results by comparing with standard solution of quercetin dimethylformamide (10 mcg/ml).

METHOD 2

Quercetin

Weigh accurately quantity of the sample equivalent to 25 mg of quercetin and extract with alcohol to get 10 mcg/ml concentration. Measure the extinction of the sample and standard (10 mcg/ml) solutions at about 372 nm using alcohol as blank and calculate the results by comparison.

Phenylbutazone

Evaporate appropriate volume of the alcoholic extract obtained in method 2 above under quercetin and extract the residue with three 25 ml portions of chloroform. Evaporate combined chloroform extract and take up the residue in 0.1 N sodium hydroxide. Measure the absorbance at 264 nm. Calculate the results taking 660 as value of A 1%, 1 cm at 264 nm.

Propyphenazone, Phenylbutazone

ESTIMATION

Propyphenazone (Isopropylphenazone)

METHOD 1

Procedure

Weigh accurately the sample equivalent to 200 mg of the compound, add 100 ml of glacial acetic acid and 10 ml of acetic anhydride. Warm for few minutes and titrate with 0.1 N perchloric acid using malachite green (0.2% w/v in acetic acid) as indicator, to a yellow end point. Each ml of 0.1 N perchloric acid is equivalent to 0.02303 g of propyphenazone.

METHOD 2

Reagent

1. Citric acid-acetic anhydride reagent : Dissolve 2 g citric acid monohydrate in 5 ml of methanol and dilute to 100 ml with acetic anhydride, prepare fresh.

Standard solution

100 mcg/ml of propyphenazone in chloroform.

Sample solution

Weigh accurately sample equivalent to 100 mg of the compound and extract with chloroform. Carry out the required dilutions with chloroform to get 100 mcg/ml.

Procedure

Evaporate 1 ml each of the sample and standard solutions to dryness, add 3 ml of citric acid reagent and 7 ml of acetic anhydride. Heat the flasks in boiling water-bath for 30 min, cool to room temperature and dilute to 25 ml with acetic anhydride. Measure the absorbance of both the solutions at about 550 nm against reagent blank. The method obeys Beer's law in the range of 1-12 mcg/ml.

Note : Aspirin, paracetamol, oxyphenbutazone and colouring agents do not interfere.

Phenylbutazone

Follow the acetone extraction and alkali titration method. For details refer to the method described in formulation 1 of this chapter.

Oxyphenbutazone, Isopropylphenazone, Paracetamol, Diazepam

ESTIMATION

Oxyphenbutazone

Accurately weighed amount of the sample equivalent to 200 mg of the compound is extracted with acetone and titrated with 0.1 N sodium hydroxide as described in formulation 3 of this chapter.

Isopropylphenazone (Propyphenazone)

Follow the non-aqueous titration method as described in formulation 9 of this chapter. Each ml of 0.1 N perchloric acid is equivalent to 0.02303 g of isopropylphenazone. The method based on reaction with citric acid-acetic anhydride as described in formulation 9 of this chapter can also be used.

Paracetamol

Follow the nitroso-derivative method described in formulation 2 of the chapter on analgesics and antipyretics.

Diazepam

Weigh accurately quantity of the sample equivalent to 2 mg of diazepam and carry out the estimation as described in formulation 25 of the chapter on analgesics and antipyretics. Alternatively, follow the method described in formulation 1 of this chapter. The yellow chromophore as a result of acid hydrolysis can be measured directly or extracted into chloroform and then measured at 410 nm.

Chlorzoxazone, Analgin, Oxyphenbutazone

ESTIMATION

Chlorzoxazone

The compound is hydrolysed by refluxing with sodium hydroxide to give p-chloro-o-aminophenol.

Standard solution

To accurately weighed 50 mg of the substance, add 20 ml of sodium hydroxide solution (20%). Reflux for 45 minutes directly on a burner, allow it to cool and dilute to 100 ml with water, 20 ml of the resulting solution is further diluted to 100 ml with dilute hydrochloric acid.

Sample solution

The sample accurately weighed equivalent to 50 mg of the compound is treated and diluted as under standard solution.

Procedure

To 5 ml each of the sample and standard solutions, add 1 ml of sodium nitrite solution (2%) and shake well for one minute. Add 2 ml of ammonium sulphamate solution (5%), shake for two minutes and adjust to 25 ml with water. Measure the extinction of both the solutions at about 405 nm against respective sample blank and calculate the results.

Note : Aspirin, phenylbutazone, paracetamol and indomethacin do not interfere.

Analgin

Follow the method involving reaction with p-dimethylaminobenzaldehyde described under formulation 32 of the chapter on analgesics and antipyretics.

Oxyphenbutazone

Follow the extraction with acetone and titration with 0.1 N sodium hydroxide as described for phenylbutazone under formulation 2 of this chapter. Each ml of 0.1 N sodium hydroxide is equivalent to 0.03424 g of oxyphenbutazone.

Chapter 10

Bronchospasm Relaxants
(Anti-asthma)

Formulation 1

Theophylline, Ephedrine hydrochloride, Phenobarbitone

ESTIMATION
METHOD A
Theophylline
METHOD 1
Standard solution

50 mcg/ml of theophylline in phosphate buffer pH 7 and 9 separately.

Sample solution

Weigh accurately a quantity of powdered tablets or capsule material equivalent to 50 mg of theophylline. Extract and adjust to 50 ml with water, filter.

   (a) Transfer 5 ml of the filtrate and adjust to 100 ml with phosphate buffer pH 7.0.
   (b) Transfer 5 ml of the filtrate and adjust to 100 ml with phosphate buffer pH 9.0.

Procedure

Measure the extinction of the sample and standard solutions in pH 9 buffer using corresponding solutions in pH 7.0 buffer as blank and calculate the results.

Note : Large amount of caffeine, if present, gives low recovery of the compound.

METHOD 2
Standard solution

Weigh accurately 60 mg of anhydrous theophylline, add 5 ml of 1 N hydrochloric acid and 25 ml of water. Shake well for 15 min and dilute to 100 ml with water. Dilute the resultant solution further to get 6 mcg/ml solution.

Sample solution

Weigh accurately a quantity of powdered tablets or capsule material equivalent to 60 mg of anhydrous theophylline and process as per standard solution.

Procedure

Measure the extinction of both the standard and sample solutions at absorption maximum at about 271 nm using water as blank. Calculate the results by comparison.

Ephedrine hydrochloride

Reagents

1. Saturated solution of sodium bicarbonate in water.
2. 2% w/v solution of sodium metaperiodate in water.

Standard solution

40 mcg/ml of ephedrine hydrochloride in water.

Sample solution

Accurately weigh a quantity of the sample equivalent to 20 mg of ephedrine hydrochloride, extract and dilute with water to get 40 mcg/ml solution.

Procedure

To 3 ml each of the sample and standard solutions, add 1 ml of saturated solution of sodium bicarbonate. After evolution of carbon dioxide has stopped, add 1 ml of sodium metaperiodate solution. Allow to stand for 15 minutes, add 20 ml of n-hexane, shake well and allow the layers to separate. Measure the extinction of the organic layer at about 242 nm using n-hexane as blank. Calculate the results by comparison.

Phenobarbitone

Reagents

1. Borate buffer, pH 9.6.
2. 0.5 N ammonium hydroxide.

Standard solution

10 mcg/ml of phenobarbitone in 0.5 N ammonium hydroxide or borate buffer, pH 9.6.

Sample solution

Weigh accurately a quantity of the sample equivalent to about 50 mg of phenobarbitone, add 10 ml of dilute hydrochloric acid and heat on water-bath for 10 min. Cool and extract with three 30 ml portions of ether. Wash combined ether extract with 20 ml of distilled water. Pass ether layer through anhydrous sodium sulphate. Evaporate the ether layer to dryness and dissolve the residue in 0.5 N ammonium hydroxide or borate buffer, pH 9.6 to get 10 mcg/ml concentration.

Concomitantly measure the extinction of sample and standard solutions at 240.5 nm using 0.5 N ammonium hydroxide as blank and calculate the results by comparisons.

Note : Usually in liquid formulations, phenobarbitone is present as sodium salt. Each mg of phenobarbitone is equivalent to 1.9047 mg of phenobarbitone sodium.

METHOD B

Theophylline

Standard solution

Weigh accurately about 140 mg of pure theophylline (anhydrous), transfer into a 500 ml volumetric flask containing 200 ml of distilled water and mix. Add few drops of methyl red solution, acidify with 1 N sulphuric acid and heat in a steam bath to effect solution. Cool to room temperature and dilute to volume with water.

Sample solution

Weigh accurately a quantity of powdered sample equivalent to about 140 mg of theophylline. Add about 200 ml of water, few drops of methyl red solution and acidify with 1 N sulphuric acid. Place the flask in a steam bath until the tablet base has completely dissolved (about 1 h is required for waxy base). Transfer the hot solution to a mechanical shaker and shake for 30 min. After shaking, allow the solution to cool to room temperature, dilute to 500 ml with water and mix well. Filter the mixture through a G₄ sintered glass funnel, discarding first 15 ml of the filtrate.

Note : Retain the remaining clear sample filtrate for the estimation of ephedrine hydrochloride.

Procedure

Dilute separately 15 ml of the clear sample filtrate and 20 ml of the standard solution to 100 ml water and mix well. Further dilute 10 ml of each solution to 100 ml with water. Concomitantly determine the absorbance of the sample and the standard solutions at the wavelength of maximum absorbance, at about 271 nm and calculate the results by comparison.

Ephedrine hydrochloride

Reagents

1. Ammoniacal copper sulphate solution : Weigh 50 g of ammonium acetate and 0.5 g of cupric sulphate, pentahydrate. Transfer to a 250 ml volumetric flask containing 75 ml of water and mix until solution is complete, cool. Dissolve 25 g of sodium hydroxide in 50 ml of water, cool, add this solution and 50 ml of ammonia solution to the above volumetric flask, mix. Dilute to volume with water and mix thoroughly (prepare fresh bi-weekly).
2. Carbon disulphide-benzene solution : Mix 5 ml of carbon disulphide with 95 ml of benzene, prepare fresh. Caution : Prepare solution in a well-ventilated area.
3. Acetic acid solution : Transfer 40 ml of glacial acetic acid into a 100 ml volumetric flask, carefully dilute to volume with water and mix thoroughly.

Standard solution

Weigh accurately, about 115 mg of ephedrine hydrochloride into a volumetric flask, add about 400 ml of water and mix. Add a few drops of methyl red solution, acidify with 1 N sulphuric acid, dilute to 1000 ml with distilled water and mix thoroughly, prepare fresh.

Procedure

Pipette 5 ml of the clear sample filtrate retained in estimation of theophylline under method B into a 100 ml volumetric flask and 5 ml of the standard solution into a second 100 ml volumetric flask. Add 15 ml of water to each flask, mix well, add 2 ml of the ammoniacal copper sulphate solution and 20 ml of the carbon disulphide-benzene solution into each flask. Mix well, stopper tightly and heat each flask in a water-bath at 45°C for 5 minutes. Remove from the bath and shake mechanically for 10 minutes. Add 2 ml of acetic acid and shake for another 5 minutes. Decant the benzene layers into separate small glass-stoppered flasks each containing a small amount of anhydrous sodium sulphate. Concomitantly determine the absorbance of benzene layer of the sample and standard solutions at about 430 nm using benzene as blank and calculate the results.

Note :   In solid dosage formulations, if lactose is present, it is likely to interfere because of its reducing action on copper sulphate. In such case, the alkaloid should be first extracted with methylene chloride from ammoniacal solution. Further, while concentrating organic layer, to avoid loss of ephedrine, add 1 ml of 1% benzoic acid solution.

Formulation 2

Dihydroxypropyltheophylline, Phenobarbitone, Chlorpheniramine maleate, Ephedrine hydrochloride

ESTIMATION

Sample

Shake an accurately weighed quantity of powdered sample equivalent to 200 mg of theophylline with 50 ml of ether. Filter, repeat the process 6-7 times. The residue thus obtained is dissolved in water to make 100 ml. This solution A is used for estimation of various ingredients of the formulation.

Dihydroxypropyltheophylline

Transfer 0.5 ml of the sample solution (A) to a 100 ml volumetric flask and make up the volume to 100 ml with water. Measure the extinction at 273 nm and calculate the contents of dihydroxypropyl-theophylline, taking 361 as the value of A 1%, 1 cm at the maximum at 273 nm.

Ephedrine hydrochloride

Reagents

1. Buffer solution, pH 10 : Dissolve 5.40 g of ammonium chloride in 50 ml water. Adjust the pH to 10.0 with ammonia solution and dilute to 100 ml with water.
2. 0.1% w/v solution of copper acetate in alcohol.
3. In a 50 ml volumetric flask, pipette out 10 ml of alcoholic solution of copper acetate, 5 ml carbon disulphide, 4 ml of glacial acetic acid and make up the volume to 50 ml with absolute alcohol.

Standard solution

80 mg of ephedrine hydrochloride is dissolved in 100 ml of distilled water.

Procedure

Appropriate volume of solution A containing 1.6 mg of ephedrine hydrochloride and 2 ml of standard solutions are taken in two separating funnels. To each, add 3 ml of 0.1 N hydrochloric acid, 10 ml buffer solution and 2 ml copper acetate solution. Mix well and allow to stand for 5 minutes. Add 15 ml chloroform and shake for one minute. Separate the chloroform layer, wash immediately with 20 ml of 0.1 N hydrochloric acid and filter through anhydrous sodium sulphate placed on filter paper into a 50 ml volumetric flask. Repeat the extraction with 15 ml, 10 ml and 10 ml portions of chloroform. Wash each chloroform extract with the same 20 ml 0.1 N hydrochloric acid and filter as described above. Adjust the combined extracts to 50 ml with chloroform. Measure the extinction of chloroform layer at 438 nm using chloroform as blank. Calculate the result by comparing with the standard.

Phenobarbitone

Follow the method described under formulation 1 of this chapter using appropriate volume of solution A.

Chlorpheniramine maleate

Reagents

1. Dilute hydrochloric acid : Dilute 1 ml of hydrochloric acid to 20 ml with water.
2. 10% w/v silicotungstic acid solution in water, filter through G_4 sintered glass funnel before use.

Procedure

Shake an accurately weighed quantity of the powdered tablets equivalent to 20 mg of the substance with 50 ml of water and filter through filter paper. Repeat this process 3 to 4 times. To the filtrate, add 2 ml of dilute hydrochloric acid and boil. To the boiling solution, add 4 ml of silicotungstic acid solution. Boil for 5-10 minutes and filter through a tared G_4 sintered glass funnel. Wash the precipitate with boiling dilute hydrochloric acid and then twice with 5 ml of water. Dry the residue at 105°C to constant weight. Each g of the precipitate is equivalent to 0.2281 g of chlorpheniramine maleate.

Dried aluminium hydroxide gel, Ephedrine hydrochloride, Theophylline, Phenobarbitone

ESTIMATION

Aluminium hydroxide gel, as aluminium oxide

Sample solution

Weigh accurately powdered tablets equivalent to 0.2 g of aluminium hydroxide and transfer to 150 ml conical flask. Add approximately 2 ml of hydrochloric acid and 50 ml of water. Boil this solution for sometime, cool, make the volume to 100 ml with water, shake and filter.

Procedure

Pipette 25 ml of the above filtrate into a 250 ml conical flask and neutralise with sodium hydroxide solution. Follow the method 3 for estimation of aluminium hydroxide described under formulation 1 of the chapter on antacids.

Ephedrine hydrochloride

Reagent

1. 50% w/v solution of potassium carbonate in water.

Procedure

Weigh accurately a quantity of sample equivalent to 50 mg of ephedrine in a dry 250 ml stoppered flask. Add 2 ml of potassium carbonate solution and 5 ml of water. Mix well and extract with five 30 ml portions of dichloromethane for fifteen minutes. Add approximately 2 g of gum tragacanth and again extract for five minutes. Filter the extract through cotton plug into a drug 250 ml conical flask. Wash the stoppered flask and funnel with sufficient dichloromethane. Add exactly 15 ml of 0.02 N sulphuric acid and evaporate the organic layer completely. Cool, add 2-3 drops of methyl red indicator and titrate against 0.05 N sodium hydroxide. Run a blank side by side. Each ml of 0.02 N sulphuric acid consumed is equivalent to 0.004033 g of ephedrine hydrochloride.

Theophylline and phenobarbitone

Follow the method for estimation of theophylline and phenobarbitone described in formulation 1 of this chapter.

Theophylline, Hydroxyzine hydrochloride, Ephedrine hydrochloride

ESTIMATION

Theophylline

Standard solution

7.5 mcg/ml of theophylline in 0.1 N sodium hydroxide.

Sample solution

Accurately weigh a quantity of powdered tablets or capsule material equivalent to 100 mg of theophylline. Add 100 ml of 0.1 N sodium hydroxide, shake for 5 min, and dilute to 200 ml with 0.1 N sodium hydroxide. Set aside for 10 min and filter through filter paper, discarding first 20-30 ml of the filtrate. Dilute 3 ml of the filtrate to 200 ml with 0.1 N sodium hydroxide.

Measure the extinction of both standard and sample solutions at the maxima at about 275 nm against 0.1 N sodium hydroxide as blank. Calculate the results by comparison (or calculate the results taking 650 as value of A 1%, 1 cm).

Hydroxyzine hydrochloride

Standard solution

15 mcg/ml of hydroxyzine hydrochloride in 0.1 N hydrochloric acid.

Sample solution

Weigh accurately a quantity of powdered material equivalent to 15 mg of hydroxyzine hydrochloride. Shake with 50 ml of chloroform for 60 min and dilute to 100 ml with chloroform. To 20 ml of the chloroform extract, add 20 ml of 1 N sodium hydroxide, shake, separate chloroform layer and pass through anhydrous sodium sulphate. Extract the alkaline layer with further 20 ml of chloroform. Combine chloroform layers and adjust to 50 ml with chloroform. Evaporate 10 ml of the chloroform layer to dryness, cool and dissolve in 0.1 N hydrochloric acid to produce 50 ml (12 mcg/ml).

Measure the extinction of standard and sample solutions at maximum at about 232 nm using 0.1 N hydrochloric acid as blank. Calculate the results by comparison.

Ephedrine hydrochloride

Reagents

1. 10% v/v methyl alcohol in water.
2. 10% v/v acetic acid in water.
3. 0.1% w/v solution of sodium bicarbonate in water.
4. Cupric chloride reagent : To 60 mg of cupric chloride, add 125 ml of water and adjust to 250 ml with pyridine.

5. Carbon disulphide-pyridine reagent : Mix 25 ml of pyridine with 65 ml of isopropyl alcohol. Immediately prior to use, add 35 ml of carbon disulphide to above mixture and mix well.

Standard solution

Weigh accurately 70 mg of pure ephedrine hydrochloride, anhydrous and dissolve in water to make 100 ml. Dilute 10 ml of this solution to 25 ml with sodium bicarbonate solution.

Sample solution

Weigh accurately a quantity of powdered material equivalent to 70 mg of ephedrine hydrochloride and shake for 15 minutes with 100 ml of 10% v/v methyl alcohol. Filter, discard first few ml and dilute 10 ml of the filtrate to 25 ml with sodium bicarbonate solution.

Procedure

To 3 ml each of sample and standard solutions, add 10 ml of carbon disulphide-pyridine reagent and then in succession, add to each 5 ml of cupric chloride reagent, 6 ml of 10% acetic acid, swirling gently after each addition. Then, add 10 ml of benzene and shake for 2-3 times. Collect benzene layer and dilute to 25 ml with isopropyl alcohol. After 35 minutes, read the absorbance of both standard and sample solutions at about 440 nm and calculate the results by comparison.

Meprobamate, Papaverine hydrochloride, Phenobarbitone

ESTIMATION

Meprobamate

Reagents

1. Acetone-glacial acetic acid mixture (3 : 1 v/v).
2. 1% w/v solution of p-dimethylaminobenzaldehyde in benzene.
3. Antimony trichloride-acetic anhydride reagent : 4 parts of antimony trichloride (25% w/v in chloroform) and one part of acetic anhydride are mixed.

Standard solution

50 mcg/ml of meprobamate in acetone.

Sample solution

Weigh accurately a quantity of powdered tablets equivalent to 100 mg of meprobamate. Add 50 ml acetone, shake for 2 minutes and dilute to 100 ml with acetone. Dilute the resulting solution appropriately with acetone to get 50 mcg/ml.

Procedure

Evaporate separately 1 ml each of sample and standard solutions on water bath, cool and add 0.5 ml of acetone-acetic acid reagent, 0.5 ml of p-dimethylaminobenzaldehyde solution and 4 ml of antimony reagent. Place the tubes in water bath maintained at 50°C for 10 minutes. Shake, cool in ice bath and dilute to 10 ml with benzene. Measure the absorbance of both the solutions at about 540 nm using benzene as blank. Deduce the results by comparison.

Papaverine hydrochloride

Weigh sample accurately equivalent to 50 mg of papaverine hydrochloride, add 40 ml of 1 N hydrochloric acid, shake and dilute to 50 ml with 1 N hydrochloric acid. Keep at room temperature for 60 min and filter. Dilute the filtrate appropriately with 1 N hydrochloric acid to get 15 mcg/ml solution. Measure the extinction at 310 nm and calculate the results using 228 as value of A 1%, 1 cm at 310 nm.

Phenobarbitone

Follow the method described under formulation 1 of this chapter.

Papaverine hydrochloride, Theophylline, Phenobarbitone

The spectrophotometric method does not require preliminary separation. For papaverine and theophylline, the sample and standard solutions are prepared in 0.1 N hydrochloric acid and for phenobarbitone solutions are prepared in borate buffer, pH 10.

The absorbance of papaverine and theophylline are measured at 309 nm (A_1) and 270 nm (A_2) and for phenobarbitone at 240 nm (A_3).

1. A_1 : Extinction value of the mixture at 309 nm is purely due to papaverine hydrochloride and there is no interference from other two components of the formulation.
2. A_2 : Extinction value of the mixture at 270 nm is due to theophylline and papaverine.
3. A_3 : Extinction value at 240 nm is mainly due to phenobarbitone, but all the three components absorb at 240 nm.

Standard solutions of pure substances (10 mcg/ml) show extinction values : papaverine—0.60 (309 nm); theophylline—0.40 (270 nm) and phenobarbitone—0.70 (240 nm).

Contents of Papaverine : Calculate by comparing with the standard solution (10 mcg/ml) of papaverine at 309 nm.

Contents of Theophylline : $(A_2 - A_1 \times 0.6)$

Contents of Phenobarbitone : $A_3 (0.4 \times A_2) - (0.7 \times A_1)$

Note : The values of A_1, A_2 and A_3 vary with the instrument and should be determined in each laboratory and on each instrument.

Papaverine hydrochloride, Caffeine citrate, Phenobarbitone

ESTIMATION

Papaverine hydrochloride and Caffeine citrate

Standard solution of papaverine and caffeine

Appropriate weight of each substance is dissolved in chloroform to get a concentration of 10 mcg/ml in respect of each substance.

Sample solution

Weigh accurately a quantity of powdered material, equivalent to 10 mg of papaverine hydrochloride. Suspend in water and basify with dilute ammonia solution. Extract with four 25 ml portions of chloroform (reserve aqueous ammonia layer for estimation of phenobarbitone). Pass each chloroform layer through anhydrous sodium sulphate and dilute with chloroform appropriately.

Measure the extinctions of both the solutions at 308 nm and 276 nm. The extinction values at 308 nm and 276 nm are used for calculations of papaverine and caffeine respectively by comparison. There is no mutual interference.

Phenobarbitone

Aqueous ammoniacal layer reserved during estimation of papaverine above is used. The solution is diluted appropriately with dilute ammonia to get a concentration of 10 mcg/ml, having absorption maxima at about 240 nm or acidify the aqueous ammoniacal layer and proceed with the method A described under formulation 1 of this chapter.

Papaverine hydrochloride, Ephedrine hydrochloride, Phenobarbitone, Theophylline

ESTIMATION

Papaverine hydrochloride and Ephedrine hydrochloride (total alkaloids)

Transfer an accurately weighed quantity of the sample powder equivalent to 50 mg of total alkaloids, to a 125 ml separator with the aid of 5 ml of water. Add 5 ml of 1 N sodium hydroxide solution and shake vigorously for 2 minutes. Extract with five quantities, each of 25 ml of chloroform. Wash the combined chloroform extracts with water till free from alkali. Add 5 g of anhydrous sodium sulphate to remove any dissolved water. Filter into a previously dried and weighed beaker through anhydrous sodium sulphate. Wash sodium sulphate with chloroform. Add 5 drops of hydrochloric acid and evaporate the chloroform. When the volume is reduced to about 5 ml, remove the beaker from the water-bath and dry residue in vacuum. Finally dry the residue at 105°C for 1 h and weigh (A). Calculate the contents of papaverine and ephedrine in each tablet.

Papaverine hydrochloride

Dissolve the above residue (A) in 1 N hydrochloric acid to get a concentration of 15 mcg/ml of papaverine hydrochloride. Measure the extinction at 310 nm and calculate the contents of papaverine hydrochloride using 228 as value of A 1%, 1 cm at 310 nm. Ephedrine hydrochloride does not interfere as it is poorly UV-absorbing compound.

Ephedrine hydrochloride

METHOD 1

Subtract the contents of papaverine as determined by the method above from the weight of residue (A) obtained in the method for total alkaloids. The difference gives the weigh of ephedrine present in the portion of the sample taken for analysis.

METHOD 2

Suspend the residue (A) obtained in the method 1 for total alkaloids in water, add 10 g of sodium chloride and 15 ml of 20% w/v solution of sodium hydroxide. Carry out the steam distillation into receiver containing 25 ml of 0.05 N sulphuric acid. Collect about 100 ml of the distillate. Titrate excess of the acid with 0.05 N sodium hydroxide using methyl red as indicator. Carry out the blank determination using same quantities of the reagents. Each ml of 0.05 N sulphuric acid neutralized by the volatile base is equivalent to 0.00826 g of anhydrous ephedrine. Multiply the results by 1.221 or 1.297 to get the contents of ephedrine hydrochloride or ephedrine sulphate respectively.

Phenobarbitone

Follow the method A for estimation of phenobarbitone described under formulation 1 of this chapter.

Aminophylline

Follow the method 2 for determination of theophylline described under formulation 1 of this chapter. Calculate the contents of aminophylline by multiplying the contents of theophylline by 1.267.

Formulation 9

Pseudoephedrine hydrochloride, Triprolidine hydrochloride, Paracetamol

ESTIMATION

Sample solution

Weigh accurately a quantity of powdered tablets equivalent to 20 mg of triprolidine hydrochloride. Add 70 ml water, shake for 15 minutes and adjust to 100 ml with water (200 mcg/ml of triprolidine hydrochloride) Solution A.

Triprolidine hydrochloride

Standard solution

25 mcg/ml of triprolidine hydrochloride in 0.1 N hydrochloric acid.

Sample solution

Weigh accurately powdered sample equivalent to 2.5 mg of the substance, dissolve in 10-15 ml water, add 5 ml of copper sulphate solution and 5 ml of strong ammonia solution. Extract with two 25 ml portions of chloroform. Wash combined chloroform layer with water and extract with 0.1 N hydrochloric acid to produce 100 ml.

Measure the extinction of sample and standard solutions at 290 nm using acid as blank, calculate the results by comparison.

Paracetamol

Follow the nitroso-derivative method described under formulation 2 of the chapter on analgesics and antipyretics diluting solution A above appropriately.

Pseudoephedrine hydrochloride

METHOD 1

Transfer 50 ml of solution A into a separator, add 5 g of sodium chloride, 3 ml of 1 N sodium hydroxide. Extract with four 100 ml portions of ether. Wash the combined ether extract with 10 ml of water. To the total ether extract, add 25 ml of 0.1 N hydrochloric acid and shake vigorously. Allow the two layers to separate and transfer the aqueous acidic layer to conical flask. Wash the ether layer with two 10 ml portions of water and combine the washings with the acidic layer. Warm the acid layer to remove trace of ether, cool and titrate with 0.1 N sodium hydroxide using methyl red as indicator.

Calculate the total volume of 0.1 N hydrochloric acid (A) consumed by pseudoephedrine and triprolidine hydrochloride. From the contents of triprolidine hydrochloride as determined above, calculate equivalent volume of 0.1 N hydrochloric acid (B) (33.29 mg of triprolidine hydrochloride is equivalent to 1 ml of 0.1 N hydrochloric acid.) Subtract the volume (ml) B from total volume A and calculate the contents of pseudoephedrine hydrochloride in the formulation by using the factor that each ml of 0.1 N hydrochloric acid is equivalent to 20.17 mg of pseudoephedrine hydrochloride.

METHOD 2

This method is based on two phase acid-base titration.

Reagents

1. Mixed indicator solution

Chlorophenol red	0.30 g
Congo red	0.15 g
Alcohol	50 ml
0.1 N sodium hydroxide	12 ml
Water to produce	500 ml

   Protect from light.

Sample solution

Weigh accurately a quantity of sample equivalent to 500 mg of pseudoephedrine, add 45 ml of water, 1 g of sodium sulphate and 5 ml of dilute sulphuric acid. Shake well and add 4 ml of 5 N sodium hydroxide. Extract with four portions of 40 ml each of chloroform, washing each extract with the same 10 ml of water. Combine chloroform layer and dilute to 200 ml with chloroform.

Procedure

Take 50 ml of the chloroform extract of the sample, add 50 ml of water and few drops of mixed indicator and titrate with 0.1 N hydrochloric acid shaking well between additions. The colour change in aqueous layer is red → colourless → yellow. The end point is taken as first appearance of yellow tinge. The colour change can be assessed without allowing the separation of phases. Each ml of 0.1 N hydrochloric acid is equivalent to 20.17 mg of pseudoephedrine hydrochloride. Or the chloroform extract may be evaporated and the residue dissolved in glacial acetic acid for non-aqueous titration (crystal violet).

Note : 1. Addition of acid before basification and extraction ensures complete dissolution of the drug.

2. Sodium sulphate minimises formation of emulsion.

3. Ephedrine does not interfere in this method.

Theophylline, Ephedrine hydrochloride, Chlordiazepoxide

ESTIMATION

Theophylline

Weigh accurately a quantity of the powdered tablets equivalent to 200 mg of theophylline, add 20 ml of water and 5 ml of dilute sulphuric acid. Extract with four 25 ml portions of chloroform-isopropyl alcohol (3 : 1 v/v) mixture. Wash the combined organic layer with 10 ml of dilute sulphuric acid. Pass organic layer through anhydrous sodium sulphate and evaporate. Find out the contents of theophylline gravimetrically. Retain the acid layer for estimation of chlordiazepoxide.

Ephedrine hydrochloride

METHOD 1

Reagents

1. 0.1% w/v solution of ninhydrin in ethyl alcohol.
2. 1% w/v potassium hydroxide solution in ethyl alcohol.

Standard solution

300 mcg/ml of ephedrine hydrochloride in water.

Sample solution

Weigh accurately a quantity of sample equivalent to 30 mg of ephedrine hydrochloride, shake with 100 ml of water and filter (300 mcg/ml).

Procedure

To 2 ml each of standard and sample solutions, add 2 ml ninhydrin solution and 0.1 ml of potassium hydroxide solution. Heat on a water bath for 30 minutes, cool and adjust the volume to 25 ml with isopropyl alcohol. Measure the absorbance of both the standard and sample solutions at about 560 nm and calculate the results by comparison.

METHOD 2

Follow the method 2 for estimation of ephedrine hydrochloride described under formulation 8 of this chapter. This is based on volatile nature of ephedrine as base.

Chlordiazepoxide and Ephedrine hydrochloride

Make the acidic layer obtained in the estimation of theophylline alkaline with 20% w/v solution of sodium hydroxide and extract with four 25 ml portions of chloroform. Pass chloroform layer through anhydrous sodium sulphate. Evaporate and dissolve the residue in 20 ml of glacial acetic acid and titrate with 0.05 N perchloric acid using crystal violet as indicator. Subtract the volume of perchloric acid equivalent to ephedrine determined earlier. The remaining volume represents chlordiazepoxide.

Each ml of 0.05 N perchloric acid is equivalent to 0.01681 g of chlordiazepoxide. Alternatively chlordiazepoxide can be subjected to acid hydrolysis and yellow colour measured at 410 nm. For details refer to estimation of diazepam in formulation 11 of the chapter on anti-inflammatory drugs.

Note :   Before proceeding with extraction, the alkaline solution may be heated on water-bath to remove ephedrine (volatile base). The volume of 0.05 N perchloric acid consumed shall correspond to chlordiazepoxide only.

Diethylcarbamazine citrate, Theophylline, Dried aluminium hydroxide gel

ESTIMATION

Diethylcarbamazine citrate

METHOD 1

Weigh a quantity of sample equivalent to 500 mg of the compound, add 50 ml of water, shake vigorously to dissolve and filter. Extract the residue with three more 50 ml portions of water and filter. Add 5 ml of 20% sodium hydroxide solution to the filtrate and extract with three 20 ml portions of chloroform. Combine chloroform layers and wash with water to get free of alkali. Extract chloroform layer with 25 ml of 0.1 N sulphuric acid and 20 ml of water. Combine acid and water extracts, warm slightly to remove traces of chloroform. Cool and titrate excess of the acid with 0.1 N sodium hydroxide using bromocresol green solution as indicator. Each ml of 0.1 N sulphuric acid is equivalent to 0.03914 g of diethylcarbamazine citrate.

METHOD 2

Reagent

1. Acetic anhydride-pyridine reagent : 57 ml of acetic anhydride is mixed with 13 ml of pyridine.

Standard solution

Prepare solution of diethylcarbamazine citrate in water (5 mg/ml). 5 ml of the resulting solution is diluted to 100 ml with glacial acetic acid (250 mcg/ml).

Sample solution

To an aliquot of composite (syrup, powder and tablets) sample equivalent to 25 mg of the compound, add 10 of water and sufficient glacial acetic acid to produce 100 ml, mix and filter (250 mcg/ml).

Procedure

To 2 ml each of sample and standard solutions, add 5 ml of the anhydride reagent. Keep at 37°C for 1 h and then allow it to come to room temperature. Measure the absorbance of both the solutions at about 428 nm and calculate the results. The method obeys Beer's law in the range of 10-100 mcg/ml. The colour of the complex is stable for 2 hours.

Note : 1. As the method involves reaction with citrate ion, it may not be applicable in syrups where citric acid has been used for pH adjustment.
2. Chlorpheniramine maleate, if present, does not interfere.

Aluminium hydroxide

Follow the method described in formulation 22 of the chapter on alimentary drugs.

Theophylline

Follow the method described in formulation 12 of this chapter.

Theophylline, Ephedrine hydrochloride, Phenobarbitone, Caffeine citrate

ESTIMATION

METHOD 1

Theophylline

Weigh accurately a quantity of powder equivalent to 250 mg theophylline, add 50 ml of water and 8 ml of dilute ammonia solution. Keep on water bath, add 50 ml of 0.1 N silver nitrate solution and warm for 15 minutes. Cool to 5-10°C for 20 minutes, filter through G$_4$ sintered funnel and wash the precipitates with three 20 ml portions of water. Acidify the combined filtrate with concentrated nitric acid, adding 3 ml of acid in excess and titrate the excess silver nitrate with 0.1 N ammonium thiocyanate using ferric ammonium sulphate solution as indicator. Perform reagent blank. Each ml of 0.1 N silver nitrate is equivalent to 18.02 mcg of theophylline, anhydrous.

Phenobarbitone

Weigh sample accurately equivalent to about 80 mg of phenobarbitone, add 10 ml of 0.1 N sodium hydroxide, shake and saturate with sodium chloride. Acidify with hydrochloric acid and extract with three 30 ml portions of ether. Reserve aqueous layer for estimation of caffeine. Wash combined ether extracts with 10 ml of dilute hydrochloric acid (1 : 1) and then with two 20 ml water. Pass ether layer through anhydrous sodium sulphate (ether washed), evaporate ether layer and dissolve the residue in 0.5 N ammonium hydroxide or borate buffer, pH 9.6 to get 10 mcg/ml. Measure the extinction at 240.5 nm and calculate the results by comparing with the standard. For further details, refer to formulation 1 of this chapter.

Caffeine citrate

Aqueous layer reserved during extraction of phenobarbitone is basified and extracted with five 20 ml portions of chloroform. Wash combined chloroform layer with ammoniacal water for 3-4 times. Filter, dry at 80°C and weigh. Weight represents the amount of caffeine present in the sample taken for analysis. Alternatively, chloroform layer may be used for spectrophotometric analysis as described in formulation 1 of the chapter on analgesics and antipyretics.

Ephedrine hydrochloride

Weigh accurately a quantity of powdered material equivalent to 100 mg of ephedrine. Suspend in water and basify with ammonia solution. Extract with four 25 ml portions of ether. Evaporate ether at low temperature and take the residue in 10 ml of 0.1 N sulphuric acid. Excess acid is titrated with 0.1 N sodium hydroxide using methyl red solution as indicator. Alternatively, wash ether layer with water till neutral. Add exactly 50 ml of 0.02 N sulphuric acid and evaporate ether layer completely. Cool, add 2-3 drops of methyl red solution and titrate with 0.02 N sodium hydroxide. Each ml of 0.02 N sulphuric acid is equivalent to 0.004033 g of ephedrine hydrochloride.

METHOD 2

Phenobarbitone

In a 150 ml separator containing about 5 ml 1 N hydrochloric acid, transfer quantity of powder accurately weighed equivalent to 100 mg of phenobarbitone and shake well. Extract with five 50 ml portions of solvent ether. Collect the ether layers. Wash the combined ether layer with 10 ml acidified water and then twice with 50 ml each of 1% w/v sodium acetate solution. Finally, wash the combined ether layer twice with 50 ml water, each. Filter the washed ether extracts into a 500 ml conical flask. Evaporate to dryness on water bath, cool, add 10 ml ethanol and 2 ml indicator (0.1% w/v thymolphthalein in ethanol). Titrate against 0.1 N alcoholic potassium hydroxide. Make the correction for blank containing 10 ml ethanol and 2 ml indicator solution. Each ml of 0.1 N alcoholic potassium hydroxide is equivalent to 0.02322 g of phenobarbitone.

Caffeine citrate

Transfer accurately weighed quantity of powdered material equivalent to 100 mg of caffeine to a separator having 15 ml water. Add about 10 ml of 1 N hydrochloric acid, shake well and extract with five 30 ml portions of chloroform. Combine the chloroform layers, add about 20 ml of 0.1 N sodium hydroxide and 15 ml of water to the combined chloroform layers. Shake well and reject aqueous layer. Then chloroform layer is washed twice with 20 ml water. Reject aqueous layer and filter chloroform layer through cotton plug into a dry 500 ml conical flask. Evaporate chloroform to dryness. Dissolve the residue in 2 ml of chloroform, add 10 ml of benzene and 10 ml of acetic anhydride. Then titrate with 0.1 N perchloric acid using 0.2 ml of solution of neutral red (0.2% w/v solution in acetic acid). Carry out the blank determination and make necessary correction.

Each ml of 0.1 N perchloric acid is equivalent to 0.01942 g of caffeine.

Aminophylline

Reagents

1. Borate buffer
   (a) 0.5% w/v solution of boric acid in water.
   (b) 1% w/v solution of sodium borate in water.
   Mix solutions (a) and (b) (1 : 1) to prepare the buffer.
2. 0.04 w/v solution of 2,6-dichloroquinone chlorimide in isopropyl alcohol.

Standard solution

Weigh accurately about 97 mg of aminophylline, transfer to a 200 ml volumetric flask and make up the volume with water.

Sample solution

Transfer accurately weighed quantity of powder equivalent to 100 mg of the compound to a 200 ml volumetric flask. Shake well with 100 ml water, make up the volume with water and filter.

Procedure

To 1 ml each of sample and standard solutions, add 5 ml of borate buffer and 2 ml of 2,6-dichloroquinone chlorimide solution. Make up the volume to 50 ml with water and keep in a refrigerator for 90 minutes. Remove and after attaining the room temperature, transfer exactly 25 ml of each of sample and standard solutions into two separating funnels and extract blue colour formed with exactly 25 ml of amyl alcohol. Reject aqueous layer and measure the optical density of the alcoholic layer at 620 nm using amyl alcohol as blank. Deduce the results by comparison.

Ephedrine hydrochloride

Standard solution

160 mcg/ml of ephedrine hydrochloride in 1 N hydrochloric acid.

Sample solution

Weigh accurately a quantity of powdered tablets equivalent to 32 mg of ephedrine hydrochloride and transfer into a 200 ml volumetric flask. Add about 100 ml of 1 N hydrochloric acid, warm on a water bath for 15 minutes, cool, make up the volume to 200 ml with 1 N hydrochloric acid and mix.

Procedure

Follow ammoniacal copper sulphate method B described in formulation 1 of this chapter.

Aminophylline, Phenobarbitone, Ephedrine hydrochloride, Codeine phosphate

ESTIMATION

Aminophylline

(a) **Ethylenediamine :** Weigh accurately a quantity of powdered material equivalent to 100 mg of aminophylline. Dissolve in 30 ml of water and titrate with 0.1 N hydrochloric acid using bromocresol green solution as indicator (colour change from blue to green). Each ml of 0.1 N hydrochloric acid is equivalent to 0.003003 g of ethylenediamine.

(b) **Theophylline :**

Reagents

1. 0.1 N silver nitrate.
2. 0.1 N ammonium thiocyanate.
3. Ferric ammonium sulphate solution (indicator).
4. Dilute solution of ammonia.

Procedure

Weigh accurately a quantity of powdered material equivalent to 150 mg of aminophylline, add 40-50 ml of water and 10 ml of dilute ammonia solution. Reflux on water bath to effect solution. Add 100 ml of 0.1 N silver nitrate, heat to boiling and boil for 5 min. Cool to 5°C for 30 minutes, dilute to 200 ml with water and filter (A). Acidify 20 ml of the filtrate (A) with nitric acid, add an excess of 3 ml of nitric acid. Cool, add 2 ml of ferric ammonium sulphate solution and titrate excess of silver nitrate with 0.1 N ammonium thiocyanate. Each ml of 0.1 N silver nitrate is equivalent to 0.01802 g of theophylline (anhydrous). From the volume of silver nitrate consumed, calculate the contents of theophylline.

Phenobarbitone

Acidify 50 ml of the filtrate (A) obtained under estimation of theophylline with dilute hydrochloric acid. Add sodium chloride to saturate it. Extract with four 20 ml portions of chloroform, washing each chloroform layer with same 10 ml of water. Filter through filter paper previously moistened with chloroform into a tared flask. Evaporate on water bath, add 2 ml of alcohol and again evaporate. Dry the residue at 105°C in an oven for 3 hours, cool and weigh. The residue is only of phenobarbitone. The residue can be dissolved in 0.5 N ammonia solution and subjected to spectrophotometric solution described in formulation 1 of this chapter.

Ephedrine hydrochloride and Codeine phosphate (as total alkaloids)

METHOD 1

Weigh accurately a quantity of powdered material equivalent to 60 mg of ephedrine hydrochloride, add

10 ml of 0.1 N hydrochloric acid, shake to suspend. Filter through G₄ glass sintered funnel. Wash sintered funnel with water. Combine the filtrate, add 12 ml 0.1 N sodium hydroxide and extract with four 50 ml portions of ether. Wash ether layer with brine solution till washings are free from alkali (use litmus). Wash brine solution with two 25 ml of ether. Mix ether layers, add 50 ml of 0.02 N hydrochloric acid to ether layer. Shake for 2-3 minutes to bring alkaloid back into acid layer. Separate acid layer quantitatively. Wash ether layer with two 10 ml portions of water to ensure quantitative removal of the acid. Add water washings to the acid layer and titrate with 0.02 N sodium hydroxide using methyl red solution as indicator. Say "A" ml of 0.02 N hydrochloric acid is consumed for titration of total alkaloids. The above titrated sample is subjected to steam distillation and ephedrine is estimated in the distillate by acid-base titration. Say "B" ml of 0.02 N hydrochloric acid is consumed for ephedrine. Volume of 0.02 N hydrochloric acid consumed by codeine = (A − B). For calculations, see formulation 2 of the chapter on expectorants and cough suppressants.

METHOD 2

The combined filtrate after basification is subjected to steam distillation and the contents of ephedrine (base) are estimated in the filtrate by acid-base titration. For details, refer to method 2 for estimation of ephedrine under formulation 8 of this chapter. The contents in the distillation flask are used for estimation of codeine phosphate as per method 1 above.

Formulation 14

Salbutamol sulphate, Theophylline

ESTIMATION

Salbutamol sulphate

METHOD 1

Reagents

1. 0.2% w/v solution of p-aminophenol in ethyl alcohol (prepare fresh).
2. 1 M solution of sodium carbonate in water.

Standard solution

100 mcg/ml of salbutamol sulphate in water.

Sample solution

Accurately weighed quantity of the sample is extracted with water to get 100 mcg/ml in respect of salbutamol sulphate.

Procedure

To 3 ml each of standard and sample solutions, add 3 ml of sodium carbonate solution, 0.2 ml of p-aminophenol reagent and volume is adjusted to 10 ml with water. After 25 min, the absorbance of both the solutions is measured at about 635 nm against blank. The method obeys Beer's law over the concentration range of 5-60 mcg/ml.

METHOD 2

Reagents

1. Borate buffer, pH 8.2.
2. 0.04% w/v solution of 3,5-dichloro-p-benzoquinone chlorimide.

Sample and standard solution

100 mcg/ml of the compound in water; see method 1 above.

Procedure

To 2 ml each of sample and standard solutions, add 1 ml of borate buffer and 1 ml of chlorimide reagent, dilute to 10 ml with water. After 20 minutes, measure the absorbance of both standard and sample solutions at about 610 nm against reagent blank. The method obeys Beer's law over the concentration range of 2-12 mcg/ml.

METHOD 3

Reagents

1. 5% w/v freshly prepared solution of sodium cobaltinitrite in water.

2. 20% w/v solution of sodium hydroxide in water.

Standard solution

500 mcg of salbutamol sulphate in water.

Sample solution

Weigh accurately a quantity of the sample equivalent to 10 mg of salbutamol sulphate and dissolve in 20 ml of water, shake, filter and discard first few ml of the filtrate.

Procedure

(A) Accurately measure 2 ml of sample and standard solutions, add 2 ml of glacial acetic acid and 2 ml of cobaltinitrite reagent. Heat on a water bath (heating should be uniform) for 15 minutes or till blank (reagents and 2 ml of water) turns bright pink. Cool and adjust to 50 ml with water. Measure the absorption of both the solutions at maximum at about 325 nm against blank. The method obeys Beer's law in the range of 10-40 mcg/ml.

(B) Follow procedure A; after heating the solutions for 15 minutes, add 10 ml of water and 20 ml of sodium hydroxide solution, filter and adjust to 50 ml with water. Measure the absorbance of both the solutions at about 412 nm against reagent blank. The method obeys Beer's law in the range of 15-40 mcg/ml. The colour is stable for 5 h. In case of coated tablets, colour of the coating should be removed to avoid interference due to the dye.

METHOD 4

Reagents

1. 1 N hydrochloric acid.
2. 3% w/v solution of sodium nitrite in water.
3. 1 N sodium hydroxide.
4. 1% w/v solution of copper acetate in water.

Standard solution

100 mcg/ml of salbutamol sulphate in water.

Sample solution

Sample accurately weighed is extracted with water to get 100 mcg/ml solution of the compound.

Procedure

(A) To 5 ml of sample and standard solutions, add 2 ml of sodium nitrite solution and 1 ml of 1 N hydrochloric acid. Allow to stand for 5 minutes and render the solutions alkaline with 3 ml of sodium nydroxide solution. Mix and allow to stand for 5 minutes and measure the absorbance of both the solutions at about 425 nm against reagent blank. The method obeys Beer's law in the range of 2-20 mcg/ml.

(B) To 10 ml each of the sample and standard solutions, add 2 ml of sodium nitrite solution and 2 ml of copper acetate solution. Mix and add 0.2 ml of 1 N hydrochloric acid. Heat on water bath for 25 minutes, cool and dilute to 25 ml with water. Measure the extinction of both the solutions at about 525 nm. Beer's law is obeyed in the range of 40-400 mcg/ml.

(C) Follow the method (A) above. After addition of hydrochloric acid, heat in a water bath for 5 min, cool and basify. Procedure (C) is more sensitive than procedure (A). Beer's law is obeyed in the range of 1-10 mcg/ml.

METHOD 5

This method is based on the reaction of phenols with 4-aminoantipyrine after oxidation with alkaline potassium ferricyanide. The following alkaline media are recommended.

Reagents

1. Alkaline solutions :
   (a) 8.4% w/v solution of sodium carbonate in water.
   (b) Buffer pH 10 : Boric acid—2.370 g, Potassium chloride—14.910 g, Water to produce 1000 ml.
       250 ml of this solution is mixed with 44 ml of 1 N sodium hydroxide and diluted to 1000 ml with water. Check pH.
   (c) Ammonia-ammonium chloride buffer : 67.5 g of ammonium chloride and 570 ml of strong ammonia solution are mixed and diluted with water to 1000 ml. 2 ml of this solution is diluted to 1000 ml with water. Any one of the alkaline solutions indicated above can be used, however alkaline solution (b) and (c) are reported to give better results.
2. 2% w/v solution of 4-aminoantipyrine in water, prepare fresh.
3. 8% w/v solution of potassium ferricyanide in water, prepare fresh.

Standard solution

400 mcg/ml of the salbutamol (base) in water (40 mg of base is equivalent to 48.2 mg of salbutamol sulphate).

Sample solution

Accurate quantity of the sample is weighed and extracted with water to get 400 mcg/ml of the base.

Procedure

To 2.5 ml each of sample and standard solutions, add 5 ml of antipyrine solution and 5 ml of ferricyanide solution. Shake and add 5 ml of alkaline solutions. Keep for 30 minutes and extract with three portions of 25 ml, 10 ml, 10 ml of chloroform. Pass each chloroform layer through anhydrous sodium sulphate, previously washed with chloroform and dilute to 50 ml with chloroform. Measure the absorbance of both the solutions at about 470 nm against reagent blank.

Theophylline

Follow the method 2 described under formulation 1 of this chapter.

Salbutamol sulphate, Choline theophyllinate

ESTIMATION

Salbutamol sulphate

Follow the method 5 described under formulation 14 of this chapter.

Choline theophyllinate

Measure sample equivalent to about 100 mg of the substance, add 25 ml of water and few drops of bromocresol solution. Add 0.5 N hydrochloric acid till the colour changes to full yellow. Add 5 g of sodium chloride and extract with four 25 ml portions of chloroform : isopropanol (3 : 1) mixture. Wash each extract with the same 10 ml of water. Pass the combined organic layer through anhydrous sodium sulphate. Wash the sodium sulphate bed with solvent mixture. Evaporate the combined extract to dryness on water bath and dry the residue to constant weight at 150°C. Cool, weigh and calculate the results.

$$\% \text{ (w/v) of choline theophyllinate} = \frac{\text{Weight (mg) of the residue} \times 1.572 \times 100}{200}$$

Alternatively, the residue obtained above after evaporation of combined organic extract may be taken up in 0.1 N hydrochloric acid and measure the absorbance at maximum at about 275 nm. Calculate the results by measuring the absorbance of standard solution at 275 nm. Or, suspend the sample in 20 ml of water and 20 ml of 0.1 N sulphuric acid, extract with 2 × 50 ml portions of ether. Collect the acidic layer and dilute with 0.1 N sulphuric acid to give a concentration of 10 mcg/ml and measure the extinction of both sample and standard (10 mcg/ml) at about 275 nm using 0.1 N sulphuric acid as blank and calculate the results.

Note : The residue may be dissolved in 50 ml of hot water, cooled and 20 ml of 0.1 N silver nitrate added and titrated with 0.1 N sodium hydroxide using bromothymol blue as indicator. Each ml of 0.1 N sodium hydroxide is equivalent to 28.33 mg of choline theophyllinate.

Salbutamol sulphate, Bromhexine hydrochloride, Hydroxyethyltheophylline

ESTIMATION

Salbutamol sulphate

Reagents

1. 5% w/v solution of sodium bicarbonate in water.
2. 1% w/v solution of 4-aminoantipyrine in alcohol.
3. 8% w/v solution of potassium ferricyanide in water.

Standard solution

20 mg/100 ml of salbutamol sulphate in water. Further dilute 10 ml of the solution to 50 ml with alcohol.

Sample solution

Weigh accurate quantity of sample equivalent to 20 mg of the substance. Add about 50 ml of water. Shake vigorously and make up to 100 ml with water. Filter and dilute 10 ml of the filtrate to 50 ml with alcohol.

Procedure

Transfer 10 ml each of the sample and standard solutions to 250 ml separator. Add 100 ml of water, 4 ml each of bicarbonate solution, antipyrine reagent and potassium ferricyanide solution. Mix and allow to stand in subdued light for 15 min. Extract with three 15 ml portions of chloroform. Pass the chloroform layer through pre-moistened anhydrous sodium sulphate layer. Make up the volume to 50 ml with chloroform and measure the absorption of both the solution at about 463 nm using chloroform as blank, deduce the results by comparison. Alternatively, method 1 described in formulation 14 of this chapter based on reaction with alkaline p-aminophenol (λ_{max} 635 nm) may be used.

Hydroxyethyltheophylline (Etofylline)

Standard solution

10 mcg/ml of hydroxyethyltheophylline in water.

Sample solution

Weigh accurately quantity of sample equivalent to 200 mg of the substance and transfer to a 100 ml volumetric flask. Add about 70-80 ml of water, shake and dissolve and make up the volume. Filter and dilute the filtrate appropriately with water to get a concentration of 10 mcg/ml. Measure the extinction of both the solutions at maxima at about 273 nm using water as blank. Calculate the results by comparison.

Bromhexine hydrochloride

Reagents

1. 5 N hydrochloric acid.
2. 2% w/v sodium nitrite solution in water.
3. 5% w/v solution of ammonium sulphamate in water.
4. 0.1% w/v solution of N-1-naphthyl-ethylene-diamine dihydrochloride (NED).

Standard solution

40 mg/ml of bromhexine in methanol. Dilute 5 ml of this solution to 100 ml with water containing 2-3 drops of dilute hydrochloric acid.

Sample solution

Weigh accurately the sample equivalent to 40 mg of substance and prepare the final solution as described under standard solution.

Procedure

To 5 ml each of sample and standard solutions, add 1 ml of 5 N hydrochloric acid, 1 ml of sodium nitrite solution. Allow to stand for 5 min, add 1 ml of ammonium sulphamate solution, allow to stand for 3 min, followed by 1 ml of NED reagent. After 10 min measure the absorption of both the solutions at about 525 nm against reagent blank. Deduce the results by comparison.

Note : For quantitative estimation, extinction of the sample (40 mcg/ml) as obtained above can directly be measured at 317 nm and results calculated by using 87 as of A 1%, 1 cm at 317 nm.

Bromhexine hydrochloride, Salbutamol sulphate, Betamethasone

ESTIMATION

Bromhexine hydrochloride

Follow the method described in formulation 16 of this chapter.

Betamethasone

Reagents

1. 0.5% w/v solution of tetrazolium blue in methanol.
2. 10% w/v solution of tetramethyl ammonium hydroxide (TMAH) solution in methanol.

Standard solution

10 mcg/ml of betamethasone in chloroform.

Sample solution

Weigh powdered sample equivalent to 1 mg of betamethasone suspended in 10 ml of water and extract with chloroform (3 × 20 ml), passing each extract through anhydrous sodium sulphate, make up the final volume to 100 ml.

Procedure

To 10 ml each of sample and standard solutions add 2 ml of tetrazolium blue solution, followed by 2 ml of TMAH solution. Keep aside for 45 min at 37°C and measure the absorbance of both the solutions at 525 nm against reagent blank. Calculate the results by comparison.

Salbutamol sulphate

Reagent

1. 0.1% w/v solution of 2,6-dichloroquinone chlorimide in isopropyl alcohol.
2. Dilute ammonia solution.
3. Isopropyl alcohol.

Standard solution

40 mcg/ml of salbutamol sulphate in water as sample solution.

Sample solution

Accurately weighed quantity of the powdered tablet equivalent to 4 mg of the substance is dissolved in water by sonication, diluted to 100 ml and filtered (40 mcg/ml).

Procedure

To 2 ml each of sample and standard solutions, add 2 ml of dilute ammonia solution, followed by 1 ml of chlorimide reagent. Make up to 25 ml with isopropyl alcohol and measure absorbance of both the solutions at 650 nm against reagent blank. To calculate amount of salbutamol (base), multiply by the factor 239.3/288.4.

Note :   In case of liquid formulations (syrups) prior extraction with ether may be necessary to remove interference due to excipients.

Hydroxyethyltheophylline (Etofylline), Theophylline

ESTIMATION

Hydroxyethyltheophylline (Etofylline)

Reagents

1. Formic acid, anhydrous.
2. 0.1 N perchloric acid.
3. Acetic anhydride.
4. Chloroform.
5. Crystal violet solution, indicator.

Procedure

Weigh sample accurately equivalent to about 250 mg of the substance, add about 75 ml of chloroform. Shake for about 15 min, filter into dry conical flask. Repeat extraction with further 25 ml of chloroform. Evaporate combined chloroform layer on water-bath. Dissolve the residue in 2 ml of formic acid, anhydrous, add 50 ml of acetic anhydride, few drops of indicator and titrate with 0.1 N perchloric acid to yellow end point. Each ml of 0.1 N perchloric acid is equivalent to 0.02242 g of etofylline.

Theophylline

METHOD 1

Reagents

1. 0.1 N sodium hydroxide.
2. Bromothymol blue solution, indicator.

Procedure

Accurately weighed quantity of the sample equivalent to 200 mg of theophylline is dissolved in about 50 ml of water by gently heating on water-bath, filter, wash the residue with water, combine the filtrate. Add 25 ml of 0.1 N silver nitrate, 1 ml of bromothymol blue solution and titrate with 0.1 N sodium hydroxide to blue end point. Each ml of 0.1 N sodium hydroxide is equivalent to 18.02 mg of theophylline (anhydrous).

METHOD 2

Reagents

1. 0.1 N silver nitrate.
2. 0.5% v/v solution of ammonium hydroxide in water.
3. 25% v/v nitric acid.
4. 0.1 N ammonium thiocyanate.

5. Ferric ammonium sulphate solution-indicator.
6. Ammonium acetate.

Procedure

Weigh accurately quantity of the sample equivalent to 200 mg of theophylline, add 50 ml of ammonia solution and shake vigorously for about 10-15 min. Centrifuge and to the clear solution, add 2 g of ammonium acetate and heat to boiling. Add 15 ml of silver nitrate solution drop-wise. Cool in ice-bath, filter, wash the precipitates with ice cold water. Dissolve the silver-theophylline precipitates in 20 ml of nitric acid (25%), cool, add 25 ml of water and 5-10 drops of indicator. Titrate with 0.1 N ammonium thiocyanate solution. Each ml of 0.1 N ammonium thiocyanate solution is equivalent to 0.0198 g of theophylline monohydrate (A).

Note : The precipitates of silver-theophylline complex should not be exposed to direct sunlight as reduction would occur.

Theophylline and Etofylline (total)

Standard solution

10 mcg/ml of etofylline in 0.1 N hydrochloric acid.

Sample solution

Weigh sample accurately equivalent to 200 mg of etofylline, add 25-30 ml of 0.1 N hydrochloric acid, heat to boiling and cool. Dilute to 100 ml with acid, filter and dilute the filtrate appropriately and step-wise with 0.1 N hydrochloric acid to get a concentration of 10 mcg/ml.

Procedure

Measure the extinction of both sample and standard solutions at maxima at about 273 nm using 0.1 N hydrochloric acid as blank. Calculate the results by comparison. This will give total (theophylline monohydrate + etofylline) = (B).

Contents of etofylline = B – (A × 1.31).

Bromhexine hydrochloride, Salbutamol sulphate, Theophylline

ESTIMATION

Bromhexine hydrochloride

METHOD 1

Follow the method described in formulation 28 of the chapter on expectorants and cough suppressants.

METHOD 2

Reagents

1. 0.04% w/v solution of p-dimethylaminocinnamaldehyde (PDAC) in methanol.
2. Trifluoroacetic acid (TFA).

Standard solution

200 mcg/ml solution of bromhexine hydrochloride in methanol.

Sample solution

Accurately weighed quantity of powdered sample equivalent to 100 mg of the substance was dissolved in methanol, filtered (for removal of the colour in coated tablets, boiling with activated charcoal is necessary) and appropriately diluted to get final concentration of 200 mcg/ml.

Procedure

To 2 ml of sample and standard solutions, add 2 ml of PDAC solution followed by 1 ml of TFA. Both the solutions were allowed to stand at room temperature for 10 min and absorbance of reddish colour was measured at 510 nm against reagent blank and results calculated by comparison.

Note : 1. The method obeys Beer's law in the concentration range of 100-1000 mcg.
2. The red colour so developed in stable for more than 60 min.

Salbutamol sulphate

The acidic extract obtained during estimation of bromhexine hydrochloride as described in formulation 28 of the chapter on expectorants is diluted appropriately and subjected to analysis as per method described in formulation 14 of this chapter.

Theophylline

Follow the method 1 described under formulation 18 of this chapter.

Bromhexine hydrochloride, Terbutaline sulphate, Guaiphenesin

ESTIMATION

Terbutaline sulphate

Follow the method described in formulation 21 of this chapter based on alkaline oxidation and coupling with 4-aminoantipyrine.

Bromhexine hydrochloride

Standard solution

50 mcg/ml of bromhexine hydrochloride in 0.1 N hydrochloric acid.

Sample solution

Suspend accurately weighed quantity of sample equivalent to 5 mg of the substance in 10 ml of water, basify with dilute ammonia solution and extract with n-hexane (4 × 25 ml). Combine the organic layer and extract with 0.1 N hydrochloric acid (4 × 20 ml). Combine the acidic layer and dilute to 100 ml. Measure the absorbance of both sample and standard solutions at 317 nm using 0.1 N hydrochloric acid as blank. Calculate the results by comparison.

Guaiphenesin

Standard solution

Dissolve 50 mg of guaiphenesin in 50 ml of water containing 1 ml of hydrochloric acid and dilute with water to produce 100 ml. Further dilutions are done with water to get working standard solution of 50 mcg/ml.

Sample solution

Accurately weighed quantity of sample is diluted as described under standard solution.

Procedure

25 ml each of sample and standard solutions are extracted with petroleum ether. The absorbance of aqueous layers is measured at 273 nm using 0.1 N hydrochloric acid as blank and results calculated by comparison.

Typical laboratory analysis

Bromhexine hydrochloride
Weight of the standard = 0.0453 g
Volume of sample = 5 ml

354 Quantitative Analysis of Drugs in Pharmaceutical Formulations

Absorbance (standard) = 0.848
Absorbance (sample) = 0.775

$$\text{Concentration of Bromhexine HCl/10 ml} = \frac{0.775}{0.843} \times \frac{\text{Weight of standard}}{\text{Volume of sample}} \times d_f$$

$$= \frac{0.775}{0.848} \times \frac{0.0453}{5} \times \frac{1}{100} \times \frac{5}{50} \times 100 \times 10$$

$$= 0.828 \text{ mg}$$

$$\text{Claim} = 8 \text{ mg}$$

$$\% \text{ claim} = 103.50\%$$

Guaiphenesin
Weight of standard = 0.0511 g
Volume of the sample = 10 ml
Absorbance (Std.) = 0.677
Absorbance (Sample) = 0.655

$$\text{Concentration of Guaiphenesin (mg/10 ml)} = \frac{0.655}{0.677} \times \frac{\text{Weight of standard}}{\text{Weight of sample}} \times d_f$$

$$= \frac{0.655}{0.677} \times \frac{0.0511}{10} \times \frac{1}{5} \times \frac{5}{100} \times \frac{100}{10} \times \frac{100}{5}$$

$$= 98.88 \text{ mg}$$

$$\text{Claim} = 100 \text{ mg}$$

$$\% \text{ claim} = 98.88$$

Terbutaline sulphate
Weight of the standard = 0.0496 g
Volume of the sample = 10 ml
Absorbance (std.) = 0.490
Absorbance (sample) = 0.495

$$\text{Concentration of Terbutaline sulphate (mg/10 ml)} = \frac{A_u}{A_s} \times \frac{\text{Weight of standard}}{\text{Weight of sample}} \times d_f$$

$$= \frac{0.495}{0.490} \times \frac{0.0496}{10} \times \frac{5}{50} \times \frac{25}{50} \times \frac{10}{1}$$

$$= 2.505 \text{ mg}$$

$$\text{Claim} = 2.5 \text{ mg}$$

$$\% \text{ claim} = 100.20$$

Theophylline or Etofylline, Terbutaline sulphate, Bromhexine hydrochloride

ESTIMATION

Terbutaline sulphate

METHOD 1

The method is based on alkaline oxidation of terbutaline (a phenol) by ferricyanide and coupling with 4-aminoantipyrine.

Reagents

1. 0.3 M tris (hydroxymethyl) amino methane buffer pH 9.5.
2. 2% w/v solution of 4-aminoantipyrine in water (prepare fresh).
3. 8% w/v solution of potassium ferricyanide in water.

Standard solution

100 mcg/ml of terbutaline sulphate in water.

Sample solution

Accurately weighed quantity of the sample equivalent to 10 mg of terbutaline sulphate is suspended in 5 ml of 0.1 N hydrochloric acid and 25 ml of water. Shake for 10-15 min and dilute to 25 ml with water. Filter and use the filtrate for analysis.

Procedure

To 5 ml each of sample, standard and blank, add 35 ml of tris buffer, 1 ml of antipyrine reagent, followed by 1 ml of ferricyanide solution. Mix and make up of the volume to 50 ml with tris buffer. Immediately measure the absorbance at 550 nm.

Note : 1. The colour is not stable but reproducible results can be obtained if time from addition of reagent and measurement of absorption is kept constant ($\not> 1$ min).
2. Theophylline gives slight colour with this reagent, it is preferable if the 'BLANK' contains appropriate quantity of theophylline.

METHOD 2

Reagents

1. 2% w/v solution of sodium metaperiodate in water.
2. Ammonium acetate solution : Dissolve 30 g of ammonium acetate in small volume of water, add 1 ml of freshly distilled acetyl acetone and dilute to 100 ml with water (pH 4.7).

Standard solution

2 mg/ml of terbutaline sulphate in water.

Sample solution

Dilute the sample appropriately with water to get solution of 2 mcg/ml.

Procedure

To 1 ml each of sample and standard solutions, add 2 ml of periodate solution and heat in water-bath (50°C) for 10 min. Then add 5 ml of ammonium acetate reagent and again heat in boiling water-bath for 10 min, cool and dilute to 100 ml with water. Measure the absorbance of both the solutions at 412 nm against reagent blank and calculate the results by comparison. The method obeys Beer's law in the concentration range of 20-160 mcg/ml.

Theophylline

Follow the method described in formulation 18 of this chapter. Alternatively, the sample may be extracted with 0.1 N hydrochloric acid (10 mcg/ml) and measure the extinction at 271 nm. Calculate the results by comparing with the standard (10 mcg/ml in 0.1 N hydrochloric acid).

Bromhexine hydrochloride

Follow the method described in formulation 16 and 19 of this chapter.

Chapter 11

Cardiovascular Drugs

Formulation 1

Dihydralazine sulphate, Hydrochlorothiazide, Reserpine

ESTIMATION

Dihydralazine sulphate

METHOD 1

Reagents

1. 1 N hydrochloric acid.
2. 2 N hydrochloric acid.
3. Methanol.
4. 2% w/v solution of 4-dimethylaminobenzaldehyde (PDAB) in methanol.

Saturated solution

100 mcg/ml of dihydralazine sulphate in 1 N hydrochloric acid.

Sample solution

Suspend accurately weighed quantity of the sample in 50 ml of 2 N hydrochloric acid and shake mechanically for 60 min, dilute to 100 ml with water (100 mcg/ml).

Procedure

To 4 ml each of sample and standard solutions, add 10 ml of methanol and 5 ml of PDAB reagent. Keep at room temperature for 30 min and dilute to 100 ml with methanol.

Measure the extinction of both sample and standard solutions at 405 nm against reagent blank and calculate the contents of dihydralazine sulphate by comparison.

METHOD 2

Reagents

1. 0.1 N hydrochloric acid.
2. Methanol.
3. 1% w/v solution of O-phenanthroline in 0.1 N hydrochloric acid (dye).
4. Methanol : 0.1 N hydrochloric acid (1 : 1) mixture (solvent).
5. 0.20 w/v solution of ferric nitrate in 0.1 N hydrochloric acid.

Standard solution

50 mcg/ml of dihydralazine sulphate in solvent.

Sample solution

Weigh accurately powdered sample equivalent to 10 mg of the substance, add 10 ml of 0.1 N hydrochloric acid and shake for 30 min, dilute to 25 ml with methanol. Filter and dilute appropriately with solvent to get solution of 50 mcg/ml.

Procedure

To 5 ml each of sample and standard solutions, add 10 ml of ferric nitrate solution and 10 ml of dye solution. Swirl the flask and warm at 60°C in water-bath for 30 min. Cool and adjust to 100 ml with water.

Measure the absorbance of both sample and standard solutions at 508 nm against solvent blank and calculate the contents of dihydralazine sulphate by comparison.

METHOD 3

Weigh accurately powdered sample equivalent to 100 mg of substance, add 50 ml of water, stir for 15 min, add 50 ml 2 N hydrochloric acid and titrate with 0.1 N sodium nitrite till blue colour is produced when a glass rod dipped into the titrated solution is streaked on the smear of starch-zinc iodide paste. Each ml of 0.1 N sodium nitrite is equivalent to 14.415 mg of dihydralazine sulphate.

Hydrochlorothiazide

METHOD 1

Reagents

1. 2 N ammonium hydroxide.
2. 2 N sodium hydroxide.
3. 2 N hydrochloric acid.
4. 0.2 N sodium nitrite.
5. 2% w/v solution of ammonium sulphamate in water.
6. 1% solution of N-(1-naphthyl)-ethylene diamine dihydrochloride (NED).

Standard solution

To 25 mg of the substance, accurately weighed, add 50 ml of 2 N ammonia and dilute to 500 ml with water (50 mcg/ml).

Sample solution

Suspend accurately weighed sample equivalent to 25 mg of the solution in 50 ml of 2 N ammonia, shake for 30 min and dilute to 500 ml with water.

Hydrolysis of sample and standard

To 20 ml each of sample and standard solutions, add 20 ml of 2 N sodium hydroxide and heat to boiling under reflux for 90 min. Cool and add 25 ml of 2 N hydrochloric acid, cool to 20-25°C, add further 25 ml of 2 N hydrochloric acid, add 1 ml of 0.2 N sodium nitrite. Mix, after 3 min add 2 ml of ammonium sulphamate solution, stir and allow to stand for 10 min, add 2 ml of NED reagent and dilute to 100 ml with water.

Measure to absorption of both sample and standard solutions at 515 nm against reagent blank and calculate the contents of hydrochlorothiazide by comparison.

METHOD 2

Standard solution

Dissolve 10 mg of the substance, accurately weighted, in 10 ml of 2 N sodium hydroxide and dilute to 100 ml with water. Further dilute 5 ml to 50 ml with water (10 mcg/ml).

Sample solution

Accurately weighed quantity of the sample equivalent to 10 mg of the substance is suspended in 20 ml of water and extracted with 4 × 15 portions of chloroform. To the aqueous layer, add 10 ml of 1 N sodium hydroxide and further extract with 4 × 15 ml portions of chloroform. Aqueous alkaline extract is diluted with water to get final concentration of 10 mcg/ml.

Concomitantly measure the absorption of both sample and standard solutions at 273 nm against reagent blank and calculate the contents of hydrochlorothiazide.

Reserpine

METHOD 1

Reagents

1. 2% w/v solution of citric acid in water.
2. 1% w/v solution of sodium bicarbonate in water.
3. 0.3% w/v solution of sodium nitrite in 50% methanol.
4. 5% w/v solution of ammonium sulphamate in water.
5. Methanol.
6. Hydrochloric acid.
7. Chloroform.

Standard solution

Dissolve 25 mg of accurately weighed substance in 1-2 drops of chloroform, mix about 30 ml of methanol (previously warmed to 50°C). Cool and dilute to 250 ml with methanol (protect this solution from light—use amber coloured glass apparatus). (Just before start of estimation, take 10 ml of the solution, add 35 ml of chloroform and dilute to 50 ml with methanol).

Sample solution

Extract accurately weighed quantity of the sample equivalent to 1 mg of the substance with 10 ml of chloroform by shaking for 5 min. Add 10 ml of citric acid and shake for 2 min, collect chloroform layer, wash citric acid layer with further 10 ml of chloroform. To the combined chloroform layer, add 10 ml of sodium bicarbonate solution, shake for 2 min. Collect chloroform layer into 50 ml flask through pre-moistened cotton plug. Extract the aqueous layer with 2 × 5 ml portions of chloroform, combine chloroform layer and dilute to 50 ml with methanol.

Procedure

To 5 ml each of sample and standard solutions, add 2 ml methanol, 1 ml of sodium nitrite solution and 5 drops of hydrochloric acid. Mix and allow to stand for 30 min. Add 0.5 ml of ammonium sulphamate solution and dilute to 10 ml with methanol. Allow to stand for 10 min. Determine the absorbance of both the solutions at 390 nm against solvent blank (chloroform-methanol-water, 3.6 + 5.4 + 1.0 v/v) and calculate the contents of reserpine.

METHOD 2

Reagents

1. To about 200 mg of vanadium pentoxide, add 20 ml of water and 200 ml of orthophosphoric acid, shake vigorously and dilute to 1000 ml with absolute alcohol. Allow to stand at room temperature for 60 min and filter.
2. Methanol-0.1 N hydrochloric acid mixture (1 : 1), solvent.

Standard solution

200 mcg/ml of reserpine in methylene chloride. Dilute 5 ml to 100 ml with solvent.

Sample solution

Suspend accurately weighed quantity of the sample equivalent to 2 mg of solution in 100 ml of 0.1 N hydrochloric acid, stir for 30 min and heat in ultrasonic water-bath for 1 min, cool and dilute to 200 ml with methanol.

Procedure

Dilute 3 ml each of sample and standard solutions to 50 ml with vanadium pentoxide reagent. Determine the contents by fluorimetry using solvent as blank.

Excitation wavelength : 400 nm

Emission wavelength : 496 nm

Calculate the contents of reserpine in the sample by comparison.

Hydrochlorothiazide, Propranolol hydrochloride

ESTIMATION

METHOD 1

Both these substances in acidic medium have iso-absorption point at 284 nm; thus could be used for total contents of hydrochlorothiazide and propranolol, whereas propranolol has no absorption at 326 nm, absorption being solely due to hydrochlorothiazide, hence at 326 nm there will be no interference from propranolol.

Standard solution

1. 2 mcg/ml of propranolol hydrochloride in 0.1 N hydrochloric acid.
2. 1 mg/ml of hydrochlorothiazide in 0.1 N hydrochloric acid.

Sample solution

Accurately weighed quantity of the sample equivalent to 40 mg of propranolol was extracted with 50 ml of methanol in ultrasonic bath and diluted to 100 ml with 0.1 N hydrochloric acid.

Both the sample and standard solutions were further diluted appropriately and absorption measured at iso-absorption point (284 nm) for total contents of both the substances and at 326 nm for hydrochlorothiazide. Thus the contents of propranolol could be obtained by difference. The method observed Beer's law with range of 10-80 mcg/ml at 284 nm for both the substances and 10-250 mcg/ml at 326 nm for hydrochlorothiazide. The melted is suitable for dissolution studies.

METHOD 2

Standard solution

1. 80 mcg/ml of propranolol hydrochloride in water.
2. 50 mcg/ml of hydrochlorothiazide in 0.04 N sodium hydroxide.

Sample solution

Accurately weighed quantity of powdered sample equivalent to 40 mg of the propranolol hydroxide was extracted with 50 ml of 0.1 N hydrochloric acid by shaking for 30 min (80 mcg/ml).

Procedure

To 6 ml each of sample and standard solutions, add 1 ml of 5 N sodium hydroxide and 25 ml of n-heptane, shake for 5 min and allow the layers to separate (reserve alkaline aqueous layer for estimation of hydrochlorothiazide).

Concomitantly measure the absorbance of n-heptane layer (test and standard—2) at 293 nm against n-heptane blank extract and calculate the contents of propranolol hydrochloride in the sample.

The absorbance of aqueous extracts (test and standard—2) is measured at 273 nm against aqueous blank extract and calculate the contents of hydrochlorothiazide in the sample.

Propranolol hydrochloride, Hydroflumethazide

ESTIMATION

Propranolol hydrochloric and Hydroflumethazide

Standard solution

1. 20 mcg/ml of propranolol in 0.1 N hydrochloric acid.
2. 10 mcg/ml of hydroflumethazide in 0.1 N sodium hydroxide.

Sample solution

Suspend accurately weighed quantity of the sample in 10 ml of water, add 25 ml of 0.1 N sodium hydroxide and extract with 3 × 50 ml portions of water-washed anaesthetic ether. Combine the ether extract and wash with 20 ml of water. Retain the main aqueous alkaline layer and the washing for estimation of hydroflumethazide.

Extract the ether layer with 3 × 50 ml portions of 0.1 N hydrochloric acid, dilute the acid layer to 200 ml with acid and mix. Dilute further 10 ml of the resultant solution to 100 ml with 0.1 N hydrochloric acid and measure the extinction of both the solutions at 290 nm using 0.1 N hydrochloric acid as blank and the contents of propranolol are calculated by comparison.

Transfer the aqueous alkaline layer to 250 ml volumetric flask and dilute to mark with 0.1 N sodium hydroxide. Further dilute 10 ml of this solution to 100 ml with 0.1 N sodium hydroxide. Measure the absorption at 275 nm and of contents of hydroflumethazide are calculated by comparison.

Propranolol hydrochloride, Hydralazine hydrochloride

ESTIMATION

Propranolol hydrochloride and Hydralazine hydrochloride

Standard solution

1. 20 mcg/ml of propranolol hydrochloride in methanol.
2. 10 mcg/ml of hydralazine hydrochloride in water.

Sample solution

Extract accurately weighed quantity of powdered sample equivalent to 200 mg of propranolol with 10 ml of absolute alcohol by shaking for 10 min. Filter, use the filtrate for estimation of propranolol and preserve the residue for estimation of hydralazine.

Dilute 2 ml of filtrate obtained above to 100 ml with methanol, mix and further dilute 5 ml to 100 ml with methanol (20 mcg/ml) and measure the absorbance of both the solutions at 290 nm using methanol as blank and contents of propranolol calculated by comparison.

Transfer the residue obtained above to 500 ml volumetric flask and dissolve in water. 5 ml of the resultant solution is further diluted to 250 ml with water.

Absorbance of both sample and standard solutions is measured at 260 nm using water as blank and contents of hydralazine calculated by comparison.

Propranolol hydrochloride, Dihydralazine sulphate, Hydrochlorothiazide

ESTIMATION

Propranolol hydrochloride

Reagents

1. 0.05 N silver nitrate.
2. 0.05 ammonium thiocyanate.
3. 10% w/v solution of ferric ammonium sulphate.
4. Dilute nitric acid.
5. Nitrobenzene.

Procedure

Accurately weighed quantity of the powdered sample equivalent to 200 mg of propranolol was suspended in 25 ml of water, shake in mechanical shaker for 30 min and dilute to 50 ml with water. To 25 ml of filtrate, add 10 ml of dilute nitric acid and 25 ml of 0.05 N silver nitrate. Titrate excess of silver nitrate with 0.05 N ammonium thiocyanate using ferric ammonium sulphate as indicator. Carry out a blank titration. Each ml of 0.05 N silver nitrate consumed is equivalent to 14.79 mg of propranolol hydrochloride.

Dihydralazine sulphate

Reagents

1. 0.1 N sulphuric acid.
2. 1 N sodium hydroxide.
3. FC phenol reagent (1 : 1).

Standard solution

250 mcg/ml of the substance in 0.1 N sulphuric acid.

Sample solution

Accurately weighed quantity of the sample equivalent to 25 mg of the substance is shaken with 50 ml of 0.1 N sulphuric acid for 50 min in mechanical shaker, make up to 100 ml.

Procedure

To 4 ml each of sample and standard solutions, add 2 ml of 0.1 N sulphuric acid, 1 ml of FC phenol reagent and 1 ml of 1 N sodium hydroxide, dilute to 100 ml with water and measure the absorbance of both sample and standard solutions at 610 nm against reagent blank and calculate the contents by comparison.

Hydrochlorothiazide

This method is based on hydrolysis, diazotization and coupling with NED.

Reagents

1. 1% w/v solution of n-(1-naphthyl)-ethylene diamine dihydrochloride in water.
2. 2 N hydrochloric acid.
3. Dimethyl sulphoxide.
4. 2% w/v solution of sulphamic acid in water.
5. 0.02 N sodium nitrite.
6. 2 N sodium acetate.

Standard solution

25 mg of a substance is suspended in 10 ml of sodium hydroxide solution and heated under reflux for 60 min, cool, add 80-100 ml of water and 20 ml of 2 N hydrochloric acid and dilute to 200 ml with water.

Sample solution

Extract the sample with 100 ml of acetone. 5 ml of acetone extract is evaporated and residue hydrolysed with 10 ml of sodium hydroxide and further proceeded as with standard solution.

Procedure

To 10 ml each of sample and standard solutions, add 1 ml of sodium nitrite solution and allow to stand for 10 min, then add 2 ml of sulphamic acid solution and after further 10 min, add 5 ml of dimethyl sulphoxide and 2 ml of 'NED' solution and make up the volume to 100 ml with sodium acetate solution and measure the absorption of both sample and standard solutions at 513 nm against reagent blank and calculate the contents by comparison.

Metoprolol tartrate, Hydrochlorothiazide

ESTIMATION

METHOD 1

Reagents

1. Carbonate buffer solution, pH 11.0 : Mix 2.5 ml of 1 M sodium bicarbonate and 65 ml of sodium carbonate and dilute to 1000 ml with water.
2. Dichloromethane, saturated with water.
3. 1 N hydrochloric acid.
4. 1 N sodium hydroxide.

Metoprolol standard solution

4 mg/ml of metoprolol tartrate in dichloromethane.

Hydrochlorothiazide standard solution

Dissolve 100 mg of the substance in 2-3 ml of 1 N sodium hydroxide and dilute to 100 ml with buffer solution, pH 11.0.

Sample solution

Accurately weighed quantity of the powdered sample is suspended in 25 ml of buffer solution, add 25 ml of dichloromethane. Shake vigorously for 30 min, centrifuge to separate to layer. Aqueous phase (upper layer) is used for estimation of hydrochlorothiazide whereas organic phase is used for estimation of metoprolol.

Metoprolol tartrate

Dilute 5 ml of organic layer to 200 ml with dichloromethane and measure the absorbance of the solution at 277 nm.

Hydrochlorothiazide

Dilute 10 ml of aqueous phase to 50 ml with water and finally 5 ml is diluted to 50 ml with 0.1 N hydrochloric acid. Measure the absorbance at 272 nm.

Note : Treat 25 ml of each standard solution with buffer and dichloromethane and treat organic layer and aqueous layer as above.

METHOD 2

Metoprolol tartrate

Standard solution

100 mcg/ml of metoprolol tartrate in 0.1 N hydrochloric acid.

Sample solution

Extract accurately weighed quantity of the sample with 0.1 N hydrochloric acid by shaking for 30 min and filtering.

Procedure

To 10 ml each of sample and standard solutions, add 2 ml of 2.5 N sodium hydroxide and extract with 3 × 25 ml portions of chloroform, passing each extract from pre-rinsed glass wool, dilute to 100 ml with chloroform and measure the absorbance of both the solutions at 276 nm using chloroform as blank.

Hydrochlorothiazide

Standard solution

50 mcg/ml of hydrochlorothiazide in methanol.

Sample solution

Accurately weighed quantity of the sample is suspended in 15 ml of water, add 60 ml of methanol and sonicate for 5 min and dilute to 100 ml with methanol. Further dilute 10 ml to 50 ml with menthol.

Concomitantly measure the absorption of both the solutions at about 316 nm using methanol as blank, and calculate the contents of hydrochlorothiazide by comparison.

Formulation 7

Frusemide, Amiloride hydrochloride

ESTIMATION

METHOD 1

Both frusemide and amiloride have iso-absorption point at 260 nm in acidic solution, whereas frusemide has no absorption at 395 nm. This property has been used for quantitative estimation of both the substances. The absorption values at iso-absorption point (260 nm) gave total concentration of both the substances, whereas at 315 nm the absorption is solely due to amiloride. Thus frusemide could be calculated by difference.

Standard solutions

1. 8 mg/ml of frusemide in 0.1 N hydrochloric acid.
2. 1 mg/ml of amiloride in 0.1 N hydrochloric acid.

Sample solution

Accurately weighed quantity of the powdered sample equivalent to 40 mg of frusemide was separately extracted with 50 ml of 0.1 N hydrochloric acid in ultrasonic bath and diluted to 100 ml with 0.1 N hydrochloric acid.

Both sample and standard solutions were further diluted appropriately and absorbance measured at 260 nm and 395 nm, and results calculated by comparison. At 260 nm, total quantity of both the substances in the sample was obtained. The amount of amiloride present in the sample is calculated from absorption values at 395 nm and subtracted to get the quantity of frusemide.

The method obeyed Beer's law in the range of 5-30 mcg/ml for both the substances at 260 nm and 5-75 mg for amiloride at 395 nm. The method is suitable for dissolution studies.

METHOD 2

The method is based on the physical property of the components. Amiloride hydrochloride is soluble in water, whereas frusemide being insoluble could thus be separated by simple extraction with water.

Accurately weighed quantity of the sample equivalent to 4 mg of amiloride (AMD) was suspended in 20 ml of water, shaken for 5 min and filtered through G_3 sintered glass funnel. The filtrate was diluted to 50 ml with water. Further dilutions were done with water to get a final solution of 10 mcg/ml in respect of AMD.

The residue thus retained on the funnel was extracted with 0.1 N methanolic sodium hydroxide and further diluted to get a solution of 10 mcg/ml in respect of frusemide (FRS). Standard solution of both the substances were prepared in water (AMD) and in methanolic sodium hydroxide (FRS).

Absorbance of both sample and standard solutions were measured at 281 nm (AMD) and 274 nm (FRS) and results calculated by comparison.

METHOD 3

Frusemide

Accurately weighed quantity of the powdered sample is extracted with 0.1 N sodium hydroxide to get solution of 10 mcg/ml. The absorbance is measured without delay at 271 nm and the results are calculated taking 580 as value of A 1%, 1 cm at 271 nm.

Amiloride hydrochloride

To accurately weighed quantity of powdered sample equivalent to 10 mg of amiloride hydrochloride, add 10 ml of methanol and dilute to 100 ml with 0.1 N sodium hydroxide. Transfer 4 ml of the resulting solution to a 50 ml stoppered centrifuge tube, add 10 ml of methanol and 20 ml of tributyl ortho-phosphate (previously washed with water) and shake vigorously for 2 min and centrifuge for 5 min. Collect the upper layer and repeat the extraction with further 20 ml of tributyl orthophosphate (water-washed). Combine the extracts, add 2 ml of methanol and dilute to 50 ml with water-washed tributyl orthophosphate. Measure the absorbance of resulting solution at 363 nm against blank (24 ml of water-washed tributyl orthophosphate and 1 ml of methanol) and calculate the results taking 692 as value of A 1%, 1 cm at 363 nm.

Spironolactone, Frusemide

ESTIMATION

METHOD 1

Accurately weighed quantity of powdered sample equivalent to 50 mg of spironolactone (SPT) was suspended in 15 mg of chloroform and filtered through G₃ sintered glass funnel. The filtrate was diluted to 50 ml with chloroform. Further dilutions were made to get concentration of 10 mcg/ml of SPT.

The residue retained on the funnel was extracted with 0.1 N methanolic sodium hydroxide and diluted to get concentration of 10 mcg/ml in respect of frusemide (FRS).

Extinction of both sample and standard solutions was measured at 244 nm for SPT and at 274 nm for FRS and results calculated by comparison.

METHOD 2

Spironolactone

Reagent

1. Isonicotonic acid hydrazide reagent.

Standard solution

40 mcg/ml of spironolactone in methanol.

Sample solution

Extract appropriate quantity of powdered sample with methanol to get concentration of 40 mcg/ml.

Procedure

Evaporate 2 ml each of sample and standard solutions to dryness, add 5 ml of INH reagent. Close the tubes and heat for 60 min at 50°C. Cool and measure the absorbance of both the solutions at 405 nm against reagent blank and calculate the results by comparison.

Frusemide

Standard solution

8 mcg/ml of frusemide in 0.1 N sodium hydroxide.

Sample solution

Accurately weighed quantity of the sample equivalent to 20 mg of the sample is extracted with three 10 portions of ethyl acetate. The combined ethyl acetate extract is shaken with five 20 ml portions of 0.1 N sodium hydroxide and finally diluted to 250 ml. 5 ml of the resultant solution is diluted to 50 ml with 0.1 N sodium hydroxide (8 mcg/ml).

Measure the absorbance of both sample and standard solutions at 272 nm using 0.1 N sodium hydroxide as blank and calculate the results by comparison.

METHOD 3

Accurately weighed quantity of powdered sample equivalent to 50 mg of spironolactone is suspended in 25-30 ml of water. Add 5 ml of sodium carbonate solution (15%) and extract with four 40 ml portions of chloroform. Combine chloroform extract and preserve for estimation of spironolactone. Aqueous alkaline layer is used for estimation of frusemide.

Spironolactone

Standard solution

0.125 mg/ml in chloroform. Evaporate 5 ml and take up the residue in 100 ml of methanol (6.2 mcg/ml).

Sample solution

Wash the chloroform extract preserved during initial extraction with 25 ml of water and dilute the organic layer to 200 ml. Evaporate 5 ml and take up the residue in 100 ml of methanol.

Blank

Prepare by evaporating 2.5 ml of chloroform to dryness and take up the residue in 50 ml of methanol.

Determine the absorbance of both sample and standard solutions at about 238 nm against blank and calculate the results by comparison.

Frusemide

Standard solution

To 20 mg of the substance add 5 ml of sodium carbonate solution (15%) and dilute to 200 ml with 0.1 N sodium hydroxide. Further dilute 10 ml with 0.1 N sodium hydroxide (20 mcg/ml).

Sample solution

Aqueous alkaline solution preserved during initial extraction is appropriate diluted to get 20 mcg/ml.

Measure the absorbance of both the solutions at 272 nm against blank and calculate the results by comparison.

Spironolactone, Hydroflumethazide

ESTIMATION

METHOD 1

Spironolactone

Follow the method 3 described in formulation 8 of this chapter.

Hydroflumethazide

The aqueous extract obtained during estimation of spironolactone is appropriately diluted and extinction measured at 274 nm. For details, see method 3 in formulation 8 of this chapter.

METHOD 2

Standard solution

10 mcg/ml each of spironolactone (SPN) and hydroflumethazide (HFT) in methanol.

Sample solution

Accurately weighed quantity of the powdered sample was extracted with methanol by vigorously shaking for 10 min and diluting appropriately to get final concentration of 10 mcg/ml.

Absorption of the sample and standard solutions was measured at 238 nm, being the absorption maximum of SPN and at 273, the absorption maximum of HFT.

The results were calculated by comparing with the standard.

Spectral measurements at respective maxima did not show any interference. The method is suitable for routine quality control.

Enalapril maleate, Amlodipine besylate

ESTIMATION

Amlodipine besylate

Reagents

1. 0.1 N sodium hydroxide in methanol.
2. Dimethyl formamide (DMF).

Standard solution

50 mcg/ml of amlodipine besylate in DMF.

Sample solution

Extract appropriate quantity of powdered sample with DMF to get concentration of 50 mcg/ml.

Procedure

To 2 ml each of sample and standard solutions, add 0.2 ml of sodium hydroxide solution and dilute to 10 ml with DMF and measure the absorption of orange chromogen at 450 nm against reagent blank. Calculate the contents of amlodipine by comparison.

Enalapril maleate and Amlodipine besylate

Both the compounds were first separated by preparative thin layer chromatography and then subjected to colour development.

Reagents

1. 1% w/v solution of bromocresol green in buffer, pH 3.1.
2. Phthalate buffer, pH 3.1.

Standard solution

1 mg/ml of amlodipine besylate and enalapril maleate prepared separately in methanol.

Sample solution

Accurately weighed quantity of the sample was extracted with methanol to get solution of 1 mg/ml. The solution was centrifuged and clear supernatant used for chromatographic separation.

   TLC plate : TLC pre-coated plates, silica gel 60F$_{254}$.
   Mobile phase : Chloroform-methanol-acetic acid (8.5 + 1.5 + 0.1, v/v).
   Sample volume : 200 µl.
   Chamber saturation : 30 min.
   Development distance : 70 mm.

Both sample and standard were simultaneously subjected to thin layer chromatography on the same plate. The spots were located under UV and area corresponding to amlodipine was scraped and collected in separate centrifuge tubes each containing 10 ml of methanol, sonicated for 5 min for complete extraction and centrifuged. Blank prepared by scraping silica gel from an equivalent area from upper part of the TLC plate and extracting with 10 ml of methanol.

Amlodipine besylate

Measure the absorption both sample and standard solutions at 237 nm against blank and calculate the results by comparison. Or follow the colour development with methanolic potassium hydroxide as described above.

Enalapril maleate

The spot corresponding to enalapril was scraped and collected in a centrifuge containing 10 ml of buffer, pH 3.1. Shake well and centrifuge. To the entire supernatant, add 1 ml of dye and extract the yellow chromogen with 10 ml of chloroform. Centrifuge the chloroform layer and measure the absorption of both sample and standard at 410 nm against blank prepared by scraping silica gel from equivalent area of the plate and suspending in buffer, followed by addition of dye and extraction.

Amlodipine besylate, Atenolol

ESTIMATION

Atenolol

Standard solution

100 mcg/ml of atenolol in 0.1 N hydrochloric acid.

Sample solution

Accurately weighed quantity of the sample equivalent to 10 mg of the substance was extracted with 0.1 N hydrochloric acid to get a solution of 100 mcg/ml, centrifuged and supernatant used for estimation.

Measure the absorbance of both sample and standard solutions at maximum at about 276 nm and calculate the results by comparison.

Amlodipine besylate

Reagent

0.1 N sodium hydroxide in methanol.

Standard solution

50 mcg/ml of amlodipine besylate in DMF.

Sample solution

Accurately weighed quantity of the sample equivalent to 50 mg of the substance extracted with DMF and diluted suitably to produce a solution of 50 mcg/ml.

Procedure

To 2 ml each of sample and standard solutions, add 0.2 ml of sodium hydroxide solution and make up to 10 ml with DMF. Measure the absorption of both sample and standard solutions at 450 nm against reagent blank and calculate the results by comparison. The chromogen is stable for 30 min. The method obeys Beer's law in the range of 25-250 mcg.

METHOD 2

This method is based on preparative thin layer chromatography.

Test plate : TLC pre-coated plate silica gel $60F_{254}$ (aluminium).
Mobile phase : Toluene-isopropyl alcohol-ammonia (7.5 + 2.5 + 0.1, v/v)
Chamber saturation : 30 min without pads
Amount spotted : 50 μl of each sample and two standards
Development distance : 100 mm

Standard solution

1. 10 mcg/ml of atenolol in methanol.
2. 1 mg/ml of amlodipine in methanol (1 mg = 1.38 mg of amlodipine besylate).

Sample solution

Powdered sample extracted with methanol by sonicating for 5 min, centrifuged and supernatant used for spotting.

Procedure

The relevant position of the spots (sample and standard) was marked under UV (254 nm), the separated spots were separately extracted with methanol by cutting the relevant portion of the plate and suspending in 5 ml of methanol, extracted by vigorously shaking. The solution was centrifuged and absorbance of solutions (both sample and two standards) was measured at 237 nm (amlodipine) and 276 nm (atenolol) and results calculated by comparison. The results were comparable with that obtained by method 1.

Atenolol, Nifedipine

ESTIMATION

Atenolol

Standard solution

20 mcg/ml of atenolol in water.

Sample solution

Accurately weighed quantity of the sample equivalent to 100 mg of the substance is suspended in 100-125 ml water and stirred for 30 min and made up to 250 ml. 5 ml is further diluted to 100 ml with water (20 mcg/ml).

Concomitantly measure the absorbance of both sample and standard solutions at the maxima at about 225 nm using water as blank and calculate the results by comparison.

Nifedipine

METHOD 1

Standard solution

50 mcg/ml of nifedipine in methanol.

Sample solution

Accurately weighed quantity of sample extracted with methanol to get solution of 50 mcg/ml.

Concomitantly measure the absorbance of both sample and standard solutions at 350 nm using methanol as blank and calculate the results by comparison.

METHOD 2

Reagent

1. 2% w/v solution of sodium hydroxide in DMF.

Standard and sample solutions

Prepare the solutions in DMF (200 mcg/ml).

Procedure

To 0.5 ml each of sample and standard solutions, add 0.1 ml of sodium hydroxide solution and dilute to 10 ml with DMF and measure the absorbance of both the solutions at 425 nm against reagent blank and calculate the results by comparison.

Note : Estimation of nifedipine in visible range should be preferred as there are chances of its decomposition in UV range.

Atenolol, Hydrochlorothiazide, Amiloride hydrochloride

ESTIMATION

Atenolol

Standard solution

100 mcg/ml of atenolol in methanol.

Sample solution

Weigh accurately powdered sample equivalent 50 mg of the substance and dry extract with 3 × 30 ml of chloroform. Evaporate the combined chloroform extract and dissolve the residue in 100 ml of methanol by shaking for 5 min. Further dilute 10 ml to 50 ml with methanol.

Determine the absorbance of the sample and standard solutions at 276 nm against blank prepared by evaporating 5 ml of chloroform and 50 ml of methanol. Calculate the results by comparison.

Hydrochlorothiazide

Standard solution

50 mg/ml of hydrochlorothiazide in methanol.

Sample solution

Extract the accurately weighed quantity of the sample equivalent to 25 mg of the substance with 3 × 30 ml acetone by shaking for 5-10 min. Evaporate the combined acetone extract and take up the residue in methanol to produce 100 ml. 10 ml is further diluted to 50 ml with methanol (50 mcg/ml).

Determine the absorbance of both sample and standard solutions at 317 nm against blank (evaporate 5 ml of acetone to dryness and take up in 50 ml of methanol) and calculate the results by comparison.

Amiloride hydrochloride

Standard solution

5 mcg/ml in 0.1 N hydrochloric acid solution is prepared by heating for 5 min, followed by shaking for 10 min.

Sample solution

Accurately weighed quantity of the sample equivalent to 50 mg of the substance was suspended in 50 ml of 0.1 N hydrochloric acid, heated in water-bath for 5 min, cooled and shaken for 10 min and diluted to 100 ml with 0.1 N hydrochloric acid. 5 ml of the resultant solution is further diluted to 50 ml with 0.1 N hydrochloric acid.

Measure the absorbance of sample and standard at 361 nm using 0.1 N hydrochloric acid as blank. Calculate the results by comparison.

Formulation 14

Captopril, Hydrochlorothiazide

ESTIMATION

Captopril

METHOD 1

Weigh accurately powdered sample equivalent to 200 mg of the substance, add 100 ml of water, warm to 70°C for 5 min with frequent shaking, cool to room temperature, add 10 ml of 3.6 N sulphuric acid and 1 g of potassium iodide and shake to dissolve. Add 2 ml of standard solution and titrate with 0.1 N potassium iodide till dark brown colour persistently for 30 seconds is observed. Each ml of 0.1 N potassium iodate is equivalent to 21.73 mg of captopril.

METHOD 2

Reagents

1. Phosphate buffer, pH 7.2.
2. 4,4-dithiopyridine solution : Dissolve 10 mg of 4,4-dithiopyridine in phosphate buffer, pH 7.2 to produce 100 ml.

Standard solution

10 mcg/ml of the captopril.

Sample solution

An accurately weighed quantity of the sample was extracted with water to get solution of 10 mcg/ml.

Procedure

To 5 ml each of sample and standard solutions, add 3 ml of the reagent and dilute to 10 ml with water. Measure the absorption of both the solutions at 324 nm against reagent blank and calculate the results. The method obeys Beer's law in the range of 0.5-20 mcg/ml.

METHOD 3

Reagent

1. Dissolve 0.5 g of citric in 4 ml of methanol and dilute to 25 ml with acetic anhydride.

Standard and sample solutions

10 mcg/ml as in method 2, but to be prepared in methanol.

Procedure

To 3 ml each of sample and standard solutions, add 1 ml of the reagent and heat in boiling water-bath for 30 min, cool and dilute to 10 ml with acetic anhydride and measure the absorbance of the chromophore at 570 nm and calculate the results by comparison.

Hydrochlorothiazide

Standard solution

10 mcg/ml of hydrochlorothiazide in 0.1 N sodium hydroxide.

Sample solution

Suspend accurately weighed quantity of the sample in 50 ml of 0.1 N sodium hydroxide, shake for 5 min and dilute to 100 ml. Filter and dilute further to get solution of 10 mcg/ml.

Measure the absorbance of both sample and standard solutions at 273 nm using 0.1 N sodium hydroxide as blank and calculate the results by comparison.

Clonidine hydrochloride, Chlorthalidone

ESTIMATION

Clonidine hydrochloride

Reagents

1. 10% w/v acetic acid in water.
2. 0.1% metanil yellow.
3. 1 N hydrochloric acid.

Standard solution

50 mcg/ml of clonidine hydrochloride in water.

Sample solution

Suspend accurately weighed quantity for the sample equivalent to 0.1 mg of the substance in 20 ml of water, add 1 ml of acetic acid and 2 ml of metanil yellow. Shake and allow to stand for 20-25 min. Extract with two 60 ml portions of chloroform. The combined chloroform layer is extracted with three 25 ml portions of 1 N hydrochloric acid (discard chloroform layer) and dilute to 100 ml with 1 N hydrochloric acid.

To 2 ml of the standard solution (100 mcg) add 20 ml of water, 1 ml of acetic acid and 1 ml of metanil yellow solution and proceed as under sample solution.

Measure the absorption of both sample and standard at 530 nm and calculate the results by comparison.

Chlorthalidone

Standard solution

1 mg/ml of chlorthalidone in water. To 5 ml add 1 ml of 2 N hydrochloric acid and dilute to 50 ml with methanol (50 mcg/ml).

Sample solution

Accurately weighed quantity of the sample is boiled with 30 ml of methanol for 30 min, and dilute to 100 ml with methanol. To 5 ml of the filtrate, add 1 ml of 2 N hydrochloric acid and dilute to 50 ml with methanol.

Measure the extinction of both the solutions at 275 nm against blank (1 ml of 1 N hydrochloric acid diluted to 50 ml with methanol) and calculate the results by comparison.

Levodopa, Benserazide hydrochloride

ESTIMATION

Levodopa

Standard solution

30 mcg/ml of levodopa in 0.1 N hydrochloric acid.

Sample solution

Suspend accurately weighed quantity of the sample in 50 ml water. Warm on a boiling water-bath for 5 min, cool and dilute appropriately with 0.1 N hydrochloric acid to get final concentration of 30 mcg/ml.

Measure the absorbance of standard and sample solutions at 280 nm against 0.1 N hydrochloric acid as blank. Calculate the results by comparison.

Benserazide hydrochloride

Suspend accurately weighed quantity of the sample equivalent to 250 mg of the substance in 20 ml of water, add 0.5 ml of nitric acid and titrate with 0.1 N silver nitrate, potentiometrically. Each ml of 0.1 N silver nitrate is equivalent to 29.37 mg of benserazide hydrochloride. 259.21 mg of benserazide ≡ 293.7 mg of benserazide hydrochloride.

Chapter 12

Expectorants & Cough Suppressants

Formulation 1

Codeine phosphate, Ephedrine hydrochloride, Sodium citrate, Alcohol

ESTIMATION

Codeine phosphate

METHOD 1

Reagents

1. 2% and 4% v/v sulphuric acid.
2. 25% w/v sodium hydroxide solution in water.
3. Hexane-chloroform (3 : 1 v/v), solvent mixture.

Standard solution

150 mcg/ml of codeine phosphate in 2% sulphuric acid.

Sample solution

Dilute accurately measured volume of the sample equivalent to 7.5 mg of codeine phosphate to 50 ml with 4% sulphuric acid (150 mcg/ml).

Procedure

Transfer 5 ml of sample solution into a 250 ml separating funnel, add 15 ml of 2% sulphuric acid and swirl to mix. Extract the acid solution with three 30 ml portions of chloroform. Combine the chloroform extracts and extract with 5 ml of 2% sulphuric acid. Discard the chloroform layer and make the total acidic solution strongly alkaline with sodium hydroxide solution. Extract the solution using gentle shaking with 50 ml of solvent mixture. Transfer the organic layer into another 250 ml separating funnel containing 50 ml 2% sulphuric acid. Continue the extraction with an additional four 25 ml portions of the solvent mixture, gently shaking each time for 10-15 seconds. Allow for a clean separation each time and transfer organic solvent through cotton plug into separating funnel containing sulphuric acid. Shake the separating funnel containing acid and solvent layers vigorously for one minute to extract codeine back into the acid layer. Allow the phases to separate and centrifuge the aqueous phase to clarify the solution. Determine the absorbance of the standard codeine phosphate solution and of the sample solution obtained above by extraction procedure at 285 and 360 nm using 285 nm to obtain the net absorbance due to codeine and calculate the results by comparing with the standard solution.

METHOD 2

The acidic extract obtained in the method 1 above can be subjected to the following method.

Reagents

1. Buffer solution : The solution is prepared by dissolving 300 g of monosodium hydrogen phosphate and 9 g of sodium hydroxide in water and the volume is made to 750 ml with water.
2. 1% w/v solution of picric acid in water.

Standard solution

10 mcg/ml of codeine phosphate in water.

Sample solution

The sample solution (acidic extract as obtained in method 1 above) is diluted appropriately with water to get a concentration of 10 mcg/ml.

Procedure

To 5 ml each of the sample and standard solutions, add 5 ml of buffer solution, 5 ml of picric acid solution and 10 ml chloroform. Shake for 5-10 seconds and allow the chloroform layer to separate. Filter organic layer through cotton plug and measure the absorbance of both the solutions at about 430 nm against reagent blank and calculate the results by comparison.

Ephedrine hydrochloride

Reagents

1. Sodium metaperiodate, 0.75 M : Dissolve 1.6 g of sodium metaperiodate in 100 ml of water, prepare each day.
2. 50% w/v solution of sodium hydroxide in water.

Standard solution

30 mcg/ml of ephedrine hydrochloride in 0.1 N hydrochloric acid.

Sample solution

Transfer aliquot of the cough syrup (sample) equivalent to 60 mg of ephedrine hydrochloride into a 500 ml separating funnel and add 10 g of sodium chloride. Shake well to dissolve sodium chloride. Make the solution alkaline with sodium hydroxide solution. Extract alkaline aqueous solution with three 50 ml portions of ether. Collect ether extracts and wash with 20 ml of saturated solution of sodium chloride. Extract the ether solution with three 50 ml portions of 0.1 N hydrochloric acid. Collect all the acid extracts in a 250 ml beaker and warm on steam-bath to expel the dissolved ether from the acid. Dilute the acid solution to 200 ml in a volumetric flask. Further dilute 10 ml of the solution to 100 ml with 0.1 N hydrochloric acid. Designate this as sample solution (30 mcg/ml).

Procedure

Transfer 5 ml each of the sample and standard solutions to 25 ml volumetric flasks. Add 2 ml of water and three drops of phenolphthalein indicator solution to the flask containing standard solution. Add 2 ml of sodium metaperiodate solution and 3 drops of phenolphthalein solution to the flask containing sample solution. Add 1 N sodium hydroxide solution dropwise to each of the flasks until a permanent pink colour appears. The alkali should be added so as not to wet the neck. Add 2 drops of excess alkali and then swirl to mix the solution. Immediately, add 10 ml of n-hexane to each flask and stopper. After 5 minutes, shake both the flasks vigorously for 15 seconds and allow the phases to separate. Carefully open the flasks and dilute to volume with hexane, stopper and mix thoroughly by shaking. Allow the phases to separate before decanting the hexane solution into a 1 cm absorption cell. Determine the differential ultraviolet absorbance of the sample solution at 240 and 260 nm using hexane layer from the standard solution in the reference cell. Absorbance due to benzaldehyde is determined by subtracting the values at 260 nm (minimum) from that observed at 240 nm (maximum). Repeat the above analytical procedure using the standard solution (30 mcg/ml) for comparative purposes. It is preferable if the standard is processed simultaneously with the sample.

Sodium citrate as total citrate

Follow methods described in formulation 6 of this chapter.

Codeine phosphate, Ephedrine hydrochloride, Potassium guaiacolsulphonate

ESTIMATION

Ephedrine hydrochloride

Weigh or measure accurately a quantity of the sample equivalent to 20 mg of ephedrine hydrochloride. Basify with dilutes solution of ammonia and extract with four 30 ml portions of ether. Reserve aqueous layer for the estimation of codeine phosphate. Evaporate the ether layer at low temperature, dissolve the residue in 40 ml of glacial acetic acid and follow the method 2 involving nonaqueous titration described for estimation of ephedrine in formulation 8 of this chapter. Each ml of 0.1 N perchloric acid is equivalent to 0.02017 g of ephedrine hydrochloride.

Codeine phosphate

This method is based on phosphate-moiety of the molecule.

Reagents

1. Molybdate reagent : To 5 g of ammonium molybdate, add 80 ml of water and 25 ml of sulphuric acid. Warm to dissolve, cool and dilute to 100 ml with water.
2. Metol-bisulphite reagent : To 50 ml of water, add 0.1 g of sodium metabisulphite and 0.35 g of metol. Shake to mix, add 20 g of sodium metabisulphite and dilute with water to 100 ml.

Standard solution

20 mcg/ml of codeine phosphate in water.

Sample solution

Take the entire aqueous layer reserved during estimation of ephedrine, warm to expel dissolved ether and adjust the volume with water to get 20 mcg/ml in respect of codeine phosphate.

Procedure

To 5 ml each of the sample and standard solutions, add 4 ml of dilute sulphuric acid, 1 ml of molybdate reagent and 1 ml of metol-bisulphite reagent. Keep at room temperature for 30 minutes and measure the extinction of both the solutions at about 725 nm against reagent blank and calculate the results by comparison.

Potassium guaiacolsulphonate

Reagents

1. Borate buffer, pH 9.4.
2. 0.04% w/v solution of 2,6-dichloroquinone chlorimide in isopropyl alcohol.

Standard solution

100 mcg/ml of potassium guaiacolsulphonate in water.

Sample solution

Dilute appropriate quantity of the sample with water to get 100 mcg/ml of the substance.

Procedure

To 1 ml each of the sample and standard solutions, add 1 ml of borate buffer solution, pH 9.4, 2 ml of isopropyl alcohol and 1 ml of water. Add 1 ml of chlorimide reagent to each tube and keep aside for 15 minutes at room temperature. Measure the absorbance of both the solutions at about 650 nm against reagent blank and calculate the results by comparison. The method obeys Beer's law in the concentration range of 10-20 mcg/ml.

Note :   1. Phenolic compounds, if present, will interfere.
2. If ascorbic acid is present, reflux the sample with 0.1 N hydrochloric acid to destroy it.
3. The colour attains its maximum intensity within 10 minutes and is stable for 20 minutes.

Codeine and Ephedrine (total alkaloids as ephedrine hydrochloride)

Weigh or measure sample accurately equivalent to 20 mg of ephedrine hydrochloride, basify with 1 N sodium hydroxide and proceed for extraction and estimation of total alkaloids as described under formulation 18 of this chapter.

Working example

Each 5 ml of the preparation contains 10 mg of ephedrine hydrochloride and 1.5 mg of codeine phosphate. Total alkaloids in term of ephedrine hydrochloride can be estimated as under. Convert the claimed contents of codeine phosphate to ephedrine and express the total alkaloids in term of ephedrine hydrochloride.

1 ml of 0.1 N sulphuric acid is equivalent to 20.17 mg of ephedrine hydrochloride.

1 ml of 0.1 N sulphuric acid is equivalent to 39.74 mg of codeine phosphate.

39.74 mg of codeine phosphate = 20.17 mg of ephedrine hydrochloride.

1.5 mg of codeine phosphate = 0.76 mg of ephedrine hydrochloride.

Total alkaloids as ephedrine hydrochloride = 10 + 0.76 = 10.76 mg

After the titration with sodium hydroxide is complete, as described in formulation 18 of this chapter, add further 5 ml of 0.1 N sodium hydroxide and subject the contents to steam distillation. Estimate ephedrine in the distillate by acid, base titration. This procedure will give the contents of ephedrine present in the sample.

Codeine phosphate, Glyceryl guaiacolate, Phenylephrine hydrochloride, Chlorpheniramine maleate

ESTIMATION

Codeine phosphate

Follow the method 1 as described under formulation 1 of this chapter.

Glyceryl guaiacolate

Reagent

1. 20% w/v solution of sodium hydroxide in water.

Standard solution

Prepare a standard solution by dissolving 300 mg of glyceryl guaiacolate in 100 ml chloroform. Pipette 2 ml aliquot into 100 ml volumetric flask and dilute to volume with anhydrous methyl alcohol (60 mcg/ml).

Sample solution

Transfer accurate volume of the sample equivalent to 300 mg of glyceryl guaiacolate into 250 ml, separating funnel. Add 10 ml of sodium hydroxide solution and extract with four 40 ml portions of petroleum ether, reject ether layer. Collect the aqueous layer and extract with four 20 ml portions of chloroform. Filter the chloroform through a small cotton pledget into a 100 ml volumetric flask. Rinse the funnel and cotton with chloroform. Dilute to volume with chloroform. Transfer 2 ml aliquot into a 100 ml volumetric flask and dilute to volume with anhydrous methanol (60 mcg/ml).

Procedure

Determine the absorbance of the sample and standard solutions at 275 nm using anhydrous methanol as blank and calculate the results by comparison.

Phenylephrine hydrochloride

METHOD 1

Follow the method based on alkaline oxidation and coupling with antipyrine. For details, refer to formulation 1 of the chapter on analgesics and antipyretics.

METHOD 2

Follow the method 2 for estimation of phenylephrine as described in formulation 9 of this chapter.

Chlorpheniramine maleate

Reagents

1. Buffered solution of sulphanilic acid : Dissolve 2.5 g of sulphanilic acid and 10 g of anhydrous sodium acetate in 40 ml methanol and make volume to 200 ml with methanol.
2. 25% w/v sodium hydroxide solution in water.
3. Saturated solution of cyanogen bromide in water.

Stock standard solution

Accurately weigh 100 mg of chlorpheniramine maleate into 100 ml volumetric flask, dissolve and dilute to volume with 0.1 N hydrochloric acid.

Working standard

Dilute 10 ml of the stock solution to 250 ml with 0.1 N hydrochloric acid (40 mcg/ml).

Sample solution

Transfer sample equivalent to 10 mg of the substance into a 250 ml separatory funnel, rinse the pipette. Add 15 ml of sodium hydroxide solution and extract with four 50 ml portions of petroleum ether. Collect and combine the ether extracts. Wash the combined ether extract twice with 25 ml water. Reject the aqueous extract and washings. Extract the combined ether extract with five 20 ml portions of 0.1 N hydrochloric acid. Collect the combined acidic extract and dilute to 250 ml with 0.1 N hydrochloric acid (40 mcg/ml).

Procedure

To 5 ml each of sample and standard solutions, add 5 ml of buffered sulphanilic acid solution, 2 ml of cyanogen bromide solution and 1 ml of 0.25 N sulphuric acid. Prepare separate sample and standard blank. Allow all the tubes to stand for 10 min, and measure the absorbance of the sample and standard solutions against respective reagent blanks at about 480 nm and calculate the amount of chlorpheniramine maleate in the sample by comparison.

Note : Ephedrine, diphenhydramine, aminophylline, pyrilamine maleate and naphazoline hydrochloride do not interfere.

Codeine phosphate, Chlorpheniramine maleate, Terpine hydrate, Potassium guaiacolsulphonate, Menthol, Tincture ipecac

ESTIMATION

Terpine hydrate

METHOD 1

Follow the method described in formulation 1 of the chapter on analgesics and antipyretics.

METHOD 2

1. 1% w/v solution of phosphomolybdic acid in water.
2. Concentrated sulphuric acid, ice cooled.

Standard solution

100 mcg/ml of terpine hydrate in chloroform.

Sample solution

Take sample equivalent to about 10 mg of terpine hydrate, add 10 ml of water and shake with 30 ml of petroleum ether (40-60°). Separate aqueous layer and then extract with four 20 ml portions of chloroform. Combine chloroform layer and dilute to 100 ml with chloroform.

Procedure

To 10 ml each of the sample and standard solutions, add 10 ml of chloroform, 5 ml of water and 2 ml of phosphomolybdic acid. Shake for 10 minutes, allow the layers to separate and discard chloroform layer. Keep aqueous layer on water-bath to remove traces of chloroform, cool and add slowly 2 ml of ice cooled sulphuric acid. Allow to remain in ice-bath for 30 minutes with occasional shaking. Now keep on water-bath for 10 minutes, cool and dilute to 25 ml with acetone. Measure the absorbance of both the standard and sample solutions at about 610 nm and calculate the results by comparison.

Chlorpheniramine maleate

Standard solution

25 mcg/ml of substance in 0.5 N sulphuric acid.

Sample solution

Take a quantity of the sample equivalent to 20 mg of the compound, acidify with hydrochloric acid and extract with three 50 ml portions of ether. Discard ether layer, make acidic layer alkaline with 5 N sodium hydroxide solution and extract with three 50 ml portions of ether. Wash combined ether extract with water till free of alkali. Extract combined ether layer with three 50 ml portions of 0.5 N sulphuric acid. Dilute the acidic extract to 200 ml (100 mcg/ml). Dilute further appropriately with 0.5 N sulphuric acid to get 20 mcg/ml.

Measure the absorbance of standard and sample solutions at maximum at about 264 nm using 0.5 N sulphuric acid as blank and calculate the contents of chlorpheniramine maleate by comparison.

Potassium guaiacolsulphonate

Follow the chlorimide reagent method for estimation of the compound as described in formulation 2 of this chapter.

Codeine phosphate

Reagents

1. Hydrochloric acid.
2. 0.1 N sulphuric acid.
3. 0.1 N sodium hydroxide.
4. 0.5 N sodium hydroxide.
5. Anhydrous sodium sulphate, granular.

Procedure

Transfer sample equivalent to 100 mg of codeine phosphate into a separatory funnel. Add 10 to 15 ml of water, 2 ml hydrochloric acid and mix well. Extract thrice each with 50 ml portions of ether and discard the ether extracts. Add 0.5 N sodium hydroxide till the aqueous layer is distinctly alkaline. Extract again with three 50 ml portions of chloroform. Wash the combined chloroform extract thoroughly with water till it is free from alkali. Filter the chloroform extract into a dry 250 ml conical flask through anhydrous sodium sulphate placed over cotton plug. Evaporate the chloroform extract to complete dryness and dissolve the residue in exactly 10 ml of 0.1 N sulphuric acid. Titrate the excess acid with 0.1 N sodium hydroxide using methyl red as indicator. Each ml of 0.1 N sulphuric acid is equivalent to 0.03974 of codeine phosphate.

Total alkaloids as emetine

Tincture ipecac contains about 0.2% of total alkaloids calculated as emetine. It has been observed that about 2 ml of tincture ipecac is usually present in 100 ml of different liquid formulations of cough mixtures.

Reagents

1. McLivaine buffer, pH 5.0 : 48.5 ml of 0.1 M citric acid monohydrate and 51.5 ml of 0.02 M disodium phosphate are mixed. Check and adjust the pH to 5.0.
2. Buffered methyl orange solution : 10 mg/100 ml of methyl orange in buffer solution, pH 5.0.
3. Acidified alcohol : To 70 ml of ethyl alcohol, add 1 ml of 1 N hydrochloric acid and dilute to 100 ml with water.

Standard solution

400 mcg/ml of emetine in buffer solution, pH 5.0.

Sample solution

Take sample equivalent to 1 ml of the tincture ipecac, basify with ammonia and extract with ether. Evaporate the ether layer and take up the residue in 5 ml of McLivaine buffer, pH 5.0.

Procedure

To 2 ml each of the standard and sample solutions, add 10 ml of the dye solution and shake with 10 ml chloroform. Allow the layers to separate. Extract aqueous layer further with three 10 ml portions of chloroform. Shake combined chloroform layer with 10 ml of 0.1 N sodium hydroxide for 15 seconds. Wash the chloroform layer with another 10 ml of 0.1 N sodium hydroxide. Combine the alkaline layers and dilute to 25 ml with 0.1 N sodium hydroxide (C). Shake chloroform layer with 10 ml of 0.1 N sulphuric acid and dilute the acid layer to 25 ml with 0.1 N sulphuric acid (D). Measure the absorbance of the sample and standard solutions (C) at about 460 nm and calculate the percentage of total alkaloids as emetine. The measurement of extinction of solutions (D) of both standard and sample at maxima at about 283 nm gives non-phenolic alkaloids calculated as emetine.

Note : Belladonna alkaloids, if present, do not interfere in this determination as at 283 nm, belladonna alkaloids have insignificant absorbance.

Menthol

Follow the method involving reaction with p-dimethylaminobenzaldehyde for estimation of menthol in formulation 5 of this chapter.

Formulation 5

Codeine phosphate, Papaverine hydrochloride, Diphenhydramine hydrochloride, Ammonium chloride, Menthol

ESTIMATION

Diphenhydramine hydrochloride

Standard solution

200 mcg/ml of diphenhydramine hydrochloride in water.

Sample solution

Weigh accurately a quantity of the sample equivalent to 20 mg of diphenhydramine hydrochloride, add 15 ml of water and make alkaline with 1 N sodium hydroxide. Extract with three 50 ml portions of petroleum ether (40-60°). Filter organic layer through sodium sulphate, anhydrous, supported on a cotton plug. Reduce the volume to 10 ml, add 10 ml of 0.1 N hydrochloric acid and evaporate ether completely. Cool and make alkaline the acidic layer with 1 N sodium hydroxide. Add 20 ml of saturated aqueous solution of ammonium reineckate. Filter through G₄ sintered funnel, wash the precipitates with water till the filtrate is colourless. Dissolve the precipitates in acetone to produce 25 ml. Take 10 ml of standard solution and process as per sample.

Measure the absorption of samples and standard solutions at about 525 nm and calculate the results. Chlorpheniramine does not interfere.

Papaverine hydrochloride

Take volume of the sample syrup, equivalent to 5 mg of papaverine hydrochloride, add 5 ml of 1 N hydrochloric acid and extract with three 25 ml portions of chloroform. Extract combined chloroform extract with 10 ml of 1 N sodium hydroxide. Reject aqueous layer, evaporate chloroform layer and dry the residue at about 75°C till free from the smell of menthol. Dissolve the residue in 1 N hydrochloric acid with the aid of slight warming to produce 250 ml. Filter and measure the extinction of the solution at 310 nm using 1 N hydrochloric acid as blank. Calculate the results using 228 as value of A 1%, 1 cm at 310 nm.

Codeine phosphate

Reagents

1. 3% w/v solution of potassium permanganate in water.
2. 5% w/v solution of sodium nitrite in water.
3. 10% w/v solution of ferrous ammonium sulphate in water, prepare fresh.
4. 15% w/v solution of sodium hydroxide in water.
5. 1% w/v solution of sodium bicarbonate in water.

6. Diazotised sulphanilic acid. To 1 g of sulphanilic acid, add 20 ml of hydrochloric acid, digest on burner for 5 minutes, cool and filter. Take 1.5 ml of the filtrate, cool in ice-bath and add 1.5 ml of sodium nitrite solution. Wait for 5 minutes, again add 5 ml of sodium nitrite solution and make up the volume to 50 ml with water.

Standard solution

2 mg/ml of codeine phosphate in water. From this solution, take 10 ml, make it alkaline with sodium hydroxide solution and proceed as under sample solution below.

Sample solution

Measure syrup (sample) equivalent to 2 mg of codeine phosphate, make it alkaline with sodium hydroxide solution. Extract with three 30 ml portions of chloroform. Filter combined chloroform extract through anhydrous sodium sulphate. Wash sodium sulphate layer with 10 ml of chloroform. Evaporate combined chloroform layer completely and take up the residue in 10 ml solution of sodium bicarbonate with slight warming for 5-10 minutes. Cool and adjust to 250 ml with water. Filter and use this solution for colour development.

Procedure

To 10 ml each of sample and standard solutions, add 1 ml of potassium permanganate solution. Keep exactly for 15 seconds, add 5 ml of ferrous ammonium sulphate solution. Keep for 3 minutes, add 5 ml of sodium hydroxide solution and 10 ml of water. After 60 minutes, filter the solution. To 10 ml of the filtrate from standard and sample solutions, add 2 ml of diazotised sulphanilic acid, shake and measure the absorbance of both the solutions at about 490 nm within 3 minutes of addition of diazotised reagent against reagent blank and deduce the results by comparison.

Menthol

Reagents

1. Dilute sulphuric acid (prepared by mixing 68 parts of sulphuric acid with water to produce 100 ml.
2. 0.5% w/v solution of p-dimethylaminobenzaldehyde in ice-cold dilute sulphuric acid. Always store in refrigerator.

Standard stock solution

1 mg/ml of menthol in methyl alcohol.

Standard working solution

5 ml of the stock solution is diluted to 100 ml with 50% v/v methanol.

Sample solution

Take syrup equivalent to about 4.5 mg of menthol, add 100 ml of water, 25 ml of methanol and glass bead to avoid bumping. Dip the tip of receiver in 25 ml of cold methanol contained in 100 ml volumetric flask. Distil slowly till 70 ml of the distillate is collected. Rinse condenser and adapter with 25 ml of methanol, add to distillate and make up the final volume to 100 ml with water.

Note : Keep the receiving flask in ice water throughout distillation.

Procedure

To 2 ml each of standard and sample solutions, add 5 ml of ice cold p-dimethylamino-benzaldehyde reagent. Heat in a boiling water-bath for exactly 2 minutes, cool and measure the absorbance of both the solutions at about 550 nm after 15 min using reagent blank and calculate the results.

Note : 1. Use phosphoric acid instead of grease for glass joints.
2. Glass joints should be air tight to avoid loss of menthol during distillation.

Ammonium chloride

Follow the ammonia distillation method or silver nitrate titration method as described in formulation 7 of this chapter.

Diphenhydramine hydrochloride, Chlorpheniramine maleate, Ephedrine hydrochloride, Ammonium chloride, Sodium citrate, Menthol

ESTIMATION

Diphenhydramine hydrochloride

METHOD 1

Reagents

1. Cobalt thiocyanate solution : Dissolve 6.8 g cobalt chloride and 4.3 g ammonium thiocyanate in sufficient water to make 100 ml. This solution should be freshly prepared.

Sample and standard solutions

750 mcg/ml of diphenhydramine hydrochloride in water.

Procedure

Transfer 10 ml each of the sample and standard solutions into a 250 ml separating funnel, add 10 ml cobalt thiocyanate solution and mix. Extract with three 25 ml portions of chloroform, filtering each chloroform extract through anhydrous sodium sulphate into 100 ml dry volumetric flask. Make up the volume to 100 ml and mix. Transfer 2 ml to a 50 ml dry volumetric flask and evaporate the chloroform to dryness. To the residue, add 10 ml concentrated sulphuric acid, mix and make up the volume to 50 ml with concentrated sulphuric acid. Measure the extinction at 430 nm using concentrated sulphuric acid as blank. Calculate the results by comparison.

METHOD 2

Follow ammonium reineckate method as described in formulation 5 of this chapter. Chlorpheniramine maleate does not interfere in this method.

METHOD 3

Reagents

1. Buffer solution, pH 3.0 : 100 ml of 0.1 N potassium hydrogen phthalate and 40.6 ml of 0.1 N hydrochloric acid are mixed and diluted to 200 ml with water, check pH with pH meter.
2. Bromocresol green solution : Dissolve 69.8 mg of the dye in 2 ml of 0.1 N sodium hydroxide and dilute to 1000 ml with water.

Standard solution

25 mcg/ml of diphenhydramine hydrochloride in water.

Sample solution

Weigh accurately a quantity of the sample equivalent to 20 mg of the compound and dissolve in water (20 mcg/ml).

Procedure

Take aliquots from sample and standard solutions equivalent to 100 mcg of the compound in separating funnel, add 20 ml of dye solution and 2-3 drops of 1 N sodium hydroxide or 1 N hydrochloric acid to obtain yellow colour. Then, add 10 ml of buffer solution and extract the yellow complex with 5, 3 and 2 ml of chloroform. Combine chloroform layers and dilute to 10 ml with chloroform (do not pass through sodium sulphate). Measure the absorption of sample and standard solutions at 415 nm against reagent blank. The complex is stable as long as 10 days.

Note : 1. Ammonium chloride, menthol, sodium citrate, paracetamol, saccharine, vitamin C, phenylephrine do not interfere.

2. Under acidic conditions, most substances with tertiary amino group or quaternary ammonium salts make yellow complex with the dye, extractable with chloroform.

Chlorpheniramine maleate

Follow the cyanogen bromide method as described in formulation 3 of this chapter.

Ephedrine hydrochloride

Follow the ammoniacal copper sulphate method as described in formulation 1 of the chapter on anti-asthma drugs.

Ammonium chloride

Follow ammonia distillation method as described in formulation 7 of this chapter. Each ml of 0.1 N hydrochloric acid is equivalent to 0.005349 g of ammonium chloride. For calculation, subtract the volume of 0.1 N hydrochloric acid equivalent to ephedrine hydrochloride present in the quantity of the sample taken for analysis. Each ml of 0.1 N hydrochloric acid is equivalent to 0.02017 g of ephedrine hydrochloride.

Sodium citrate

METHOD 1

Reagent

1. 0.05 M calcium chloride solution.

Procedure

Take sample equivalent to 120 mg of sodium citrate in a beaker and dissolve in 20 ml water. Add 25 ml of calcium chloride solution and adjust the pH of the mixture between 7.0 to 7.5 by pH meter. Add a volume of alcohol approximately equal to that of the solution in the beaker and digest the precipitates on boiling water-bath for 30 minutes covering the beaker with a watch glass. Cool and filter the precipitates through a Whatman filter paper No. 1 or 4, wash with four 10 ml portions of 50% v/v alcohol and dry carefully. Carbonise the residue in silica dish first on low flame and then strongly. Cool, add 50 ml of 0.1 N hydrochloric acid, boil and filter through a plug of cotton wool. Wash the dish 2 to 3 times each with 20 ml water and filter the washings through the same cotton wool. Add 3-4 drops of methyl red, indicator and titrate the excess acid against 0.1 N sodium hydroxide. Perform blank with 50 ml of acid. Each ml of 0.1 N hydrochloric acid is equivalent to 0.0098 g of sodium citrate.

If ammonium chloride is present in the formulation along with sodium citrate, above method with slight modification may be used.

METHOD 2

Add calculated amount of 0.1 N silver nitrate equivalent to chloride of ammonium chloride to precipitate chloride as silver chloride. Filter and wash the precipitates. Evaporate the filtrate to dryness and carbonise. Take the residue in known volume of 0.1 N hydrochloric acid (50 ml), boil and cool. Titrate the excess acid with 0.1 N sodium hydroxide using methyl red as indicator. Each ml of 0.1 N hydrochloric acid consumed is equivalent to 0.0108 g of potassium citrate, 0.0098 g of sodium citrate, or 0.0064 g of total citrates.

METHOD 2 (a)

Take accurately 2 ml of the sample preparation in a platinum crucible and heat gently with care, then heat to a temperature not exceeding 450°C until free from carbon. Cool and boil the residue with about 50 ml of water. Cool and filter the solution into a 100 ml volumetric flask. Wash the platinum crucible and the filter paper with water until the last washing is neutral to litmus. Combine the washings with main filtrate. Make up the volume to 100 ml with water, mix and mark the solution as sample solution.

Solution 1 : Take 50 ml of the sample solution and titrate with 0.1 N sulphuric acid using methyl red-methylene blue solution (Teshiro's indicator). Each ml of 0.1 N sulphuric acid is equivalent to 0.0098 g of sodium citrate.

Solution 2 : Take 25 ml of the sample solution, add 3 ml of nitric acid, 5 ml of nitrobenzene and 25 ml of 0.1 N silver nitrate solution. Shake vigorously for one minute and titrate with 0.1 N ammonium thiocyanate, using solution of ferric ammonium sulphate as indicator. Each ml of 0.1 N silver nitrate is equivalent to 0.0098 g of sodium citrate.

Calculations

Amount of sodium citrate (g/5 ml) = $X \times 0.0098 \times 5$ (a)—from solution 1
X = Volume (ml) of 0.1 N sulphuric acid consumed in the titration.

Amount of sodium citrate (g/ml) = $Y \times 0.0098 \times \dfrac{5}{0.5}$ (b)—from solution 2

Y = Volume (ml) of 0.1 N silver nitrate used in the titration.
Total sodium citrate = (a) + (b)

Note : 1. Other sodium salts of the substances usually present in the formulation such as sodium benzoate, methyl paraben, propyl paraben (sodium salt) will interfere as they will finally get converted into sodium hydroxide on ignition as described in method 1 (a) and will get titrated with sulphuric acid.
2. However, citric acid usually added to adjust the pH of the preparation will not interfere in this method.

METHOD 3
Reagent ‚

1. Pyridine-acetic anhydride (3 : 1) mixture.

Standard solution

1 mg/ml of sodium citrate in water.

Sample solution

Measure accurately the volume of the sample and dilute with water to get a concentration of 1 mg/ml of sodium citrate.

Procedure

Take 3 test tubes and mark them as standard, sample and sample blank. Pipette out 1 ml each of standard and sample solutions in respective tubes, add 2 ml water in each tube. Cool the tubes and the pyridine-acetic anhydride mixture to 5 to 10°C. Add 10 ml of pyridine-acetic anhydride mixture each to standard and sample tubes and 10 ml water to sample blank tube. Mix gently and measure absorbance of both the solutions at 450 nm against reagent blank between 3 to 4 minutes after the addition of reagent and calculate the results.

Note : 1. Higher results are obtained due to presence of citric acid in the formulation.

  2. Temperature should not exceed 10°C during the entire experiment.

METHOD 4

Reagent

  1. 0.05% w/v solution of ferric chloride in 0.1 N hydrochloric acid (freshly prepared).

Standard solution

1 mg/ml of sodium citrate in water, prepare fresh.

Sample solution

Dilute the sample appropriately with water to get 1 mg/ml concentration.

Procedure

To 2 ml each of the sample and standard solutions, add 10 ml of 0.01 N hydrochloric acid and 5 ml of ferric chloride solution and dilute to 25 ml with 0.01 N hydrochloric acid. Mix and measure absorbance of standard and sample solutions at about 380 nm against blank prepared with 2 ml of sample solution but without ferric chloride solution.

Note : This method measures total citrate including citric acid present in the sample.

METHOD 6

Reagent

  1. 0.25% w/v solution of ferric nitrate in 1% nitric acid.

Standard solution

  (a) 1.7 mg/ml of sodium citrate in water.
  (b) 1 mg/ml of salicylic acid : Dissolve 100 mg of salicylic acid accurately weighed in 20 ml of methanol and dilute to 100 ml with water.

Sample solution

Dilute sample appropriately with water to get a solution of 1 mg/ml.

Procedure

Pipette 5 ml each of salicylic acid and ferric nitrate in 2 test tubes. Allow to stand for 2 min. To each tube add 10 ml each of sample and standard solutions respectively. Dilute to 50 ml with water and measure the absorption of both the solutions at 525 nm against reagent blank (dilute 10 ml of the sample solution to 50 ml with water) and calculate the results by comparison.

METHOD 7

Procedure

Measure sample accurately equivalent to 100 mg of the substance, add three drops of bromothymol blue indicator and titrate with 0.1 N sodium hydroxide till bluish green colour is produced. Add 35 ml of 0.1 N silver nitrate and heat on a water-bath for complete coagulation. Add 30 ml of acetone to help in coagulation. Filter through Whatman No. 1 filter paper, wash the residue with acetone. Dissolve the residue in 10 ml of concentrated nitric acid and titrate with 0.1 N ammonium thiocyanate using ferric ammonium sulphate as indicator. Carry out blank titration with 35 ml of 0.1 N silver nitrate.

Each ml of 0.1 N silver nitrate is equivalent to 9.804 mg of sodium citrate.

Menthol

Follow the method for estimation of menthol involving reaction with p-dimethylamino-benzaldehyde as described in formulation 5 of this chapter.

Formulation 7

Noscapine, Chlorpheniramine maleate, Ephedrine hydrochloride, Ammonium chloride

ESTIMATION

Noscapine and Chlorpheniramine maleate

Procedure

Weigh sample accurately, equivalent to 10 mg of noscapine, add 20 ml of water and adjust the pH to 9.0 with dilute solution of ammonium hydroxide. Extract the alkaline solution with four 25 ml portions of chloroform. Combine chloroform layers and evaporate on water-bath. Dissolve the alkaloidal residue in 0.1 N hydrochloric acid to make 250 ml (A). Shake the total acidic extract with 50 ml of ether. Methyl and propyl parabens present as preservatives which absorb at 265 nm and 310 nm get removed by this step. Measure the extinction of acidic extract at 265 nm and 310 nm and calculate the content of noscapine and chlorpheniramine maleate (CPM) by the following method.

$$\text{Noscapine (mg)/15 ml of the sample} = \frac{A_{310}}{89.4} \times \frac{\text{Weight per ml}}{\text{Weight of sample taken}} \times 15$$

Extinction of "CPM" at 310 nm is negligible i.e. 0.03. Correction, if necessary, can be applied.

$$\text{CPM (mg)/15 ml of the sample} = \frac{(A_{265} - A_{310}) \times 0.413}{212} \times \frac{\text{Weight per ml}}{\text{Weight of sample taken}} \times 15$$

89.4 = E 1%, 1 cm of Noscapine at 310 nm, reported value is 90.7.
212 = E 1%, 1 cm of 'CPM' at 265 nm.
0.413 = It is the ratio between A_{310} and A_{265} of Noscapine and 'CPM'.

Chlorpheniramine maleate (CPM)

Use appropriate volume of the solution (A) obtained above for estimation of 'CPM' by cyanogen bromide method as described in formulation 3 of this chapter.

Ephedrine hydrochloride

Follow the periodate oxidation method as described in formulation 1 of this chapter.

Ammonium chloride

METHOD 1

Transfer volume of the sample equivalent to 100 mg of ammonium chloride in a conical flask. Add 100 ml of 0.1 N silver nitrate solution, 30 ml of water and 3 ml of nitric acid. Boil for ten minutes or until the solution turns yellow. Cool, add 10 ml of nitrobenzene and titrate with 0.1 N ammonium thiocyanate, using ferric alum as indicator. Each ml of 0.1 N silver nitrate is equivalent to 0.005349 g of ammonium chloride.

METHOD 2

Reagents

1. 4% w/v solution of sodium hydroxide in water.
2. Indicator solution : 80 mg of methylene blue and 125 mg of methyl red are dissolved in alcohol to produce 100 ml. (This is called Teshiro's indicator solution.)

Procedure

Transfer volume of the sample equivalent to 100 mg of ammonium chloride into a Kjeldahl distillation flask. Add through the funnel about 70 ml of sodium hydroxide solution, rinse the funnel with a small portion of water. Tightly close the flask and start distillation. Collect the distillate in about 50 ml of boric acid (5%) solution containing few drops of indicator solution. Add sufficient water to cover the end of the condensing tube. Continue the distillation until the distillate measures about 200 ml. Remove the absorption flask, rinsing the end of the condensing tube with a small quantity of water. Titrate the distillate (ammonia-boric acid complex) with 0.1 N hydrochloric acid. The end point is the first persistent purple colour that follows a grey colour.

Each ml of 0.1 N hydrochloric acid is equivalent to 0.005349 g of ammonium chloride.

Note : Necessary correction for ephedrine solution be made both in method 1 and 2.

Each ml of 0.1 N hydrochloric acid is equivalent to 0.02017 g of ephedrine hydrochloride.

METHOD 3

Procedure

Measure sample accurately equivalent to about 150 mg of the substance, add 50 ml of water and 10 ml of dilute sulphuric acid. Add potassium permanganate solution (0.1 N) dropwise till solution is colourless or pale yellow. Neutralize (phenolphthalein) with 5 N sodium hydroxide. Add 1 ml of excess 5 N sodium hydroxide and neutralize with 0.1 N sulphuric acid. Add 25 ml of previously neutralized (phenolphthalein) formaldehyde solution and titrate with 0.1 N sodium hydroxide. Each ml of 0.1 N sodium hydroxide is equivalent to 5.349 mg of ammonium chloride.

Noscapine, Ephedrine hydrochloride, Potassium guaiacolsulphonate

ESTIMATION

Ephedrine hydrochloride

METHOD 1

Follow the method as described in formulation 1 of chapter on anti-asthma drugs or in formulation 1 of this chapter.

METHOD 2

Weigh sample accurately equivalent to 20 mg of ephedrine hydrochloride, basify with dilute solution of ammonia and extract with four 25 ml portions of ether. Evaporate ether layer, take up the residue in 40 ml of glacial acetic acid and add 10 ml of 10% w/v solution of mercuric acetate. Titrate with 0.1 N perchloric acid using crystal violet as indicator. Each ml of 0.1 N perchloric acid is equivalent to 0.02017 g of ephedrine hydrochloride.

Noscapine

Reagents

1. Hydrochloric acid-sodium chloride buffer solution, pH 1.0 : Mix 50 ml of 0.2 M solution of sodium chloride with 97 ml of 0.2 N solution of hydrochloric acid and dilute to 200 ml with water.
2. Citrate-phosphate buffer solution : Mix 39.8 ml of 0.1 M solution of citric acid and 10.2 ml of 0.2 M solution of disodium phosphate and dilute to 100 ml with water.
3. Dye solution : Dissolve 54 mg of bromocresol purple (acid form) in citrate-phosphate buffer solution and dilute to 100 ml.
4. 1% v/v solution of hydrochloric acid in water.

Standard solution

Dissolve 30.0 mg of noscapine in hydrochloric acid-sodium chloride buffer solution to produce 250 ml (120 mcg/ml).

Sample solution

Accurately weigh the sample equivalent to 30 mg of noscapine and dilute to 250 ml with hydrochloric acid-sodium chloride buffer solution.

Procedure

Take .1 ml each of sample and standard solutions in a 50 ml stoppered cylinder. Add 50 ml of hydrochloric acid-sodium chloride buffer solution, 5 ml of dye solution and 10 ml of benzene. Shake for 1 minute and centrifuge about 7.5 ml portion of benzene layer rapidly to effect complete clarification. Measure the absorbance of the supernatant layer at 410 nm against reagent blank prepared following the same procedure but without sample preparation. The result may be obtained by comparing.

Potassium guaiacolsulphonate

Reagents

1. 1% v/v trihexylamine in chloroform.
2. Citrate buffer, pH 4.2 : Prepare by mixing equal volumes of 0.5 M citric acid and 0.5 M sodium citrate, adjust the pH to 4.2 with citrate.
3. Adsorbent, celite-545, acid washed.
4. 0.1 M phosphoric acid.
5. Chloroform, saturate with water before use.

Standard solution

20 mcg/ml of substance in 0.1 N sodium hydroxide.

Sample solution

Dilute the sample with citrate-buffer, pH 4.2 to get 2.5 mg/ml of the compound.

Preparation of column : Mix 2 g of celite-545 with 1 ml of phosphoric acid, transfer to the column with tempering using gentle pressure. Take 2 ml of the sample solution (5 mg), add 5 mg of sodium hydrosulphite and 3 g of celite. Mix and transfer to the column by tapping with light pressure. Scrap beaker with 1 g of celite and 2-3 drop of buffer and transfer to the column. Cover the top of the column with a pad of cotton wool.

Procedure

Pass 100 ml chloroform, water saturated and discard the eluate. Elute the column with 100 ml of trihexylamine solution. Collect the eluate in separating funnel containing 25 ml of 0.1 N sodium hydroxide, previously saturated with chloroform. Shake the total eluate and allow to stand for 10 minutes for complete separation. Dilute 10 ml of the aqueous phase to 100 ml with 0.1 sodium hydroxide (20 mcg/ml).

Record the extinction of both sample and standard solutions at maximum at about 290 nm using 0.1 N sodium hydroxide as blank and compare the results.

Note : Dextromethorphan, codeine, morphine, noscapine, antihistamines, diphenhydramine, phenyl-ephrine, alcohol and glycerin do not interfere.

Noscapine, Chlorpheniramine maleate, Phenylephrine hydrochloride, Ephedrine hydrochloride, Ascorbic acid

ESTIMATION

Noscapine

To volume of the syrup equivalent to 40 mg of noscapine, add 25 ml of water, 2.0 g of sodium chloride and make the solution alkaline with sodium hydroxide solution. Extract with anaesthetic ether thrice each with 50 ml. Combine the ether extract and wash with water till free from alkali (test with litmus paper). Evaporate the ether and to the residue, add 50 ml of 0.1 N hydrochloric acid, warm to dissolve. Transfer to a 100 ml volumetric flask and make up the volume with water. Further dilute 5 ml to 50 ml with water and measure the extinction at 310 nm against the blank. Calculate the results taking 90.7 as valve of E 1%, 1 cm at 310 nm.

Ascorbic acid

Weigh accurately, syrup equivalent to 150 mg of ascorbic acid. Add to this, 10 ml acetic acid and 20 ml water. Titrate with 0.1 N iodine using starch as indicator. Each ml of 0.1 N iodine is equivalent to 0.008806 g of ascorbic acid.

Chlorpheniramine maleate

Follow cyanogen bromide method as described in formulation 3 of this chapter.

Phenylephrine hydrochloride

METHOD 1

The method is based on alkaline oxidation of phenolic group and then coupling with 4-aminoantipyrine as described in formulation 1 of the chapter on analgesics and antipyretics. Ascorbic acid present in this formulation will interfere as it is a strong reducing agent. However, the use of 10% w/v solution of potassium ferricyanide will overcome this problem.

METHOD 2

Reagents

1. 1% w/v solution of sodium carbonate in water.
2. 0.1% w/v solution of p-aminophenol in ethyl alcohol, prepare fresh.

Standard solution

250 mcg/ml of phenylephrine hydrochloride in water.

Sample solution

Dilute accurately measured volume of the sample with water to get 250 mcg/ml concentration of phenylephrine hydrochloride.

Procedure

To 2 ml each of sample and standard solutions, add 5 ml of sodium carbonate solution, 0.5 ml of p-aminophenol solution and dilute to 10 ml with water. Mix and allow to stand for 25 minutes. Read the absorbance of both the standard and sample solution at about 640 nm. The colour is stable up to 50 min and obeys Beer's law in the concentration range of 10-80 mcg/ml.

Note : Caffeine, paracetamol, pheniramine maleate and chlorpheniramine maleate do not interfere in this method.

Ephedrine hydrochloride

Follow the method described in formulation 8 of this chapter.

Promethazine hydrochloride, Noscapine, Codeine phosphate, Ephedrine hydrochloride

ESTIMATION

Promethazine hydrochloride

Reagents

1. 0.01 N hydrochloric acid.
2. Buffer solution, pH 2.0 : Dissolve 10 g of sodium acetate in about 50 ml of water and 80 ml of 1 N hydrochloric acid and dilute to 200 ml with water.
3. Palladous chloride reagent.

Standard solution

300 mcg/ml of promethazine hydrochloride in 0.01 N hydrochloric acid.

Sample solution

To accurately measured volume of the sample equivalent to 30 mg of promethazine hydrochloride, add 15 ml of 0.1 N hydrochloric acid and warm on water-bath for 5 minutes and extract with three 15 ml portions of cyclohexane. Separate acid layer (lower layer) and rinse the total cyclohexane layer with 10 ml of 0.01 N hydrochloric acid. Combine the acid layer and adjust to 100 ml with 0.01 N hydrochloric acid.

Procedure

To 2 ml each of the standard and sample solutions, add 1 ml of 0.01 N hydrochloric acid and 20 ml of buffer solution (pH 2.0). Mix well, add 2 ml of palladous chloride reagent and allow to stand at room temperature for 15 minutes. Measure the absorbance of both the solutions at about 470 nm against reagent blank (3 ml of water, 20 ml of buffer and 2 ml of palladous chloride reagent) and calculate the results.

Noscapine

Reagents

1. Chloroform, water saturated.
2. Chloramine-T, 2% w/v solution in water.
3. 30% w/v solution of sodium sulphite in water, prepare fresh each day.
4. 5% w/v solution of sodium hydrogen phosphate in water.
5. 2.5 N hydrochloric acid, approximately.

Standard solution

0.3 mg/ml of pure noscapine in water saturated chloroform. 5 ml of this solution is transferred to a 50 ml graduated flask and evaporated to dryness on water-bath. Dissolve the residue in 5 ml of methanol.

Sample solution

Weigh/measure accurately, a quantity of the sample equivalent to 30 mg of noscapine, evaporate to dryness and dry at 105°C for 1 hour. Extract the residue with four 20 ml portions of anhydrous cyclohexane. Discard the cyclohexane layer and dry the residue in vacuum for 15 minutes to remove traces of cyclohexane. Extract the dried residue with four 20 ml portions of water saturated chloroform and adjust the volume with same solvent. Evaporate 5 ml of this solution on water-bath and dissolve residue in 5 ml of methanol.

Blank solution

To 5 ml of methanol, add 5 ml of 2.5 N hydrochloric acid, 5 ml of chloramine-T solution and 15 ml of sodium sulphite solutions, dilute to 50 ml with sodium hydrogen phosphate solution.

Procedure

Store sample, standard and blank solutions throughout colour development at 20°C. To 5 ml each of sample and standard solutions, add 5 ml of 2.5 N hydrochloric acid. Mix well and after 5 minutes, add 5 ml chloramine-T solution. Mix and after 15 minutes, add freshly prepared solution of sodium sulphite and finally adjust the volume to 50 ml with disodium hydrogen phosphate solution. Exactly after 5 minutes after the addition of sodium sulphite, measure the extinction of both the solutions at about 505 nm against blank solution as prepared above and calculate the results by comparison.

Ephedrine hydrochloride

Follow the ammoniacal copper sulphate method as described in formulation 1 of the chapter on bronchospasm relaxants (anti-asthma). Alternatively, the method based on distillation of volatile base (ephedrine) as described in formulation 8 of the chapter on anti-asthma drugs.

Codeine phosphate

Reagents

1. Phosphate buffer, pH 5.7 : Dissolve 0.5 g of potassium dihydrogen phosphate in 50 ml of water and adjust the pH to 5.7 and make up volume to 100 ml with water.
2. Buffered dye solution : 0.0030% w/v solution of bromothymol in phosphate buffer, pH 5.7.
3. 0.05 N sodium hydroxide solution.

Standard solution

750 mcg/ml of codeine phosphate in water.

Sample solution

Extract accurately weighed quantity of the sample equivalent to 70 mg of the compound with water and adjust to 100 ml.

Procedure

Take 2 ml each of sample and standard solutions in a separator, add 10 ml of water and make alkaline with dilute solution of ammonia. Extract with three 25 ml portion of chloroform, washing each chloroform layer with the same 20 ml of water. Add 25 ml of buffered dye solution to chloroform layer and shake vigorously for 2 minutes. Allow the layers to separate and discard the aqueous layer. Filter chloroform layer through a filter paper moistened with chloroform. Shake the filtered chloroform layer with 40 ml of sodium hydroxide solution. Separate alkaline aqueous layer, filter and adjust to 100 ml with sodium hydroxide solution. Measure the extinction of both the solutions at 617 nm and calculate the results by comparison. Alternatively follow the method described in formulation 2 of this chapter based on colour reaction with metol-bisulphite reagent.

Dextromethorphan hydrobromide, Ephedrine hydrochloride, Cetylpyridinium chloride, Benzocaine, Menthol

ESTIMATION

Dextromethorphan hydrobromide

Reagents

1. 0.2 N sodium hydroxide.
2. 25% w/v solution of sodium hydroxide in water.
3. 0.1 N hydrochloric acid.

Standard solution

100 mcg/ml of standard dextromethorphan hydrobromide in 0.1 N hydrochloric acid.

Sample solution

Weigh accurately, powdered lozenges equivalent to 10 mg of dextromethorphan, add 15 ml of 0.1 N sodium hydroxide and swirl to dissolve. Heat on a water-bath for 20 minutes. Cool and extract with five 35 ml portion of ether. Combine ether extract and wash the combined ether extract with 5 ml of 0.1 N sodium hydroxide. Extract ether layer with 20 ml, 15 ml, 10 ml portions of 0.1 N hydrochloric acid. Combine acid layer and make strongly alkaline with sodium hydroxide solution and extract with four 25 ml portions of n-hexane. Extract the combined hexane extract with 40, 20, 20 ml portions of 0.1 N hydrochloric acid and dilute the acid layer to 100 ml with 0.1 N hydrochloric acid.

Determine the extinction of sample and standard solutions at maximum at about 278 nm using 0.1 N hydrochloric acid as blank and deduce the results. Use 0.733 as factor to convert dextromethorphan hydrobromide to the base.

Cetylpyridinium chloride

Reagents

1. 2 N hydrochloric acid.
2. 0.1% w/v picric acid in water.
3. Sodium sulphate anhydrous, granular.
4. Ammonium hydroxide solution.

Standard solution

30 mcg/ml of cetylpyridinium chloride, in water.

Sample solution

Accurately weigh a quantity of the sample equivalent to 500 mcg of the compound, transfer to 125 ml separatory funnel containing 15 ml of 2 N hydrochloric acid. Stopper the funnel and shake to dissolve the sample, adjust the volume to 25 ml with water.

Procedure

Transfer 15 ml of the sample and standard solutions to a separatory funnel. Add 2 ml of picric acid solution and 2 ml of ammonium hydroxide solution. Swirl to mix the contents and extract with four 10 ml portions of chloroform. Pass the chloroform extract through a small pledget of cotton contained in a funnel into a 50 ml volumetric flask, dilute to the mark with chloroform, mix. Determine the absorbance of the sample and standard solutions at 365 nm using chloroform as blank.

Note :   The chloroform solutions should be absolutely clear. If either of the chloroform solutions is hazy, the solutions should be rapidly filtered through 5 g of anhydrous sodium sulphate, supported in a funnel by a pledget of cotton, directly into a 5 ml glass stoppered flask. Both standard and sample solutions should be treated similarly. Calculate the contents by comparison.

Benzocaine

Reagents

1. 0.1 N hydrochloric acid.
2. Hydrochloric acid, dilute.
3. 0.1% w/v sodium nitrite solution in water, prepare weekly.
4. 0.5% w/v sulphamic acid solution in water, prepare weekly.
5. Bratton-Marshall reagent : Dissolve 100 mg of N-1-naphthyl-ethylenediamine dihydrochloride in 100 ml of water. Store the solution in a dark bottle, prepare weekly.
6. 10% v/v ammonium hydroxide solution.
7. Sodium sulphate anhydrous, granular.

Standard solution

10 mcg/ml of benzocaine in 0.1 hydrochloric acid.

Sample solution

To accurately weighed powdered sample equivalent to 1 mg of benzocaine, add about 10 ml of water and shake until the sample is dissolved. Make the solution alkaline to phenolphthalein, using ammonia solution. Without delay, extract the aqueous solution with four 25 ml portions of ether. Pass the ether extracts through 20 g of anhydrous sodium sulphate supported on a funnel by a pledget of cotton into a 400 ml beaker. Rinse the sodium sulphate layer with two 20 ml portions of ether. Add 35 ml of dilute hydrochloric acid, and several non-porous boiling chips. Heat on the water-bath until free from ether, cover with a watch glass and heat for an hour. Remove the beaker from the water-bath and cool to room temperature. Quantitatively transfer the solution to a 100 ml volumetric flask using water, dilute to volume with water and mix well.

Procedure

Transfer 5 ml each of standard and sample solutions to 50 ml flasks. Add 10 ml of dilute hydrochloric acid and heat on a water-bath for 1 hour. Cool the solution to room temperature. To each flask, add 5 ml of sodium nitrite solution, swirl to mix, and allow to stand for 3 minutes. Add 5 ml of sulphamic acid solution and swirl to mix. Stopper securely and shake to remove most of the gas bubbles. Add 5 ml of Bratton-Marshall reagent to each flask, dilute to volume with water and mix well. Determine the absorbance of the standard and sample solutions at about 550 nm using the reagent blank. Calculate the contents of benzocaine in each lozenge.

Menthol

Follow the method involving reaction with p-dimethylaminobenzaldehyde as described in formulation 5 of this chapter.

Ephedrine hydrochloride

Follow the ammoniacal copper sulphate method. For details refer to method under formulation 1 of the chapter on anti-asthma drugs. Alternatively, follow the method described in formulation 1 of this chapter.

Dextromethorphan hydrobromide, Ephedrine hydrochloride, Ammonium chloride, Liquid extract of ipecac

ESTIMATION

Dextromethorphan hydrobromide

Reagents

1. Buffer solution, pH 4.0 : Dissolve 5.25 g of citric acid monohydrate in 50 ml of 1 N sodium hydroxide in a 250 volumetric flask, add water to volume and mix. On the day of the use, combine 55 ml of this solution with 45 ml of 0.1 N hydrochloric acid. Check pH and adjust with acid or alkali.
2. Bromocresol purple solution : Dissolve 150 mg of bromocresol purple and 150 mg of anhydrous sodium carbonate in water to make 100 ml.
3. Chloroform-butanol solution : Mix 1 ml of n-butanol with chloroform to make 100 ml.

Standard solution

7.5 mcg/ml of dextromethorphan hydrobromide in water.

Sample solution

Transfer volume of the sample equivalent to 100 mg of the compound into a 100 ml volumetric flask and make to volume with water and mix. Transfer 10 ml of this solution into a separator, add about 40 ml of 1 N hydrochloric acid and extract with six 15 ml portions of chloroform. Wash the combined chloroform extract with 20 ml of 1 N hydrochloric acid. Discard the wash and filter the chloroform extract through a pledget of glass wool overlaid with about 5 g of anhydrous sodium sulphate into a 100 ml volumetric flask. Dilute to volume with chloroform. Dilute 4 ml of the chloroform solution to 50 ml with chloroform-butanol solution (8 mcg/ml).

Procedure

Pipette 5 ml of the sample preparation into a 30 ml glass-stoppered centrifuge tube and add 5 ml of water. Pipette 5 ml of the standard preparation into a second centrifuge tube and 5 ml of water into a third centrifuge tube to serve as a blank. Add to these two tubes 15 ml of chloroform-butanol solution. Now treat the three tubes concurrently in the following manner :

Add 5 ml of pH 4.0 buffer solution and 1 ml of bromocresol purple solution. Stopper the tubes and shake vigorously for 2 minutes. Centrifuge, and remove the aqueous layer by aspiration. Determine the absorbance of the sample and standard solutions at 415 nm using reagent solution as blank and calculate the results.

Ephedrine hydrochloride

Follow the ammoniacal copper sulphate method as described in formulation 1 of chapter on anti-asthma drugs.

Ammonium chloride

Follow the ammonia distillation method as described in formulation 7 of this chapter.

Ipecac liquid extract

Follow the method as described for tincture ipecac under formulation 4 of this chapter.

Dextromethorphan hydrobromide, Pseudoephedrine hydrochloride, Chlorpheniramine maleate, Menthol

ESTIMATION

Dextromethorphan hydrobromide

Follow the method described in formulation 12 of this chapter.

Pseudoephedrine hydrochloride

Follow the method described in formulation 19 of this chapter.

Chlorpheniramine maleate (CPM)

Reagent

1. 1% w/v solution of bromothymol blue.

Standard solution

1 mg/ml of CPM in water.

Sample solution

Directly take the sample (usually liquid) of standard solution. Add 1 ml of dye solution and extract with 25 ml of chloroform. Pass the chloroform layer through anhydrous sodium sulphate and measure the absorbance at about 420 nm using chloroform as blank.

Menthol

Follow the method described in formulation 5 of this chapter.

Dextromethorphan hydrobromide, Ephedrine hydrochloride, Paracetamol, Potassium guaiacolsulphonate

ESTIMATION

Dextromethorphan hydrobromide

METHOD 1

Follow the method for estimation of dextromethorphan described in formulation 12 of this chapter.

METHOD 2

Reagents

1. Bromothymol blue solution : Triturate 100 mg of bromothymol blue with 1.6 ml of 1 N sodium hydroxide, then dilute with about 200 ml of water. Boil, filter it after cooling and dilute to 250 ml with water.
2. Phosphate buffer solution, pH 7.5 : Dissolve 17 g of potassium dihydrogen phosphate in little water, add 105 ml of 1 N sodium hydroxide and dilute to 500 ml with water, check pH.

Standard stock solution

Weigh accurately 25 mg of dextromethorphan hydrobromide, monohydrate and dilute to 100 ml with water. This may be used as stock solution. If stored in refrigerator, it is stable for quite some time.

Working standard

Dilute 10 ml of the stock solution to 100 ml with water (25 mcg/ml).

Sample solution

Weigh accurately, appropriate quantity of the sample equivalent to 25 mg of dextromethorphan hydro-bromide and transfer to a separating funnel. Add 5 ml of dilute hydrochloric acid and 30 ml of water. Extract with four 25 ml portions of chloroform. Wash combined chloroform extracts with 30 ml of 0.1 N hydrochloric acid and evaporate chloroform layer. Dissolve the residue in 100 ml of water and 10 ml of the resultant solution is diluted to 100 ml with the same solvent to get sample solution (25 mcg/ml).

Procedure

Take 5 ml each of sample, standard and water (blank). To each tube, add 5 ml of buffer solution, 5 ml dye solution and 15 ml of benzene. Shake for 15 min, centrifuge to separate the layers. Measure the absorbance of benzene layer at about 405 nm using benzene layer of blank in reference cell and calculate the results.

Paracetamol

Reagents

1. 10% w/v solution of α-naphthol in methanol, prepare fresh.
2. 4% w/v solution of sodium hydroxide in water.

Standard solution

0.5 mg/ml of paracetamol in water.

Sample solution

Accurately measured/weighed quantity of the sample is appropriately diluted with water to get 0.5 mg/ml concentration.

Procedure

To 2 ml each of sample, standard and water, add 15 ml of hydrochloric acid, 25 ml of water and heat on boiling water-bath for 2 hours. Cool to room temperature and dilute to 50 ml with water and proceed as under :

Take 5 ml each of hydrolysed sample and standard solutions in 25 ml volumetric flasks. To each, add 0.5 ml of α-naphthol solution and 5 ml of sodium hydroxide solution. Mix well after the addition of each reagent and dilute to 25 ml with methanol. After 30 min, measure the absorbance of both the solutions at 620 nm against the reagent blank. Calculate the contents of paracetamol by comparison.

Potassium guaiacolsulphonate

Reagents

1. 1% w/v solution of 4-aminoantipyrine in water.
2. 2% w/v solution of potassium ferricyanide in water.
3. Phosphate buffer solution : 11.88 g of disodium hydrogen phosphate dissolved in water to produce 1000 ml.

Standard solution

40 mcg/ml of potassium guaiacolsulphonate in water.

Sample solution

Weigh accurately sample equivalent to 40 mg of the compound and dilute appropriately with water to get 40 mcg/ml.

Procedure

To 10 ml each of the sample and standard solutions, add 15 ml of buffer solution and 2 ml of aminoantipyrine reagent. Shake to mix, add about 15 ml of water, 2 ml of potassium ferricyanide solution and dilute to 50 ml with water. After 10 min, measure the extinction of both the solutions at 550 nm against reagent blank.

Note : Codeine phosphate, promethazine, diphenhydramine and ammonium chloride do not interfere. Phenylephrine will interfere.

Ephedrine hydrochloride

Follow the method as described in formulation 8 of the chapter on bronchospasm relaxants. Ephedrine, a volatile base is subjected to distillation and then estimated by acid-base titration; refer to formulation 8 of the chapter on bronchospasm relaxants.

Dextromethorphan hydrobromide, Pseudoephedrine hydrochloride, Azatadine maleate

ESTIMATION

Dextromethorphan hydrobromide

Follow the method described in formulation 12 or 14 of this chapter.

Pseudoephedrine hydrochloride

Follow the method described in formulation 19 of this chapter.

Azatadine maleate

Follow the method described in formulation 27 of the chapter on analgesics and antipyretics.

Dextromethorphan hydrobromide, Bromhexine hydrochloride, Ammonium chloride, Menthol

ESTIMATION

Dextromethorphan hydrobromide

Follow the method described in formulation 12 or 14 of this chapter.

Menthol

Follow the method described in formulation 5 of this chapter. Use distillate for the colour development.

Bromhexine hydrochloride

Follow the method described in formulation 26 of this chapter.

Ammonium chloride

Follow the method described in formulation 7 of this chapter.

Pheniramine maleate, Ammonium chloride, Sodium citrate, Menthol

ESTIMATION

Pheniramine maleate

Reagents

1. 0.02 N perchloric acid.
2. 10% w/v solution of sodium hydroxide in water.

Procedure

Transfer equivalent to 60 mg of pheniramine maleate into a separating funnel. Dilute with 20 ml water. Make alkaline with sodium hydroxide solution and extract with three 20 ml portions of solvent ether. The combined ethereal extracts are dried over anhydrous sodium sulphate. Evaporate the ether extract carefully. The residue is dissolved in previously neutralised glacial acetic acid and titrated with 0.02 N perchloric acid, using crystal violet as indicator. Each ml of 0.02 N perchloric acid is equivalent to 0.003564 g of pheniramine maleate.

Ammonium chloride

Transfer the preparation equivalent to 100 mg of ammonium chloride into a conical flask, dilute with 20 ml water. Titrate with 0.1 N silver nitrate using solutions of fluorescein sodium as indicator. The end point is detected by the appearance of a pronounced pink tint of the precipitates. 1 ml of 0.1 N silver nitrate is equivalent to 0.00535 g of ammonium chloride.

Sodium citrate

Follow the calcium chloride precipitation method as described in formulation 6 of this chapter.

Menthol

Follow the method involving reaction with p-dimethylaminobenzaldehyde. For details refer to formulation 5 of this chapter.

Ephedrine hydrochloride, Ethylmorphine hydrochloride

ESTIMATION

Total alkaloids

To accurately measured volume of the sample equivalent to 100 mg of ephedrine hydrochloride, add 50 ml of normal saline and 5 ml of 4% w/v aqueous solution of sodium hydroxide. Add sufficient sodium chloride powder to saturate. Extract with three 50 ml portions of ether. Wash ether layer with the same 10 ml of brine solution. Extract ether layer with exactly 20 ml of 0.1 N sulphuric acid. Warm the acid extract (A) to dispel dissolved ether and titrate excess acid with 0.1 N sodium hydroxide using bromothymol blue as indicator. Each ml of 0.1 N sulphuric acid is equivalent to 0.02017 g of total alkaloids calculated as ephedrine hydrochloride. For calculations, refer to formulation 2 of this chapter.

Ephedrine hydrochloride

As ephedrine (base) is volatile, follow the distillation method as described in formulation 8 of the chapter on bronchospasm relaxants. Alternatively, follow the general ammoniacal copper sulphate method.

Ethylmorphine hydrochloride

METHOD 1

Follow the method described in formulation 29 of the chapter on analgesics and antipyretics.

METHOD 2

Dilute part of acid extract obtained under total alkaloids approximately with 0.1 N sulphuric acid and measure the absorbance at about 284 nm and calculate the results taking 42.5 as value of A 1%, 1 cm at 284 nm for ethylmorphine.

Note : Ephedrine has negligible absorbance at 284 nm, hence no interference.

Pseudoephedrine hydrochloride, Diphenhydramine hydrochloride, Ammonium chloride, Menthol, Sodium citrate

ESTIMATION

Pseudoephedrine hydrochloride

Reagents

1. Benzene-carbon disulphide (3 : 1) mixture.
2. 5% w/v solution of copper sulphate in water.

Standard solution

100 mcg/ml of pseudoephedrine hydrochloride in water.

Sample solution

Take appropriate quantity of the sample equivalent to 25 mg of pseudoephedrine hydrochloride and dilute to 250 ml with water to get 100 mcg/ml.

Procedure

Transfer 2 ml each of standard, sample and water into respective tubes. Into each tube, add 2 ml strong ammonia solution, 2 ml copper sulphate solution and shake it gently. Then, to each tube add 10 ml of mixture of benzene-carbon disulphide, stopper the tubes and shake it for one minute. Collect the organic phase, filter through filter paper and measure the absorption immediately against reagent blank at 440 nm and calculate the results.

Diphenhydramine hydrochloride

Follow the cobalt thiocyanate method as described in formulation 6 of this chapter. Alternatively, follow ammonium reineckate precipitation method as described in formulation 5 of this chapter.

Sodium citrate, Menthol, Ammonium chloride

Follow the methods described in formulation 5, 6 and 7 respectively of this chapter.

Dextromethorphan hydrobromide, Guaiphenesin, Phenylpropanolamine hydrochloride

ESTIMATION

Dextromethorphan hydrobromide

Follow the method described in formulation 12 or 14 of this chapter.

Guaiphenesin

Standard solution

30 mcg/ml of guaiphenesin in chloroform.

Sample solution

To accurately weighed/measured aliquot of the sample equivalent to 75 mg of the compound, add 10 ml of saturated solution of sodium bicarbonate and extract with four 25 ml portions of chloroform. Wash the combined chloroform layer with 15 ml of 1 N hydrochloric acid. Combine the aqueous acidic layer and preserve for assay of phenylpropanolamine. Dilute the chloroform layer to 100 ml and carry out further dilution appropriately to get a solution of 30 mcg/ml.

Concomitantly measure the extinction of both the solutions at maxima at 276 nm with chloroform as blank.

Phenylpropanolamine hydrochloride

Reagents

1. Saturated solution of sodium bicarbonate in water.
2. 2.5% w/v solution of sodium carbonate in water.
3. 0.2% w/v solution of sodium metaperiodate in water.
4. Methylene chloride.
5. 1 N hydrochloric acid.

Standard solution

0.2 mg/ml of the compound in water. To 10 ml of above solution, add 10 ml of saturated solution of sodium bicarbonate and 45 ml of 1 N hydrochloric acid and dilute to 200 ml with water (10 mcg/ml).

Sample solution

Dilute the aqueous layer reserved during estimation of guaiphenesin to 200 ml with water.

Procedure

To 10 ml each of sample and standard solutions, add 10 ml of sodium carbonate solution and 10 ml of sodium metaperiodate solution. Allow to stand for 15 min, and extract with three 30 ml portions of methylene chloride. Dilute organic layer to 100 ml with the same solvent and measure the extinction at 242 nm using solvent as blank.

Diethylcarbamazine citrate, Glyceryl guaiacolate (Guaiphenesin), Chlorpheniramine maleate

ESTIMATION

Diethylcarbamazine citrate

Take sample accurately measured/weighed equivalent to 50 mg of the compound and carry out non-aqueous titration using thymol blue as indicator. Each ml of 0.1 N perchloric acid is equivalent to 0.03914 g of diethylcarbamazine citrate.

Note : The reaction based on citrate moiety of the molecule can be used for quantitative estimation of the compound. For details, refer to method 2 for estimation of sodium citrate described under formulation 6 of this chapter.

Guaiphenesin

Dissolve or dilute the sample with water to get a concentration of 15 mcg/ml. Measure the extinction at maxima at about 275 nm and calculate the result by comparing with the standard (15 mcg/ml).

Chlorpheniramine maleate

Carry out the cyanogen bromide method as described in formulation 3 of this chapter.

Mepyramine maleate, Pheniramine maleate, Phenylpropanolamine hydrochloride

ESTIMATION

Mepyramine maleate

Standard solution

25 mcg/ml of mepyramine maleate in 0.1 N hydrochloric acid.

Sample solution

Measure appropriate portion of the sample equivalent to 5 mg of the compound. Make it alkaline with ammonia and extract with four 30 ml portions of solvent ether. Wash the combined ether layer with 20 ml of water and reject the aqueous layer. Extract the base back into acid from ether layer using four 25 ml portions of 0.1 N hydrochloric acid. Remove the traces of ether from acid layer by slight warming and make the volume to 250 ml.

Measure the extinction of both the sample and standard solutions at maximum at about 316 nm and calculate the results by comparison.

Pheniramine maleate

Follow the cyanogen bromide method as described in formulation 3 of this chapter under chlorpheniramine maleate. Use a solution of 25 mcg/ml and measure the chromogen at 480 nm.

Phenylpropanolamine hydrochloride

Measure appropriate portion of the sample equivalent to 60 mg of the compound. Make it alkaline with dilute ammonia and extract with four 25 ml portion of chloroform. Wash the combined chloroform extract with water and pass the organic layer through anhydrous sodium sulphate. Evaporate chloroform layer, dissolve the residue in glacial acetic acid and carry out the non-aqueous titration. From the total volume of perchloric acid consumed in the above titration, subtract the volume of the acid equivalent to the estimated contents of mepyramine maleate and pheniramine maleate and calculate the contents of phenylpropanolamine hydrochloride from the remaining volume using a factor of 0.003754 g for each ml of 0.02 N perchloric acid.

Diphenhydramine hydrochloride, Ephedrine hydrochloride, Noscapine, Ammonium chloride, Sodium citrate

ESTIMATION

Diphenhydramine hydrochloride

Follow the cobalt thiocyanate method as described under formulation 6 of this chapter.

Ephedrine hydrochloride

Follow the ammoniacal copper sulphate method as described under formulation 1 of the chapter on bronchospasm relaxants.

Ammonium chloride

Follow the ammonia distillation, followed by acid-base titration as described under formulation 7 of this chapter.

Sodium citrate

Follow the method 4 involving colour with ferric chloride as described under formulation 6 of this chapter.

Noscapine

Measure 10 ml of the sample, basify with ammonia solution and extract with chloroform. Evaporate chloroform layer which contains all the three bases i.e. ephedrine, diphenhydramine and noscapine. Carry out non-aqueous titration with perchloric acid using crystal violet as indicator. This gives the total volume of perchloric acid required for three bases. Subtract the volume of perchloric acid equivalent to the amount of ephedrine and diphenhydramine as determined by the method described above. The remaining volume of perchloric acid is equivalent to the amount of noscapine present in 10 ml of the sample.

Typical laboratory analysis

Each 10 ml of the sample is labelled to contain 21 mg of diphenhydramine hydrochloride, 11 mg of ephedrine hydrochloride and 20 mg of noscapine.

1. Total volume of 0.01102 N perchloric acid consumed by three bases in non-aqueous titration

    = 15.8 ml   ...(A)

2. Volume of 0.01102 N perchloric acid equivalent to 21 mg of diphenhydramine hydrochloride

    $$= \frac{0.021 \times 0.01}{0.01102 \times 0.002918} = 6.5 \text{ ml} \qquad \qquad \text{...(a)}$$

    (each ml of 0.01 N perchloric acid is equivalent to 0.002918 g of diphenhydramine hydrochloride)

3. Volume of 0.01102 N perchloric acid equivalent to 11 mg of ephedrine hydrochloride

$$= \frac{0.011 \times 0.01}{0.01102 \times 0.002017} = 4.9 \text{ ml} \qquad \qquad \text{...(b)}$$

(each ml of 0.01 N perchloric acid is equivalent to 0.002017 g of ephedrine hydrochloride)

4. Volume of 0.01102 N perchloric acid consumed by noscapine present in 10 ml of the sample

$$= A - (a + b)$$
$$= 15.8 - (6.5 + 4.9) = 4.4 \text{ ml}$$

(each ml of 0.01 N perchloric acid is equivalent to 0.004134 g of noscapine)

$$\text{Total amount (mg) of Noscapine/10 ml} = \frac{4.4 \times 0.01102 \times 0.004134 \times 10}{0.01}$$

$$= 20.02 \text{ mg}$$
$$\text{Claim} = 20 \text{ mg}$$

Salbutamol sulphate, Bromhexine hydrochloride, Guaiphenesin

ESTIMATION

Salbutamol sulphate

METHOD 1

Follow the method 5 described in formulation 14 of the chapter on bronchospasm relaxants.

METHOD 2

Reagents

1. 8% w/v solution of potassium ferricyanide in water.
2. 0.1% w/v solution of N,N-dimethyl-p-phenylene-diammonium sulphate.
3. 5% w/v solution of sodium carbonate in water.

Standard solution

40 mcg/ml of salbutamol as salbutamol sulphate in water.

Sample solution

Dilute sample equivalent to 2 mg of salbutamol to 50 ml with water.

Procedure

To 5 ml each of sample and standard solutions, add 50 ml of water, 5 ml of sodium bicarbonate solution and 4 ml of N,N-dimethyl reagent, shake to mix, add 4 ml of potassium ferricyanide solution. Allow to stand for 15 minutes and then extract with 10, 5, 5 ml portions of chloroform. Pass chloroform layer through a layer of anhydrous sodium sulphate and make up to 25 ml with chloroform. Measure the extinction of each solution at about 620 nm using chloroform as blank. Calculate the results by comparing with standard.

Bromhexine hydrochloride

Reagents

1. Dilute ammonia solution : Dilute 210 ml of ammonia solution to 500 ml with distilled water.
2. 0.1 N methanolic hydrochloric acid : To 20 ml of water, add 5 ml of hydrochloric acid and dilute to 500 ml with methanol.

Standard solution

Weigh accurately 40 mg of bromhexine hydrochloride and transfer to a separating funnel, basify with 5 ml of dilute ammonia solution. Add 25 ml of water and extract with four 25 ml portions of chloroform.

Pass combined chloroform layer through anhydrous sodium sulphate previously washed with chloroform. Evaporate chloroform layer and dissolve the residue in 0.1 N methanolic hydrochloric acid to produce 100 ml (400 mcg/ml). Further dilutions may be done appropriately with methanolic hydrochloric acid to get 40 mcg/ml.

Sample solution

Measure accurately sample equivalent to 4 mg of the substance, add 25 ml of water and continue with the procedure as described under preparation of standard solution.

Measure the extinction of the standard and sample solutions at 317 nm using 0.1 N methanolic hydrochloric acid as blank. Calculate the results by comparison.

Alternatively, to 2 ml of standard and sample solutions prepared above, add 8 ml of p-dimethyl-aminobenzaldehyde solutions (10% w/v in methanol) and 5 ml of hydrochloric acid. Mix and allow to stand for 10 minutes and make up the volume to 25 ml with water. Measure the absorption at 425 nm against reagent blank and calculate the results by comparison with standard.

Guaiphenesin

Standard solution

Weigh accurately 100 mg of guaiphenesin, transfer to a separating funnel. Add 20 ml of water and 5 ml of sodium hydroxide solution (20% w/v). Extract with four 40 ml portions of petroleum ether (60-80°C). Discard ether layer, collect the aqueous layer and extract four 20 ml portions of chloroform. Pass combined chloroform layer through anhydrous sodium sulphate and make up to 100 ml with chloroform. Evaporate 5 ml of the above solution, take up the residue in methanol to produce 100 ml (50 mcg/ml).

Sample solution

Measure accurately sample equivalent to 100 mg of the substance, add 20 ml of water and continue the procedure as described under preparation of standard solution. Alternatively further dilute chloroform solution appropriately (50 mcg/ml) with chloroform and concomitantly determine the absorption of sample and standard solutions at 276 nm.

Measure the extinction of the standard and sample solutions at 275 nm using methanol as blank. Calculate the results by comparison.

Bromhexine hydrochloride, Pseudoephedrine hydrochloride, Chlorpheniramine maleate

ESTIMATION

Bromhexine hydrochloride

METHOD 1

Reagents

1. Dilute ammonia solution : Dilute 15 ml of strong ammonia solution to 100 ml with water.
2. 0.1 N methanolic hydrochloric acid : Dilute 8 ml of hydrochloric acid to 1000 ml with methanol.

Standard solution

Prepare 30 mcg/ml solution of bromhexine hydrochloride in 0.1 N methanolic hydrochloric acid.

Sample solution

Take the sample equivalent to 8 mg of bromhexine hydrochloride in a 250 ml separating funnel, add 10 ml of water and 15 ml of dilute ammonia solution. Extract with four 20 ml portions of chloroform. Evaporate the chloroform layer, dissolve the residue in 0.1 N methanolic hydrochloric acid and make up the volume to 50 ml. Dilute 10 ml to 50 ml with the same solvent (32 mcg/ml).

Procedure

Measure the absorbance of both standard and sample solutions at the maximum at about 317 nm using 0.1 N methanolic hydrochloric acid as the blank and deduce the results by comparison.

METHOD 2

Follow the method described in formulation 26 of this chapter involving diazotization and coupling with n-naphthyl-ethylenediamine dihydrochloride.

Pseudoephedrine hydrochloride

METHOD 1

Reagents

1. Saturated sodium carbonate solution.
2. 2% w/v solution of sodium metaperiodate in water.
3. n-hexane or petroleum ether (40-60°C).

Standard solution

Prepare 30 mcg/ml solution of pseudoephedrine hydrochloride in water.

Sample solution

Weigh the sample accurately equivalent to 60 mg of pseudoephedrine hydrochloride and dilute to 100 ml with water. Further dilutions are made with water appropriately and step-wise to get a solution of 30 mcg/ml.

Procedure

To 5 ml each of standard and sample solutions add 4 ml of sodium carbonate solution and 2 ml of sodium metaperiodate solution. Mix, allow to stand for 10 minutes, add 20 ml of n-hexane or petroleum ether and shake for 30 seconds. Measure the absorbance of both standard and sample solutions (organic layer) at the maximum at about 242 nm. Deduce the results by comparison.

METHOD 2

Reagents

1. Phosphate buffer, pH 7.5 : Mix 45 ml of 0.2 N sodium hydroxide and 50 ml of 0.2 N potassium dihydrogen phosphate, dilute to 200 ml with water.
2. Bromothymol blue solution : 1 mg/ml solution of dye in phosphate buffer, pH 7.5.

Standard solution

500 mcg/ml of pseudoephedrine hydrochloride in water.

Sample solution

Extract accurately weighed quantity of the powdered sample with water to produce concentration of 500 mcg/ml.

Procedure

To 10 ml each of sample and standard solutions, add 10 ml of phosphate buffer, 25 ml of bromothymol blue solution. Make it alkaline (litmus) with sodium hydroxide (20%). Extract with benzene (3 × 30 ml), pass combined benzene extract through anhydrous sodium sulphate and extract with 50% sodium hydroxide solution (4 × 25 ml). Combine the alkaline layer and dilute to 200 ml. Further, dilute 5 ml to 50 ml with 5% sodium hydroxide solution and measure the absorption of both sample and standard solutions at about 620 nm with 5% solution of sodium hydroxide as blank. Calculate the results by comparison.

Chlorpheniramine maleate

Reagents

1. 1% w/v solution of sodium dithionate in water.
2. 4% v/v solution of aniline (distilled) in methanol.
3. 10% w/v solution to potassium cyanide in water.
4. 10% w/v solution of cyanogen bromide in water.

Standard solution

Prepare 20 mcg/ml solution of chlorpheniramine maleate in water.

Sample solution

Dilute the sample appropriately with water to get 20 mcg/ml in water.

Procedure

To 10 ml each of standard and sample solutions, add one or two drops of dithionate solution, 5 ml of aniline and 2 ml of cyanogen bromide solution. Shake and allow to develop the golden yellow colour. Measure the absorbance of standard and sample solutions at the maximum at about 430 nm using a blank prepared in the same manner omitting the substance to be analysed. Deduce the results by comparison.

Amoxycillin, Bromhexine hydrochloride

ESTIMATION

Amoxycillin

METHOD 1

Follow the method described under formulation 8 of the chapter on antibiotics. The method is based on alkaline oxidation of phenolic group and coupling with 4-aminoantipyrine.

METHOD 2

Follow the method described under formulation 8 of the chapter on antibiotics. Each ml of 0.1 N sodium hydroxide is equivalent to 0.03654 g of amoxycillin.

Note : The method official in Indian Pharmacopoeia based as reaction with imidazole mercury reagent can be used in such combinations.

Bromhexine hydrochloride

METHOD 1

Standard solution

50 mcg/ml in 0.1 N methanolic hydrochloric acid.

Sample solution

Weigh accurately quantity of the sample equivalent to about 12 mg of substance and transfer to a separating funnel. Add about 15 ml of water; basify with dilute solution of ammonia and extract with three 25 ml portions of n-hexane. Combined organic layer is extracted with three 25 ml portions of 0.1 N hydrochloric acid ensuring complete separation of layers after each extraction. Dilute the acidic layer to 250 ml with 0.1 N methanolic hydrochloric acid.

Measure the extinction of both sample and standard solutions at 317 nm using 0.1 N methanolic hydrochloric acid as blank. Calculate the results by comparison.

METHOD 2

Reagents

1. 1 N hydrochloric acid.
2. 1% w/v solution of sodium nitrite in water.
3. 0.5% w/v solution of ammonium sulphamate in water.
4. 0.1% w/v solution of N-naphthyl ethylenediamine dihydrochloride (NED) in water.
5. 2% w/v solution of resorcinol in water.

Standard solution

Weigh accurately about 25 mg of bromhexine hydrochloride. Add about 40 ml of alcohol, shake for 5 minutes and dilute to volume with 1 N hydrochloric acid. Further dilution is done with 1 N hydrochloric acid to get a concentration of 40 mcg/ml.

Sample solution

Prepare the sample as under method 1 above. Filter, if necessary.

Procedure

Take 3 ml each of sample and standard solutions in 25 ml volumetric flask. Cool in ice-bath for about 10 minutes. Add 1 ml each of sodium nitrite solution, ammonium sulphamate solution and 'NED' reagent at an interval of 2 minutes. Mix and dilute to 25 ml with water. Measure the absorbance of both sample and standard solutions at about 500 nm against reagent blank. Calculate the contents of bromhexine hydrochloride in the sample by comparison.

Note :   Instead of 'NED' reagent, add 1.2 ml of resorcinol solution and dilute to 25 ml. The chromophore exhibits absorption maximum at about 435 nm.

Betamethasone, Bromhexine hydrochloride, Salbutamol sulphate

ESTIMATION

Betamethasone

Reagents

1. 10% v/v solution of tetramethyl ammonium hydrochloride (TMAH) in methanol.
2. 0.5% w/v solution of tetrazolium blue in methanol.

Standard solution

10 mcg/ml of betamethasone in chloroform.

Sample solution

Accurately weighed quantity of the sample equivalent to 1 mg of the substance is extracted with 3 × 20 ml portions of chloroform and chloroform layer passed through anhydrous sodium sulphate kept on cotton plug and made up to 100 ml with chloroform (10 mcg/ml).

Procedure

To 10 ml each of sample and standard solutions, add 2 ml of tetrazolium blue solution and 2 ml of TMAH. Keep for 45 min at 37°C and dilute to 25 ml with chloroform. Measure absorbance of both the solutions at 525 nm using chloroform as blank and calculate the results by comparison.

Bromhexine hydrochloride

Follow the method 2 described in formulation 26 of this chapter.

Salbutamol sulphate

Follow the method 2 described under formulation 14 of the chapter on bronchospasm relaxants.

Bromhexine hydrochloride, Cephalexin

ESTIMATION

Bromhexine hydrochloride

Accurately weighed quantity of the sample equivalent to 4 mg of bromhexine hydrochloride is suspended in 10 ml of 0.1 N hydrochloric acid and extracted with three 25 ml portions of chloroform (retain aqueous layer for estimation of cephalexin). The combined chloroform layer diluted to 100 ml with chloroform. Further dilutions are done appropriately and stepwise to get a concentration of 20 mcg/ml. Measure extinction of the solutions at maximum at about 317 nm. Calculate the results by comparing with the standard solution of bromhexine hydrochloride in chloroform (20 mcg/ml). Alternatively, evaporate appropriate volume of above solution and take up the residue in 0.1 N methanolic hydrochloric acid and measure the extinction at 317 nm. Alternatively, follow the method described in formulation 16 of the chapter on bronchospasm relaxants.

Cephalexin

The aqueous acidic extract retained during estimation of bromhexine hydrochloride is diluted appropriately with 0.1 N methanolic hydrochloric acid to get a concentration of 20 mcg/ml. Measure extinction of the solution at maxima at about 258 nm. Calculate the results by comparing with the standard (20 mcg/ml).

Note : Cephalexin and other antibiotics as tetracycline, oxytetracycline, phenoxymethyl penicillin exhibit maxima at about 260 nm, 280 nm and 340 nm. Bromhexine hydrochloride shows zero absorbance above 330 nm. It is therefore preferable to estimate cephalexin and other antibiotics at 340 nm instead of 258 nm as indicated above. This will eliminate the possibility of interference, if any, due to bromhexine hydrochloride.

Alternatively, sample equivalent to 250 mg of cephalexin is dissolved in 20 ml of neutral methanol and titrated with 0.1 N sodium hydroxide using bromothymol blue as indicator, perform blank for necessary correction. Each ml of 0.1 N sodium hydroxide is equivalent to 0.03474 g of cephalexin.

Bromhexine hydrochloride, Erythromycin estolate

ESTIMATION

Bromhexine hydrochloride

Follow the method described in formulation 26 of this chapter.

Erythromycin estolate

Reagents

1. 0.4% w/w solution of O-nitro-benzaldehyde in glacial acetic acid.
2. Concentrated hydrochloric acid.

Standard solution

250 mcg/ml of erythromycin (base) in glacial acetic acid.

Sample solution

Accurately weighed quantity of powdered sample equivalent to 100 mg of erythromycin (base) is suspended in glacial acetic acid to make 100 ml. Filter and dilute appropriately to get solution of 250 mcg/ml.

Procedure

To 2 ml each of sample and standard solutions, add 2 ml of benzaldehyde reagent and 3 ml of concentrated hydrochloric acid. Keep at room temperature for 15 minutes and dilute to 25 ml with glacial acetic acid. Measure the absorbance of both sample and standard solutions within 10 min at 490 nm, and calculate the results by comparison.

Bromhexine hydrochloride, Guaiphenesin, Pseudoephedrine hydrochloride

ESTIMATION

Bromhexine hydrochloride

Follow the method described in formulation 26 of this chapter.

Pseudoephedrine hydrochloride

Follow the method described in formulation 25 of this chapter.

Guaiphenesin

Reagents

1. Formaldehyde methanol reagent : Prepared by diluting 30 ml of formaldehyde solution (38-40% w/v) to 1000 ml with absolute methanol.
2. Solvent : Cautiously add 600 mg of concentrated sulphuric acid to 400 ml of methanol-water (1 + 1) mixture previously cooled in ice-bath.

Standard solution

80 mcg/ml of guaiphenesin in solvent.

Sample solution

To accurately measured quantity of sample equivalent to 100 mg of guaiphenesin, add 10 ml of water and 10 ml of 1 N sodium hydroxide, mix and extract with chloroform (3 × 25 ml). Combined chloroform layer is in turn extracted with the solvent (3 × 25 ml). The combined acidic layer is made up of 100 ml with the solvent and 2 ml of the resultant solution is further diluted to 25 ml with the solvent and used for analysis (80 mcg/ml).

Procedure

To 5 ml each of sample and standard solution, add 15 ml of solvent and 1 ml of formaldehyde methanol reagent, mixed and diluted to 25 ml with the solvent. Measure absorbance of sample and standard solutions at maxima at about 550 nm against reagent blank and calculate the results by comparison.

Salbutamol sulphate, Bromhexine hydrochloride, Phenylephrine hydrochloride

ESTIMATION

Salbutamol sulphate

Follow the method described in formulation 14 of the chapter on bronchospasm relaxants.

Bromhexine hydrochloride

Follow the method described in formulation 26 of this chapter.

Phenylephrine hydrochloride

Follow the method 1 described in formulation 1 of the chapter on analgesics and antipyretics.

Bromhexine hydrochloride, Diphenhydramine hydrochloride, Guaiphenesin, Ammonium chloride, Menthol

ESTIMATION

Bromhexine hydrochloride

Follow the method described in formulation 26 of this chapter. Sample and standard solution are prepared in methanol.

Ammonium chloride

Follow the method 2 described in formulation 7 of this chapter.

Diphenhydramine hydrochloride

Follow the method described in formulation 6 of this chapter based on coloured complex formation with cobalt thiocyanate.

Guaiphenesin

Follow the method described in formulation 17 of this chapter. Alternatively, follow the method given below :

This method is based on oxidation of terminal vicinal hydroxyl group, liberating formaldehyde which reacts with acetyl acetone in presence of ammonium acetate to give yellow coloured chromogen (λ_{max} 412 nm).

Reagents

1. 0.214% w/v solution of sodium periodate in water.
2. 30% w/v solution of ammonium acetate.
3. 1% v/v solution of acetyl acetone in ammonium acetate solution.
4. Saturated solution of sodium bicarbonate.
5. 1 N hydrochloric acid.

Standard solution

150 mcg/ml of guaiphenesin in 5% acetic acid.

Sample solution

To the sample equivalent to 100 mg of the add 10 ml of saturated solution of sodium bicarbonate and extract with 25 ml portions of chloroform, washing each layer with 5 ml of 1 N hydrochloric acid.

Combine layers and make up to 100 ml with chloroform (1 mcg/ml). Evaporate 15 ml of chloroform by and take up the residue in 5 ml of glacial acetic acid and dilute to 100 ml with water (150 mcg/ml).

Procedure

To 2 ml each of sample and standard solutions, add 2 ml of sodium periodate solution and allow to stand at room temperature for 5 minutes with occasional stirring. Add 5 ml of acetyl acetone reagent and retain at room temperature for 30 min, dilute to 25 ml with water. Measure the absorbance of both the solution at 412 nm against reagent blank and calculate the results by comparison.

Menthol

Follow the method described in formulation 5 of this chapter.

Formulation 33

Ibuprofen, Pseudoephedrine hydrochloride

ESTIMATION

Ibuprofen

To accurately weighed quantity of a sample equivalent to 150-200 mg of the substance, add 4-5 ml of water and acidify with 0.1 N hydrochloric acid. Extract with four 25 ml portions of chloroform. Pass the chloroform layer through anhydrous sodium sulphate, placed on a copper plate. Evaporate the chloroform extract till there is no precipitate smell of chloroform. Dissolve the entire residue in 50 ml of neutral (phenolphthalein) methanol and dilute with 0.1 N sodium hydroxide. Each ml of 0.1 N sodium hydroxide is equivalent to 0.020639 g of ibuprofen.

Pseudoephedrine hydrochloride

Pipette out appropriate volume of the uniformly suspended sample representing 90-100 mg of the substance, add 4-5 ml of water and basify distinctly with dilute solution of ammonia. Extract with four 25 ml portions of ether, passing each ether layer through cotton plug. Evaporate the combined ether extract till no precipitate smell of ether.

To the residue, add 40 ml of glacial acetic acid, 10 ml of acetic anhydrite and titrate with 0.1 N perchloric acid using crystal violet as indicator.

Each ml of 0.1 N perchloric acid is equivalent to 0.02017 g of pseudoephedrine hydrochloride.

Amoxycillin, Carbocysteine (S-Carboxymethyl cysteine)

ESTIMATION

Amoxycillin and Carbocysteine

Reagents

1. Dimethyl sulphoxide (DMSO).
2. 1% w/v solution of nickel (II) nitrate in DMSO.

Standard solution

50 mcg/ml each drug in water.

Sample solution

Accurately weighed or measured aliquot of the sample equivalent to 5 mg of, the drug was extracted with water to produce 100 ml. The filtrate was used for analysis.

Procedure

To 5 ml of sample and standard solutions, add 2 ml nickel nitrate solution, mix and after 30 min (optimum time for complete complexation) measure the absorbance of solutions at 259 nm (for carbocysteine) and 327 nm (for amoxycillin). The results were calculated by comparison. The method obeys Bear's law in the range of 5-50 mcg/ml. The complexes were stable for at least 3 hrs.

After complexation with nickel (II), significant improvement in spectral characteristics was observed with both chromic and hyperchromic shift. Molar absorptivity increases by 3-4 folds for amoxycillin and 6-7 folds for carbocysteine.

Amino and ketonic functions present in the molecule appear to be responsible for complexation. DMSO plays important role as nickel formed complex only in DMSO and not in water by coordinate bond through ion-pairs of electrons on oxygen.

METHOD 2 (for carbocysteine)

Accurately weighed quantity of sample equivalent to 300 mg of carbocysteine is suspended in 25 ml of 0.1 N sodium hydroxide and stirred for 45 min (use magnet stirrer). Filter and wash the flask and filter paper with water (3 × 50 ml). Combine both the aqueous washings with the filtrate and titrate with 0.1 N hydrochloric acid (methyl red). Carry out the blank titration or carry out potentiometric titration.

Each ml of 0.1 N hydrochloric acid is equivalent to 17.92 mg of carbocysteine.

Note : Amoxycillin interference is in the range of 5-7.5%.

METHOD 3 (for carbocysteine)

Dissolve the sample in 10 ml of formic acid (98-100%) and add further 50 ml of formic acid and titrate with 0.1 N perchloric acid using 0.05 ml of oracet blue B solution (0.5% solution of the dye in glacial acetic acid) as indicator (change from blue to clear purple). Each ml of 0.1 N perchloric acid is equivalent to 17.92 mg of carbocysteine.

Chapter 13

Eye, Ear & Nasal Preparations

Formulation 1

Domiphen bromide, Boric acid, Borax, Salicylic acid, Zinc sulphate, Allantoin, Chlorbutol

ESTIMATION

Domiphen bromide

Reagents

1. Sodium lauryl sulphate solution, 0.00025 M : Dissolve 360 mg of pure sodium lauryl sulphate which has been previously dried at 105°C and cooled, in 100 ml of water. Dilute 10 ml of this to 500 ml. Standardise this solution against dicyclomine hydrochloride.
2. 0.003% w/v solution of methylene blue in water.

Procedure

Transfer sample equivalent to 2 mg of domiphen bromide into dry separating funnel and extract with three 10 ml portions of chloroform, allowing each extract to separate fully before proceeding with the next. Combine the chloroform extract in a 250 ml stoppered measuring cylinder and to this, add 25 ml of methylene blue solution and 50 ml of water. Stopper and shake the cylinder. The colour remains in the aqueous phase. Titrate with small addition of 0.00025 M sodium lauryl sulphate shaking after each addition until the colour is of equal intensity in both the phases. Each ml of 0.00025 M sodium lauryl sulphate is equivalent to 0.000208 g of domiphen bromide.

Borax

Measure accurately aliquot of the sample equivalent to 100 mg of borax and titrate with 0.1 N hydrochloric acid using methyl orange or methyl red as indicator. Each ml of 0.1 N hydrochloric acid is equivalent to 0.09536 g of borax.

Total boric acid

Transfer the sample equivalent to 100 mg of boric acid into 250 ml conical flask, and neutralise it with 0.1 N sulphuric acid using methyl orange as indicator to a faint pink colour. Add about 10 g of mannitol, warm to dissolve and titrate against 0.1 N sodium hydroxide solution using phenolphthalein as indicator. Each ml of 0.1 N sodium hydroxide is equivalent to 0.006183 g of boric acid.

Salicylic acid

Reagents

1. Ammonium ferric sulphate solution : Dissolve 8 g of ferric ammonium sulphate in 100 ml of water and warm on a water-bath. Filter, if necessary, to remove any precipitate that might have formed.
2. Acidic ammonium ferric sulphate solution : To 2 ml of ammonium ferric sulphate solution, add 1 ml of 1 N hydrochloric acid and make up the volume to 100 ml with distilled water, solution to be freshly prepared.

Standard solution

25 mcg/ml of salicylic acid in water.

Sample solution

Dilute sample equivalent to 2.5 mg of salicylic acid with water to produce 100 ml (25 mcg/ml).

Procedure

Take 5 ml each of sample and standard solutions in two test tubes, add 2 ml of acidic ferric ammonium sulphate solution and mix thoroughly. Measure the absorption of both the solutions against water as blank at about 540 nm and calculate the results by comparison.

Zinc sulphate

Reagents

1. Zincon reagent : Dissolve 60 mg of 'Zincon' in 2 ml of 0.2 N sodium hydroxide and 10 ml distilled water. Dilute to 50 ml with water, stable only for 2 days at room temperature.
2. Buffer solution, pH 9.2 : Dissolve 12.4 g of boric acid and 15 g of potassium chloride in 86 ml of 1 N sodium hydroxide. Dilute to 1000 ml with water.

Standard solution

40 mcg/ml of zinc sulphate in water.

Procedure

To accurately measured volume of sample containing 200 mcg of zinc sulphate and 5 ml of standard solution, add 50 ml of buffer solution, 2 ml of zincon reagent and dilute to 100 ml with buffer. Mix and measure the absorbance of sample and standard solutions at about 625 nm against reagent blank and compare the results.

Allantoin

In alkaline medium, allantoin is hydrolysed to allantoic acid, then in acidic medium to glyoxylic acid and urea. Glyoxylic acid reacts with phenylhydrazine to give hydrazone which is converted to coloured chromophore (λ_{max} 520 nm) on oxidation with potassium ferricyanide.

Reagents

1. 1% w/v solution of phenylhydrazine hydrochloride in water.
2. 1% w/v solution of potassium ferricyanide in water, stable for 1 day only.
3. 12.5% w/v solution of oxalic acid in water.

Standard solution

2.5 mcg/ml of allantoin in water.

Sample solution

Dilute sample appropriately with water to get 2.5 mcg/ml.

Procedure

Transfer 5 ml each of sample and standard solutions, and 5 ml of distilled water in 25 ml boiling tubes. To each tube, add 1 ml of 0.5 N sodium hydroxide and heat in boiling water-bath for exactly 5 minutes. Remove from heat and add 2 ml of oxalic acid solution and 1 ml of phenylhydrazine solution. Heat the tubes in boiling water for exactly 2 minutes. Cool, add 4 ml of hydrochloric acid, boil for 2 min, cool and add 0.5 ml of potassium ferricyanide solution. Mix well and measure the extinction of the solutions after 5 minutes against water as blank at about 520 nm and calculate the results by comparison.

Chlorbutol (Chlorbutanol)

Reagents

1. 10% w/v solution of ferric ammonium sulphate in water.
2. 10% w/v solution of sodium hydroxide in water.

Procedure

Transfer sample equivalent to 30 mg of chlorbutol into a flask. Add 5 ml of sodium hydroxide solution. Reflux for 30 minutes and cool. Add 5 ml of concentrated nitric acid, 2 ml of nitrobenzene and 10 ml of 0.1 N silver nitrate solution. Shake the contents vigorously for one minute. Add 1 ml of ferric ammonium sulphate solution and titrate excess of silver nitrate with 0.1 N ammonium thiocyanate to a pale red end point. Carry out the blank. Each ml of 0.1 N silver nitrate is equivalent to 0.005917 g of chlorbutol.

Benzocaine, Antipyrine, Hexylresorcinol

ESTIMATION

Benzocaine

METHOD 1

Take 5 ml each of sample and standard solutions (15 mcg/ml in water) and follow the method described in formulation 11 of the chapter on expectorants and cough suppressants.

METHOD 2

Reagents

1. 0.1% w/v solution of p-dimethylaminocinnamaldehyde in methanol.
2. 50% w/v solution of trichloroacetic acid in methanol.
3. Methyl alcohol, acetone free.

Standard solution

10 mcg/ml of benzocaine in methyl alcohol.

Sample solution

(a) Ear drops, creams and ointments (water soluble bases) : Weigh or measure accurately sample equivalent to 10 mg of benzocaine, suspend or dissolve in methanol and dilute to 100 ml with methyl alcohol. Filter through dry filter paper and discard first 5 ml of the filtrate. Dilute 1 ml of the filtrate to 50 ml with methyl alcohol.

(b) Ointment (water insoluble bases) : Dissolve accurately weighed or measured quantity of the sample equivalent to 10 mg of substance in 15 ml of cyclohexane. Transfer to 100 ml volumetric flask, rinse the beaker thrice with 2 ml portions of cyclohexane and transfer to the flask. Shake vigorously for 2-3 minutes and make up the volume with methyl alcohol. Filter through dry filter paper and carry out further dilutions for preparation of sample solutions as under (a) above.

(c) Lozenges : Powder finely and weigh accurately equivalent to 10 mg of benzocaine. Add 75 ml of methyl alcohol and shake for 30 minutes, dilute to 100 ml with methyl alcohol. Carry out further dilutions with methanol as described under (a) above for preparation of sample solution.

Procedure

To 2 ml each of the sample and standard solutions, add 4 ml of p-dimethylaminocinnamaldehyde reagent, followed by 2 ml of trichloroacetic acid solution. Keep at room temperature for 10 minutes and record the absorbance of both the solutions at about 545 nm against reagent blank.

Note : 1. The red Schiff's base produced in anhydrous medium is stable for 2 h. This reaction is more sensitive than the reaction with p-dimethylaminobenzaldehyde (yellow colour).
2. Menthol, camphor, benzalkonium chloride do not interfere.
3. Pink dye, usually present in lozenges, does not interfere.

Hexylresorcinol

METHOD 1

Reagents

1. Dilute hydrochloric acid.
2. Molybdo-phosphotungstate solution.
3. 10% w/v solution of sodium carbonate in water.

Standard solution

Weigh accurately 250 mg of standard hexylresorcinol and transfer to a 250 ml volumetric flask. Add 10 ml of alcohol to dissolve and dilute to volume with water. Dilute 10 ml of this solution to 100 ml with water (100 mcg/ml).

Sample solution

Accurately weigh, a quantity of the sample equivalent to 5 mg of hexylresorcinol and transfer to 50 ml volumetric flask. Dilute to volume with water and filter.

Procedure

Transfer 10 ml each of standard, water and sample solutions into separate 100 ml volumetric flasks. Add 2 ml of dilute hydrochloric acid, 1 ml of molybdo-phosphotungstate solution, about 60 ml of water and allow to stand for 10 minutes. Add 25 ml of sodium carbonate solution and dilute to volume with water. Mix thoroughly and allow to stand for 1 hr. Filter through a dry filter paper, rejecting the first portion of the filtrate. Determine the absorbance of the standard and the sample at about 640 nm using blank in the reference cell. Calculate the contents of hexylresorcinol by comparison.

METHOD 2

Reagents

1. 0.5 N ammonium hydroxide.
2. 0.5% w/v solution of 1,2-naphthoquinone-4-sulphonic acid (sodium salt) in water.

Standard solution

7.5 mcg/ml of hexylresorcinol in water.

Sample solution

Weigh accurately, a quantity of the sample equivalent to about 7.5 mg of hexylresorcinol, extract with water and make up to 100 ml with water. Further dilution is done with water to obtain solution of 7.5 mcg/ml.

Procedure

To 1 ml each of the standard and sample solution, add 0.5 ml of naphthoquinone reagent, 1.5 ml of 0.5 N ammonium hydroxide and dilute to 10 ml with water. Mix and read immediately (within 5 minutes) at 580 nm against reagent blank. Calculate the results by comparison. The method obeys Beer's law in the range of 2.5 to 7.5 mcg/ml.

Note : 1. The colour of the complex is stable for 5 minutes.
2. The method can be directly applied to lozenges without isolation.

Antipyrine

Reagent

1. 5% w/v solution of ferric chloride in water.

Standard solution

1 mg/ml of antipyrine in water.

Sample solution

Dilute an accurately weighed quantity of the sample equivalent to 100 mg of antipyrine to 100 ml with water.

Procedure

Transfer 1 ml each of the standard, sample and water into three separate test tubes. Add 5 ml of water into each tube followed by 1 ml of ferric chloride solution and mix well. Determine the absorbance of the sample and standard solutions at 540 nm using the blank in the reference cell and calculate the results by comparison.

Pilocarpine nitrate, Benzalkonium chloride, Potassium chloride, Boric acid, Polyvinyl alcohol

ESTIMATION

Pilocarpine nitrate

Reagents

1. McLivaine's buffer solution, pH 6.0 : 36.85 ml of 0.1 M citric acid and 63.15 ml of disodium hydrogen phosphate are mixed and adjusted to pH 6.0.
2. Bromocresol purple solution : It is prepared by dissolving 30 mg of bromocresol purple in 500 ml of chloroform.

Standard solution

1 mg/ml of pilocarpine nitrate in buffer, pH 6.0.

Sample solution

The sample is appropriately diluted with pH 6.0 buffer to get 1 mg/ml concentration of pilocarpine nitrate.

Procedure

To 1 ml each of sample and standard solutions, add 10 ml of dye solution and 10 ml of buffer, pH 6.0. Shake for 2 minutes and allow the layers to separate. Transfer the chloroform layer to a separator containing 10 ml of 0.1 N sodium hydroxide and shake for 15 seconds to liberate the dye. Dilute the alkaline layer to 10 ml with water or 0.1 N sodium hydroxide and measure the absorption of standard and sample solutions at about 580 nm against reagent blank.

Note : This method is quite suitable for estimation of pilocarpine in presence of its degradation product, pilocarpic acid.

Benzalkonium chloride

METHOD 1

Reagents

1. Dye solution : 0.06 w/v solution of bromothymol blue in ethyl alcohol.
2. Buffer solution, 0.05 M and 0.25 M, pH 7.5 : 0.05 M and 0.25 M solutions of dibasic and monobasic potassium phosphate are mixed to get buffer solutions of pH 7.5 with different molarity.

Standard solution

100 mcg/ml of benzalkonium chloride in water.

Sample solution

Dilute sample approximately with water to get concentration of 100 mcg/ml of the compound.

Procedure

To 3 ml each of the sample and standard solutions, add 25 mg of sodium chloride and 10 ml of 0.05 M buffer solution and 5 ml of dye solution. Shake and then add sufficient buffer to produce 25 ml. Measure the absorbance of both the solutions at about 610 nm against reagent blank.

Note : 1. When pilocarpine hydrochloride or epinephrine bitartrate are present in the formulation, 0.25 M buffer should be used as these salts are more acidic and buffer of higher buffering capacity is required to maintain pH at 7.5 as pH of the medium is very critical for complex formation.

2. The above method is suitable for estimation of chlorhexidine gluconate.

METHOD 2

Follow the method as described under formulation 15 of this chapter.

Polyvinyl alcohol

Reagents

1. 3.5 N sodium hydroxide solution.
2. 2.5 N hydrochloric acid.
3. 0.5 N ferric chloride solution in 0.1 N hydrochloric acid.
4. 1% w/v hydroxylammonium chloride solution, to be prepared fresh every day.

Standard solution

Dissolve 200 mg of the compound in 50 ml of water by warming at 70-80°, cool and dilute with water to 100 ml (2 mg/ml).

Sample solution

Dilute appropriate volume of the eye drops with water to get 2 mg/ml solution.

Procedure

To 5 ml each of the sample and standard solutions, add 1 ml of hydroxylammonium chloride solution and 1 ml of the sodium hydroxide solution. Allow to stand for 10 minutes, acidify with 2 ml of 2.5 N hydrochloric acid and add 1 ml of ferric chloride solution. After a period of minimum of 10 minutes, measure the absorbance at about 500 nm against a reagent blank. The method obeys Beer's law in the range of 1-20 mcg/ml.

Note : Preservatives (chlorhexidine salts, benzalkonium chloride, mercury salts), surface active agents, electrolytes, buffering agents, acetic acid and its salts, viscosity-binders (polyvinyl pyrrolidine and cellulose derivatives) do not modify the absorption of the chromophore. Homatropine hydrobromide, chloramphenicol and sulphacetamide do not interfere. The potential interference by pilocarpine and other alkaloidal salts, local anaesthetics (benzocaine) often used in eye drops can be eliminated by extraction with chloroform prior to analysis by the above method.

Alternatively, polyvinyl alcohol is quantitatively precipitated by using 4% w/v aqueous solution of boric acid and the precipitates are taken up in water and analysed by above method.

Boric acid

Follow the method as described in formulation 1 of this chapter.

Chlorpheniramine maleate, Naphazoline hydrochloride, Boric acid, Zinc sulphate, Chlorbutol

ESTIMATION

Chlorpheniramine maleate

Follow the method described in formulation 1 of the chapter on rubefacients.

Naphazoline hydrochloride

Follow the method described in formulation 11 or 12 of this chapter.

Boric acid

Follow the method described in formulation 1 of this chapter.

Chlorbutol

Follow the method described in formulation 1 of this chapter.

Zinc sulphate

Take sample equivalent to 100 mg of zinc sulphate, add 2 ml of strong ammonia-ammonium chloride buffer solution and 2 drops of eviochrome black solution and dilute with 0.05 M EDTA to a deep blue end point. Each ml of 0.05 M EDTA is equivalent to 0.01438 g of zinc sulphate ($ZnSO_4 \cdot 2H_2O$). Perform blank.

Typical laboratory analysis

Chlorpheniramine maleate
(Follow the cyanogen bromide method, see formulation of the chapter on expectorants)
Weight of the standard = 0.106 g
Volume of the sample = 4 ml of 0.01%

$$\text{Contents of chlorpheniramine} = \frac{A_u}{A_s} \times \frac{10}{4} \times \frac{0.106}{100} \times \frac{4}{100} \times 100$$

$$= \frac{0.194}{0.199} \times \frac{0.106}{10}$$

$$= 0.01035$$

$$\% \text{ claim} = \frac{0.01035}{0.01} \times 100 = 103.5$$

Naphazoline hydrochloride
Weight of the standard = 0.103 g

Volume of the sample = 3.6 ml of 0.056%

$$\text{Contents of naphazoline hydrochloride} = \frac{A_u}{A_s} \times \frac{0.103}{100} \times \frac{2}{100} \times \frac{100}{3.6} \times 100$$

$$= 0.0538$$

$$\% \text{ claim} = \frac{0.0538}{0.056} \times 100 = 95.99$$

Choline salicylate, Benzalkonium chloride

ESTIMATION

Benzalkonium chloride

Follow the ion-pair complex method described in formulation 3 of this chapter.

Choline salicylate

Follow the method described under formulation 5 of this chapter and enzymes & digestives for choline dihydrogen citrate. Each g of the residue (as reineckate) is equivalent to 0.241 g of choline salicylate ($C_{12}H_{19}NO_4$).

On acidification of aqueous solution, free salicylic acid is produced. This can be quantitatively estimated. For details refer to estimation of salicylic acid under formulation 1 of this chapter.

Formulation 6

Phenazone, Benzocaine, Potassium hydroxyquinoline sulphate, Chlorbutol

ESTIMATION

Phenazone

Procedure

Transfer the sample solution equivalent to 200 mg of phenazone to a 250 ml separating funnel, add 100 ml water and extract the solution with three 30 ml portions of chloroform. Transfer the chloroform extracts to a 250 ml conical flask and evaporate the chloroform. Add to the residue, 20 ml sodium acetate solution (10%), 40 ml 0.1 N iodine and leave the solution for 20 minutes in a cool dark place. Then, add 10 ml chloroform and shake vigorously. Titrate the excess of iodine with 0.1 N sodium thiosulphate using starch solution as indicator. Repeat the procedure omitting the sample (blank titration). Each ml of 0.1 N iodine is equivalent to 0.09412 g of phenazone.

Benzocaine

Transfer sample solution equivalent to 100 mg of benzocaine to a 100 ml separating funnel, add 20 ml water and extract with three 25 ml portions of ether. Wash the combined ether extracts thrice with 30 ml water each. Evaporate the combined ether extracts to dryness. Add 30 ml water and 10 ml hydrochloric acid to the residue. Titrate the solution with 0.1 M sodium nitrite at temperature not exceeding 15°C till a blue colour is produced using starch iodide paper as indicator. The titration is complete when the end point is reproducible after leaving the titrated solution for one minute. Repeat the procedure omitting the sample for blank titration.

Each ml of 0.1 M sodium nitrite is equivalent to 0.01652 g of benzocaine.

Chlorbutol

Follow the method described in formulation 1 of this chapter. Each ml of 0.1 N silver nitrate is equivalent to 0.005917 g of chlorbutol.

Sulphacetamide sodium, Phenylephrine hydrochloride, Boric acid

ESTIMATION

Sodium sulphacetamide

Reagents

1. 3% w/v solution of sodium nitritc in water.
2. 2% w/v solution of urea in water.
3. 3% ethanolic solution of ethyl aceto-acetate.
4. 20% w/v solution of sodium hydroxide in water.

Standard solution

15 mcg/ml of sodium sulphacetamide in water.

Sample solution

Dilute appropriate volume of the sample with water to get 15 mcg/ml of sodium sulphacetamide.

Procedure

To 1 ml each of the sample and standard solutions, add 1 ml of 1 N hydrochloric acid and 1 ml of sodium nitrite solution. Cool in ice-bath and allow to stand for 2 minutes. Add 2 ml of urea solution, shake and allow to stand for 2 minutes. Then, add 1 ml of ethyl aceto-acetate solution, 2 ml of sodium hydroxide solution and dilute to 25 ml with water. Measure the absorbance of both the solutions at about 400 nm against reagent blank. Calculate the results by comparison.

Phenylephrine hydrochloride

Follow the method involving alkaline oxidation with potassium ferricyanide, followed by coupling with 4-aminophenazone. For details, refer to method described in formulation 1 of chapter of analgesics and antipyretics.

Boric acid

Follow the method described in formulation 1 of this chapter. Each ml of 0.1 N sodium hydroxide is equivalent to 0.006183 g of boric acid.

Dexamethasone sodium phosphate, Bacitracin, Benzalkonium chloride

ESTIMATION

Dexamethasone sodium phosphate

Reagents

1. Phenylhydrazine reagent : Dissolve 65 mg of phenylhydrazine hydrochloride in 40 ml of water. Add 60 ml of phosphoric acid and 50 ml of isopropyl alcohol, prepare fresh.
2. 1 N sodium hydroxide.
3. 10% w/v sodium chloride solution in water.
4. Methylene chloride.

Standard solution

Weigh accurately 100 mg of dexamethasone sodium phosphate, add 1 ml of 1 N sodium hydroxide and dilute to 100 ml with water. 10 ml of the resulting solution is further diluted with water to 100 ml (100 mcg/ml).

Sample solution

Weigh or measure accurately, a portion of ointment, cream or solution equivalent to 1 mg of the compound. Add 10 ml of sodium chloride solution and 25 ml of methylene chloride. Agitate to disperse the cream. Allow the organic layer to separate and discard it. Extract with further 25 ml of methylene chloride and discard organic layer. Dilute aqueous layer to 10 ml with water (100 mcg/ml).

Procedure

To 2 ml each of the sample and standard solutions, add 5 ml of freshly prepared phenylhydrazine reagent. Insert the stopper loosely and maintain at 60°C for 2 h. Cool and measure the absorbance of both the solutions at about 410 nm and calculate the results by comparison.

Benzalkonium chloride

Follow the method described in formulation 3 or 15 of this chapter.

Bacitracin

METHOD 1

Reagents

1. Sodium hypobromite solution : Dissolve 2 g of bromide in 100 ml volumetric flask which has been previously half-filled with 1 N sodium hydroxide solution. Dilute to volume with the same solvent.

2. Phloroglucinol reagent : Dissolve 0.5 g of phloroglucinol in 15 ml of distilled water by warming in hot water and shaking. Dilute to 50 ml with hydrochloric acid.

Standard solution

200 mcg/ml of bacitracin in water.

Sample solution

Weigh accurately, a quantity of the sample of the ointment, equivalent to approximately 10 mg (650 units) of bacitracin into a 50 ml centrifuge tube with ground glass joint. Add 2 ml of petroleum ether (40-60°), warm slightly in a water-bath at 40°C, and shake briefly until the contents of the tube become a homogenous viscous mass. Add 4 ml of distilled water and shake mechanically for one hour. To assist solution of the active compounds, interrupt the shaking two or three times for 1 minute intervals and place the tube briefly in the water-bath each time. Finally, centrifuge for 5 minutes at 4000 rpm. Remove the aqueous (lower phase) layer with the help of a pipette, and filter it through a filter paper previously washed with distilled water and dried. Dilute the filtrate appropriately with water to get 200 mcg/ml.

Procedure

Transfer 4 ml of above aqueous solutions of both sample and standard into 20 ml test tubes and add 1 ml of sodium hypobromite solution. Place the tubes in a boiling water-bath for 5 minutes and then add 3 ml of phloroglucinol reagent. Stir and again place the tubes in the bath for a further 10 minutes, a stable pink colour is developed. Cool the tube in cold water (20°C) for about 10 minutes. Add 2 ml of 25% aqueous ethanol into each tube (occasionally an opalescence develops which disappears when ethanol is added and shaken well). Determine the absorbance of both the solutions at about 505 nm against a reagent blank. Calculate the amount (mg) of bacitracin. To convert the weight into units, multiply by the factor (i), microbiological potency of standard bacitracin in units per mg.

Note : Microbiological assay for potency is the method of choice.

Pilocarpine nitrate, Phenylephrine hydrochloride

ESTIMATION

Pilocarpine nitrate

METHOD 1

Reagent

1. 1% w/v solution of chromotropic acid in sulphuric acid.

Standard solution

2 mg/ml of pilocarpine nitrate in water.

Sample solution

Eye drops : Transfer sample equivalent to 20 mg of pilocarpine nitrate, basify with 1 N sodium hydroxide and extract with four 10 ml portions of chloroform. Wash combined chloroform layer with 1 ml of water and evaporate chloroform to dryness. Dissolve the residue in acidified water to produce 10 ml (2 mg/ml).

Eye ointment : Weigh accurately ointment equivalent to 20 mg of the substance, add 20 ml of chloroform-water (1 : 1) mixture, shake and separate chloroform layer. Extract water layer with further quantities of chloroform till fatty base is completely removed. Wash the combined chloroform layer with 5 ml of water and add this aqueous wash to the original aqueous liquid. Make the aqueous layer alkaline and extract with four 10 ml portions of chloroform. Evaporate the combined chloroform layer and take up the residue in 10 ml of acidified water.

Procedure

Transfer accurately measured volume of the sample and standard solutions equivalent to 4 mg of pilocarpine nitrate to 250 ml distillation flask. Add 20 ml of water, 25 g of sodium chloride and 5 g of purified sand, previously pulverized and mixed. Start distillation by rapidly heating to boiling. Collect 20 ml of the distillate and adjust to 25 ml with water. To 2 ml distillate of the sample and standard solutions, add with caution 3 ml of chromotropic acid reagent by letting the reagent run down the side of the tubes and mix thoroughly by gentle swirling. Allow to stand for 10 minutes at room temperature and then measure the absorbance of both the solutions at about 545 nm against reagent blank. The method obeys Beer's law in the concentration range of 20-100 mcg/ml.

METHOD 2

Reagents

1. 0.1 N sulphuric acid.
2. 2% w/v sodium nitroprusside in water.
3. 1 N sodium hydroxide.
4. 0.01 N solution of potassium permanganate.
5. Dilute sulphuric acid.

Standard solution

800 mcg/ml of pilocarpine nitrate in water.

Sample solution

Take sample preparation equivalent to 20 mg of pilocarpine nitrate in 25 ml volumetric flask and dilute to volume with 0.1 N sulphuric acid (800 mcg/ml).

Procedure

To 5 ml each of sample and standard solutions, add 1 ml each of sodium nitroprusside solution and 0.1 N sodium hydroxide solution. Allow to stand for 5 minutes, then add 5 ml of 0.01 N potassium permanganate, followed immediately by 3 ml of dilute sulphuric acid. Dilute to volume (25 ml) and measure the absorbance of both the solutions at about 520 nm against reagent blank. The absorbance should be measured within 5 minutes.

Phenylephrine hydrochloride

Follow the method as described in formulation 1 of the chapter on analgesics and antipyretics.

Proflavine hemisulphate, Acriflavine hydrochloride, Methylene blue

In a mixture of dyes, whenever their absorption spectra is well separated, it is one of the convenient methods for analysis of individual dye. Proflavine and acriflavine exhibit maxima at about 450 nm, whereas methylene blue shows maxima at about 665 nm. It has been observed that absorbance of one compound at the maxima of other is almost nil, hence there is no mutual interference while estimating the above compounds in combination.

Total acridines

As both acriflavine and proflavine exhibit maxima at about the same wavelength i.e. 450 nm, it is only possible to estimate total acridines whenever they are in combination. Proflavine is usually the major component, hence is used for preparation of standard solution.

Standard solution of proflavine hemisulphate : 5 mcg/ml of proflavine hemisulphate in water.
Standard solution of methylene blue : 5 mcg/ml of methylene blue in water.

Sample solution

The sample is appropriately diluted with water to get a concentration of 5 mcg/ml of each substance.

Procedure

For total acridines, the absorbance of one part of the sample solution is measured at 450 nm and results calculated by measuring the absorbance of the respective standard solution at the same wavelength. For methylene blue, measure the absorbance of both sample and standard solutions at 665 nm.

Note : Buffering agents and plant extracts, usually present in such formulation, do not interfere.

Formulation 11

Naphazoline nitrate (Privine nitrate), Antazoline sulphate (Antistine sulphate)

ESTIMATION

Naphazoline nitrate

Reagents

1. 0.5% w/v solution of chloranil in chloroform (chloranil may be purified by crystallization from double distilled benzene before use).
2. 10% w/v solution of sodium carbonate in water.

Standard solutions

Solutions of both the pure compounds (as their salts) are separately basified with dilute ammonia solution and extracted with chloroform. Pooled chloroform layer is dried over anhydrous sodium sulphate and diluted to get required concentrations (10 mcg/ml for naphazoline nitrate and 100 mcg/ml for antazoline sulphate).

Sample solution

An accurately measured aliquot of the sample equivalent to 0.25 mg of naphazoline nitrate is taken and to this add about 10 ml of water, add slowly and with stirring 5 ml of solution of sodium carbonate. Allow to stand for 10 minutes and filter. Wash the precipitate with three 10 ml portions of water. Extract the combined filtrate with two 10 ml portions of chloroform and final volume is adjusted to 25 ml with chloroform.

Procedure

Take 4 ml each of chloroform extract of sample and standard solutions, add 5 ml of solution of chloranil. Maintain at 40°C in a water-bath for 45 minutes, cool and adjust to 10 ml with chloroform. Measure the absorbance of both the solutions at about 515 nm against blank prepared by diluting 5 ml of chloranil solution to 10 ml with chloroform. The above colour is stable for 1 h. The method obeys Beer's law in the concentration range of 16-50 mcg/ml.

Note : 1. After precipitation with sodium carbonate, some amount of antazoline salt still remains in assay solution with no loss of naphazoline. This residual antazoline forms no complex with chloranil in chloroform due to basicity.

2. Substances present as preservatives, antioxidants or buffering agents exhibit no interference during assay procedure as it is based on the extraction of free base prior to complexation.

Antazoline sulphate

METHOD 1

Reagent

1. 0.001 M iodine solution in chloroform.

Standard solution

100 mcg/ml; for preparation, refer to the method under naphazoline nitrate.

Sample solution

Portion of the sample equivalent to 10 mg of antazoline sulphate is processed for preparation of sample solution as described for naphazoline nitrate.

Procedure

To 5 ml each of sample and standard solutions, add 2 ml of iodine solution, mix and dilute to 25 ml with chloroform. Allow to stand at room temperature for 30 minutes and measure the extinction at 300 nm and 365 nm against a blank prepared by diluting 2 ml of iodine solution to 25 ml with chloroform. Calculate the absorbance value at 300 nm and 365 nm. Compare with the standard and calculate by subtracting extinction value at 365 nm from that at 300 nm.

METHOD 2

Reagents

1. Cerric sulphate reagent : Dissolve by slight warming 50 mg of dried cerric sulphate in 50 ml of concentrated sulphuric acid, cool and dilute to 100 ml with formate free acetic acid. The reagent is quite stable at room temperature.
2. Acetic acid, formate free.
3. Perchloric acid, 70%.

Standard solution

50 mcg/ml of antazoline sulphate in acetic acid.

Sample solution

Accurately measured aliquot of the sample is approximately diluted with acetic acid to get 50 mcg/ml.

Procedure

To 1 ml of the cerric sulphate solution, add 2 ml of perchloric acid, mix and then add 1 ml each of sample and standard solution and dilute to 10 ml with acetic acid. Measure the absorbance of both the solutions at about 505 nm against acetic acid as blank. Naphazoline and tolazoline do not interfere. Deduce the results by comparison.

Phenylephrine hydrochloride, Naphazoline hydrochloride, Diphenhydramine hydrochloride

ESTIMATION

Phenylephrine hydrochloride

Follow the method described in formulation 1 of the chapter on analgesics and antipyretics.

Naphazoline hydrochloride

METHOD 1

Reagents

1. 4.0% w/v solution of sodium hydroxide in water.
2. 5.0% w/v solution of sodium nitroprusside in water, freshly prepared.
3. 8.4% w/v solution of sodium bicarbonate in water.

Standard solution

Dissolve 0.025 g of naphazoline hydrochloride, 0.25 g of phenylephrine hydrochloride and 0.1 g of diphenhydramine hydrochloride, 0.25 g phenylephrine hydrochloride and 0.1 g of diphenhydramine hydrochloride in a 100 ml volumetric flask and dilute with water up to the mark. 5 ml of the solution is treated in the same way as the sample according to the following procedure.

Procedure

Take 5 ml of standard and 5 ml of sample containing 1.25 mg of the substance, add 1 ml of sodium hydroxide solution to each, followed by 1 ml sodium nitroprusside solution. After 10 minutes, add 2 ml of solution of sodium bicarbonate and shake. Dilute with water up to 50 ml and after 30 min, determine the absorption of both the solutions at about 575 nm against the reagent blank. Calculate the percentage of naphazoline hydrochloride in the sample by comparison.

METHOD 2

Follow the method described in formulation 11 of this chapter.

Diphenhydramine hydrochloride

Follow the method described in formulation 6 of the chapter on expectorants and cough suppressants.

Domiphen bromide, Xylometazoline hydrochloride

ESTIMATION

Domiphen bromide

Reagents

1. 2 N ammonia solution.
2. 0.1% w/v solution of bromocresol purple in ethanol.
3. Titrating solution : Dissolve 0.5 g sodium lauryl sulphate in water to make 1000 ml. Dilute 20 ml to 100 ml with water.

Standard solution

100 mcg/ml of domiphen bromide in water.

Procedure

Use stoppered test tube of 30 ml capacity as titrating vessel. Introduce sample aliquot equivalent to 0.4 mg of domiphen bromide into titrating vessel, add 10 ml water, 5 ml chloroform and 4 drops of bromocresol purple solution. Then add 1 ml of 2 N ammonia solution, thus causing the indicator to turn violet. Shake and titrate by adding the titrating solution from a 10 ml microburette and shaking slowly for 1 minute after each addition and waiting until the phases have separated.

The end-point is reached when the chloroform phase is colourless. In the vicinity of the end-point, add titrating solution slowly in portions of 0.1 ml. 4 ml of standard solution is titrated under similar conditions with sodium lauryl sulphate. From the volume of sodium lauryl sulphate used for sample and standard solutions, calculate the amount of domiphen bromide in the sample.

Xylometazoline hydrochloride

Reagents

1. 1 N sulphuric acid.
2. 2 N sodium acetate.
3. Benzene or chloroform.
4. 0.1% w/v solution of sodium lauryl sulphate in water.
5. Potassium cobalt thiocyanate reagent : Dissolve 10 g of cobalt (II) nitrate hexahydrate and 13.5 g of potassium thiocyanate in water to produce 100 ml.

Standard solution

1 mg/ml of xylometazoline hydrochloride in water.

Sample solution

The sample is appropriately diluted with water to get 1 mg/ml concentration of the substance.

Procedure

Transfer 5 ml each of sample and standard solutions into two separatory funnels. To each, add 5 ml sodium lauryl sulphate solution, and 20 ml of potassium cobalt thiocyanate reagent. Extract twice each with 20 ml of benzene and one with 10 ml of benzene. Combine benzene extract and dilute to 50 ml with benzene. Clear the solution by adding about 2 g anhydrous sodium sulphate, filter if necessary. Measure the absorption of clear sample and standard solutions at about 620 nm against solvent blank and calculate the results.

Isoprenaline sulphate, Atropine methonitrate, Papaverine hydrochloride, Sodium metabisulphite

ESTIMATION

Isoprenaline sulphate

Reagents

1. 20% w/v solution of sodium hydroxide in water.
2. Sodium phosphate-tungstate reagent : Boil gently under reflux for 90 minutes 10 g of sodium tungstate with 75 ml of water and 8 ml of phosphoric acid (88% w/w), cool and dilute to 100 ml with water.

Standard stock solution of isoprenaline sulphate

Dissolve 0.1 g of isoprenaline sulphate, accurately weighed, and 0.515 g of sodium metabisulphite in water in a 100 ml volumetric flask, dilute to volume with water and mix.

Working standard solution

Immediately before use, dilute 5 ml of stock standard isoprenaline sulphate solution to 100 ml with water (50 mcg/ml).

Sample solution

Dilute appropriate volume of the sample with water to get 50 mcg/ml.

Procedure

Transfer 5 ml each of sample and standard solutions to a 100 ml volumetric flasks. To both the flasks, add the following reagents in the order given below :

1 ml of sodium phosphotungstate reagent, 30 ml of water and 1 ml of sodium hydroxide solution. Dilute the contents of both the flasks to volume with water and mix well. Immediately measure the absorption of both the solutions at about 730 nm using water in the reference cell and calculate the results by comparison.

Atropine methonitrate

Reagent

1. Atropine methoreineckate wash solution : Mix equal volumes of 1% w/v solution of atropine methonitrate and solution of ammonium reineckate and acidify with dilute sulphuric acid. Wash the precipitates with water till washings are free from sulphate. Shake the precipitates with water to get saturated solution, filter and use as wash solution.

Procedure

Transfer sample solution equivalent to about 10 mg of the substance into a 150 ml separator; add 2 ml of dilute sulphuric acid. Extract with three 50 ml portions of chloroform, washing each extract with the same 10 ml portions of 0.1 N sulphuric acid. Discard the chloroform layer. Combine the aqueous acidic solutions, rinse the separator with 25 ml of dilute sulphuric acid and add the rinsing to the main aqueous solution. Add 30 ml of a freshly prepared and filtered solution of ammonium reineckate. Allow to stand for 30 minutes and filter through a weighed G_4 porosity sintered glass crucible. Wash the residue with four 5 ml quantities of atropine methoreineckate wash solution, followed by 3 ml of water. Dry the residue to a constant weight. Each g of the residue is equivalent to 0.5884 g of atropine methonitrate.

Papaverine hydrochloride

Dilute sample solution equivalent to 100 mg of papaverine hydrochloride to 100 ml with water. Dilute further 10 ml of this solution to 100 ml with water. Transfer 20 ml of this solution into a 100 ml volumetric flask, add 1 ml of hydrochloric acid and dilute to volume with water (20 mcg/ml of papaverine hydrochloride). Measure the extinction of this solution at 310 nm using 0.1 N hydrochloric acid in the reference cell. Calculate using 228 as value of E 1%, 1 cm of papaverine hydrochloride at 310 nm.

Sodium metabisulphite

Transfer the sample solution equivalent to about 25 mg of the compound to a 150 ml conical flask. Add approximately 10 ml of chloroform and titrate with 0.05 N iodine till both layers have the same pale yellow colour. During the titration, stopper the flask and shake vigorously intermittently.

Each ml of 0.05 N iodine is equivalent to 0.002376 g of sodium metabisulphite.

Triamcinolone acetonide, Thiomersal, Phenylephrine hydrochloride, Neomycin sulphate, Benzalkonium chloride

ESTIMATION

Triamcinolone acetonide

Reagent

1. Isoniazid reagent : Dissolve 500 mg of isoniazid in 250 ml of methanol, add 0.63 ml of hydrochloric acid and adjust to 500 ml with methanol.

Standard solution

40 mcg/ml of triamcinolone acetonide in chloroform.

Sample solution

Accurately weigh the sample equivalent to 1 mg of triamcinolone acetonide in a 25 ml volumetric flask. Add about 15 ml of chloroform and shake well for about 10 minutes. Make up to the mark with chloroform. Filter, if necessary, through a No. 42 Whatman paper.

Procedure

Transfer 5 ml each of sample and standard solutions into 25 ml volumetric flasks. To each of two flasks, add 10 ml of isoniazid reagent. Place the flasks in a water-bath at 55°C (± 2°C) for 45 minutes. Cool the flasks to room temperature and make up to volume with chloroform and mix. Measure the absorbance of both the solutions at 415 nm and calculate the results.

Note : 1. Prevent incorporation of moisture as it reduces the intensity of the final colour.
2. Addition of hydrochloric acid (0.63 ml) to the isoniazid reagent should be accurate as excessive acid reduces the sensitivity of the method.
3. Instead of heating, the solution after addition of isoniazid reagent can be kept at room temperature for 45 min and then made up the volume.

Thiomersal

Note : All glassware must be rinsed with warm dilute nitric acid (1 : 2) and then rinsed with distilled water before using. The titration must be performed in one continuous operation.

Reagents

1. Dilute hydrochloric acid.
2. Strong dithizone solution : Dissolve 50 mg of dithizone (diphenylthiocarbizone) in 100 ml of chloroform.

3. Dilute dithizone solution : Transfer 25 ml of strong dithizone solution to a 250 ml volumetric flask, dilute to volume with chloroform and mix well.
4. 30% hydrogen peroxide.
5. Acidic potassium permanganate solution. Add 3 ml of sulphuric acid to 100 ml of 0.1 N potassium permanganate.
6. Dilute nitric acid : Dilute 3 ml of nitric acid to 100 ml with distilled water.
7. 1% w/v solution of hydroxylamine hydrochloride in water.

Standard mercury solution

Accurately weigh 80 mg of reagent grade mercuric oxide and transfer to a 250 ml volumetric flask, add sufficient dilute nitric acid to dissolve the powder. Dilute to volume with distilled water and mix well. Dilute 10 ml to 500 ml with distilled water and mix well. Calculate the amount of mercury.

$$\text{Mercury, mcg/ml} = \frac{A \times 0.9261 \times 1000 \times 10}{250 \times 500} = A \times 0.0741$$

where A = weight (mg) of sample taken for analysis; 0.9261 is factor to convert mercuric oxide to mercury.

Procedure

Transfer 10 ml of the sample and 15 ml of standard mercury solution into 500 ml standard joint flasks, add 40 ml of dilute hydrochloric acid, 2 ml of hydrogen peroxide and a few glass beads to each flask. Insert a reflux condenser and reflux on a hot plate for 2 h. Raise the temperature gradually as the sample solution may form foam as it starts to boil. Allow to cool to room temperature, then wash the condensers with distilled water, collecting the washings in the flasks. Quantitatively, transfer the contents to 125 ml separatory funnels with the aid of distilled water. Add 10 ml of dithizone solution to each and shake vigorously for 3 min. Allow the layers to separate, then transfer the chloroform layer to a 100 ml separatory funnel. Add 10 ml of acid potassium permanganate and 10 ml of distilled water. Shake vigorously for 3 minutes and allow the layers to separate. Drain off the chloroform layer and discard. Add 3 ml of hydroxylamine hydrochloride solution and shake until the solution is completely colourless. If an emulsion persists, add 1 ml more of hydroxylamine solution and mix well. Combine the resultant aqueous phase with the main. Add dilute dithizone solution from a burette in small volumes with shaking until the green colour turns to orange colour. Draw off each portion of dithizone before adding the next one. When a green tinge appears in the orange, use 0.2 ml at a time until completely green colour persists. Perform blank, not more than 1 ml should be required for the blank. Calculate thiomersal as under :

$$\text{Thiomersal (mg/ml)} = \frac{A \times C \times 15 \times 2.018}{B \times 10}$$
$$= \frac{A \times C \times 3.027}{B}$$

where A = volume (ml) of dithizone required for the sample (corrected for blank);
B = volume (ml) of dithizone required for the standard, corrected for the blank;
C = amount of mercury (mcg/ml) in standard solution.

Phenylephrine hydrochloride

Follow the method 1 for estimation of phenylephrine described under formulation 4 of the chapter on analgesics and antipyretics.

Benzalkonium chloride

Reagents

2. Buffer solution, pH 10 : Dissolve 3.09 g of boric acid, 3.725 g of potassium chloride and 1.75 g of sodium hydroxide in water to produce 1000 ml.
3. Methyl orange, test solution.

Standard solution

12.5 mcg/ml of benzalkonium chloride in water.

Sample solution

Transfer sample equivalent to 1.25 mg of the substance into 100 ml volumetric flask and dilute to volume with water (12.5 mcg/ml).

Procedure

Add 15 ml of pH 10 buffer and 1 ml methyl orange solution to two separating funnel. Shake well and let stand for two minutes. Pipette 3 ml of each sample, standard and water into separating funnels. Add 10 ml chloroform to each funnel and shake for two minutes. Separate chloroform layer and repeat the extraction procedure with another 10 ml portion of chloroform. To the combined chloroform extracts, add 10 ml of 1 N hydrochloric acid and shake for two minutes. Allow the phases to separate and determine the absorbance of the aqueous phase of both sample and standard solutions at 510 nm using the blank solution in the reference cell and calculate the results.

Neomycin sulphate

Follow the method described under formulation 5 of the chapter on topical antifungal drugs involving the use of ninhydrin reagent.

Naphazoline hydrochloride, Phenylephrine hydrochloride, Sulphacetamide sodium, Boric acid

ESTIMATION

Phenylephrine hydrochloride

Follow the method as described in formulation 1 of the chapter on analgesics and antipyretics.

Naphazoline hydrochloride

Follow the method as described in formulation 11 of this chapter. Alternatively, method described in formulation 17 of this chapter may be used.

Sulphacetamide sodium

Transfer accurately measured aliquot of the sample equivalent to 250 mg of sulphacetamide sodium, add 10 ml of hydrochloric acid and about 50 ml of water. Shake and cool to 15°C. Titrate against 0.1 M sodium nitrite. Each ml of 1 N sodium hydroxide is equivalent to 0.02362 g of sulphacetamide sodium.

Boric acid

Follow the method described in formulation 1 of this chapter.

Naphazoline nitrate, Betamethasone sodium phosphate, Neomycin sulphate

ESTIMATION

Naphazoline nitrate

Reagents

1. Dye solution : Dissolve 200 mg of bromophenol blue in 100 ml of distilled water and 6 ml of 0.1 N sodium hydroxide. Dilute to 250 ml with water.
2. Buffer solution : Dissolve 10.93 g of anhydrous disodium hydrogen phosphate and 10.93 g of anhydrous citric acid in water to make 1000 ml, adjust to pH 4.0.

Standard solution

50 mcg/ml of naphazoline nitrate in water.

Sample solution

Dilute accurately measured aliquot of the sample equivalent to 2.5 mg of the substance to 50 ml with water (50 mcg/ml).

Procedure

Into each of the three separating funnels, add 20 ml of buffer solution and 5 ml of dye solution. Add 5 ml of standard naphazoline nitrate solution, 5 ml aliquot of the sample solution and 5 ml of water (blank). To each separator, add 25 ml of chloroform and shake gently for one minute. Allow the layers to separate and collect the chloroform into 50 ml volumetric flasks. Repeat the extraction using 20 ml and 5 ml of chloroform. Adjust the volume to 50 ml with chloroform. Measure the absorption of the sample and standard solutions against the blank and calculate the naphazoline nitrate content in the sample by comparison.

Betamethasone sodium phosphate

Follow the method described for estimation of dexamethasone sodium phosphate in formulation 8 of this chapter.

Neomycin sulphate

Follow the method described in formulation 5 of the chapter on topical antifungal involving colour with ninhydrin.

Chapter 14

Keratolytics & Cleansers

Formulation 1

Resorcinol (Resorcin), Sulphur, Alcohol base

ESTIMATION

Resorcino!

METHOD 1

Reagents

1. 0.1 N hydrochloric acid.
2. Chloroform.

Standard solution

25 mcg/ml resorcinol in 0.1 N hydrochloric acid.

Sample solution

Weigh into a stoppered conical flask sample equivalent to 10 mg of resorcinol and add 100 ml of chloroform. Add 50 ml of 0.1 N hydrochloric acid to the above flask. Shake the mixture thoroughly for at least one minute. After the sample is well shaken, decant the acid layer and filter. Transfer 5 ml of the clear filtrate to a 50 ml volumetric flask and dilute to volume with 0.1 N hydrochloric acid.

Procedure

Determine the extinction of the standard and the sample solutions at about 273 nm using 0.1 N hydrochloric acid as reference solvent and calculate the results by comparison.

METHOD 2

The method is based on the formation of indophenol by reacting resorcinol with 2,6-dibromoquinone-4-chlorimide in alkaline medium.

Reagents

1. 1% w/v sodium borate solution in water, prepare daily.
2. Borate buffer, pH 9.4.
3. 2,6-dibromoquinone-4-chlorimide solution : This solution is prepared daily by dissolving 40 mcg/ml of chlorimide in 10 ml of methanol.

Standard solution

10 mcg/ml of resorcinol in water, prepare weekly.

Sample solution

The sample equivalent to 25 mg of resorcinol is accurately weighed and dissolved in water to produce 25 ml and filtered. 1 ml of this solution is further diluted with water to produce 100 ml.

Procedure

To 2.5 ml each of the standard and sample solutions, add 2 ml of borate buffer and dilute to 10 ml with water. Then, add 0.1 ml of chlorimide solution, mix and measure the absorbance after 50 seconds but before 100 seconds at 530 nm, against a reagent blank.

Note : 1. Full resorcinol colour develops in about 50 seconds and after that phenol and salicylic acid begins to react with the chlorimide reagent and will cause positive interference after 120 seconds as with compounds having one phenolic group, the reaction is delayed and this will not interfere if the colour is measured well within 120 seconds.
2. The method obeys Beer's law in the concentration range of 20-25 mcg/ml.
3. Boric acid, phenol and salicylic acid do not interfere in the proposed method.

Sulphur

Reagents

1. 5% w/v sodium sulfite solution, freshly prepared.
2. Formaldehyde solution.
3. 0.1 N iodine solution.
4. Silicone oil, defoamer.

Procedure

Weigh and transfer sample equivalent to approximately 50 mg of sulphur into a 250 ml round bottom flask. Add 40 ml solution of sodium sulphite, small piece of paraffin and few drops of silicone oil, defoamer. Stopper the flask and shake well to disperse the sample. Remove the stopper, rinse with several small portions of distilled water. Attach the flask to a reflux condenser and reflux until the sulphur is completely dissolved. Cool the solution and rinse inside of condenser with a small quantity of water. Add 10 ml of formaldehyde solution and 6 ml of glacial acetic acid. Titrate the solution immediately with freshly standardized 0.1 N iodine solution using starch solution as the indicator. Prepare blank in the same manner using all ingredients except sample. Each ml of 0.1 iodine is equivalent to 0.003207 g of sulphur.

Alcohol

Transfer appropriate volume of the sample into 500 ml round bottom flask. Add about 200 ml of distilled water and shake well. Attach to a condenser and distil slowly. Collect distillate in a 100 ml volumetric flask, collecting slightly less than 100 ml. Bring distillate to a temperature of 25°C and dilute to volume with distilled water. Determine the specific gravity at 25°C and calculate per cent alcohol by weight or in terms of % v/v by referring to alcohol table.

Buclosamide, Hydrocortisone acetate, Salicylic acid

ESTIMATION

Chlorohydroxybenzoic acid butylamide (Buclosamide)

Reagents

1. 5% w/v solution of sodium bicarbonate in water.
2. 1 N sodium hydroxide.

Procedure

Ointment is extracted with methanol in the centrifuge, using 25 ml at a time. The ointment is brought into contact with the alcohol in the centrifuge tube, by cautious warming on the steam-bath while stirring, and subsequently resolidifying in ice-water. The combined alcoholic extract is made up to 100 ml with alcohol (use appropriate volume for estimation of hydrocortisone acetate). 20 ml of the alcoholic extract is cautiously dried on the steam-bath at low temperature. The residue is transferred into a separating funnel, using 50 ml of ether and is shaken with five 20 ml portions of sodium bicarbonate solution. The combined aqueous extract is made up to 100 ml with sodium bicarbonate solution and retained for assay of salicylic acid. The ethereal layer remaining in the separating funnel is extracted with five 20 ml portions of 1 N sodium hydroxide solution. The alkaline extracts are combined and made up to 100 ml with 1 N sodium hydroxide solution. 20 ml is further diluted to 100 ml with water.

Maximum absorption of alkaline solution is observed at 325 nm which is characteristic of chlorohydroxybenzoic acid butylamide. Results are calculated by comparing with the standard.

Salicylic acid

10 ml of sodium bicarbonate extract obtained during estimation of buclosamide is made up to 100 ml with water. This solution exhibits maximum absorption at 295 nm which is characteristic for salicylic acid in sodium bicarbonate solution. Salicylic acid contents can be determined by comparison with standard solution of salicylic acid.

Hydrocortisone acetate

Reagents

1. 0.5% w/v solution of tetrazolium blue in alcohol.
2. Tetramethylammonium hydroxide-alcohol (1 : 9) mixture.

Standard solution

Weigh accurately 10 mg of hydrocortisone acetate in a dry 100 ml volumetric flask, dissolve in methanol and make to 100 ml with methanol.

Sample solution

25 ml of alcoholic solution obtained in assay of buclosamide is passed through aluminium oxide (6 g) column. Collect the eluate in a dry 25 ml volumetric flask for estimation.

Procedure

To 2 ml each of sample and standard solutions, add 2 ml of tetrazolium blue solution and mix. Then to each flask, add 2 ml of tetramethyl ammonium hydroxide-alcohol mixture, mix and allow to stand in the dark for 90 minutes. Without delay, make up the volume with methanol and measure the absorbance of the assay and standard solutions at about 525 nm against the blank. Calculate the results by comparison.

Betamethasone dipropionale, Salicylic acid

ESTIMATION

Betamethasone dipropionale

Follow the method described in formulation 4 of the chapter on topical antifungal. The method involves reaction with isoniazid.

Salicylic acid

Follow the method described in formulation 2 or 5 of this chapter.

Alternatively, suspend the sample (cream) equivalent to 150 mg salicylic acid in 50% aqueous methanol by slight warming to ensure complete suspension. Cool and titrate with 0.1 N sodium hydroxide (phenol red). Perform blank, if necessary. Each ml of 0.1 M sodium hydroxide is equivalent to 0.01381 g of salicylic acid.

Chloretone, Salicylic acid, Benzoic acid, Alcohol base

ESTIMATION

Chloretone

Measure sample equivalent to 50 mg of chloretone, subject to general steam distillation process, dipping the end of condenser to the bottom of a flask dipped in ice and containing 30 ml of alcoholic potassium hydroxide solution (35% w/v in alcohol). Collect the distillate and reflux on the steam-bath for 1 hr. Remove from the bath and allow to cool before opening. Transfer the contents to a 500 ml iodine flask. Rinse several times with small quantities of distilled water sufficient to remove all the chloride and add the washings to the iodide flask. Add about 50 ml of distilled water and slowly neutralize with nitric acid using phenolphthalein solution as indicator, and add 2 ml of excess acid. Add enough water to dissolve any precipitated salt and allow to cool. Add 50 ml of 0.1 N silver nitrate and swirl to mix completely. Then, add 10 ml of nitrobenzene, stopper the flask and shake. Titrate with excess silver nitrate with 0.1 N ammonium thiocyanate using ferric alum as indicator, shaking the flask vigorously as the end point is approached. Each ml of 0.1 N silver nitrate is equivalent to 0.005916 g of chloretone.

Alcohol

Transfer appropriate volume of the sample and follow the method described in formulation 1 of this chapter.

Salicylic acid and Benzoic acid

Suspend 5 ml of the sample in 100 ml of ether and extract the ethereal layer with four 20 ml portions of 0.5 N sodium hydroxide. Combine the alkaline extract and shake with 10 ml of ether, make up the volume to 100 ml. Carry out the subsequent dilutions with 0.5 N sodium hydroxide to get a solution of 20 mcg/ml in respect of salicylic acid. Carry out the quantitative determination by iso-absorption method as described in formulation 4 of this chapter.

Formulation 5

Salicylic acid, Benzoic acid, Menthol, Thymol, Camphor, Dusting powder base

ESTIMATION

METHOD 1

Salicylic acid (SA) and Benzoic acid (BA)

1. 1 g of the sample accurately weighed is extracted with three 10 ml portions of isopropyl alcohol at 90°C and cooled. Combined organic extract is extracted with four 10 ml portions of 1 N sodium hydroxide and combined alkaline extract is diluted with water to get a concentration of 20 mcg/ml of salicylic acid. Measure the extinction at 298 nm which corresponds only to salicylic acid.
2. Calculate total acids (BA and SA) by the UV spectrophotometric method described in method 4 of this formulation. By subtracting the contents of salicylic acid obtained by the method 1 above, we can find out the contents of benzoic acid in the sample under analysis.

Total acids

Accurately weigh the sample, add 30 ml of 50% v/v neutral alcohol, warm gently to melt the ointment base and titrate when still warm with 0.1 N sodium hydroxide using phenolphthalein solution as indicator. After determining the end point, add 2 to 3 ml of the 0.1 N sodium hydroxide and reserve this solution for the determination of salicylic acid.

Calculations

Volume of 0.1 N sodium hydroxide used in titration (V) =

$$= \frac{\text{Titre value} \times \text{Normality of sodium hydroxide}}{0.1}$$

ml of 0.1 N sodium hydroxide equivalent to total acid in 1 g of the sample = $\dfrac{V}{a}$

where 'a' is weight (g) of the sample taken for analysis.

Salicylic acid

Cool and filter the titrated solution obtained in the assay for total acids through Whatman filter paper No. 1. Wash the filter paper with several small portions of water and add washing to the main filtrate. Collect the filtrate in a 150 ml beaker and evaporate the filtrate in order to completely remove alcohol present in the solution. Transfer this solution to a 250 volumetric flask with the aid of small portion of water and make up the volume. Transfer 50 ml of this solution to an iodine flask and exactly add 25 ml of 0.1 N bromine solution, 5 ml of hydrochloric acid and immediately insert the stopper. Shake the flask for 30 minutes, add quickly 5 ml of potassium iodide solution (1 in 5). Shake thoroughly, remove the stopper and rinse it and the neck of the flask with little water, so that the washings flow into the flask. Add 1 ml of chloroform, shake the mixture well and titrate the liberated iodine with 0.1 N sodium thiosulphate using solution of starch as indicator, to be added when the end point is almost near. Run a blank side by side.

Calculations

1. Salicylic acid (mg)/g of the sample $(B) = \dfrac{(A - a) \times 2.3 \times 250}{w \times 50}$

   where A = ml of 0.1 N bromine added,

   a = ml of 0.1 N sodium thiosulphate required titrate the excess bromine,
   w = weight (g) of the sample taken for analysis.
2. Benzoic acid : Volume (ml) of 0.1 N sodium hydroxide equivalent to the salicylic acid present
   in 1 g of the sample $(v) = \dfrac{B}{13.81}$

   B = mg of salicylic acid present in 1 g of the sample found by the method
   for salicylic acid.

   Volume (ml) of 0.1 N sodium hydroxide equivalent to benzoic acid present in 1 g of sample
   $(c) = (V - v)$; where V is the volume (ml) of 0.1 N sodium hydroxide equivalent to total acids.

METHOD 2

(a) Weigh accurately the sample equivalent to 25 mg of salicylic acid and add 100 ml of hot water
    (75°C) and 2 drops of phenolphthalein solution. Then, add enough 0.1 N sodium hydroxide so
    that the mixture is light pink. Heat to 85°C and add more sodium hydroxide to get clear pink
    colour. Cool the solution and dilute to 250 ml with distilled water. Filter, reject first few ml of
    the filtrate. Take 15 ml of this solution, add 5 ml of ferric nitrate solution (0.1% in 1% nitric
    acid) and dilute to 50 ml and read the pink colour at 525 nm. Compare with the standard solution
    processed by the above method. This method gives the amount of salicylic acid (% w/v) present
    in the sample.

(b) Suspend the sample accurately weighed in 200 ml of alcohol and estimate the total acid
    (salicylic acid and benzoic acid) as per method given under total acids. Subtract the volume of
    0.1 N sodium hydroxide equivalent to the amount of salicylic acid to calculate the contents of
    benzoic acid as per method given above.

METHOD 3

In this method, iso-absorption point for the two compounds is determined using standard solutions of
salicylic acid (40 mcg/ml) and benzoic acid (40 mcg/ml) in 0.5 N sodium hydroxide. Record the UV
spectra of both the standard solutions separately on the same graph to get iso-absorption point and
maxima for salicylic acid.

Iso-absorption point = 267 nm
Absorption maxima for salicylic acid = 299 nm

	Absorption value at		Ratio 299/267
	299 nm	267 nm	
Salicylic acid (40 mcg/ml)	0.930	0.190	4.94 (Q_1)
Benzoic acid (40 mcg/ml)	0.00	0.190	0.00 (Q_2)
Standard mixture (40 mcg/ml of each acid)	0.940	0.380	2.47 (Q_M)

Absorptivity (g/lit) at 267 nm = 4.75 (A)

C_1 [amount (g) of salicylic acid/L] $= \dfrac{Q_M - Q_2}{Q_1 - Q_2} \times \dfrac{a}{A}$ ...(1)

$$C_2 \text{ [amount (g) of benzoic acid/L]} = \frac{Q_M - Q_2}{Q_2 - Q_1} \times \frac{a}{A} \qquad \qquad \dots(2)$$

where a = absorption of the mixture at iso-absorption point, A = absorptivity.

Typical laboratory analysis

A formulation contains 7% w/w salicylic acid, 3% w/w benzoic acid, 5% boric acid and 0.5% w/w thymol.

Procedure

Take sample accurately weighed (0.71 g), add 20 ml of ether and suspend the contents by slight warming. Extract the ether layer with four 10 ml portions of 0.5 N sodium hydroxide. Shake the combined alkaline extract with 10 ml of ether, reject ether layer and adjust the alkaline layer to 50 ml. Dilute 2 ml of this solution to 50 ml with 0.5 N sodium hydroxide and read at 267 nm and 299 nm.

Absorption of the mixture at 267 nm = 0.27 $\qquad \qquad \dots$(a)

Absorption of the mixture at 299 nm = 0.92

Value for $Q_M = \dfrac{0.92}{0.27} = 3.40$

Substitute the standard values and the values obtained for the sample in analogous equations, 1 and 2 described above.

$Q_1 = 4.92$

$Q_2 = 0.00$

$Q_M = 3.40$

Absorptivity (A) = 4.75

Amount of salicylic acid (g %) $= \dfrac{Q_M - Q_2}{Q_1 - Q_2} \times \dfrac{a}{A}$

$\qquad = 0.0394 \text{ g/L}$

$\qquad = \dfrac{0.0394 \times 50 \times 50}{0.71 \times 2 \times 10} = 7.2\% \text{ w/w}$

Claim = 7.0% w/w

Amount of benzoic acid (g %) $= \dfrac{Q_M - Q_1}{Q_2 - Q_1} \times \dfrac{a}{A}$

$\qquad = \dfrac{4.92 - 3.40}{0.00 - 4.92} \times \dfrac{0.27}{4.75}$

$\qquad = \dfrac{1.5}{3.92} \times \dfrac{0.27}{4.75} = 0.0176 \text{ g/L}$

$\qquad = \dfrac{0.0176 \times 50 \times 50}{0.71 \times 2 \times 10} = 3.0\% \text{ w/w}$

Claim = 3.0% w/w

METHOD 4

Total acids (BA and SA)

This iso-absorption method can be applied efficiently for determination of total acids. By taking the values obtained for Q_M in the above formulation, the total acids can easily be calculated.

Total acids (g/L) $= \dfrac{a}{A} = \dfrac{0.27}{4.75}$

$\qquad = 0.057 \text{ g/L}$

$$\text{Total acids (g \%)} = \frac{0.057 \times 50 \times 50}{0.71 \times 2 \times 10}$$

$$= 10.2\% \text{ w/w}$$

Claim for total acid = 10% w/w (7% + 3%)

Total volatile contents

Weigh the sample accurately and follow the method 1 or 2 as described under formulation 4 of chapter on rubefacient.

Thymol

Follow the method 1 for determination of thymol as described under formulation 4 of the chapter on rubefacients.

Menthol

Follow the method described in formulation 1 of the chapter on rubefacients.

Note : Carry out the distillation of volatile material as described in formulation 4 of the chapter on rubefacients under method 1 for estimation of total volatile contents and use the distillate for estimation of menthol and thymol. Since salicylic acid and benzoic acid present in the formulation are volatile, the contents should be suspended in 1 N sodium hydroxide before subjecting to distillation.

Identification of Camphor

Follow the method described in formulation 3 of the chapter on rubefacients.

Formulation 6

Salicylic acid, Benzoic acid, Boric acid, Soft paraffin base

ESTIMATION

METHOD 1

Benzoic acid and Salicylic acid

Procedure

Extract the sample with five 40 ml portions of ether (retain the residue for determination of boric acid). Evaporate the ether layer on water-bath at low temperature. Add about 20 ml of alcohol, while nearing complete evaporation and titrate the alcoholic extract with 0.1 N sodium hydroxide using phenol-phthalein as indicator. Each ml of 0.1 N sodium hydroxide is equivalent to 0.01301 g of combined salicylic acid/benzoic acid (total acids).

Boric acid

The residue reserved for boric acid in the above method is suspended in 50 ml mixture of water-glycerin (1 : 1) by slight warming. The contents are titrated with 0.1 N sodium hydroxide using phenolphthalein as indicator. Each ml of sodium hydroxide is equivalent to 0.006183 g of boric acid. From the volume of 0.1 N sodium hydroxide consumed in the titration, the total amount of boric acid is calculated. Determine the contents of salicylic acid by bromination as described in the formulation 4 of this chapter. Deduct the amount of salicylic acid thus determined from the total acids to get the amount of benzoic acid in the formulation.

Note : For extraction, chloroform can be used.

METHOD 2

(a) Take 10 g of the sample accurately weighed and suspend in 40 ml of ethyl alcohol by slight warming. Add 20 ml of water and warm for complete suspension. Make up the volume to 100 ml with distilled water. Take 50 ml of the solution and titrate with 0.1 N sodium hydroxide using phenolphthalein solution as indicator. Calculate the amount of combined salicylic acid/benzoic acid (total acids) from the volume of 0.1 N sodium hydroxide consumed in above titration as explained in method 1 above.

(b) As soon as the above titration for total acids is complete, add 25 ml of glycerin and continue titration to pink end point. From the amount of sodium hydroxide consumed in the second titration, boric acid contents are calculated as discussed above.

(c) The remaining portion of the sample solution is appropriately diluted with 0.1 N sodium hydroxide to get a solution of 20 mcg/ml of salicylic acid and measure the extinction at about 298 nm, specific for salicylic acid (see method under formulation 4 of this chapter). Benzoic acid does not absorb at 298 nm.

METHOD 3

Take sample accurately weighed, suspend in ether by slight warming and extract with fine 20 ml portions of 0.1 N sodium hydroxide. Shake the combined alkaline extract with 5 ml of ether. Adjust the alkaline layer to get concentration of 10 mcg/ml of salicylic acid. Carry out the quantitative determination of salicylic acid and benzoic acid by iso-absorption method as described in formulation 4 of this chapter. Boric acid does not interfere.

Boric acid

The ether layer obtained under method 3 above is evaporated and suspended in 50 ml of water-glycerin mixture (1 : 1) by slight warming. Carry out the titration and calculation as per method 1 discussed above.

Salicylic acid, Benzoic acid, Resorcinol

Combined (Salicylic acid and Benzoic acid) acids—Total acids

Take 25 ml of water in a separator and volume of the sample equivalent to 175 mg of salicylic acid. Add 30 ml of petroleum ether (40-60°C), shake well and run the aqueous solution to another separator. Wash petroleum ether with 10 ml of water. Mix the aqueous layers and extract with four 25 ml portions of solvent ether. Wash each ether extract with same 10 ml of water and make up the volume to 100 ml with solvent ether. Evaporate 25 ml of ether extract below 40°C, cool and dissolve the residue in 20 ml of alcohol, warm the alcohol if necessary. Cool and titrate with 0.1 N sodium hydroxide using phenol red as indicator. Each ml of 0.1 N sodium hydroxide is equivalent to 0.01381 g of salicylic acid and 0.01221 g of benzoic acid. After finding out the contents of salicylic acid, salicylic acid should be deducted from combined acids to know the amount of benzoic acid present in the sample taken for analysis.

Salicylic acid

The aqueous solution obtained above is made alkaline and filtered. The filtrate is acidified with hydrochloric acid extracted with four 25 ml portions of chloroform. The combined chloroform layer is extracted with five 20 ml portions of saturated solution of sodium bicarbonate, washing each extract with the same 20 ml of ether. Acidify the bicarbonate extract with hydrochloric acid and extract with four 25 ml portions of solvent ether. Combine ether layer and make up to 100 ml. Evaporate 25 ml of the ether extract and take up the residue in 5 ml of 0.5 N sodium hydroxide and carry out the bromination method described in formulation 4 of this chapter. Each ml of 0.1 N bromine is equivalent to 0.002302 g of salicylic acid.

Resorcinol

METHOD 1

Take sample accurately weighed equivalent to 20 mg of resorcinol and evaporate to about 2 ml. Transfer into a separator, wash the beaker two times with 5 ml of water and extract with 25 ml of chloroform. Run the aqueous layer to another separator. Wash the chloroform layer with 10 ml of water and mix washing with the aqueous layer and make up the volume to 100 ml with water. To 25 ml, add 50 ml of 0.1 N bromine, 10 ml of hydrochloric acid and shake vigorously. Allow to stand for 15 minutes, then add 10 ml of potassium iodide solution. Shake vigorously and titrate with 0.1 N sodium thiosulphate using towards end starch mucilage as indicator. Each ml of 0.1 N bromine is equivalent to 0.001835 g of resorcinol. Run blank side by side. Salicylic acid and benzoic acid remain in chloroform layer.

METHOD 2

Reagents

1. About 0.12% w/v solution of iodine in chloroform. The standardization of this reagent is not necessary.

2. Acetate buffer, pH 5.7.
3. 1% w/v solution of starch.
4. 0.5% w/v solution of potassium iodide in water.
5. 0.001 and 0.01 N sodium thiosulphate solution. This may be standardized against potassium iodate solution of similar normality.
6. The bromine water, saturated.

Standard solution

1 mg/ml solution of resorcinol in water. The solution may be diluted as required.

Sample solution

The sample may be dissolved/extracted with water and diluted appropriately to get a concentration of 1 mg/ml.

Procedure

(a) **Titrimetric method :** In a 100 ml separating funnel, place a suitable volume of the sample representing 500 mcg of the resorcinol. Add 10 ml buffer solution, pH 5.7 and 10 ml of iodine solution. Shake exactly for 1 minute and separate the organic layer. Remove the last traces of iodine from aqueous layer by extraction with 10 ml of chloroform. Transfer quantitatively the aqueous phase into conical flask. Add 2 ml of bromine water, shake for 3 minutes and destroy excess of bromine with 1 ml of formic acid. Add about 2.5 g of potassium iodide and titrate the liberated iodine with 0.01 N sodium thiosulphate solution using starch as indicator. Run a blank determination. If the sample under estimation contains less than 500 mcg of the compound, preferably use 0.001 N sodium thiosulphate solution. Each ml of 0.01 sodium thiosulphate solution is equal to 61.17 mcg of resorcinol.

(b) **Spectrophotometric method :** Carry out the extraction procedure as described under titrimetric method with about 100 mcg of resorcinol. Transfer the iodide formed into 50 ml volumetric flask, add 1 ml of 0.5 N sulphuric acid and 0.5 ml of bromine water. Shake for 2 minutes, add 1 ml of formic acid, shake for 2 minutes and add 2 ml of potassium iodide solution, 2 ml of starch solution and dilute with water. Measure the extinction of blue solution at 600 nm against reagent blank and calculate the results.

Note : 1. Iodination time should not be allowed to exceed one minute as excessive time gives higher results.
2. pH higher than 5.7 usually gives higher results.
3. Phenol, salicylic acid, hydroquinone and cresol do not interfere even when present 25 folds.

Formulation 8

Salicylic acid, Benzoic acid, Ichthammol, Triamcinolone acetonide

ESTIMATION

Salicylic acid

Follow the method described in formulation 4 of this chapter.

Benzoic acid

Follow the method described in formulation 4 of this chapter for estimation of salicylic acid and benzoic acid as total acids by titrating with 0.1 N sodium hydroxide. Then deduct the volume of 0.1 N sodium hydroxide required for salicylic acid contents as estimated above taking each ml of 0.1 N sodium hydroxide as equivalent to 0.01381 g of salicylic acid. Excess volume of sodium hydroxide consumed will be due to benzoic acid. Each ml of 0.1 N sodium hydroxide is equivalent to 0.01221 g of benzoic acid.

Triamcinolone acetonide

Follow the method described in formulation 7 of the chapter on topical antifungal preparations under fluocinolone acetonide.

Note : Separation by preparative thin layer chromatography using dichloromethane-diethyl ether-methanol (77 + 15 + 8%) as mobile phase, elution of separated spot with methanol as subsequent colour development with tetrazolium blue has seen found to give more satisfactory results.

Ichthammol

The method is based on estimation of organically combined sulphur contents. Accurately weighed quantity of sample taken in crucible is mixed with 1 g of analysing sodium carbonate, add 2-3 ml of chloroform and heat gently on water-bath with constant stirring till no smell of chloroform. Add 2 g of cupric nitrate and heat on a gas burner. Cool and place the crucible in a 500 or 1000 ml beaker. Add drop by drop 20 ml of concentrated hydrochloric acid. After the reaction has stopped, add 100 ml of water and boil for 15-20 minutes for copper oxide to dissolve. Filter and heat the filtrate gently for about 15 minutes. Add 20 ml of barium chloride solution (20%) and set aside for complete precipitation. Filter through fine filter paper to collect the precipitates. Ignite the precipitate at 800°C till constant weight. Each g of the residue so obtained is equivalent to 0.1374 g of combined sulphur.

Dithranol, Salicylic acid

ESTIMATION

Salicylic acid

Reagents

1. Phosphate solution : 5% w/v solution of sodium phosphate in water.
2. 5% w/v solution of potassium iodide in water.

Procedure

Weigh accurately sample (ointment) equivalent to 50 mg of salicylic acid, disperse in chloroform and extract with phosphate solution (3×20 ml). Collect the aqueous layer. Wash the chloroform layer further with water (2×20 ml) and add the washings to the main aqueous layer (combined aqueous layer may be warmed to remove dissolved chloroform). Transfer the entire aqueous solution to iodine flask, make it slightly acidic (hydrochloric acid), add 30 ml of 0.1 N bromine and 10 ml of concentrated hydrochloric acid. Shake intermittently during 45 min, add 10 ml of potassium iodide solution and titrate with 0.1 N sodium thiosulphate using starch as indicator. Carry out the blank titration without the sample. Each ml of 0.1 N bromine is equivalent to 0.0023 g of salicylic acid.

Dithranol

Standard solution

30 mcg/ml of dithranol in glacial acetic acid.

Sample solution

To accurately weighed quantity of the sample equivalent to 15 mg of the substance, add 20-30 ml of glacial acetic acid, warm in water-bath for 5 min with stirring. Cool and make up the volume to 50 ml. Filter and dilute 5 mg of the filtrate to 50 ml with glacial acetic acid.

Procedure

To 5 ml each of sample and standard solutions, add 1 ml of sodium nitrite solution (5%), keep in boiling water-bath for 2 min, cool and dilute to 25 ml with glacial acetic acid. Measure the absorbance of both the solutions of 460 nm against reagent blank within 10 min. Calculate the results by comparison.

Note : 1. Maximum colour intensity is observed within 2 min of heating, it tends to fade if heating is continued.
2. One may be confronted with formation of turbidity on addition of sodium nitrite solution; the solution is clear on dilution.

Salicylic acid, Lactic acid

ESTIMATION

METHOD 1

Salicylic acid and Lactic acid (total acids)

Weigh accurately about 0.5 g of the sample containing about 170 mg of total acids, add 30 ml of water and shake for 5-10 min. Add 25 ml of 0.1 N sodium hydroxide and allow to stand at room temperature in a stoppered flask for 30 min (this is sufficient for complete hydrolysis of lactic anhydride to lactic acid usually present in lactic acid and subsequent neutralization with sodium hydroxide). Titrate the excess alkali with 0.1 N hydrochloric acid using phenolphthalein as indicator.

Record the volume of 0.1 N sodium hydroxide consumed by both the acids—X ml.

Salicylic acid

Follow the method described in formulation 4 of this chapter. Alternatively, extract the sample with 0.1 N sodium hydroxide and dilute to get final solution of 10 mcg/ml. Measure the absorption of both sample and standard solution (10 mcg/ml) at 298 nm and calculate the amount of salicylic acid present in the sample. Lactic acid does not absorb at 298 nm. From the amount of salicylic acid so determined, calculate the equivalent volume of 0.1 N sodium hydroxide (13.80 mg of salicylic acid represents 1 ml of 0.1 N sodium hydroxide—Y ml.

Lactic acid

Determine the volume of 0.1 N alkali consumed by lactic acid (X − Y) and calculate the contents of lactic acid in the sample. Each ml of 0.1 N sodium hydroxide consumed for estimation of lactic acid is equivalent to 9.008 mg of lactic acid.

METHOD 2

Reagent

1. 0.1% w/v solution of ferric chloride : To 100 mg of ferric chloride, add 5 ml of methanol and dilute to 100 ml with water, prepare fresh.

Standard solution

100 mcg/ml each of lactic acid and salicylic acid in water.

Sample solution

Extract accurately weighed quantity of the sample with slightly warm water to get final concentration of 100 mcg/ml in respect of both the acids.

Procedure

To 10 ml each of sample and standard solutions, add 1 ml of ferric chloride reagent and immediately measure the absorption at 370 nm (lactic acid) and at 530 nm (salicylic acid) against reagent blank.

Typical laboratory analysis

Weight of lactic acid taken for standard solution = 0.1 g

Weight of salicylic acid taken for standard solution = 0.1230 g

	Absorption value	
	530 nm	370 nm
Sample	0.452	0.232
Standard	0.585	0.223

$$\text{Salicylic acid (\%)} = \frac{0.452}{0.585} \times d_f \times \frac{0.1230}{100} \times \frac{0.9575 \times 100}{16.7}$$

$$= 107\% \text{ of claim } (16.7\%)$$

$$\text{Lactic acid (\%)} = \frac{0.232}{0.223} \times d_f \times \frac{0.1}{100} \times \frac{0.9575 \times 100}{16.7}$$

$$= 103.46\% \text{ of claim } (16.7\%)$$

(0.9575 is the weight/ml)

Zinc undecenoate, Zinc naphthenate, Mesulphan, Methyl salicylate, Terpineol, Chlorocresol

ESTIMATION

Total zinc

Transfer 5-10 g of the sample accurately weighed to silica dish. Add 10 ml of alcohol and evaporate with constant stirring to remove alcohol. Repeat this process 2-3 times till water is removed. Ignite the contents of the dish, cool, add 3 ml of concentrated nitric acid and ignite again carefully. Cool, dissolve the residue in 15 ml of 30% sulphuric acid. Transfer to a conical flask with the aid of 100 ml water. Add 5 g of ammonium sulphate and titrate the solution with 0.1 N potassium ferrocyanide using 2-4 drops of 1% w/v diphenylbenzidine solution in concentrated sulphuric acid (colour change from blue to green). Each ml of 0.1 N potassium ferrocyanide is equivalent to 0.003269 g of zinc.

Methyl salicylate and Chlorocresol

Procedure

(a) Take 5 g of the sample accurately weighed and suspend in 20 ml of dilute hydrochloric acid. Reflux for 30 minutes and extract the acidic layer with four 25 ml portions of ether. The combined ether layer (A) is shaken with four 20 ml portions of 5% solution of sodium bicarbonate. The combined alkaline extract is diluted to get a solution of 20 mcg/ml of salicylic acid. Read at 298 nm which is characteristic for salicylic acid. By comparing with standard solution (20 mcg/ml) of salicylic acid in 5% sodium bicarbonate, the results are deduced.

(b) Evaporate the ether extract (A) at low temperature of water-bath. Dissolve the residue in water to get a solution of 200 mcg/ml of chlorocresol and determine the contents of chlorocresol by 4-aminophenazone method as described below :

Chlorocresol

Reagents

1. 2% w/v 4-aminoantipyrine is distilled water. Protect from light. It is stable only for 2-3 days.
2. Strong ammonia buffer : Dissolve 67.5 g of ammonium chloride in 570 ml of strong ammonia and dilute to 1000 ml with distilled water.
3. Dilute ammonia buffer : 2 ml of strong ammonia buffer is diluted to 1000 ml with distilled water.
4. 8% w/v potassium ferricyanide solution in water.

Procedure

Volume of the sample and standard equivalent to 200 mcg of chlorocresol are taken. To this, add 1 ml of antipyrine reagent, followed by 1 ml of potassium ferricyanide solution and 1 ml of dilute ammonia buffer. The coloured complex is extracted with three 15 ml portions of chloroform and final volume is adjusted to 50 ml with chloroform. Measure the absorption at about 450 nm and calculate the contents of chlorocresol by comparing with the standard.

Chapter 15

Rubefacients

Formulation 1

Chlorpheniramine maleate, Methyl nicotinate, Methyl salicylate, Mephenesin, Menthol, Turpentine oil

ESTIMATION

Chlorpheniramine maleate

Reagents

1. 0.2 M phosphate buffer, pH 7.0.
2. Saturated solution of cyanogen bromide in water (prepare fresh).
3. Aniline solution : 4% v/v solution of aniline (freshly distilled) in methanol.

Standard solution

Prepare a 40 mcg/ml solution of chlorpheniramine maleate in water.

Sample solution

Weigh accurately sample equivalent to 4 mg of chlorpheniramine maleate in a 100 ml dry beaker. Add 20 ml of phosphate buffer, stir well and transfer to a 100 ml volumetric flask and make up the volume with phosphate buffer and filter.

Procedure

Take 5 ml each of sample and standard solutions in two separate 50 ml volumetric flasks. To each flask add 20 ml of phosphate buffer, 2 ml of aniline solution and 3 ml of cyanogen bromide solution. Measure the absorbance of both the solutions, exactly at 5th minute after the addition of cyanogen bromide solution to each flask, against water.

Note : Colour of the solutions reaches maximum in about five minutes after the addition of cyanogen bromide solution and then fades away slowly. Prepare the blank in a similar manner except addition of cyanogen bromide solution. The solution exhibits absorption maximum at about 430 nm. Deduce the results by comparison.

Methyl nicotinate

Reagents

1. Cyanogen bromide solution : Prepare as mentioned above in the determination of chlorpheniramine maleate.
2. Buffer solution, pH 6.6 : Mix 2.5 ml of phosphoric acid (85%), 87.5 ml of methanol with 350 ml of water and sufficient 20% sodium hydroxide to give a pH of 6.6 and dilute to 500 ml with water. Check the final pH.
3. 10% procaine hydrochloride : Dissolve 10 g of procaine hydrochloride in 30 ml of hydrochloric acid and make up to 100 ml with water.
4. Concentrated hydrochloric acid.

Standard solution

Prepare 1 mg/ml solution of methyl nicotinate in distilled water.

Sample solution

Weigh accurately about 2 g of sample in 100 ml dry beaker. Add 2 ml of hydrochloric acid and about 20 ml of distilled water and warm. Transfer this to a 100 ml volumetric flask and sufficient washings to make up the volume with distilled water and filter.

Procedure

Take sample and standard solutions equivalent to 1 mg of methyl nicotinate in two different test tubes and adjust the volume to 10 ml. To each test tube, add 2 ml of hydrochloric acid and water. Keep the test tubes in a boiling water-bath for one hour. Adjust the pH of the standard and sample preparations to 6.5 ± 0.1 and dilute to 100 ml with water. Prepare a set of four test tubes marked S, SB, T and TB. To the tubes marked S and SB, add 5 ml of hydrolysed standard preparation and to the tubes marked T and TB, add 5 ml of hydrolysed sample preparation. Add to each tube, 5 ml of buffer. Then to S and T tubes add 5 ml of cyanogen bromide solution and to tubes marked SB and TB, add 5 ml of water. After 20 minutes, add 1 ml of procaine hydrochloride solution to each tube. After further 5 minutes measure the absorbance at about 430 nm. Deduce the results by comparison.

Menthol

Reagents

1. Dilute sulphuric acid : Prepared by mixing 61 parts of sulphuric acid with 39 parts of water (v/v).
2. 0.5% w/v solution of paradimethylaminobenzaldehyde (PDAB) in dilute sulphuric acid.
3. 5% w/v solution of sodium hydroxide.
4. Methyl alcohol.

Standard solution

50 mcg/ml of menthol in methyl alcohol.

Sample solution

Suspend an accurately weighed quantity of sample equivalent to 5 mg of menthol in 100 ml of sodium hydroxide solution. Distil and collect about 50 ml of distillate, cool and extract the distillate with ether. Pass ether extract through sodium sulphate (anhydrous). Evaporate ether layer to dryness at a very low temperature and dissolve the residue in methanol to get 50 mcg/ml solution.

Procedure

To 5 ml each of sample and standard solutions, add 2 ml of 'PDAB' reagent, dilute to 10 ml with methanol. Keep in boiling water-bath for 2-3 min, cool and measure the absorbance of both the solutions at the maximum at about 545 nm against reagent blank.

Note : This test will serve as identification test for menthol as well.

Mephenesin

METHOD 1

Reagents

1. Periodic-acetic acid solution : Dissolve 0.215 g of sodium metaperiodate in 25 ml of water in a 250 ml volumetric flask, make up to the mark with glacial acetic acid and mix well.
2. 0.01 N sodium thiosulphate solution.
3. Starch mucilage as indicator.
4. Chloroform.
5. Glacial acetic acid.
6. Saturated sodium chloride solution.
7. 1% w/v solution of potassium iodide in water.

Sample preparation

Weigh accurately about 0.2 g of sample in a dry 100 ml beaker. Add 10 ml of water and stir well with a glass-rod to disperse the sample in water. Transfer the solution, carefully, to a separating funnel. Rinse the beaker twice with 5 ml portions of water and transfer to the separating funnel. Rinse the beaker with 50 ml of chloroform and add to the separating funnel. Shake well for two minutes and allow the layers to separate. Extract the sample with further 50 ml of chloroform. Combine chloroform layers, add 10 ml of saturated solution of sodium chloride. Shake well and allow the layers to separate. Transfer the chloroform layer to 500 ml iodine flask through funnel fitted with cotton-plug (sodium chloride layer may be extracted with 10 ml of chloroform and after separation, transfer the chloroform layer to iodine flask).

Add exactly 15 ml of periodic-acetic acid solution to the chloroform in the iodine flask, mix and add sufficient glacial acetic acid to get clear solution. Keep aside for 30 minutes. Add 100 ml of potassium iodide solution and titrate the liberated iodine with 0.01 N sodium thiosulphate using starch mucilage as indicator to be added towards the end of the titration. Continue titration till both the aqueous and chloroform layers become colourless. Shake the flask vigorously towards the end of the titration and carry out the blank titration with the sample. Each ml of 0.01 N sodium thiosulphate is equivalent to 0.00912 g of mephenesin.

Typical laboratory analysis

Mephenesin (by iodometric method)
Wt. of a sample taken = 2.75 g
Blank value = 22.65 ml
Sample value = 6.80 ml
Volume of sodium thiosulphate consumed by the sample = 15.85 ml

$$\text{Mephenesin (\% w/w)} = \frac{\text{Volume of 0.1 N Na}_2\text{S}_2\text{O}_3 \text{ consumed} \times \text{Factor}}{\text{Wt. of the sample taken for analysis}}$$

$$= \frac{15.85 \times 0.00912}{2.75}$$

$$= 5.26$$

$$\text{Claim} = 5.00$$

$$\% \text{ claim} = 105.10\%$$

METHOD 2

Reagents

1. Phosphate buffer, pH 7.4 : Dissolve 6.805 g of potassium dihydrogen phosphate in 250 ml of water, add 195.5 ml of 0.2 N sodium hydroxide and dilute to 1000 ml. Check the final pH.
2. Diazotised 2,4-dinitroaniline : Dissolve 1 g of dinitroaniline in 5 ml of concentrated sulphuric acid by gentle warming on water-bath. Cool to 0°C in ice-bath (A). Separately dissolved 0.5 g of sodium nitrite in 5 ml of concentrated sulphuric acid and cooled to 0°C (B). Mix solutions (A) and (B) and to this add some of phosphoric acid (85%). Just before use, dilute 1 : 1 with phosphoric acid.

Standard solution

To 100 mg of the working standard of mephenesin, add 2 ml of methanol and dilute to 100 ml with buffer solution. 25 ml of this further diluted to 100 ml with buffer (250 mcg/ml).

Sample solution

Accurately weighed quantity of cream or any other semisolid preparation equivalent to 100 mg of substance is extracted and diluted as under standard solution.

Procedure

To 2 ml each of sample and standard solutions, add 5 ml of phosphoric acid and 1 ml of diluted reagent. Heat on boiling water-bath for 20 min, cool in ice-bath and dilute to 50 ml with phosphoric acid (85%). Measure the absorption of both sample and standard solutions at about 510 nm using phosphoric acid as blank. Calculate the results by comparison.

METHOD 3

Standard solution

150 mcg/ml of mephenesin in water.

Sample solution

Suspend the sample (ointment, cream) in 20 ml of water by warming and extract with six 15 ml portions of chloroform. Wash the combined chloroform layer with 2 × 10 ml portions of water and dilute the organic layer to 100 ml. Evaporate 15 ml of chloroform layer to dryness on water-bath, take up the residue in 20 ml of ethanol and dilute to 100 ml with water.

Procedure

Follow the method described for guaiphenesin under formulation 32 of the chapter on expectorants.

Note : The method is based on oxidation of terminal vicinal hydroxyl group with sodium periodate to liberate formaldehyde, followed by coupling with acetyl acetone in presence of ammonia.

Methyl salicylate

METHOD 1

Reagents

1. Ferric ammonium sulphate solution.
2. 1 N and 0.02 N hydrochloric acid.

Standard solution

150 mcg/ml solution of salicylic acid in 0.02 N hydrochloric acid.

Sample solution

Take sample accurately weighed equivalent to 2 mg of total salicylate, add 30 ml of 0.5 N sodium hydroxide and 20 ml of methyl alcohol, mix and reflux for one hour on steam-bath to saponify and hydrolyse. Cool, add 20 ml of hydrochloric acid (resulting solution should be distinctly acidic) and dilute to 250 ml with water and filter.

Procedure

Take 15 ml of sample filtrate and 15 ml of standard solution. Extract each with 25 ml of chloroform, separate chloroform layer. To 5 ml of chloroform layer add 10 ml of ferric ammonium sulphate reagent. Centrifuge and separate the aqueous layer. Measure the extinction of aqueous layers at the maximum at about 530 nm. Deduce the results by comparison.

METHOD 2

Weigh sample accurately equivalent to about 100 mg of the substance in a beaker, add about 15-20 ml of cyclohexane. Stir to dissolve the substance. Make up the volume to 100 ml with cyclohexane. 1 ml of the resulting solution is further diluted with cyclohexane to 100 ml. Measure the extinction of the solution at the maximum at about 308 nm. To convert methyl salicylate (v/v) to w/w, multiply by the factor 1.182. For calculations use 357 as value of A 1%, 1 cm at 308 nm.

Total volatile contents (Menthol, Methyl salicylate, Oil of turpentine)

For details, refer to formulation 4 of this chapter.

Glycol monosalicylate, Histamine dihydrochloride, Methyl nicotinate, Capsaicin

ESTIMATION

Glycol monosalicylate

Reagents

1. Alcohol.
2. Potassium hydroxide.
3. Ferric ammonium sulphate solution.
4. Dilute acetic acid.

Standard solution

20 mcg/ml of salicylic acid in alcohol.

Sample solution

Take sample equivalent to 5 mg of the substance, add 25 ml of alcohol and 2 g of potassium hydroxide. Reflux for 1 h to saponify the material, cool and dilute to 250 ml with alcohol.

Procedure

To 2.5 ml each of sample and standard solutions, add 1 ml of dilute acetic acid, 15 ml of ferric ammonium sulphate solution and dilute to 100 ml with distilled water. Measure the absorption of both the solutions at about 530 nm. Compare the results for calculations.

Histamine dihydrochloride

Reagents

1. 0.1% w/v sodium nitrite solution in water.
2. Sulphanilic acid solution : To 300 mg of sulphanilic acid, add 2.5 ml hydrochloric acid and dilute to 100 ml with water.
3. 4% w/v sodium hydroxide solution in water.

Standard solution

15 mcg/ml of histamine dihydrochloride in water.

Sample solution

Take sample accurately weighed equivalent to about 12.5 mg of the compound, add 30 ml of distilled water, 50 ml of alcohol and 5 g of potassium hydroxide. Reflux on boiling water-bath for about 1 h. Cool and transfer the contents to a volumetric flask with the aid of 50 ml of alcohol and dilute to 500 ml. Add 10 ml of hydrochloric acid, mix and make up the volume to 1000 ml with distilled water and filter (A). 50 ml of the filtrate is extracted with four 25 ml portions of chloroform. Discard chloroform layer, filter aqueous layer and use as sample for estimation of histamine.

Procedure

To 2 ml each of sample and standard solutions, add 2 ml of sodium nitrite solution. Wait for 2 min, add 4 ml of sulphanilic acid solution. After 3 min, add 4 ml of sodium hydroxide solution and dilute to 25 ml with water. Measure the absorption of both the solutions at 420 nm against reagent blank. Deduce the results by comparison.

Methyl nicotinate

Take 10 ml of the filtrate (A) obtained during estimation of histamine and dilute to 100 ml. Proceed as per method described for this compound under formulation 1 of this chapter.

Capsaicin

METHOD 1

Reagent

1. 0.5% w/v vanadium oxytrichloride solution in ethyl acetate.

Standard solution

100 mcg/ml of capsaicin in ethyl acetate.

Sample solution

Take sample accurately weighed equivalent to 10 mg of capsaicin, extract the material with ethyl acetate for 24 h in cold or reflux for 2 h and filter. Dilute to 50 ml with ethyl acetate.

Procedure

Take 5 ml each of the sample and standard solutions and just before absorption measurement, add 0.5 ml of vanadium oxytrichloride solution. Shake to mix and immediately measure the absorption at about 720 nm. Run the blank prepared by using 0.5 ml of the reagent and 5 ml of ethyl acetate.

Note : 1. Although the colour fades away in 1 to 1.5 min, but 30 seconds elapse between the time the reagent is added and the absorbance is measured.

2. Use of acetone as extracting solvent is not recommended as due to its hygroscopic nature, it produces turbid solution.

METHOD 2

To accurately weighed quantity of sample equivalent to 2 mg of capsaicin (oleoresin capsicum containing about 8% of capsaicin), add 2 ml of anaesthetic ether and dilute to 50 ml with methanol. Add 2-3 g of sodium chloride, 10 ml of water and basify with 5 ml of 0.1 N sodium hydroxide. Extract with petroleum ether 80-100°C (4 × 10 ml). Combine the ether extract and wash with 60% methanol (3 × 25 ml). The combined hydroalcoholic layer is evaporated to about 5 ml. Add 30-40 ml water and adjust to pH 7.2 ± 0.2 (phenol red) with 0.1 N sodium hydroxide or 0.1 N hydrochloric acid as the case may be. The entire solution in turn is extracted with anaesthetic ether (4 × 50 ml). The combined ethereal layer is evaporated and residue taken up in 50 ml of methanol (decolourise with charcoal if the solution is coloured). To one 10 ml portion of alcoholic solution, add 5 ml of 0.1 N sodium hydroxide, cool and dilute to 25 ml with methanol, whereas to another 10 ml portion, add 5 ml of 0.05 N hydrochloric acid, cool and dilute to 25 ml with methanol. Measure extinction of alkaline solution at 248 nm against reagent blank. Calculate the results using 313 as value of A 1%, 1 cm for capsaicin.

Note : 1. Addition of alkali or acid and subsequent spectrophotometric reading should be made very fast and first instrumental reading should be taken for calculations.

2. From the contents of capsaicin so estimated, calculate the amount of oleoresin capsicum present in the sample (oleoresin capsicum containing about 8% of capsaicin).

Typical laboratory analysis (based on capsaicin assay value of 8.0% of raw material)

Weight of the sample taken for analysis = 12.75 g

A_s at 248 nm = 0.298

A_u at 248 nm = 0.245

$$\text{Capsaicin (contents) } \% = \frac{A_u}{A_s} \times \frac{d_f \times 100}{\text{Weight of the sample taken}}$$

$$= \frac{245}{298} \times \frac{1.25 \times 100}{12.75 \times 8}$$

$$\% \text{ claim} = 100.75$$

Benzyl nicotinate, Salicylamide, Methyl salicylate, Camphor, Oil of turpentine

ESTIMATION

Benzyl nicotinate

Reagents

1. Saturated solution of cyanogen bromide in water (prepare fresh).
2. Aniline solution : 4.0% v/v solution of aniline (freshly distilled) in methanol.

Sample solution

2 ml of liniment is boiled with about 30 ml of methanol for 5 minutes. Cool and filter into 100 ml volumetric flask. Wash the filter paper with methanol and make up the volume to 100 ml with methanol. 2.5 ml of this solution is further diluted to 50 ml with methanol.

Procedure

2 ml of the above solution is taken into 50 ml conical flask, add 10 ml of methanol and 5 ml of cyanogen bromide solution. Allow the solution to stand for 5 minutes, then add 5 ml of alcoholic aniline solution and keep aside for further 5 minutes. The extinction of yellow colour is measured at 436 nm using alcohol as a blank. The quantity of benzyl nicotinate in the sample is calculated by comparing with the standard processed similarly.

Salicylamide and Methyl salicylate (Total salicylic acid)

Reagents

1. Dilute hydrochloric acid (10% v/v).
2. 1% and 10% w/v solution of sodium hydroxide in water.
3. 2% w/v solution of ferric chloride in water.

Standard solution

20 mcg/ml of salicylic acid in water.

Sample solution

An accurately weighed amount of the sample equivalent to 5 mg of total salicylates is heated with 10 ml of dilute hydrochloric acid for 30 minutes on a boiling water-bath in order to destroy the emulsion. Add 30 ml of 10% sodium hydroxide solution and saponify for one hour while boiling under reflux. Transfer the solution into a separating funnel and shake twice with 50 ml solvent ether. The ether extract is discarded. The aqueous phase is acidified with hydrochloric acid and extracted with five 20 ml portions of ether. The combined ether extracts are shaken four time with 30 ml of 1% sodium hydroxide solution and 50 ml of water each. Slightly acidify the alkaline solution, make up the volume to 250 ml with water and filter.

Procedure

1 ml each of sample and standard solutions are taken in 10 ml volumetric flask, two drops of dilute hydrochloric acid and 0.2 ml of ferric chloric solution are added and the solution is made up to the volume with water. Measure the absorption of both solutions at about 550 nm against solution of 0.2 ml of ferric chloride solution in 10 ml water as blank. The amount of total salicylic acid is calculated by comparing with the standard.

Alternatively, follow the method for estimation of total salicylic acid described in formulation 3 of this chapter.

Menthol, Thymol, Camphor, Methyl salicylate, Oil of turpentine, Oil of eucalyptus, Oil of lemon-grass

ESTIMATION

Total volatile contents

Procedure

1. Place in a one litre round bottom flask about 70 g of the sample accurately weighed and add 300-400 ml of water, add few pieces of pumice stone to avoid bumping. Connect the flask to a special reflux still fitted with oil-trap. Heat the contents to boiling in a heating mantle. Continue distillation for about 2 h. Cool the distillate (volatile contents) collected in the trap and measure the volume. Calculate the volume in terms of ml/100 g (% v/w) of the sample.

2. In a previously dried and weighed china dish, take an accurately weighed quantity of the sample, keep the china dish on a boiling water-bath for 30 minutes or till there is no aromatic odour. Then transfer the china dish to an oven and dry it to a constant weight at 105°C for 4 h. Transfer to desiccator to cool and weigh the residue. Calculate the total volatile matter from the loss in weight of the sample.

Thymol

METHOD 1

Reagent

1. Para-aminophenol solution, 0.1% w/v : Dissolve 10 mg of pure and freshly sub-limed p-amino-phenol in 10 ml of alcohol, prepare fresh.

Standard solution

100 mg of pure thymol, accurately weighed, is dissolved in 100 ml of alcohol. 5 ml of this solution is further diluted to 100 ml distilled water to give a solution of 50 mcg/ml.

General procedure for preparation of standard curve

An aliquot of standard solution ranging from 1 to 5 ml is taken in graduated stoppered 10 ml centrifuge tubes. Add 2.5 ml of 2 N ammonium hydroxide solution and 0.3 ml of p-aminophenol solution (0.1%) to each tube and dilute to 10 ml with distilled water. Shake and keep for 5 minutes and read the absorbance of blue complex at 600 nm against reagent blank. The standard curve against concentration of thymol is prepared.

Formulations

Generally three different types of formulations containing thymol are available in the market :

1. Creams and ointments.

2. Solutions (such as gum paints, mouth wash).

3. Powders and tablets (lozenges).

Creams and ointments : Accurately weighed quantity of the preparation is mixed with 10 ml of 10% sodium hydroxide solution and the mixture is heated on water-bath to melt. The wax is separated by cooling. Neutralise the solution with dilute hydrochloric acid and dilute to produce a solution of 50 mcg/ml. Take 1 ml of this solution and follow the general procedure and calculate the amount from the standard curve.

Solutions : Known volume of the sample solution is diluted with distilled water to produce a solution of 50 mcg/ml. Use 1 ml of this solution for estimation of thymol by the general method. If the sample contains iodine, it should be removed with sodium thiosulphate before proceeding with the estimation by general method.

Tablets or powders : Extract the powder or powdered tablets with 50 ml of alcohol and dilute with water to produce a solution containing 50 mcg/ml. Take 1 ml of the solution and proceed with the estimation by general method.

Note : 1. The method obeys Beer's law over a concentration of 1.8 mcg/ml of the final solution.

2. Menthol, camphor, turpentine oil, cinnamon oil, methyl salicylate, salicylic acid, benzoic acid and boric acid do not interfere in this method.

METHOD 2

A simple colorimetric method by coupling thymol with chlorimide reagent is described.

Reagents

1. 0.4% w/v solution of 2,6-dichloroquinone chlorimide in methanol.
2. Alkaline borate buffer, pH 9.4.

Stock solution of thymol

1 mg/ml of thymol in methanol.

Working solution of thymol

1 ml of stock solution is diluted to 100 ml water (10 mcg/ml).

Preparation of standard curve

Take aliquot containing 10-70 mcg of thymol and dilute each of them to 10 ml with water. Add 2 ml of buffer solution and 0.1 ml of chlorimide reagent. Mix and measure the absorbance at 600 nm within 15 minutes. Prepare standard curve against concentration of thymol. The sample solutions of different types of formulations are prepared as described under method 1 and subjected to analysis as per method described under preparation of standard curve. Amount of thymol in the sample is calculated from the standard curve.

Note : 1. The colour is stable for 15 minutes; measure the extinction as quickly as possible.

2. The method obeys Beer's law in the range of 10-70 mcg/ml of thymol. Menthol, camphor, salicylic acid, benzoic acid, methyl salicylate, cinnamon oil, turpentine oil, lemon grass oil, borax, sodium bicarbonate, iodine, potassium iodide, tannic acid and oleoresin capsicum in the concentration of 1 mg/ml do not give colour with this reagent. However, eucalyptus oil gives green and clove oil produces blue colour with this reagent.

METHOD 3

A colorimetric method involving reaction of thymol with diazotised 4-nitroaniline-2-sulphonic acid is described.

Reagents

1. 4-nitroaniline-2-sulphonic acid solution : 0.158 g of the compound is dissolved and made up to 100 ml with dilute hydrochloric acid.
2. 0.2% w/v sodium nitrite solution in water.
3. Diazotised reagent : 18 ml of solution (1) is cooled to 5°C and completely diazotised with solution (2) using starch-iodide paste as external indicator. The final solution should be clear and colourless. It should be kept in cold and protected from light. Diazotised reagent should always be freshly prepared. Usually 1 ml of solution (2) is required for 4.5 ml of solution (1) for complete diazotization.
4. Alkaline borate buffer, pH 10.0.

Stock solution of thymol

1 mg/ml of thymol in ethyl alcohol.

Working solution of thymol

Stock solution is approximately diluted with water to obtain a concentration of 100 mcg/ml of thymol.

Standard curve

Take aliquot containing 10 to 60 mcg of thymol. Add 10 ml of water, 1 ml of 0.1 N sodium hydroxide and 6 ml of alkaline borate buffer solution to each and cool to about 5°C. Then, add 0.5 ml of freshly prepared diazotised reagent and dilute the contents to 25 ml with water and set aside for 15 minutes. The absorbance of the coloured product is measured at 520 nm and standard curve against the concentration of thymol is prepared. For estimation of thymol in analgesic balms, the following procedure is recommended for preparation of sample solution :

About 0.5 g of the balm is accurately weighed in a 50 ml capacity platinum dish containing 10 ml of 10 per cent sodium hydroxide solution and 25 ml distilled water. To this, add 5 mg thymol in alcoholic solution and mix. The dish is heated on a boiling water-bath and heating is continued till there is no easily perceptible camphoracious odour. The solution in the dish is not allowed to evaporate to less than 20 ml. The water lost is replaced from time to time. The solution is then chilled and the clear liquid is filtered into a 100 ml volumetric flask. The residue left in the dish is heated with about 25 ml of water three times on a water-bath and the extractives filtered into the volumetric flask. The solution in the flask is made up to volume with distilled water. One ml of this solution is taken for analysis. The amount of thymol is calculated from the standard curve.

Note : 1. The method obeys Beer's law in the range of 10-60 mcg/ml.
      2. Colour of the complex is stable for 24 hrs.

Methyl salicylate

METHOD 1

Take 2 g of the sample accurately weighed and suspend in 10 ml dilute hydrochloric acid by warming for about 15 minutes. Add 30 ml of 1 N sodium hydroxide and saponify by refluxing for 1 h. Carry out the extraction and colour development as described in formulation 3 of this chapter.

METHOD 2

Weigh accurately sample equivalent to 100 mg of methyl salicylate in a 100 ml beaker and add about 10 ml of cyclohexane. Stir the mixture thoroughly to effect the solution and then transfer quantitatively into 100 ml dry volumetric flask with the aid of cyclohexane. Finally make up the volume. Filter and dilute 1 ml of the filtrate to 100 ml with cyclohexane. Measure the extinction of the resulting solution at the maxima at 308 nm. Calculate the percentage of methyl salicylate (v/v) taking 357 as the value of E (1 per cent, 1 cm) v/v. To convert the so obtained percentage of methyl salicylate in v/v into w/w, multiply by 1.182 which is weight per ml of methyl salicylate.

Menthol

Follow the method described in formulation 1 of this chapter.

Oxyphenbutazone, Phenylbutazone, Methyl salicylate, Mephenesin, Menthol

ESTIMATION

Oxyphenbutazone/Phenylbutazone

Follow the method described under formulation 2 of the chapter on anti-inflammatory drugs.

Methyl salicylate

Weigh the sample (cream) accurately equivalent to about 100 mg methyl salicylate, transfer to a volumetric flask, add about 25 ml of cyclohexane. Heat on a water-bath to effect solution. Cool and make up to 100 ml with cyclohexane. Further dilutions may be done with cyclohexane to get final concentration of 10 mcg/ml. Measure the extinction at 308 nm using cyclohexane as blank. Calculate the results using 357 as value of A 1%, 1 cm, at 308 nm. Also refer to formulation 3 of this chapter.

Mephenesin

Weigh the sample (cream) accurately equivalent to 100 mg of mephenesin. Suspend in water by slight warming and add 5 ml of ammonia solution. Extract with four 25 ml portions of chloroform. Wash the combined chloroform layer with 10 mg each of 0.02 N sodium hydroxide and water and then pass through a layer of anhydrous sodium sulphate. Evaporate the combined chloroform layer and take up the residue in water to get volume of 200 ml. Dilute further appropriately with water to get final concentration of 25 mcg/ml. Measure the absorbance of the resulting solution at maximum at about 270 nm. Calculate the contents of mephenesin taking 80 as value of A 1%, 1 cm at 270 nm. Alternately, the chloroform layer can be directly used for estimation by using a standard (25 mcg/ml) in chloroform for comparison.

Menthol

Suspend adequate quantity of the sample equivalent to 1 mg of menthol in water and distil. For details, refer to the method described under formulation 1 of this chapter.

Ibuprofen, Methyl salicylate, Mephenesin, Menthol

ESTIMATION

Ibuprofen

Follow the method described in formulation 34 of the chapter on analgesic and antipyretic drugs. Each ml of 0.1 N sodium hydroxide is equivalent to 0.02063 g of ibuprofen or 0.02543 g of ketoprofen. Alternatively, suspend accurately weighed quantity of the sample in water by slight warming, add 1 ml of dilute hydrochloric acid and extract the precipitated ibuprofen with n-hexane (3 × 25 ml), passing each extract through anhydrous sodium sulphate. Evaporate the combined chloroform layer in water-bath and take up the residue in 0.1 N sodium hydroxide to produce 100 ml (50 mcg/ml). Measure the absorbance of sample and standard solutions (processed as per sample) at 264 nm and calculate the results by comparison.

Methyl salicylate

Follow the method described in formulation 1 and 4 of this chapter.

Menthol

Follow the method described in formulation 1 of this chapter.

Mephenesin

Follow the method described in formulation 1 and 5 of this chapter.

Formulation 7

Diethylamine salicylate, Methyl nicotinate

ESTIMATION

Diethylamine salicylate

Reagents

1. Ferric chloride solution : To 5.5 g of ferric chloride, add 2.5 ml of concentrated hydrochloric acid and dilute to 100 ml with water.

Standard solution

80 mcg/ml of diethylamine salicylate in water.

Sample solution

The sample is extracted with water by slight warming, subsequently cooled and filtered. Further dilutions are done with water and kept cool while filtering.

Procedure

To 4 ml each of sample and standard solutions, add 0.5 ml of ferric chloride solution, mix and make up to 50 ml with water.

Measure the absorbance of both sample and standard solutions at about 540 nm against reagent blank and calculate the results by comparison.

Methyl nicotinate

Follow the method described in formulation 1 of this chapter.

Piroxicam, Capsaicin, Methylsalicylate, Menthol

ESTIMATION

Piroxicam

The method is based on differential spectroscopy.

Reagents

1. 0.01 N methanolic hydrochloric acid.
2. 0.01 N methanolic sodium hydroxide.

Standard solution

10 mcg/ml of piroxicam in 0.01 N methanolic hydrochloric acid and methanolic sodium hydroxide.

Sample solution

Accurately weighed quantity of the sample equivalent to 10 mg of the substance was extracted with methanol to get solution of 100 mcg/ml. Further dilutions were done as given under standard solution.

Procedure

Measure the absorbance of acidic solutions of both sample and standard at 326 nm using respective alkaline solutions as blank and calculate the results by comparison. The method obeys Beer's law in the concentration range of 4-22 mcg/ml.

Capsaicin

Follow the method described in formulation 2 of this chapter.

Methylsalicylate

Follow the method described in formulation 3 of this chapter.

Menthol

Follow the method described in formulation 1 of this chapter.

Chapter 16

Sedatives & Tranquillisers

Formulation 1

Chlordiazepoxide hydrochloride, Clidinium bromide

ESTIMATION

Chlordiazepoxide hydrochloride

METHOD 1

Standard solution

20 mcg/ml of chlordiazepoxide hydrochloride in 0.1 N hydrochloric acid.

Sample solution

Shake a quantity of the sample powder equivalent to 20 mg of chlordiazepoxide hydrochloride with 150 ml of 0.1 N hydrochloric acid, make volume to 200 ml and filter. Dilute 10 ml of the filtrate to 50 ml with 0.1 N hydrochloric acid (20 mcg/ml).

Measure the extinction of standard and sample solutions at the maximum at about 308 nm. Calculate the content of chlordiazepoxide hydrochloride by comparison.

METHOD 2

Reagents

1. 1% w/v solution of vanillin in acetone.
2. Hydrochloric acid.

Standard solution

100 mcg/ml of the compound in glacial acetic acid.

Sample solution

Extract accurately weighed quantity of the sample with glacial acetic acid and dilute to get 100 mcg/ml.

Procedure

To 2 ml of the sample and standard solutions, add 2 ml of vanillin reagent and 2 ml of hydrochloric acid. Heat on water-bath for 10 minutes, cool to room temperature and dilute to 10 ml with water. Measure the absorbance of both the solutions at about 530 nm. The method obeys Beer's law in the range of 40-200 mcg/ml.

METHOD 3

Reagents

1. Dilute hydrochloric acid.
2. 0.5% w/v hydrochloric acid.
3. 2% w/v solution of p-dimethylaminobenzaldehyde in methanol.

Standard solution

Weigh accurately 100 mg of the compound, add 50 ml of dilute hydrochloric acid and heat on water-bath for 40 minutes. Cool and dilute to 100 ml with water. 5 ml of the resultant solution is further diluted with water to 100 ml.

Sample solution

Weigh accurately aliquot of the sample equivalent to 100 mg of the compound and proceed as per standard solution.

Procedure

To 1 ml of sample and standard solutions, add 1.5 ml of dilute hydrochloric acid and 1.5 ml of p-dimethylaminobenz aldehyde reagent. Shake and dilute to 10 ml with water. The absorbance of both the solutions is measured at about 452 nm against blank (0.5% hydrochloric acid). The method obeys Beer's law in the range of 2.5 to 7 mcg/ml.

Clidinium bromide

METHOD 1

Reagents

1. Buffer solution, pH 7.0 : To 104.5 ml of 0.2 M sodium phosphate, dibasic, add 85.5 ml of 0.2 M potassium phosphate, monobasic and water to make 1000 ml.
2. Bromocresol purple solution (buffered) : Weigh about 80 mg of the bromocresol purple and dissolve in few drops of methyl alcohol. Add 50 ml of buffer solution and make up the volume to 100 ml with water. Wash the dye solution with chloroform till chloroform washings are colourless. This treatment reduces the blank values.

Standard solution

100 mcg/ml clidinium bromide in water.

Sample solution

Transfer the powdered sample accurately weighed equivalent to 10 mg of the compound to a 100 ml volumetric flask. Shake with 50 ml of water for five minutes, add sufficient water to produce 100 ml and filter.

Procedure

Transfer 10 ml aliquot of the standard and sample solutions to separating funnel and add 10 ml of buffered bromocresol purple solution. Extract it with three 25 ml portions of chloroform. Pass the chloroform into a 50 ml dried volumetric flask through a cotton plug previously moistened with chloroform. Add sufficient chloroform to make the volume. Measure the absorbance of the standard and test solutions at about 420 nm using chloroform as blank and calculate the results by comparison.

METHOD 2

Reagents

1. Buffer solution, pH 8.8 : Dissolve 26.8 g of dibasic sodium phosphate in 200 ml of water, adjust pH with 0.1 N sodium hydroxide.
2. Thymol blue : Dissolve 100 mg of the dye in 100 ml of water with the aid of 1 ml of 1 N sodium hydroxide.

Standard and sample solution

See method 1 above.

Procedure

As described under method 1 above. Absorption maxima of the complex is observed at about 410 nm.

Note : Centrifugation of chloroform layer gives consistent results.

Imipramine hydrochloride, Diazepam

ESTIMATION

Imipramine hydrochloride

METHOD 1

Weigh accurately powdered tablets equivalent to about 25 mg of imipramine hydrochloride and extract and adjust the volume to 50 ml with ether saturated water. Shake total aqueous extract with 10 ml of ether. Allow the layers to separate. Retain ether layer for estimation of diazepam. Dilute aqueous layer with 0.1 N sulphuric acid to get 20 mcg/ml and measure the extinction at about 251 nm. Calculate the contents of imipramine hydrochloride taking 264 as value of A 1%, 1 cm. Alternatively, the sample equivalent to 300 mg of the substance is suspended in 2 ml sodium hydroxide and extracted with 50 ml of ether. The ether layer is dissolved in 20 ml of methanol and titrated with 0.1 N hydrochloric acid using bromothymol blue as indicator. Each ml of 0.1 N hydrochloric acid is equivalent to 31.69 mg of imipramine HCl.

METHOD 2

Reagents

1. Cobalt thiocyanate reagent : Dissolve 4.3 g of ammonium thiocyanate and 6.8 g of cobalt chloride in 100 ml of water.
2. Britton and Robinson buffer, pH 2.0.

Standard solution

1 mg/ml of imipramine hydrochloride in water.

Sample solution

Transfer powdered sample accurately weighed equivalent to 100 mg of the compound into a 100 ml volumetric flask. Shake with water, filter and adjust to volume.

Procedure

Transfer 10 ml of standard and the sample solutions into separatory funnels. Add 1 ml of buffer solution, followed by 5 ml of cobalt thiocyanate reagent. Extract the aqueous layer with 10, 5 and 5 ml of benzene. Measure the absorbance of blue coloured chromogen at about 625 nm against reagent blank. The method obeys Beer's law in the concentration range of 20-560 mcg/ml.

METHOD 3

Reagents

1. Brilliant blue solution : 0.1% w/v solution of the dye in water.

Standard solution

50 μg/ml of the substance in water.

Sample solution

Accordingly weighed quantity of the powdered sample was extracted with water to get final concentration of 50 μg/ml of the substance.

Procedure

To 2 ml each of sample and standard solutions, add 3 ml of dye solution and make up to 10 ml with water. Add 10 ml of chloroform to each and shake for not less than 2 min. Allow the layers to separate and centrifuge. Measure the absorbance of chloroform layer at 620 nm chloroform using chloroform as blank. The method following linearity with range of 2-20 μg.

Note :   1.   Common excipients present in tablets, capsules did not interfere.

2.   Diazepam did not interfere.

Diazepam

METHOD 1

Evaporate the ether layer as obtained in method 1 and dissolve the residue in 0.1 N sulphuric acid to get a solution of about 3 mcg/ml. Measure the extinction at about 241 nm and calculate the contents of diazepam taking 1402 as A 1%, 1 cm.

METHOD 2

A slight variation in the above extraction procedure has been tried and found to give satisfactory results :

Weigh sample accurately equivalent to about 25 mg of imipramine hydrochloride. Add 10 ml of ether saturated water and 10 ml of ether (water saturated). Shake vigorously for 5 minutes in a tightly stoppered separating funnel. Allow the two layers to separate and proceed for determination of each component as per procedure given in method A above.

METHOD 3

The sample was suspended in 20 ml of ether, and filtered through G₄ sintered funnel. The filtrate was evaporated and residue taken up in methanol to get solution of 5 mcg/ml in respect of diazepam. The absorbance of both sample and standard solutions (5 mcg/ml in methanol) was measured at 245 nm and results calculated by comparison.

To residue retained on the sintered funnel was extracted and diluted with water to get 10 mcg/ml of imipramine. The absorbance of both sample and standard was measured at 250 nm and results deduced by comparison.

Trifluoperazine hydrochloride, Trihexyphenidyl

ESTIMATION

Trifluoperazine hydrochloride

Reagents

1. 0.1% w/v ammonium vanadate solution (slight warming is necessary to get quick solution).
2. Dilute hydrochloric acid (1 : 1 and 1 : 4 v/v).

Standard solution

200 mcg/ml of authentic trifluoperazine hydrochloride in 0.1 N hydrochloric acid.

Sample solution

Accurately weigh powdered tablets equivalent to about 10 mg of trifluoperazine hydrochloride, add 25 ml of 0.1 N hydrochloric acid. Shake and adjust the volume to 50 ml with 0.1 N hydrochloric acid (200 mcg/ml).

Procedure

To each 25 ml volumetric flask, add 0.5 ml of ammonium vanadate solution and 1 ml of dilute hydrochloric acid (1 : 1). Mix and allow to stand for 1 minute. Add 5 ml of standard and sample solutions to each flask and make up the volume with dilute hydrochloric acid (1 : 5). Concomitantly measure the absorbance of both the solutions at absorption maximum at about 525 nm against reagent blank. Calculate the results by comparison.

$$\text{Trifluoperazine (mg/tab)} = \frac{A_u}{A_s} \times \frac{W_s}{W_u} \times d_f \times \text{Av. wt.} \times 1000 \times 0.85$$

$$= \frac{0.294}{0.288} \times \frac{0.1001}{0.076} \times 0.256 \times \frac{1}{20} \times 1000$$

$$= 1.03$$

Claim = 1.0 mg as base

Multiply with 0.85 to convert salt and base.

Trihexyphenidyl

Its determination requires thin layer chromatographic separation, followed by colour complex with bromocresol purple.

Reagents

1. Phosphate buffer solution, pH 5.3.
2. 0.4% w/v solution of bromocresol purple in water.
3. Chloroform.

4. TLC glass plates (20 × 20 cm), coated (0.25 mm) with silica gel G and activated at 105°C for 20 minutes.
5. Developing solvent.
    (i) Benzene : Acetone : Strong ammonia (8 : 4 : 1 v/v).
    (ii) Chloroform : Methyl alcohol (9 : 1 v/v).
    (iii) Acetone-water (85 + 15 v/v).

Standard solution

100 mcg/ml of pure trihexyphenidyl in chloroform.

Sample solution

Weigh accurately powdered tablets equivalent to about 10 mg of the compound, add 25 ml of chloroform, shake and filter. Wash the residue with chloroform and adjust the filtrate to 100 ml.

Procedure

Apply with the help of a microsyringe 4 μl each of standard and sample solutions, 1.5 cm from the lower edge of the plate and 1.5 cm apart. Apply also 1 μl of the standard solution to serve as a guide. The plate is developed in either of the solvents to a distance of 10 cm. The plates are dried and spot obtained with 1 μl of standard solution is located with the help of Dragendorff's reagent. Using this as a guide, the corresponding areas of standard as well as sample are marked and extruded on a butter paper. To each extruded portion, add 5 ml of phosphate buffer solution, pH 5.3 and 5 ml of bromocresol purple solution and shake. It is then shaken with 10 ml of chloroform. Chloroform layer is allowed to separate and absorbance of the yellow complex in organic layer is measured at absorption maximum at about 410 nm. The results are calculated by comparison.

Diazepam, Diphenhydramine hydrochloride

ESTIMATION

Diazepam

Standard solution

5 mcg/ml of diazepam in methanol.

Sample solution

Accurately weighed quantity of the powdered sample equivalent to 5 mg of diazepam extracted with 20 ml of dry ether by shaking for 5 min. The ether layer evaporated to dryness and residue taken up in methanol to get a solution of 5 mcg/ml.

The absorbance of both sample and standard solutions measured at 245 nm and results calculated by comparison.

Diphenhydramine hydrochloride

Standard solution

200 mcg/ml of diphenhydramine hydrochloride in methanol.

Sample solution

The residue left after extraction of the powdered sample with dry ether as under estimation of diazepam was taken up in methanol and diluted to get final concentration of 200 mcg/ml in respect of the substance.

The absorbance of both sample and standard was measured at 255 nm using methanol as blank and results calculated by comparison.

Formulation 5

Haloperidol, Trihexyphenidyl

ESTIMATION

Haloperidol

Accurately weighed quantity of powdered sample is suspended in 30 ml of ether (saturated with water). Extract with 4 × 15 ml portions of 0.25 M sulphuric acid. Combine the acid extracts and heat in a water-bath till there is no perceptible odour of ether. Dilute to 100 ml with 0.25 M sulphuric acid. To 25 ml of the sample, add 5 ml of methanol and sufficient 0.25 M sulphuric acid to get 50 ml.

Measure the absorbance of a resulting solution at 245 nm and calculate the results using 340 as value of A 1%, 1 cm.

Trihexyphenidyl

Reagents

1. Phosphate buffer solution, pH 5.3 ± 0.1 : To 55 ml of solution of dipotassium hydroxide phosphate (8.7%), add 20 ml of citric acid solution (9.6%).
2. Bromocresol purple solution : Dissolve 400 mg of 30 ml of the dye in 30 ml of water, add 6.3 ml of 0.1 N sodium hydroxide and dilute to 500 ml with water.

Standard solution

10 mcg/ml of the substance in water (solution is usually affected by heating).

Sample solution

Accurately weighed quantity of the powdered sample equivalent to 2 mg of the substance is suspended in 40 ml of hot water. Heat slightly with swirling and make up the volume to 100 ml.

Procedure

To 2 ml each of sample and standard, add 5 ml of buffer and 5 ml of dye solution, shake to mix and to each add 10 ml of chloroform. Shake and allow the layers to separate. Measure the absorbance of chloroform layer at 420 nm using chloroform as blank.

Haloperidol, Propantheline bromide

ESTIMATION

Haloperidol

Standard solution

200 mcg/ml of haloperidol in methanol. 5 ml of this solution is diluted to 100 ml with 1 N sulphuric acid (10 mcg/ml).

Sample solution

Weigh accurately powdered sample equivalent to 1 mg of the substance and suspend in 20 ml of 1 N sulphuric acid. Make it distinctly alkaline with 1 N sodium hydroxide and extract with 5 × 40 ml of chloroform, washing each chloroform layer with same 2 × 25 ml of water. Discard the aqueous layer and extract the organic layer with 4 × 20 ml of 1 N sulphuric acid, collecting the acid extract in 100 ml volumetric flask. Add 5 ml of methanol and dilute to volume with 1 N sulphuric acid.

Measure the absorbance of both sample and standard solutions at about 248 nm using 5% v/v methanol or 1 N sulphuric acid as blank. Calculate the results in term of mg/tablet.

Propantheline bromide

Transform accurately weighed quantity of the powdered sample equivalent to 250 mg of propantheline bromide to a G₃ sintered glass funnel. Water the powdered material with 4 × 20 ml portions of anaesthetic ether, removing ether each time by mild suction. Extract the powder on sintered funnel with 6 × 25 ml chloroform. Evaporate the combined chloroform layer and take up the residue in 50 ml of glacial acetic acid. Warm gently to affect the solution. Add 6 ml of mercuric acetate (6%) and dilute with 0.05 N perchloric acid using crystal violet as indicator. Carry out the blank titration. Each ml of 0.05 N perchloric acid is equivalent to 14.948 of propantheline bromide.

Formulation 7

Trifluoperazine, Isopropamide iodide

ESTIMATION

Isopropamide

Standard solution

100 mcg/ml of isopropamide iodide in 0.1 N sulphuric acid.

Sample solution

Weigh accurately powdered sample equivalent to 10 mg of isopropamide iodide, suspend in 60-70 ml of 0.1 N sulphuric acid, shake for 20 min and dilute to 100 ml with 0.1 N sulphuric acid (100 mcg/ml).

Methyl orange buffer solution

Dissolve 200 mg of methyl orange in phosphate-sodium carbonate buffer (pH 10.2) by heating in steam-bath and constant stirring and finally diluting to 200 ml with buffer.

Procedure

To 5 ml each of sample and standard solutions, add 60 ml of chloroform and 30 ml of methyl orange buffer solution. Shake well for 3-4 min and allow to stand to ensure complete separation of two phases. Separate chloroform layer and repeat the extraction with 2 × 50 ml of chloroform. Combine the chloroform layer and extract with 3 × 25 ml of 10% hydrochloric acid. The acid layers are separated and diluted to 10 ml.

Measure the absorbance of both sample and standard at 510 nm using 10% hydrochloric acid as blank.

Trifluoperazine

Accurately weighed quantity of the sample is suspended in 0.1 N hydrochloric acid to get final solution of 10 mcg/ml in respect of trifluoperazine. Measure the absorption of the solution at about 256 nm and calculate the results.

Note : Isopropamide has negligible absorbance at 256 nm (A 1%, 1 cm = 9.1) and interferes to the extent of about 5%.

Alternatively, 25 ml of the solution is made alkaline with 2 N sodium hydroxide (about 1.5 ml) and extracted with 3 × 25 ml of ether. The combined ether layer is in turn extracted with 0.1 N hydrochloric acid (3 × 25 ml) and diluted to 100 ml.

The absorption of both sample and standard (100 mcg/ml in 0.1 N hydrochloric acid) may be measured at 256 nm for final calculation.

METHOD 2

Reagents

1. 0.04% solution of bromophenol blue in water.

2. Buffer, pH 3.5, potassium hydrogen phthalate.

Standard solution

100 mg of trifluoperazine (base) and 40 mg of trihexyphenidyl is diluted in 50 ml of methanol. 10 ml of the resultant solution is diluted to 50 ml with methanol.

Sample solution

Accurately weighed quantity of the powdered sample equivalent to 20 mg of trifluoperazine is suspended in 30-35 ml of methanol. Shake vigorously for 15-20 min and make up to 50 ml with methanol, centrifuge.

Chromatographic parameters

TLC plates (aluminium) pre-coated with silica gel 60F$_{254}$.
Mobile phase : Acetone-water (85 + 15 v/v)
Development distance : 100 mm
Amount spotted : 80 μl of both sample and standard
Detection : Iodine chamber
After developing, the plate was dried and evaporated to iodine vapours. The spots were marked and plate was slightly heated to remove iodine. The separated marked spots to trifluoperazine and trihexyphenidyl were separately extracted with 5 ml of phosphate buffer (pH 3.5). To this add 5 ml of dye solution and 10 ml of chloroform. Shake and then allow the layers to separate. Measure the absorption of chloroform layer at 410 nm using chloroform as blank.

Trifluoperazine, Chlordiazepoxide hydrochloride

ESTIMATION

Trifluoperazine

Follow the method for determination of trifluoperazine described under formulation 3 of this chapter. It has been experimentally observed that chlordiazepoxide hydrochloride does not interfere in the assay of trifluoperazine even when present 10 times its concentration.

Chlordiazepoxide hydrochloride

METHOD 1

Weigh powdered tablets accurately, equivalent to 100 mg of chlordiazepoxide. Extract and adjust the volume to 100 ml with 0.1 N hydrochloric acid. Dilute the resultant solution appropriately with 0.1 N hydrochloric acid to get a concentration of 5 mcg/ml. Measure the extinction at about 246 nm and calculate the results taking 1020 as value of A 1%, 1 cm.

Note : Trifluoperazine is normally present 1/10th of chlordiazepoxide in formulations and in such concentration, it has been observed that interference by trifluoperazine is even less than 3%.

METHOD 2

Being 1,4-benzodiazepines derivative, the compound can be subjected to acid hydrolysis (6 N hydrochloric acid) and the resulting yellow colour can be measured at about 410 nm. For details, refer to the method as described for diazepam in formulation 1 of the chapter on anti-inflammatory drugs.

Typical laboratory analysis

Chlordiazepoxide

Average weight of the tablet = 0.256 g

$$\text{Chlordiazepoxide mg/tab} = \frac{A_v}{A_s} \times \frac{W_s}{W_u} \times d_f \times Av.\ wt. \times 1000$$

$$= \frac{0.407}{0.406} \times \frac{0.1011}{0.2561} \times \frac{1}{10} \times 0.256 \times 1000$$

$$= 10.14 \text{ mg}$$

$$\text{Claim} = 10 \text{ mg}$$

Diazepam

Average weight of the tablet = 0.276 g

$$\text{Diazepam (mg/ml)} = \frac{A_u}{A_s} \times \frac{W_s}{W_u} \times d_f \times Av.\ wt. \times 1000$$

$$= \frac{0.230}{0.235} \times \frac{0.1018}{0.545} \times \frac{1}{20} \times \frac{0.276}{1} \times 1000$$

$$= 2.52 \text{ mg}$$

$$\text{Claim} = 2.52 \text{ mg}$$

Propranolol hydrochloride

$$\text{Propranolol hydrochloride (mg/tab)} = \frac{0.490}{0.460} \times \frac{0.1004}{0.1432} \times \frac{1}{10} \times 0.276 \times 1000$$
$$= 20.74 \text{ mg}$$
$$\text{Claim} = 20 \text{ mg}$$

Diazepam, Propranolol hydrochloride

ESTIMATION

Diazepam

This method is based on acid hydrolysis of diazepam to 2-methylamino-5-chlorobenzophenone and the resultant yellow colour is measured at 410 nm. Methanolic solution of sample and standard (200 mcg/ml) is used for the acidic hydrolysis. For details refer to formulation 1 of the chapter on anti-inflammatory drugs.

Propranolol hydrochloride

Standard solution

10 mcg/ml of propranolol hydrochloride in methanol.

Sample solution

Accurately weighed quantity of the powdered sample is extracted with methanol to get a concentration of 10 mcg/ml.

Measure the extinction of both sample and standard at 290 nm using methanol as blank.

Note : Interference due to diazepam in this method is less than 4%.

Chapter 17

Topical Antifungal & Anti-infective Preparations

Boric acid, Sulphanilamide, Acriflavine or Euflavine

ESTIMATION

Boric acid

Follow the method described in formulation 1 of the chapter on eye, ear & nasal preparations.

Sulphanilamide

Weigh accurately, a quantity of the sample equivalent to 200 mg of sulphanilamide and dissolve in 75 ml of water and 10 ml of hydrochloric acid. Cool and titrate slowly with 0.1 M sodium nitrite at a temperature not above 15°C. The titration is complete when the end point is reproducible after the titrated solution has been allowed to stand for one min. Each ml of 0.1 M sodium nitrite is equivalent to 0.01722 g of sulphanilamide.

Acriflavine

METHOD 1

Standard solution

10 mcg/ml of acriflavine in methyl alcohol.

Sample solution

Weigh accurate quantity of the aliquot equivalent to 2.5 mg of acriflavine, add 10 ml of methyl alcohol (in case of ointments and creams, heat on a boiling water-bath till base fully melts, cool) and dilute to 25 ml with methyl alcohol. An appropriate quantity of the above solution is further diluted with methyl alcohol to produce a concentration of 10 mcg/ml.

Procedure

Measure the absorption of the solutions at maximum at about 450 nm against methyl alcohol as blank. Calculate the results by comparing with the standard.

METHOD 2

Reagents

1. 1 N hydrochloric acid.
2. 0.05 M sodium nitrite in water.

Sample solution

100 mcg/ml of pure acriflavine in water.

Sample solution

Accurately weighed quantity of the sample is either diluted (in case of liquid preparation) or extracted with water by warming on water-bath to produce 100 mcg/ml concentration.

Procedure

To 2.5 ml each of the sample and standard solutions, add 5 ml of 1 N hydrochloric acid and 1.5 ml of 0.05 M sodium nitrite and dilute to 25 ml with water. Measure the extinction at maximum at about 580 nm and deduce the results by comparison.

Euflavine

Reagent

1. Methanolic hydrochloric acid : Dilute 100 ml of 0.5 N hydrochloric acid to 500 ml with methanol.

Standard solution

Dissolve about 25 mg of the euflavine accurately weighed (it is preferable to use the same batch of euflavine which is used to prepare the formulation) in 250 ml methanolic hydrochloric acid. Dilute 10 ml of the solution to 100 ml with the same solvents (10 mcg/ml).

Sample solution

Disperse accurate weight of the sample equivalent to 2.5 mg of euflavine in 50 ml of light petroleum ether (40-60°C). Extract the euflavine by shaking the mixture with 50, 20 and 20 ml volumes of methanolic hydrochloric acid, washing each extract with the same 20 ml of light petroleum and filtering it through a cotton wool plug into a 100 ml volumetric flask. Dilute the extracts to volume with methanolic hydrochloric acid. Dilute further with the solvent to get 10 mcg/ml concentration.

Procedure

Transfer 5 ml each of the sample and standard solutions into 50 ml volumetric flasks, dilute to 50 ml with methanolic hydrochloric acid. Measure the absorption of the solutions at about 462 nm with methanolic hydrochloric acid as blank, calculate the results by comparison.

Benzocaine, Benzyl benzoate, Dicophane (DDT)

ESTIMATION

Benzocaine

Take accurately weighed quantity of the sample equivalent to 200 mg of benzocaine in beaker. Add 10 ml of water and 15 ml of hydrochloric acid. Heat to dissolve the benzocaine, cool the solution in an ice-bath to about 10°C and titrate with 0.1 M sodium nitrite until a blue colour is produced immediately, with starch iodide paste as an external indicator. Each ml of 0.1 N sodium nitrite is equivalent to 0.01652 g of benzocaine. Calculate the results from the volume of 0.1 M sodium nitrite consumed in the titration using the above factor.

Benzyl benzoate

Weigh accurately, quantity of the sample equivalent to 2 g of benzyl benzoate and dissolve in 10 ml of neutralised alcohol. Neutralise the free acid with 0.1 N alcoholic potassium hydroxide using 0.2 ml solution of phenolphthalein as indicator. Add 50 ml of 0.5 N alcoholic potassium hydroxide, attach the flask to a reflux condenser, boil on water-bath for one hour. Add 20 ml of water and titrate the excess of alkali with 0.5 N sulphuric acid, using a further 0.2 ml of solution of phenolphthalein as indicator. Repeat the experiment with the same quantities of the reagents omitting the sample. The difference between the two titrations is equivalent to the alkali required to saponify benzyl benzoate. Each ml of 0.5 N alcoholic potassium hydroxide is equivalent to 0.1061 g of benzyl benzoate. Results are deduced by applying the above factor.

DDT (Dicophane)

Weigh accurately sample equivalent to 250 mg of DDT and boil under a reflux condenser for thirty minutes with 20 ml of alcohol and 1 g of sodium hydroxide. Add 20 ml of water, 15 ml of dilute nitric acid and 20 ml of 0.1 N silver nitrate, shake vigorously and titrate with 0.1 N ammonium thiocyanate using ferric alum as indicator. Perform the blank experiment with the same quantities of the reagents omitting the sample. Each ml of 0.1 N silver nitrate is equivalent to 0.00709 g of DDT.

Urea, Glycine, Ammonium chloride, Sodium chloride, Potassium chloride, Magnesium chloride, Sodium acid phosphate, Calcium lactate, Lactic acid, Hydrocortisone acetate

ESTIMATION

Urea

METHOD 1

Weigh accurately a quantity of the sample equivalent to 0.5 g of urea, add about 50 ml of water and extract with four 30 ml portions of chloroform. Wash the combined chloroform layer with 20 ml of water and add the water washing to the aqueous extract. Dilute aqueous extract to 250 ml with water (solution A).

To 20 ml of the solution A, add 90 ml of glacial acetic acid and 10 ml of xanthydrol solution (10% w/v in methanol). Mix and allow to stand at room temperature for 60 minutes. Filter through previously weighed G_3 sintered glass crucible. Wash the precipitates with 20-25 ml methanol and dry at 105°C to constant weight. Each g of the residue is equivalent to 0.1425 g of the urea.

METHOD 2

Standard solution

2 mg/ml of urea in water.

Sample solution

Weigh accurately sample equivalent to 500 mg of urea and suspend in 100-150 ml of water, warm gently in water-bath till uniform suspension is obtained. Cool and dilute to 250 ml with water, filter and use the filtrate as sample solution for analysis.

Procedure

To 7.5 ml each of sample and standard solutions, add 200 mg of urease dissolved in 50 ml of water and incubate at 37°C for 45 min. Run individual blanks (sample and standard), adding 50 ml of water instead of urease solution. Cool all the four flasks to room temperature and add to each 2 ml of 0.05 M zinc sulphate solution and 1 ml of 1 N sodium hydroxide solution and finally dilute to 250 ml with water, mix and filter. To 2 ml each of the four filtrates, add 30 ml of water and 2 ml of Nessler's reagent and dilute to 50 ml. Keep at room temperature for 10 min and measure the absorbance of both sample and standard solutions at 400 nm against respective blanks and calculate the results by comparison.

Total chlorides

Take 100 ml of the solution A, add 10 ml of nitric acid and boil. Add 25 ml of 0.1 N silver nitrate to the boiling solution. Digest the precipitates for 30 minutes on water-bath. Filter and wash the precipitates 4-5 times with water. The combined filtrate is titrated with 0.1 N ammonium thiocyanate using 2 ml solution of ferric alum as indicator, run blank. Each ml of 0.1 N silver nitrate is equivalent to 0.003545 g of chloride.

Total nitrogen

Take 10 ml of solution A in 500 ml Kjaldahl flask, add about 10 g of anhydrous potassium sulphate, 0.5 g of copper sulphate and 20 ml of sulphuric acid. Heat till the solution is green or blue. Cool and attach to ammonia distillation apparatus. The receiving flask should contain 50 ml of 1% boric acid. Add 100 ml of 3% w/v sodium hydroxide solution and heat. Collect about 125 ml of distillate and titrate the distillate with 0.1 N hydrochloric acid. Calculate nitrogen contents as under :

$$\% \text{ of total nitrogen} = \frac{\text{Titre value (ml)} \times 0.001402 \times 100 \times \text{dilution factor}}{\text{Weight of the sample (g) taken for analysis}}$$

Hydrocortisone acetate

Follow the method described in formulation 2 of the chapter on keratolytics and cleansers.

Glycine

Reagent

Indicator solution : 75 mg of phenolphthalein and 25 mg of thymol blue are dissolved in sufficient alcohol (50% v/v) to produce 100 ml.

Procedure

Weigh accurately a quantity of the sample equivalent to 100 ml of glycine, add 50 ml of water and shake. Filter, add 10 ml of formaldehyde previously neutralised to pH 9.0 and 4-5 drops of indicator solution. Titrate with 0.1 N sodium hydroxide until the yellow colour disappears and a faint violet colour appears. Each ml of 0.1 N sodium hydroxide consumed is equivalent to 0.007507 g of glycine.

Sodium acid phosphate, Calcium lactate, Magnesium chloride

Follow the method described in formulation 35 of the chapter on alimentary drugs.

Note : Conventional method of estimation by EDTA titration is not possible in presence of phosphate, as both calcium and magnesium get precipitated out with ammonia.

Clotrimazole/Econazole nitrate, Betamethasone dipropionate, Gentamicin sulphate

ESTIMATION

Clotrimazole

METHOD 1

Suspend accurately weighed quantity of sample in 100 ml of warm water, cool and extract with chloroform (3 × 25 ml), passing each extract through anhydrous sodium sulphate. Evaporate combined chloroform extract to dryness at 105°C. Dissolve the residue in previously neutralized glacial acetic acid (0.02 M perchloric acid). Carry out non-aqueous titration with 0.02 M perchloric acid using α-naphtholbenzein solution as indicator. Each ml of 0.02 M perchloric acid is equivalent to 6.896 mg of clotrimazole or 8.894 mg of econazole nitrate.

METHOD 2

Reagents

1. 0.1 N citric acid in water.
2. 0.1% w/v solution of acid orange 4S in 40% aqueous methanol.

Standard solution

100 mcg/ml in 0.1 N hydrochloric acid.

Sample solution

100 mcg/ml in 0.1 N hydrochloric acid (see formulation 5 of this chapter).

Procedure

To 1 ml each of sample and standard solutions, add 3 ml of citric acid solution and 2 ml of dye solution. Extract the colour with three 8 ml portions of chloroform. Make up the volume to 25 ml and pass through anhydrous sodium sulphate. The solution has absorption maxima at 422 nm. It follows Beer's law in the range of 2-14 mcg/ml, with detection limit of 0.05 µg/ml.

Note : Hydrolytic product of clotrimazole, betamethasone, lignocaine do not interfere. The method was found to be suitable for vaginal tablets, creams and optical solutions.

Betamethasone dipropionate

METHOD 1

Follow the method described in formulation 6 of this chapter for beclomethasone dipropionate.

METHOD 2

Reagents

1. Acidic methanol : Dilute 1.2 ml of hydrochloric acid to 1000 ml with methanol.
2. 0.5 M sodium chloride solution in water.
3. INH reagent : Dissolve 50 mg of isonicotinic acid hydrazide in 200 ml of acidic methanol.

Standard solution

20 mcg/ml of betamethasone dipropionate in chloroform.

Sample solution

Suspend accurately weighed quantity of the sample (cream) equivalent to 2 mg of betamethasone dipropionate in 30 ml of methanol (90%) and 50 ml of n-hexane, shake till cream is completely dispersed. Transfer the contents to a separating funnel and shake vigorously. Separate lower layer (methanol-water), extract organic layer with quantity of acid-methanol (2 × 20 ml). Combine the aqueous layer and discard the n-hexane layer. Add 100 ml of 0.5 M sodium chloride solution and extract with chloroform (3 × 30 ml), passing each extract through a bed of anhydrous sodium sulphate. Make up the volume to 100 ml with chloroform (20 mcg/ml).

Procedure

Evaporate 20 ml each of sample and standard solutions to dryness in water-bath at 60°C, cool and add 25 ml of INH reagent to each and keep in water-bath (50°C) for 90 min. Cool and measure the absorbance of both the solutions at 405 nm against reagent blank and calculate the results by comparison.

Gentamicin

Follow the microbiological method for antibiotics.

Miconazole nitrate, Neomycin sulphate, Betamethasone valerate

ESTIMATION

Miconazole nitrate

Reagents

1. Bromothymol blue solution : Dissolve 50 mg of water in 2 ml of 0.05 N sodium hydroxide and dilute to 500 ml with potassium biphthalate buffer, pH 3.5.
2. Potassium biphthalate buffer, pH 3.5.

Standard solution

400 mcg/ml of miconazole nitrate in chloroform.

Sample solution

Use chloroform extract reserved during estimation of neomycin sulphate.

Procedure

To 2 ml each of sample and standard solutions, add 10 ml of bromothymol blue solution and 50 ml of chloroform. Shake and transfer the chloroform layer to a 100 ml volumetric flask through a layer of anhydrous sodium sulphate. Make up the volume and measure the absorbance of both sample and standard solutions at 410 nm against reagent blank and calculate the results by comparison.

Neomycin sulphate

Reagents

1. Phosphate buffer, pH 8.0 : Dissolve 16.73 g of dipotassium hydrogen phosphate (anhydrous) and 0.523 g of potassium dihydrogen phosphate (anhydrous) in water to produce 1000 ml, adjust pH to 8.0.
2. Citrate buffer, pH 5.0 : Dissolve 2.94 g of sodium citrate, monohydrate in 100 ml of water, add 2.10 g of citric acid, dilute to 200 ml, adjust pH to 5.0.
3. Ninhydrin reagent :
   (a) 80 mg of chloride is dissolved in titrate buffer to produce 50 ml (heating may be required to dissolve).
   (b) 4.0% w/v solution of ninhydrin in water or methanol. Mix equal volumes of (a) and (b) just before estimation.

Standard solution

100 mcg/ml of neomycin sulphate in phosphate buffer.

Sample solution

Weigh sample (cream) equivalent to 10.0 mg of neomycin sulphate, suspend in 25 ml of phosphate buffer and extract with chloroform (3 × 30 ml). Collect chloroform in a dry 100 ml volumetric flask filtering each layer through same anhydrous sodium sulphate bed. Rinse sodium sulphate layer with chloroform, the combined chloroform layer is made up of volume (reserve chloroform layer for estimation of miconazole nitrate and Betamethasone valerate). Aqueous buffered layer heated in water-bath till no perceptible smell of chloroform is diluted to 100 ml with phosphate buffer and used for estimation of neomycin sulphate.

Procedure

To 5 ml each of sample, standard and buffer solutions add 5 ml of freshly prepared ninhydrin reagent and heat in water-bath for 20 min, cool, add 2 ml of methanol and dilute to 50 ml with phosphate buffer. Measure the absorbance of sample and standard against reagent blank at 570 nm and calculate the results by comparison.

Betamethasone valerate

Follow the general method for assay of steroids based on reaction with tetrazolium blue. Colour development may be carried out in chloroform. For details, refer to formulation 6 of this chapter.

Miconazole nitrate, Beclomethasone dipropionate or Hydrocortisone acetate, Chlorocresol

ESTIMATION

Miconazole nitrate

Reagents

1. Solochrome dark blue : 0.1% w/v solution of the dye in distilled water. The dye solution should be prepared immediately before use.
2. Buffer, pH 4.0 : Weigh and dissolve 5.1 g of potassium hydrogen phthalate in distilled water to make 500 ml.

Standard solution

Transfer accurately weighed about 50 mg of miconazole nitrate to volumetric flask containing about 50 ml of chloroform, warm in hot water-bath till a clear solution is obtained. Cool and dilute to 100 ml with chloroform. Further dilution of the standard solution may be done appropriately with chloroform to get a working standard of 100 mcg per ml.

Sample solution

Transfer accurately weighed quantity of the sample (cream) containing about 10 mg of the miconazole nitrate to a beaker, add about 50 ml of chloroform, warm for dissolving the substance. Transfer the contents to a 100 ml volumetric flask and dilute to the mark with chloroform.

Procedure

Transfer 10 ml each of the sample and standard solutions to 125 ml separating funnels. To each funnel, add 50 ml of chloroform, 5 ml of buffer solution and 5 ml of dye solution, shake gently and allow the layers to separate. Pass the chloroform layer through a bed of anhydrous sodium sulphate into dry flask. Measure the absorption of the coloured complex at about 513 nm against reagents blank prepared simultaneously. Calculate the results by comparison.

Beclomethasone dipropionate

METHOD 1

Reagents

1. Tetrazolium blue : 0.5% w/v solution in alcohol.
2. Tetramethyl ammonium hydroxide solution 10% v/v solution in ethanol.

Standard solution

10 mcg per ml beclomethasone dipropionate in (TMAH) alcohol.

Sample solution

Weigh accurately the quantity of the sample (cream) equivalent to 2.5 mg of beclomethasone dipropionate and transfer to a separating funnel containing 50 ml methanol, shake for few minutes, add 100 ml cyclohexane and shake vigorously. Allow the layer to separate and transfer the lower layer (methanolic) to a separating funnel containing about 50 ml of brine solution. Extract the cyclohexane layer with further two 10 ml portions of brine solution. Extract the cyclohexane layer with further 2 × 10 ml portions of alcohol and collect the alcohol layer into a separating funnel containing brine solution. Shake vigorously to mix the contents. The aqueous layer is extracted with four 20 ml portions of chloroform. The combined chloroform extract is evaporated and the residue is taken in alcohol. Filter through cotton plug if necessary and make up the volume to 50 ml. Further dilution of the sample solution may be carried out with alcohol to get a solution of 20 mcg/ml.

Procedure

10 ml each of standard and sample solutions is taken in 25 ml volumetric flask. Add 2 ml of tetrazolium blue solution and 2 ml of tetramethyl ammonium hydroxide, shake gently and allow to stand in water-bath at 25-35°C for 90 min and measure the absorption of resulting solutions at 525 nm against the reagent blank (chloroform + both the reagents) and calculate the results by comparing with standard.

Note : It is always preferable to carry out the above procedure using aldehyde-free ethyl alcohol. As ethyl alcohol is not easily available, the following alternative methods based on practical experience are suggested to give excellent reproducible results.

The standard solution should be initially prepared in methanol and further diluted appropriately with chloroform to get working standard (10 mcg/ml).

The chloroform extract of the sample need not be evaporated, instead can be further diluted to get appropriate final concentration (comparable with standard—10-20 mcg/ml).

Solutions of TMAH and tetrazolium blue may be prepared in methanol.

This modified procedure is suitable for most of the steroidal compounds.

METHOD 2

Reagents

1. 0.05% w/v solution of tetrazolium blue (BTZ) in methanol (stable for 7 days).
2. 0.1 N tetrabutyl ammonium hydroxide (TBAH) in methanol.
3. Glacial acetic acid.
4. Methanol.

Standard solution

10 mcg/ml of beclomethasone dipropionate in methanol.

Sample solution

Suspend an accurately weighed quantity of the sample (cream) containing 0.5 mg of the substance in 20 ml of methanol, dissolve by gentle stirring and filter through G_3 sintered glass funnel, wash the residue on funnel with methanol and adjust the filtrate to 25 ml with methanol. Further dilutions are made to get solution of 10 mcg/ml.

Procedure

To 1 ml each of sample and standard solutions, add 6 ml of TBAH reagent and 2 ml of BTZ solution. Heat on water-bath at 70°C for 15 min, cool to room temperature and dilute to 10 ml with glacial acetic acid. Measure the absorbance of both the solutions at 515 nm against reagent blank and calculate the results by comparison.

Note : 1. The method obeys Beer's law in the concentration range of 2-50 mcg/ml.
2. Clotrimazole and neomycin commonly present in antifungal formulations do not interfere.
3. As the reaction is specific for α-ketol group, other non-steroidal drugs do not interfere.
4. Rate and extent of formazan formation bears inverse relationship with dielectric constant of the solvent used in the reaction, the formazan formation is faster in methanol than in ethanol (solvent in official method). In chloroform, though the reaction is faster, but has lower sensitivity.

Chlorocresol

Follow the method described in formulation 11 of the chapter on keratolytics and cleansers.

Miconazole nitrate, Fluocinolone acetonide

ESTIMATION

Miconazole nitrate

METHOD 1

Follow the methanol described in formulation 4 of this chapter or titration with sodium lauryl sulphate using dimethyl yellow as indicator (see formulation of the chapter on analgesics and antipyretics under dicyclomine HCl).

METHOD 2

Follow the non-aqueous titration method determining the end point potentiometrically or using crystal violet as indicator. Each ml of 0.01 M perchloric acid is equivalent to 0.004792 g of miconazole nitrate.

METHOD 3

Reagents

1. 1 mg/ml of tropactin in water : Dissolve the dye in water by slight warming. Wash the dye solution with chloroform (1 × 25 ml), discard chloroform layer.
2. pH 3.0 phosphate buffer : Dissolve 1.67 g of citric acid monohydrate and 1 g of sodium phosphate, dibasic in 100 ml of water.
3. Acidified methanol : 1 ml of sulphuric acid in 100 ml of methanol.

Standard solution

400 mcg/ml of miconazole nitrate in chloroform.

Sample preparation

Disperse accurately weighed quantity of sample (cream, ointment) equivalent to 4 mg of miconazole nitrate in water and extract with chloroform (3 × 25 ml), passing each extract through anhydrous sulphate placed in a funnel over cotton plug and make up the volume.

Procedure

To 15 ml each of sample and standard solutions add 3 ml of dye solution, 10 ml of phosphate buffer, pH 3.0 and 15 ml of chloroform. Shake for about 2-3 min and allow the layers to separate. Collect chloroform layer and repeat the extraction with chloroform (2 × 30 ml). Combine the chloroform layers, add 3 ml of acidified methanol and dilute to 100 ml with chloroform. Concomitantly measure the absorbance of solutions at about 540 nm and calculate the results by comparison.

Fluocinolone acetonide

Follow the method described in formulation 8 of this chapter.

Fluocinolone acetonide, Iodochlorhydroxyquinoline (Chinoform), Tolnaftate

ESTIMATION

Fluocinolone acetonide

Reagent

1. Dehydrated alcohol, aldehyde free.
2. Methanolic sodium chloride : Dilute 20 mg of 10% sodium chloride solution (aqueous) to 100 ml with methanol.
3. Tetrazolium blue solution : 0.5% w/v solution in aldehyde free alcohol.
4. Dilute tetramethyl ammonium hydroxide solution (TMAH) : Dilute 1 ml of 10% sodium to 10 ml with aldehyde free alcohol.
5. Saturated solution of sodium chloride in water.
6. 5% w/v solution of aluminium potassium sulphate in water.

Standard solution

20 mcg/ml of fluocinolone acetonide in aldehyde free alcohol.

Sample solution

To accurately weighed quantity of sample (cream, ointment) equivalent to 0.5 g of fluocinolone acetonide, add 50 ml of cyclohexane, 25 ml of methanol and 1 ml of saturated solution of sodium chloride. Shake and allow the layers to separate. Cyclohexane layer is extracted with 10-15 ml of methanolic sodium chloride solution and aqueous layer is combined with the first extract. Dilute the combined methanolic extract to 100 ml with aluminium potassium sulphate solution and extract with chloroform (4 × 20 ml), passing each chloroform extract through anhydrous sodium phosphate. Evaporate combined chloroform layer and dissolve the residue in aldehyde free alcohol to get solution of 20 mcg/ml.

Procedure

To each 10 ml of sample and standard solutions, add 10 ml of aldehyde free alcohol, 2 ml of tetrazolium blue solution and 2 ml of dilute TMAH solution. Keep in dark for 60 min and measure the absorbance of both the solutions at maximum at about 525 nm against reagent blank and calculate the results by comparison.

Iodochlorhydroxyquinoline (Chinoform)

Reagent

1. 10% w/v solution of copper sulphate in water.

Standard solution

100 mcg/ml of chinoform in chloroform.

Sample solution

To accurately weighed quantity of the sample equivalent to 100 mg of iodochlorhydroxyquinoline, add 50 ml of ethyl acetate, keep on water-bath and dissolve the residue obtained in chloroform to get a solution of 100 mcg/ml.

Procedure

To 10 ml each of sample and standard solutions, add 10 ml of copper sulphate solution, shake vigorously and allow the layers to separate. Pass chloroform layer through anhydrous sulphate and measure the absorbance of both sample and standard solutions at 430 nm against reagent blank and calculate the results by comparison.

Note : If aldehyde free alcohol is not easily avoidable then colour development of both standard and sample can be carried out with chloroform solution. For details refer to formulation of this chapter.

Tolnaftate

Transfer portion of the sample (semi-solid) equivalent to 10 mg of the substance to a separator, add 70-80 ml of chloroform and wash successively with 0.1 N sodium hydroxide (2 × 25 ml) and 0.1 N hydrochloric acid (2 × 25 ml). Dilute chloroform layer to 100 ml (10 mcg/ml). Measure the absorbance at maximum at about 250 nm and compare the results with standard solution (10 mcg/ml in chloroform).

Clobetasol propionate, Miconazole nitrate

ESTIMATION

Clobetasol propionate

METHOD 1

Follow the methanol described in formulation 8 of this chapter.

METHOD 2

Reagents

1. 0.05% w/v solution of blue tetrazolium (BTZ) in methanol. The solution is stable for 7 days.
2. 0.1 N tetrabutyl ammonium hydroxide (TBAH).
3. Glacial acetic acid.
4. Methanol.
5. Toluene.

Standard solution

50 mcg/ml of clobetasol propionate in methanol.

Sample solution

Suspend accurately weighed quantity of the sample equivalent to 50 mg of the substance in 25 ml of methanol, filter and use the filtrate for analysis.

Procedure

To 1 ml each of sample and standard solutions, add 2 ml of tetrazolium blue reagent and 6.5 ml of TBAH reagent. Heat on water-bath (80°C) for 5 min, cool to room temperature and dilute to 10 ml with glacial acetic acid. Measure the absorbance of red-coloured complex at 513 nm against reagent blank and calculate the results by comparison. The method obeys Beer's law in the concentration range of 5-40 mcg/ml and red-coloured complex is stable up to 2 hrs.

Miconazole nitrate

Follow the method 2 (non-aqueous titration) described in formulation 7 of this chapter.

Halcinonide, Econazole nitrate

ESTIMATION

Halcinonide

Standard solution

30 mcg/ml of halcinonide in chloroform.

Sample solution

Weigh accurately sample (cream) equivalent to 30 mg of halcinonide, add 60 ml of chloroform, warm to disperse the sample, cool and make up to 100 ml with chloroform, pass through anhydrous sodium sulphate and use for estimation.

Procedure

To 10 ml each of sample and standard solutions in chloroform, add 10 ml of isoniazid reagent, shake and keep in water-bath (55 + 1°C) for 30 min, cool and dilute to 25 ml with chloroform. Measure the absorbance of sample and standard solutions at about 390 nm against reagent blank and calculate the results by comparison.

Econazole nitrate

Weigh accurately sample (cream) equivalent to 50 mg of econazole nitrate acid and extract with chloroform (3 × 30 ml), passing each extract through same bed of anhydrous sodium sulphate. Dry the combined chloroform extract in vacuum oven at 60°C. Cool and take up the residue in 50 ml of glacial acetic acid by slight warming. Titrate with 0.01 N perchloric acid (violet). Carry out the blank titration for final calculations. Each ml of 0.01 N perchloric acid is equivalent to 4.447 mg of econazole nitrate.

Hydrocortisone acetate, Lidocaine, Allantoin, Zinc oxide

ESTIMATION

Hydrocortisone acetate

Follow the method for estimation of steroids using tetrazolium blue or triphenyl tetrazolium chloride. The absorption of the resulting coloured solution is measured at 550 nm or 490 nm depending on nature of tetrazolium salt used.

Lidocaine

Accurately weighed quantity of the sample (ointment) is suspended in water with slight warming. Extract with chloroform (3 × 50 ml). Wash the combined chloroform layer with 25 ml of water (discard the aqueous layer). Evaporate chloroform layer to dryness and carry non-aqueous titration by titrating with 0.1 N perchloric acid (crystal violet or brilliant green). Each ml of 0.1 N perchloric acid is equivalent to 23.43 mg of lidocaine.

Allantoin

Reagents

    (a) 2.5 w/v solution of dimethylglycoxime in concentrated hydrochloric acid.
    (b) To 1 g of thiosemicarbazide, add 100 ml of hydrochloric acid (1 : 1), heat in water-bath for 15 min, cool and filter.

    Mix 10 ml each of solution (a) and (b), add sufficient hydrochloric acid (1 : 1) and produce 100 ml, prepare the reagent fresh on the day of use.

Standard solution

50 mcg/ml of allantoin in 0.1 N hydrochloric acid, gentle warming may be necessary to effect the solution.

Sample solution

Accurately weighed quantity of sample (ointment) equivalent to 15 mg of the substance is suspended in 50 ml of 0.1 N hydrochloric acid with the aid of heating in a water-bath. Cool and shake with 20 ml of chloroform. Reject organic layer and dilute the acid layer to 100 ml. Filter and dilute appropriately to get final concentration of 30 mcg/ml for analysis.

Procedure

To 5 ml each of sample, standard and blank solutions, add 10 ml of the dimethylglycoxime-thiosemicarbazide reagent. Heat on a water-bath at 90°C for 30 min, cool and dilute to 50 ml with hydrochloric acid (1 : 1). Measure the absorbance of both test and standard solutions at about 525 nm against reagent blank and calculate the results by comparison.

Note : Entire procedure is carried out in actinic liquid (use of amber coloured flasks).

Zinc oxide

Ignite sample equivalent to about 150 mg of zinc oxide in a platinum crucible at 700°C. Cool, add few drops of concentrates sulphuric acid and 20 ml of water, warm to dissolve and transfer the contents to a conical flask. Wash the crucible with water and transfer the washings to the conical flask. Adjust the pH to 10.5 with ammonia-ammonium chloride buffer and titrate with 0.05 M EDTA (Eviochrome Black T). Each ml of 0.05 M EDTA is equivalent to 4.069 mg of zinc oxide.

Clotrimazole, Lignocaine hydrochloride

ESTIMATION

Clotrimazole

Transfer accurately weighed sample (ear drops) equivalent to 100 mg of clotrimazole to a separating funnel containing about 20 ml of water. Extract with solvent ether (3 × 40 ml). Wash the combined ethereal layer with 20 ml of water and pass through anhydrous sodium sulphate (pressure the combined aqueous layer for estimation of lignocaine hydrochloride). Evaporate ether layer on water-bath, cool and add 5 ml of acetic anhydride and 15-20 ml of dioxane. Carry out the non-aqueous titration using α-naphtholbenzein indicator (end point, pink to green). Each ml of 0.02 N perchloric acid is equivalent to 6.896 g clotrimazole.

Lignocaine hydrochloride

Titrate the entire aqueous layer preserved during estimation of clotrimazole with 0.1 N silver nitrate using potassium chromate as indicator. Each ml of 0.1 N silver nitrate is equivalent to 28.88 mg of lignocaine hydrochloride.

Formulation 13

Tinidazole, Miconazole nitrate

ESTIMATION

Tinidazole

Follow the method described in formulation 14 of this chapter.

Miconazole nitrate

Reagents

1. Cobalt thiocyanate reagent : To 20 g of ammonium thiocyanate in 100 ml of water, add 5 g of cobalt nitrate, shake to dissolve. Add sufficient sodium chloride to saturate the solution.

Standard solution

Treat 40 mg of miconazole nitrate as described under preparation of sample solution.

Sample solution

An accurately weighed quantity of powdered sample equivalent to 50 mg of miconazole nitrate is suspended in 10 ml of water, basify with ammonia solution and extract with chloroform (4 × 50 ml). Combined chloroform layer is shaken with 15-20 ml of saturated solution of sodium chloride, separated, passed through anhydrous sodium sulphate, concentrated to about 60-70 ml and then finally adjusted to 100 ml.

Procedure

To 25 ml each of sample and standard solutions, add 10 ml of cobalt thiocyanate reagent, shake for 5 min. Separate organic layer, pass through anhydrous sodium sulphate, measure the absorbance at about 617 nm against regent blank processed similarly.

Note : 1. Solutions may sometime develop haziness if the laboratory working temperature is below 20°C.
2. Both the components can be identified by TLC by applying methanolic solution and n-hexane-chloroform-methanol-ammonia (60 + 30 + 10 + 1) as mobile phase, detection by exposing to iodine vapours.

Tinidazole, Clotrimazole

ESTIMATION

Tinidazole

Standard solution

20 mcg/ml of tinidazole in water (slight warming may be necessary to aid the solution).

Sample solution

Accurately weighed quantity of the finely powdered sample equivalent to 50 mg of tinidazole is suspended in 70-80 ml of water and heated in a water-bath for about 15 min, cooled, filtered and diluted to 100 ml with water/methanol. 2 ml of the filtrate is further diluted with water/methanol to 100 ml (20 mcg/ml).

Measure the extinction of both sample and standard solutions at about 310 nm and calculate to results by comparison.

Clotrimazole

Suspend accurately weighed quantity of powdered sample equivalent to 100 mg of the substance in 10-15 ml of water. Add 10 ml of 1 N sulphuric acid and shake to obtain a uniform suspension. Add 30 ml of chloroform, 0.2 ml of indicator solution (dimethyl yellow), shake vigorously and titrate with 0.02 N sodium lauryl sulphate (SLS), shaking vigorously after each addition.

Each ml of 0.02 M SLS is equivalent to 6.987 mg of clotrimazole.

Clotrimazole, Sulphamethoxazole

ESTIMATION

Clotrimazole

Standard solution

100 mcg/ml of clotrimazole in 0.1 N hydrochloric acid.

Sample solution

Accurately weighed quantity of the sample equivalent to 100 mg of the substance was shaken with 50-60 ml of 0.1 N hydrochloric acid and placed in a shaker at 37°C for 2 hrs. The volume was adjusted to 100 ml with acid and filtered through G_3 sintered funnel.

Procedure

To 2 ml each of sample and standard solutions, add 8 ml of perchloric acid (70%), mix and place in boiling water-bath for 5 min. The orange yellow colour formed was measured at about 440 nm after cooling to room temperature against reagent blank. Deduce the results by comparison.

Clotrimazole in the formulation can be estimated by titration with sodium lauryl sulphate. Equivalent factor for sodium lauryl sulphate can be determined by titration with clotrimazole of known purity using methyl yellow as indicator. Refer to the procedure for dicyclomine in formulation 10 of the chapter on analgesics and antipyretics.

Sulphamethoxazole

Weigh accurate quantity of the sample equivalent to 500 mg of the sample, add 20 ml of glacial acetic acid, 40 ml water and 15 ml hydrochloric acid. Shake to dissolve and carry out sodium nitrite titration. Each ml of 0.1 M sodium nitrite is equivalent to 0.02533 g of sulphamethoxazole.

Cetrimide, Chlorhexidine gluconate

ESTIMATION

Cetrimide

Reagents

1. Bromophenol blue solution : Prepare a 0.04% w/v solution of bromophenol blue in 20% v/v isopropyl alcohol in distilled water.
2. 0.001 M sodium lauryl sulphate solution : Dissolve about 0.3 g of sodium lauryl sulphate in 1000 ml of water. To stabilize the solution, see formulation 10 of the chapter on analgesics and antipyretics.
3. 0.001 M cetrimide solution : Dissolve 0.35 g of cetrimide of known strength in a small amount of warm distilled water, cool and dilute to 1000 ml.

Sample solution

Dilute the sample equivalent to 0.3 g of cetrimide to 100 ml with distilled water. Further dilute 10.0 ml of the above solution to 100 ml with distilled water.

Procedure

Pipette a 25.0 ml aliquot of the sample solution into a tall, narrow-necked, glass-stoppered bottle of 250 ml, add 50 ml of chloroform, 50 ml of 0.001 M sodium lauryl sulphate solution and 5-10 drops of bromophenol blue solution. Make the contents of the bottle alkaline with sodium carbonate solution (10%). Prepare a blank in the same manner omitting the substance to be analysed.

Titrate both blank and sample solutions with 0.001 M cetrimide solution shaking after each addition of titrant. The end-point is indicated by the appearance of the permanent blue colour in the chloroform layer.

Note : The solution should remain alkaline during titration. The method utilises the stochiometric reaction between cetrimide and sodium lauryl sulphate. An excess of the reactant is added to the diluted sample followed by back titration of the excess sodium lauryl sulphate with a standard cetrimide solution.

Chlorhexidine gluconate

METHOD 1

Reagents

1. Alkaline sodium hypobromite solution : Dissolve 10 g of sodium hydroxide in 400 ml of distilled water and add, in small portions, 2.75 ml of bromine until the bromine is completely dissolved. Adjust the volume of the solution to 500 ml and standardize the solution as follows :

Pipette 10.0 ml of the solution into a 250 ml conical flask and add 25 ml of distilled water, 2 g of potassium iodide and 10 ml of glacial acetic acid. Titrate the liberated iodine with 0.1 N sodium thiosulphate solution. Each ml of 0.1 N sodium thiosulphate solution is equal to 0.0080 g of bromine. Based on the figure obtained, adjust the sodium hypobromite solution with distilled water to contain 1.5% w/v of available bromine. The reagent is then prepared by mixing 66 ml of the latter solution with 33 ml of 3 N sodium hydroxide solution.

Standard solution

Weigh accurately about 300 mg of chlorhexidine gluconate into a 100 ml volumetric flask, dissolve and dilute to volume with distilled water. Dilute 10 ml of this to 100 ml with water.

Sample solution

Dilute sample equivalent to 30 mg of chlorhexidine gluconate to 100 ml with water.

Procedure

To 5 ml each of standard and sample preparations, add 70 ml of water, 5 ml of cetrimide solution and 1 ml of isopropyl alcohol. Maintain the solutions at 20°C and add 2.0 ml of sodium hypobromite solution. Adjust to volume with distilled water and after 25 minutes measure the absorbance of both the solutions at about 480 nm using a reagent blank prepared in the same manner omitting the substance to be analysed.

METHOD 2
Reagents

1. Phosphate buffer, pH 5.7 : 100 ml of 0.1 M citric acid and 140 ml of 0.2 M disodium hydrogen phosphate are mixed to get the buffer of pH 5.7.
2. Bromocresol green solution : 0.03% solution in phosphate buffer, pH 5.7.

Standard solution

50 mcg/ml of chlorhexidine in water.

Sample solution

Accurately measured volume of the sample (lotions, shampoos, viscous solutions), equivalent to 10 mg of the substance is basified with 10 N sodium hydroxide and extracted with chloroform (2 × 20 ml), combine chloroform layer and dilute to 50 ml.

Procedure

To 1 ml each of sample and standard solutions, add 3 ml of dye solution and 5 ml of chloroform. Shake for 3 min and centrifuge. Measure the absorbance of chloroform layer at 410 nm against reagent blank and calculate the results by comparison.

Silver sulphadiazine, Chlorhexidine gluconate

ESTIMATION

Silver sulphadiazine

Standard solution

To 50 mg of silver sulphadiazine, add 100 ml of water and 25 ml of concentrated hydrochloric acid, shake well and dilute to 250 ml. Filter and dilute to 10 ml of the filtrate to 100 ml with water (20 mcg/ml).

Sample solution

Accurately weighed amount of sample (cream) equivalent to 50 mg of the substance is heated as under standard solution.

Procedure

Take 10 ml each of sample and standard solutions and proceed with diazotization and colour development as described under formulation 1 of the chapter on anti-malarials.

Chlorhexidine gluconate

Suspend the sample in 20 ml of water, add 10 ml of 1 N hydrochloric acid and shake with chloroform (3 × 25 ml), reject the chloroform layer and dilute the aqueous layer to get 300 mcg/ml.

Procedure

To 100 ml each of sample and standard solutions (300 mcg/ml) add to each 10 ml of sodium hydroxide (10%), 5 ml of cetrimide solution (2%), 1 ml of isopropyl alcohol and 2 ml of bromine water, dilute to 100 ml and allow to stand for 20 min. Measure the absorbance at 480 nm and calculate the results by comparison or by taking 214 as value of A 1%, 1 cm at 480 nm.

Paraformaldehyde, Formaldehyde

ESTIMATION

Paraformaldehyde in tooth paste

Reagents

1. 0.01 N sodium hydroxide.
2. 0.002 N sodium hydroxide.
3. 2 N sodium hydroxide.
4. 1% w/v phenylhydrazinium hydrochloride solution.
5. 5% w/v potassium ferricyanide solution, to be prepared just before use.
6. Hydrochloric acid, concentrated.

Linearity curve

Standard solution

Dissolve 100 mg of paraformaldehyde in 10 ml of 2 N sodium hydroxide and dilute to 100 ml with distilled water. Dilute suitably with distilled water to get 25 mcg/ml solution of paraformaldehyde.

To series of 50 ml volumetric flasks, transfer accurately 0.5, 1.0, 1.5, 2.0, 3.0, 4.0, 5.0, 6.0, 7.0 and 8.0 ml of standard solution. Add appropriate amount of 0.002 N sodium hydroxide to produce 10 ml of total volume in each flask. Add 5 ml of phenylhydrazinium hydrochloride reagent to each flask followed by 5 ml of 0.5 N hydrochloric acid and 1 ml of potassium ferricyanide reagent. Mix well and add 10 ml of hydrochloric acid to each flask, keep aside for 30 minutes. Measure the absorption of the resulting solutions at about 520 nm using a reagent blank prepared in the same manner omitting the substance (paraformaldehyde). Draw the standard curve to check the linearity.

Sample solution

Dissolve 1 g of the paste in 5 ml of 0.1 N sodium hydroxide, dilute to 100 ml with distilled water. Centrifuge in stoppered centrifuge tube for 20 minutes at 3000 rpm.

Take 5.0 ml each of standard (25 mcg/ml solution as prepared under linearity studies) and sample solution and proceed with colour development as described under general procedure for linearity studies.

The method obeys Beer's law in the range of 25-200 mcg/ml.

Formaldehyde in tooth paste

Standard solution

Dilute 5 ml of formaldehyde solution (40% w/v) to 100 ml with water. Further dilutions are done with 0.2 N sodium hydroxide to get a concentration of 25 mcg/ml.

For sample preparation and procedure for estimation, refer to the method described above for paraformaldehyde.

Clotrimazole, Selenium sulfide

ESTIMATION

Clotrimazole

METHOD 1

Follow the method described in formulation 4 of this chapter.

METHOD 2

Reagents

1. Phthalate buffer, pH 2.5.
2. 0.1% w/v solution of bromocresol in water.

Standard solution

200 mcg/ml of clotrimazole in isopropyl alcohol.

Sample solution

Weigh accurately sample equivalent to 25 mg of the substance, add 25 ml of isopropyl alcohol, slightly warm, vortex for 2 min and make up the volume to 100 ml.

Procedure

To 5 ml each of sample and standard solutions, add 5 ml of buffer solution and 2.5 ml of the dye and 10 ml of chloroform. Shake vigorously and allow the layers to separate. Measure the absorption of chloroform layer at 430 nm and calculate the results by comparison.

METHOD 3

Reagents

1. 1% w/v solution p-chloranil in 1,4-dioxane.
2. 1,4-dioxane.
3. 0.1 N hydrochloric acid.

Standard and sample solutions

As described under method 2.

Procedure

To 5 ml each of sample and standard solutions, add 2 ml of chloranil reagent and keep in boiling water-bath for 60 min, cool, add 15 ml of dioxane to dissolve the residue completely. Add 2 ml of 0.1 N hydrochloric acid, shake well and dilute to 25 ml with isopropyl alcohol. Concomitantly measure the absorbance of both sample and standard solutions at 475 nm against reagent blank prepared by taking 5 ml of isopropyl alcohol and calculate the results by comparison.

Selenium sulfide

Reagent

Fuming nitric acid : To 250 ml concentrated nitric acid, add slowly and carefully 3 ml of formaldehyde. When the reaction is completed, close it properly. This addition should be done in fuming chamber.

Procedure

Accurately weighed quantity to the sample (semi-solid) equivalent to 100 mg of the substance is digested with 25 ml of nitric acid for 2 hours at hot plate, cool and dilute to 250 ml with water. To 50 ml of this solution, add 20 ml water, 10 g urea and heat to boiling till volume is reduced to almost half. Cool, add 10 ml of dilute sulphuric acid and 10 ml of potassium iodide (10%) and titrate with 0.05 N sodium thiosulphate using starch as indicator. End point is reddish brown. Each ml of 0.05 N sodium thiosulphate is equivalent to 987 µg of selenium (Se) or 1.789 mg of selenium sulfide (SeS_2).

Cetrimide, Calcium pantothenate

ESTIMATION

Cetrimide

Reagents

1. 0.1 N sodium hydroxide.
2. 5% w/v solution of potassium iodide in water.
3. 0.05 M potassium iodate.

Procedure

Measure accurately quantity of the sample containing about 2.0 g of cetrimide, dilute to 100 ml with water. To 25 ml of the solution, add 10 ml of 0.1 N sodium hydroxide and 10 ml of freshly prepared solution of potassium iodide. Extract with four 20 ml portions of chloroform. Discard the chloroform layer. To the aqueous layer, add 50 ml of hydrochloric acid and titrate with 0.05 M potassium iodate till the solution is pale brown, add 2 ml of chloroform and continue titration, shaking well between each addition, until the chloroform layer is colourless. Carry out blank titration with 25 ml of water, 10 ml of potassium iodide. Difference between the two titrations represents the volume of 0.05 M potassium iodate consumed by the sample actually taken for analysis. Each ml of 0.05 M potassium iodate is equivalent to 0.03364 g of cetrimide.

Calcium pantothenate

Follow the method 1 for estimation of calcium pantothenate under chapter on vitamins.

Typical laboratory analysis

Cetrimide
Volume of the sample taken for analysis = 25 ml
Volume of 0.05 M potassium iodate consumed by the sample = 16.1 ml
Volume of 0.05 M potassium iodate consumed in blank titration = 30.3 ml
Net volume of potassium iodate consumed by the sample = 14.2 ml
Each ml of 0.05 M potassium iodate is equivalent to 0.03364 g of cetrimide.

$$\text{Contents of cetrimide (\%)} = \frac{14.2 \times 0.03364 \times 100 \times 100}{25 \times 40}$$

$$= 4.78 \text{ g}$$
$$\text{Claim} = 5.0 \text{ g}$$
$$\% \text{ claim} = 95.54$$

Calcium pantothenate
Weight of standard taken = 0.151 g
Volume of the sample taken = 7.5 ml (wt./ml = 1.02)

Contents of calcium pantothenate (%) $= \dfrac{A_u}{A_s} \times \dfrac{0.151}{100} \times \dfrac{5}{50} \times \dfrac{100}{7.5} \times \dfrac{50}{5} \times \dfrac{1.02}{1} \times 100$

$= \dfrac{0.286}{0.298} \times \dfrac{0.151}{7.5} \times \dfrac{1.02}{1} \times \dfrac{100}{1}$

$= 98.55\%$ of claim (2%)

Nitrofurantoin, Deglycyrrhizinised liquorice, Trimethoprim

ESTIMATION

Nitrofurantoin

METHOD 1

Reagents

1. Dimethylformamide (DMF).
2. Buffer solution : It contains 1.8% w/v sodium acetate and 0.14% v/v glacial acetic acid in water. It has approximately pH of 5.50.

Procedure

To a quantity of the powdered sample equivalent to 30 mg of nitrofurantoin, add 50 ml of dimethyl-formamide, shake for 5 minutes and add sufficient water to produce 500 ml, mix thoroughly. Dilute 10 ml of the above solution to 100 ml (6 mcg/ml) with the buffer solution and filter through G_4 sintered glass funnel. Collect 20 ml portion after discarding first 15 to 20 ml of the filtrate. Measure the absorption at 367 nm using 1% v/v solution of dimethylformamide as blank. Calculate the contents of nitrofurantoin per tablet by taking 765 as the value of A 1%, 1 cm at 367 nm.

METHOD 2

Reagents

1. 0.1% w/v solution of resorcinol in water.
2. 1.5 N sodium hydroxide.

Standard solution

100 mcg/ml of nitrofurantoin in water.

Sample solution

Accurately weighed or measured quantity of the sample (tablets, capsule or suspension) equivalent to 10 mg of nitrofurantoin is shaken with 50-60 ml of water, filtered and volume adjusted to 100 ml with water.

Procedure

To 1 ml each of the standard and sample solutions, add 1.5 ml of resorcinol reagent and 1 ml of 1.5 N sodium hydroxide. Immerse the flask in boiling water-bath for 15 minutes, cool and adjust to 10 ml with water. The absorption of pink colour is measured at 535 nm against reagent blank. The method obeys Beer's law in the range of 2-14 mcg/ml.

METHOD 3

Reagents

1. 0.05 w/v solution of isoniazid in water.
2. 0.1 N sodium hydroxide.

Standard solution

100 mcg/ml of nitrofurantoin in water.

Sample solution

Weigh accurately sample equivalent to 10 mg of nitrofurantoin, add 50 ml of water, shake for 5 minutes and filter. Wash the residue twice with 25 ml of water, mix the filtrate and dilute to 100 ml with water.

Procedure

To 0.5 ml each of the sample and standard solutions add 0.5 ml of isoniazid reagent and 2.0 ml of 0.1 N sodium hydroxide and dilute to 10 ml with water. Measure the absorbance of the colour after 5 minutes at 390 nm against reagent blank. The method obeys Beer's law in the concentration range of 1-10 mcg/ml of the final solution. Yellow colour is stable for 30 minutes.

METHOD 4

Reagents

1. Dimethylformamide (DMF) : Before use treat with activated charcoal (2 g/100 ml) for 5 min and filter.
2. 0.1 M tetraethylammonium hydroxide in methyl alcohol (TEAH).
3. 0.1% v/v acetone in DMF.

Standard solution

20 mcg/ml of nitrofurantoin in DMF.

Sample solution

Sample equivalent to 50 mg of nitrofurantoin is extracted with DMF and suitably diluted with DMF to get a concentration of 25 mcg/ml.

Procedure

To 1 ml each of sample and standard solutions, add 8 ml of DMF, 0.2 ml acetone solution, 0.5 ml of 'TEAH' reagent and dilute to 10 ml with DMF. Measure the absorbance of both the solutions after 8 minutes at about 540 nm against reagent blank. The method obeys Beer's law in the concentration range of 1-60 mcg/ml.

Note : 1. The entire method should be carried out in low actinic light, for which amber coloured glass apparatus is recommended.
2. The method can also be applied to creams, ointments and dusting powder containing nitrofurantoin.

Liquorice deglycrrhizinated (estimated as glycyrrhizic acid)

METHOD 1

Reagent

1. 3% w/v solution of trichloro-acetic acid in acetone.

Procedure

Weigh a portion of the sample equivalent to 1 g of liquorice and transfer to a 250 ml beaker. Add 50 ml, hot trichloroacetic acid solution and keep for 20 minutes, stir with glass rod. Allow the mixture to stand for 3 minutes and decant the liquid into filter paper No. 41. Repeat the extraction two more times by adding 25 ml of hot trichloroacetic acid solution and steeping for 15 minutes each time. With the third extraction, transfer the solids and liquid to the filter paper. Wash the beaker and filter paper containing residue with 25 ml of acetone. Collect the extracts in 250 ml beaker, add drop by drop strong ammonia solution and stir until an abundant cheesy precipitates are formed. Adjust pH to 8.3 to 8.6, transfer the precipitates together with the mother liquor to a sintered glass funnel. Wash the residue with 50 ml of acetone in 3-4 stage. Pass water through sintered funnel in which precipitation is made and transfer the resultant solution quantitatively to 250 ml volumetric flask. Dilute 20 ml of the resulting solution to 100 ml with water and determine the absorption at 248 nm against water as blank.

Content of glycyrrhizic acid (glycoside of glycyrrhetinic acid) (X) =

$$= \frac{D \times 822.92 \times 100 \times 100 \times 250}{a \times b \times 11400 \times 1000}$$

where X = glycyrrhizic acid content;

     D = absorption of the final solution at 258 nm;

     a = weight of the sample taken for analysis;

     b = volume (ml) of final solution taken for analysis;

822.92 = molecular weight of glycyrrhizic acid ($C_{42}H_{62}O_{16}$);

11400 = molar index of absorption.

Note : Do not use filter paper, as it is difficult to wash the residue free of nitrofurantoin which will otherwise contribute to absorption at 258 nm.

METHOD 2

The method is based on coupling of acidic genin, 18β-glycyrrhetinic acid obtained after acid hydrolysis with a basic dye, methylene blue to yield a blue coloured complex.

Reagents

1. 0.1% w/v solution of methylene blue in water.
2. Citrate-phosphate-borate buffer, pH 9.2.
3. 6 N sulphuric acid.
4. Ethyl alcohol.

Standard solution

500 mcg/ml glycyrrhetinic acid in chloroform.

Sample solution

Weigh sample accurately equivalent to 1 g of liquorice, add 20 ml of boiling water. Transfer the contents to a separating funnel and wash the residue with further two 10 ml portions of boiling water, cool, add 5 ml of ethyl alcohol and 1 ml of 6 N sulphuric acid. Shake gently with three 20 ml portions of chloroform. Discard chloroform layer, transfer aqueous phases and the residue to boiling flask with the help of 5 ml of water and 10 ml of 6 N sulphuric acid. Heat in boiling water-bath for 20 minutes. While hot, transfer to a separator and extract with four 20 ml portions of chloroform. Pass chloroform through 2 g of anhydrous sodium sulphate and dilute to 100 ml with chloroform.

Procedure

To 20 ml of chloroform layer of sample solution, add 20 ml of buffer, pH 9.2 and 2 ml of dye solution.

Shake for 1 minute and allow to separate (after separation, the aqueous layer must be blue in colour, if it has greenish or yellow colour, add 1 ml more of dye solution and re-shake). Separate chloroform layer and shake with 5 ml of pH 9.2 buffer and separate chloroform layer. Continue the extraction of the dye complex with further 10, 5, 5 ml portions of chloroform, shaking each layer in turn with the same 5 ml of pH 9.2 buffer solution. All chloroform layers are combined (do not pass chloroform extract through sodium sulphate at this stage) and diluted to 100 ml with ethanol. To 5 ml of the standard solution, add 15 ml of chloroform, 20 ml of buffer solution, pH 9.2 and 2 ml of dye solution and proceed as above. The absorbance of the extracted ion-pair complex of both standard and sample solutions is measured at about 640 nm against a blank prepared by same coupling procedure but with 20 ml of chloroform. The method obeys Beer's law in the range of 5-10 mcg/ml.

Calculations

$$\% \text{ glycyrrhizic acid} = \frac{A_u}{A_s} \times \frac{1.75 \times \text{Average weight of the tablet}}{\text{Weight of sample taken for analysis}}$$

1.75 = transformation factor of glycyrrhetinic acid to glycyrrhizic acid.

(400 mg of glycyrrhetinic acid is equal to 700 mg of glycyrrhizic acid).

Note : The first chloroform extraction in the procedure for sample preparation ensures elimination of free acidic constituent such as simple organic acid, sugar acid and free glycyrrhetinic acid. The further procedure ensures complete glycyrrhizic acid hydrolysis and extraction of liberated glycyrrhetinic acid.

Trimethoprim

Weigh accurate quantity of the sample equivalent to 200 mg of trimethoprim. Extract with three 50 ml portions of boiling chloroform, filtering through sintered glass funnel (G_4). Evaporate the combined chloroform extract to 20 ml and titrate with 0.05 N perchloric and using α-naphtholbenzein as indicator. Each ml of 0.05 N perchloric acid is equivalent to 0.01451 g of trimethoprim.

Identification of glycyrrhizic acid in liquorice

Adsorbent : HPTLC pre-coated plates, coated with Silica gel 60F$_{254}$ (20 × 10 cm).
Solvent : Chloroform : Acetone (9 : 1 v/v).
Development distance : 50 mm.

Standard solution

50 mcg/ml of glycyrrhetinic acid in chloroform : methanol (1 : 1) v/v.

Sample solution

Sample equivalent to 1 g of liquorice is refluxed with 40 ml of 1 N hydrochloric acid for 2 hours. Cool and extract with five 20 ml portions of chloroform. Evaporate the combined chloroform extract at low temperature and make up to 25 ml with chloroform-methanol (1 : 1 v/v).

Amount spotted : 5 μl.
Detection : UV (short).

Alternatively, the following method based on differential solvation properties may be employed. The result has been found reasonably acceptable for routine quality control.

Standard solution

(a) 10 mcg/ml of trimethoprim (TMP) in chloroform.
(b) 5 mcg/ml of nitrofurantoin (NFT) in acetone.

Procedure

An accurately weighed quantity of finely powdered sample equivalent to 40 mg of trimethoprim was suspended in 15 ml of chloroform and filtered through sintered glass funnel (G₃). The filtrate was diluted with chloroform to get a concentration of 10 mcg/ml in respect of TMP. Absorbance of both sample and standard solutions was measured at 242 nm and results calculated by comparison.

The residue retained on the funnel was extracted with dry acetone by slowly pouring 20 ml of the solvent along the sides of the funnel. The acetone extract was diluted (5 mcg/ml) and absorbance of sample and standard solutions measured at 365 nm for calculation of results.

The residue still left on the sintered funnel was extracted with hot water and diluted to get concentration of 200 mcg/ml in respect of DGL. Follow the method 1 described above.

Nalidixic acid, Metronidazole/Metronidazole benzoate

ESTIMATION

METHOD 1

Nalidixic acid

Standard solution

12 mcg/ml of nalidixic acid in 0.1 N sodium hydroxide.

Sample solution

Shake the sample gently and then transfer accurately measured volume of the sample equivalent to 300 mg of nalidixic acid to separating funnel. Add 10 ml of 1 N sodium hydroxide and extract with four 25 ml portions of chloroform. Wash the combined chloroform layer with 15 ml of water containing 0.1 ml of 0.1 N sodium hydroxide (reserve the chloroform layer for estimation of metronidazole). Transfer the alkaline layer and washings to a 250 ml volumetric flask and dilute to volume with water. Further dilutions are done appropriately with 0.1 N sodium hydroxide to get a concentration of 12 mcg/ml in respect of nalidixic acid.

Measure the extinction of both sample and standard solutions at maxima at about 228 nm and calculate the results by comparing or use 1120 as value of A 1%, 1 cm.

Metronidazole benzoate

Standard solution

Dissolve accurately weighed quantity of metronidazole benzoate in 0.1 N methanolic sulphuric acid to get a solution of 15 mcg/ml in respect of metronidazole.

Sample solution

Transfer the combined chloroform extract reserved in the estimation of nalidixic acid to a dry 100 ml volumetric flask by passing through anhydrous sodium sulphate. Dilute to volume. Further dilutions are done with 0.1 N methanolic sulphuric acid to get a concentration of 15 mcg/ml in respect of metronidazole.

Measure the extinction of both sample and standard solutions at maxima at about 277 nm using 0.1 N methanolic sulphuric acid as blank. Calculate the results by comparison.

Metronidazole benzoate may be converted to metronidazole by applying the factor $\dfrac{171.2}{275.3}$.

METHOD 2

This method is used when metronidazole is present as base (not as benzoate) as in solid dosage forms.

Metronidazole

Standard solution

1 mg/ml of metronidazole in 0.1 N hydrochloric acid. Further dilution is done quantitatively with 0.1 N hydrochloric acid to get a solution of 15 mcg/ml of metronidazole.

Sample solution

Transfer accurately weighed quantity of the sample equivalent to 45 mg of metronidazole to a separator. Add 25 ml of 0.1 N hydrochloric acid and extract with four 25 ml portions of chloroform. Wash the combined chloroform layer with three 30 ml portions of 0.1 N hydrochloric acid (reserve the chloroform layer for estimation of nalidixic acid). Dilute the combined acid layer and washings to 250 ml with 0.1 N hydrochloric acid. Filter and dilute further appropriately with 0.1 N hydrochloric acid to get a concentration of 15 mcg/ml in respect of metronidazole.

Measure the extinction of both sample and standard solutions at maximum at about 277 nm using 0.1 N hydrochloric acid as blank and calculate the results by comparison.

Nalidixic acid

Standard solution

About 9.5 mcg/ml of nalidixic acid in chloroform.

Sample solution

Pass the combined chloroform layer reserved in the estimation of metronidazole through anhydrous sodium sulphate (pre-moistened with chloroform) and make up to 100 ml with chloroform. Dilute further appropriately with chloroform to get a concentration of about 10 mcg/ml.

Measure the extinction of both sample and standard solutions at maxima at about 334 nm using chloroform as blank and calculate the results by comparison.

Note : Nalidixic acid exhibits the same maxima i.e. 334 nm both in alkaline medium as well in chloroform.

METHOD 3

In case of solid dosage forms (capsules and tablets), the following simple and inexpensive method can be used with reasonable accuracy and precision.

Metronidazole

Standard solution

15 mcg/ml of metronidazole in water.

Sample solution

Weigh accurately a quantity of the sample equivalent to 150 mg of metronidazole. Extract the dry powder with three 25 ml portions of water, filtering each through the same G_2 sintered glass funnel. Dilute the combined filtrate to 100 ml with water.

Measure the extinction of both the solutions at about 320 nm using water as blank. Deduce the results by comparison.

Nalidixic acid

Use the entire residue left after the extraction of metronidazole as above. Dissolve the residue left in sintered funnel in 2 N sodium hydroxide and follow the procedure described under method 1 of this formulation. Alternatively, the residue is taken up in neutral (phenolphthalein) methanol and titrated with 0.1 N sodium hydroxide. Each ml of 0.1 N sodium hydroxide is equivalent to 0.02322 g of nalidixic acid.

Phenazopyridine hydrochloride, Nalidixic acid

ESTIMATION

METHOD 1

Phenazopyridine hydrochloride

Standard solution

6 mcg/ml of phenazopyridine hydrochloride in chloroform.

Sample solution

Transfer accurately weighed sample equivalent to 100 mg of phenazopyridine hydrochloride to a separator, add 50 ml of 1 N sodium hydroxide solution. Extract with four 50 ml portions of chloroform. (reserve alkaline layer for estimation of nalidixic acid). Pass organic layer through anhydrous sodium sulphate and make up the volume of 250 ml with chloroform. Transfer 3 ml of the solution and dilute to 200 ml with chloroform (6 mcg/ml).

Measure the extinction of both the solutions at maxima at about 390 nm using chloroform as blank. Calculate the results by comparison.

Nalidixic acid

Standard solution

8 mcg/ml of nalidixic acid in 1 N sodium hydroxide.

Sample solution

Dilute sodium hydroxide layer obtained during the estimation of phenazopyridine above appropriately with 1 N sodium hydroxide to get 8 mcg/ml.

Measure the extinction of both sample and standard solutions at maxima at about 258 nm and calculate the results by comparison.

Note : These two compounds PPZ and NLA are usually formulated in the ratio of 1 : 10 and there is no mutual interference at their respective maxima.

The following simple method can also be applied to such formulations without prior separation or extraction of each ingredient.

Nalidixic acid and phenazopyridine hydrochloride are usually present in the ratio of 10 : 1.

METHOD 2

Common sample solution

Weigh accurately the powdered sample equivalent to 25 mg of nalidixic acid and transfer to 100 ml volumetric flask. Add 70-80 ml of chloroform : methanol (80 : 20) mixture, warm gently to ensure complete solution of both the ingredients, cool and dilute to 100 ml with above solution.

Nalidixic acid

Standard solution

7.5 mcg/ml of nalidixic acid in chloroform-methanol (80 : 20) v/v mixture.

Sample solution

Dilute the common sample solution prepared above appropriately with the solvent to get final concentration of 7.5 mcg/ml of the substance.

Measure the extinction of both the sample and standard solutions at maxima at about 258 nm against solvent blank and calculate the results by comparison.

Phenazopyridine hydrochloride

Standard solution

7.5 mcg/ml of substance in chloroform : methanol (80 : 20) mixture.

Sample solution

Dilute the common sample solution prepared above appropriately with the solvent to get final concentration of 7.5 mcg/ml of the substance.

Measure the extinction of both the sample and standard solutions at maxima at about 390 nm and calculate the results by comparison.

Note : At their respective maxima, there is no significant interference by the other component, so estimation can be done without prior separation or extraction.

Alternatively, the following method is recommended.

METHOD 3

Nalidixic acid

Standard solution

Weigh accurately about 85 mg of nalidixic acid and transfer to a separating funnel containing about 25 ml 1 N hydrochloric acid.

Sample solution

Weigh accurately quantity of the sample equivalent to 85 mg of nalidixic acid and transfer to separating funnel. Add 25 ml of 1 N hydrochloric acid and shake to disperse the powder.

Extract both sample and standard solutions with three 25 ml portions of chloroform. Wash combined chloroform layer with 25 ml of 1 N hydrochloric acid and use the combined acidic layer for estimation of phenazopyridine hydrochloride by spectrophotometric analysis.

Extract the washed chloroform layer with five 20 ml portions of 1 N sodium hydroxide. Combine the alkaline aqueous layer and dilute to 100 ml with 1 N sodium hydroxide.

Solutions of both sample and standard in 1 N sodium hydroxide are further diluted appropriately to get a concentration of 5 mcg/ml.

Measure the extinction of resulting solutions at maxima at about 258 nm using water as blank. Calculate the contents of nalidixic acid by comparison.

Phenazopyridine hydrochloride

METHOD 1

Standard solution

Accurately weigh and transfer about 50 mg of phenazopyridine hydrochloride to a 250 ml separating funnel containing 25 ml of 1 N sodium hydroxide.

Sample solution

Transfer accurately weighed quantity of the sample equivalent to 50 mg of the substance to a separating funnel containing 25 ml of 1 N sodium hydroxide. Shake to disperse. Saturate both sample and standard solutions placed in separating funnel with sodium chloride. Extract with three 25 ml portions of chloroform. Combine the chloroform layer and wash with 25 ml 0.1 N sodium hydroxide. Extract the combined chloroform layer with five 20 ml portions of 0.1 N hydrochloric acid and filter the acid layer through filter paper and make up to 100 ml with the acid. Solutions of both sample and standard are further diluted appropriately with the acid to get final concentration of 7.5 mcg/ml.

Measure the extinction of resulting solutions at maxima at about 390 nm using acid as blank, calculate the results by comparison.

Reagents

1. 2% w/v solution of sodium nitrite in water.
2. 5% w/v solution of ammonium sulphamate in water.
3. 0.1% w/v solution of N-(1-naphthyl)-ethylenediamine dihydrochloride (NED).
4. 1 N hydrochloric acid.

Standard solution

50 mcg/ml of phenazopyridine hydrochloride in water.

Sample solution

An accurately weighed quantity of powdered sample equivalent to 5 mg of the substance was extracted with water and diluted to 100 ml, filtered.

Procedure

To 5 ml each of sample and standard solutions, add 1 ml of 1 N hydrochloric acid and 2 ml of sodium nitrite solution. Keep aside for 10 min, then add 2 ml of ammonium sulphamate solution. Keep aside for 5 min and add 1 ml of 'NED' reagent. Dilute to 25 ml with water. Measure the absorbance of both the solutions at about 550 nm after 15 min against reagent blank prepared by taking 5 ml of water instead of sample. Deduce the results by comparison.

Trimethoprim, Sulphadiazine

ESTIMATION

Trimethoprim

Weigh accurately a quantity of the sample equivalent to 50 mg of trimethoprim. Add about 30 ml of 0.1 N sodium hydroxide, mix to suspend. Extract with four 50 ml portions of chloroform, washing each extract with the same two 10 ml portions of 0.1 N sodium hydroxide, wash the combined chloroform layer with water till washings are neutral. (Combine the alkaline layer and washings and reserve for estimation of sulphadiazine). Evaporate chloroform layer to dryness, take up the residue in glacial acetic acid with the aid of gentle heat. Titrate with 0.1 N perchloric acid using crystal violet as indicator. Each ml of 0.1 N perchloric acid is equivalent to 0.02903 g of trimethoprim. Alternatively, take up the residue in dilute acetic acid and dilute appropriately and step-wise to get concentration of 15 mcg/ml. Measure the extinction of the solution at 271 nm and calculate the contents of trimethoprim taking 204 as value of E 1%, 1 cm at 271 nm.

Sulphadiazine

Standard solution

5 mcg/ml of sulphadiazine in 0.1 N sodium hydroxide.

Sample solution

Combine the alkaline aqueous layer and the washings reserved during estimation of trimethoprim and dilute with 0.1 N sodium hydroxide to produce 100 ml. Dilute further appropriately with 0.1 N sodium hydroxide to get concentration of 5 mcg/ml. Measure the extinction of both the solutions at about 240 nm and calculate the results by comparison. Alternatively, the sample can be taken up in water and hydrochloric acid and titrated with 0.1 M sodium nitrite. Each ml of 0.1 M sodium nitrite is equivalent to 0.02503 g of sulphadiazine.

Chapter 18

Vitamins, Minerals & Digestive Enzyme Preparations

This chapter describes the general methods for the assay of individual vitamin in solutions and liquid dosage forms of multivitamin formulations. These methods have been found to give reproducible and reliable results in many formulations with varying composition and different vitamin levels. However, as there are innumerable possibilities to formulate multivitamin preparations, the determination of each vitamin in such preparations is a complex problem for the analysts. This problem is further complicated due to instability of vitamins during storage and owing to interaction of vitamins amongst themselves leading to interference in many procedures. It may therefore be practically impossible to establish many procedures which could be generally applied to all kinds of formulations. The suitability and accuracy of a method is largely dependent on the composition of the product to be analysed and on the type and level of various vitamins present in the formulation. Vitamin B$_{12}$ is present at microgram level and forms minor component of the formulation. Difficulty has often been encountered in its extraction from formulations. It is always preferable to extract it with dilute alcohol (25% v/v) instead of water and buffer usually employed.

Extraction of folic acid particularly in presence of iron salts poses serious problem and addition of internal standard is always recommended.

Generally, the methods described in this chapter are quite suitable, however in case of difficulty, their applicability must be validated.

Thiamine hydrochloride (Vitamin B₁)

METHOD 1

Reagents

1. 0.04% w/v solution of p-aminophenol in ethyl alcohol, prepare fresh.
2. 0.1 M ammonium hydroxide solution.

Standard solution

Dissolve 100 mg of thiamine hydrochloride (previously dried at 100°C) in distilled water to produce 100 ml. Dilute this solution suitably with water to give a concentration of 20 mcg/ml.

Sample solution

Dissolve and dilute suitably with water to give a concentration of 20 mcg/ml. In case of tablets having coloured coating, remove the colour by rubbing with cotton wetted with water or organic solvent.

Procedure

To 3 ml each of sample and standard solutions, add 3 ml of 0.1 M ammonium hydroxide solution and 0.5 ml of p-aminophenol reagent. Wait for 5 minutes and extract the coloured complex with 10 ml of chloroform. Measure the absorption of organic layer at about 430 nm against reagent blank. The contents of thiamine are calculated by comparison. The method obeys Beer's law in the concentration range of 3-12 mcg/ml in final solution.

The following compounds do not interfere in the above method. The figures in bracket indicate the number of folds excess the compounds can be tolerated. Pyridoxine (5), Niacinamide (20), Riboflavin (1), Vitamin B₁₂ (0.05), Ascorbic acid (2), Folic acid (1), Menadione (15), Calcium glycerophosphate (25), Magnesium glycerophosphate (5), Dried yeast (10), Calcium pantothenate (1), Ferrous sulphate (100), Sodium glycerophosphate (75), Potassium glycerophosphate (50).

If the preparations contain high percentage of minerals, they form hydroxides and get precipitated in ammoniacal medium. It is therefore necessary to centrifuge the alkaline solution before proceeding with addition of the reagent and colour development.

Precautions

1. p-aminophenol should be freshly sublimed or freshly prepared.
2. The reagent should be prepared fresh before use.
3. Concentration of the reagent should not be more than 0.04%, otherwise the reagent blank is very high, sometime even the solution turns black.
4. Reagent blank and sample blank should be prepared simultaneously.
5. When ascorbic acid is present in the formulation, a slightly longer time is required (10 min) to get the full intensity of the colour.
6. When ascorbic acid is present in the formulation, add 6-7 ml of 0.1 M ammonium hydroxide instead of usual 3 ml.

If ascorbic acid is present in the formulation, the following treatment of the sample is suggested before proceedings with method 1 above.

To 10 mg of vitamin B_1, add 5 ml of hydrochloric acid and 200 ml of water. Warm to dissolve, cool and dilute to 250 ml with water (40 mcg/ml). To 25 ml of this solution, add 10 ml of 1 N sodium hydroxide, mix and add 200 mg of manganese dioxide. Heat on water-bath for 30 minutes with frequent agitation, cool and dilute to 50 ml with water and filter. Take 3 ml of the filtrate and follow method 1 as described above.

Preparation of p-aminophenol

To procure p-aminophenol as a white crystalline powder is quite difficult. Para-aminophenol, a raw material for synthesis of paracetamol is usually available as black crystalline powder. To get the desired grade of purity for use in estimation of various drug substances, the commercially available p-amino-phenol can be purified by sublimation. However, an easier and cheaper method for its preparation is described which involves the acid-hydrolysis of paracetamol.

Dissolve paracetamol in minimum amount of 4 N hydrochloric acid by slight warming in boiling water-bath (usually for every 1 g of paracetamol, 3-4 ml of 4 N hydrochloric acid is required). Reflux on boiling water-bath under water condenser in a fume cup board for 30-40 minutes, allow it to cool. Crystals of p-aminophenol separates out. Filter through G_3 sintered funnel under vacuum. Wash the crystals with small amount of water to remove traces of acid. Collect the crystals, dry them between folds of filter paper and store in amber coloured bottle. Prepare fresh stock when crystals develop more than slightly brown colour. The compound is stable for about 2 months if stored under proper conditions.

METHOD 2

The method based on pH induced spectral change is suitable in the presence of vitamin B_6 and B_{12}.

Standard solution

(a) 16 mcg/ml thiamine hydrochloride in 0.1 N sulphuric acid.
(b) 16 mcg/ml thiamine hydrochloride in 0.01 N sodium hydroxide.

Sample solution

Extract the sample with water and then 2 equal volumes are diluted separately with 0.1 N sulphuric acid and 0.01 N sodium hydroxide to get a concentration of 16 mcg/ml.

The absorbance of the acid solution is measured at 265 nm using alkaline solution in the reference cell. The method obeys Beer's law in the concentration range of 8 to 56 mcg/ml.

METHOD 3

This method is based on simultaneous spectrophotometric determination of thiamine (B_1) and pyridoxine (B_6) in presence of vitamin B_{12}, using iso-absorption point method. Record the spectra of standard solutions of vitamin B_1 (20 mcg/ml) and vitamin B_6 (20 mcg/ml) in 0.1 N hydrochloric acid. The solutions exhibit iso-absorption point at 276 nm and maximum for vitamin B_6 at 291 nm and for vitamin B_1 at 247 nm.

By applying absorbance ratio method and using two analogous equations, the amount of both the vitamins can be estimated.

$$C_1 = \frac{Q_0 - Q_2}{Q_1 - Q_2} \times \frac{A_1}{a_1} \qquad \qquad \text{...(i)}$$

$$C_2 = \frac{Q_0 - Q_1}{Q_2 - Q_1} \times \frac{A_1}{a_1} \qquad \qquad \text{...(ii)}$$

where C_1 = concentration (g/L) of thiamine hydrochloride in the sample;

C_2 = concentration (g/L) of pyridoxine hydrochloride in the sample;

Q_0 = ratio of absorbance value of unknown binary mixture at two wavelengths (291 : 276);

Q_1 = ratio of absorbance values of thiamine hydrochloride (20 mcg/ml) at two wavelengths (291 : 276);

Q_2 = ratio of absorbance values of pyridoxine hydrochloride (20 mcg/ml) at two wavelengths (291 : 276);

A_1 = absorbance values of the sample at iso–absorption point (276 nm);

a_1 = absorptivity of components at iso–absorption point (276 nm).

Absorptivity (a_1) at 276 nm	21
Q_1 (Vitamin B_6) (291 : 276)	2.0
Q_2 (Vitamin B_1) (291 : 276)	0.119
Q_0 (Sample) 291 : 276	to be determined

Note : 1. The values of Q_1, Q_2 and a_1 as noted above are mean of 5 determinations on standard solutions of both vitamins (20 mcg/ml).

2. These values are likely to differ from laboratory to laboratory, hence these values are required to be determined on the available instrument and placed in record for future use.

Several market preparations, tablets and injections, containing three vitamins were analysed. Lignocaine, common preservatives and excipients do not interfere. Analgin present in one of the formulations along with three vitamins interfere in this method.

Working example

Each ml of the formulation is labelled to contain :

Vitamin B_1	50 mg
Vitamin B_6	25 mg
Vitamin B_{12}	500 mcg
Lignocaine	1% w/v

1 ml of the above formulation was diluted to 100 ml with 0.1 N hydrochloric acid and 2 ml was subsequently diluted to 100 ml with 0.1 N hydrochloric acid. Absorbance of the resultant solution was measured at 276 and 291 nm and absorbance ratio of the mixture calculated.

Q_2 (vitamin B_6) = 2.00

Q_1 (vitamin B_1) = 0.110

Absorbance of the mixture at 291 nm = 0.265

Absorbance of the mixture at 276 nm = 0.395

$$Q_0 = \frac{0.295}{0.395} = 0.670$$

Absorptivity at 276 nm = 21

Calculations

$$\text{Amount of vitamin } B_1 \text{ (mg/ml)} = \frac{Q_0 - Q_2}{Q_1 - Q_2} \times \frac{A_{276}}{21}$$

$$= \frac{0.67 - 2.00}{0.119 - 2.00} \times \frac{0.395}{21}$$

$$= 13.30 \times \text{dilution factor}$$

$$= 13.30 \times \frac{100}{1} \times \frac{100}{2} \times \frac{1}{1000}$$

$$= 66.5 \text{ mg}$$

$$\text{Claim} = 50 \text{ mg}$$

Usually 20% overages of the vitamins are added.

$$\text{Amount of vitamin B}_2 \text{ (mg/ml)} = \frac{Q_0 - Q_1}{Q_2 - Q_1} \times \frac{0.395}{21}$$

$$= \frac{0.67 - 0.119}{1.881} \times \frac{0.395}{21}$$

$$= \frac{0.55}{1.881} \times \frac{0.395}{1} \times \frac{100}{1} \times \frac{100}{2} \times \frac{1}{1000}$$

$$= 27.5 \text{ mg}$$

$$\text{Claim} = 25.0 \text{ mg}$$

The method was tried on several formulations with satisfactory results.

METHOD 4

This is based on the formation of coloured ion-pair complex between vitamin B_1 and alizarin-violet-3B in buffer of pH 4.5, which is extractable into chloroform.

Reagents

1. Potassium acid phthalate-sodium hydroxide buffer, pH 4.5.
2. 0.2% w/v solution of alizarin-violet-3B (Cl No. 60725).

Standard solution

200 mcg/ml of thiamine hydrochloride in water.

Sample solution

Different solid and liquid formulations are either diluted or extracted with water to get a concentration of 200 mcg/ml.

Procedure

To 0.5 ml each of the sample and standard solutions, add 2 ml of dye solution, 6 ml of buffer solution and water to get 10 ml. Add 25 ml of chloroform. Shake for 2 minutes, separate chloroform layer and measure its absorbance at about 575 nm against reagent blank. Vitamins and other ingredients usually present along with vitamin B_1 do not interfere even where present 15 folds excess.

Choline chloride, panthenol, pantothenyl alcohol, riboflavin, nicotinic acid, nicotinamide, ascorbic acid, folic acid, pyridoxine, vitamin B_{12}, sodium chloride, glucose, sucrose, gelatin, urea and lignocaine do not interfere.

METHOD 5

Reagents

1. 0.05% w/v solution p-N,N-dimethyl phenylenediamine, dihydrochloride (DMPD).
2. 0.1% w/v solution of chloramine-T.
3. Glycine-sodium hydroxide buffer, pH 8.5-10.

Standard solution

500 mcg/ml of thiamine hydrochloride in water.

Sample solution

(a) Tablets : Powdered sample material equivalent to 50 mg of vitamin B_1 is dissolved in water, filtered and diluted to 100 ml with water (500 mcg/ml).

(b) Syrups, liquids and injections : An appropriate aliquot of the composite sample is diluted with water to produce 500 mcg/ml.

Procedure

To 2 ml each of the sample and standard solutions, add 10 ml of buffer solution, 2 ml of 'DMPD' solution and 2 ml of chloramine-T solution. Keep aside for 5 minutes and dilute to 25 ml with buffer solution. Measure the absorbance of the coloured complex at about 450 nm against reagent blank. The method obeys Beer's law over a concentration range of 10-80 mcg/ml. The coloured complex is stable for at least 5 hours. Water soluble vitamins, choline chloride do not interfere in this method.

METHOD 6

Reagents

1. Bromothymol blue solution : 62.44 mg of the dye is dissolved in chloroform to make 250 ml.
2. Buffer solution, pH 6.6 : To 50 ml of 0.2 M potassium hydrogen phosphate add appropriate volume of 0.2 M sodium hydroxide and dilute to 20 ml with water.

Standard solution

Stock solution of thiamine hydrochloride or thiamine mononitrate is prepared in water. Working standards may be prepared freshly in phosphate buffer, pH 6.6 (20 mcg/ml).

Sample solution

Appropriate quantity of the sample is extracted or diluted with buffer to get concentration of 20 mcg/ml.

Procedure

To 10 ml each of sample and standard solution add 10 ml of dye. Shake vigorously and separate chloroform layer. The aqueous layer is further extracted with three 10 ml portions of chloroform. Combine the chloroform layer and make up to 50 ml. Centrifuge and measure the absorbance of clear solution at about 420 nm. Calculate the results by comparison.

Note : 1. The method obeys Beer's law in the concentration range of 5-20 mcg/ml.
2. Decomposition products of thiamine and other vitamins likely to be present do not interfere.
3. In liquid formulations, if alcohol is present it should be removed by gently heating the sample before assay as alcohol will interfere in assay.

METHOD 7

Reagents

1. 4.5% w/v solution of sodium nitrite in water.
2. Phenol buffer : 0.85 ml of phenol diluted to 100 ml with methanol.
3. 1% w/v solution of thymol blue in methanol (indicator).
4. Sodium bicarbonate-sodium hydroxide solution : 2.88 g of sodium bicarbonate and 2.0 g of sodium hydroxide are dissolved in water to produce 100 ml.
5. 2 N sodium hydroxide.
6. 0.635% w/v solution of 4-aminoacetophenone in 0.1 N hydrochloric acid.
7. Diazotizing reagent : To 1.66 ml of 4-aminoacetophenone solution, add 1.66 ml of sodium nitrite solution. Wait for 15 min and dilute to 10 ml with sodium nitrite solution.

Standard solution

100 mcg/ml of thiamine mononitrate/hydrochloride in water.

Sample solution

Extract accurately weighed quantity of powdered sample with water to get solution of 100 mcg/ml in respect of thiamine mononitrate/hydrochloride.

Procedure

To 5 ml each of sample and standard solutions, add 30 ml of buffer solution, 0.9 ml of indicator, 0.9 ml of 2 N sodium hydroxide, 75 ml of sodium bicarbonate-sodium hydroxide solution and 7.5 ml of diazotizing reagent. Then add 25 ml of xylene or toluene and shake vigorously for 10 min. Allow the layers to separate and measure absorbance of xylene layer at about 550 nm against blank prepared by using water instead of sample/standard.

Note : 1. If the sample is not coloured, extraction with xylene is not necessary; the solution after reaction with diazotized reagent may be diluted with isopropyl alcohol for measurement at 550 nm.

2. Common water soluble vitamins and iron do not interfere.

Riboflavin (Vitamin B$_2$)

Usually vitamin B$_{12}$ is first incorporated on an adsorbent before mixing with other vitamins. The absorbent so used is likely to adsorb riboflavin and other vitamins. It is therefore essential to have riboflavin in the free form before analysis. To accurately weighed or measured sample, add 10 times the volume of extracting solvent (methanol-glacial acetic acid-pyridine-water—30 : 01 : 10 : 10 v/v) to produce solution containing 100 µg/ml in respect of riboflavin. Reflux for 60 min, cool, centrifuge. Further dilutions are done with water depending upon the sensitivity of the method to be used. This extraction method has been employed for extracting riboflavin from multivitamin tablets, capsules and liquids.

METHOD 1

Reagents

1. 0.1% w/v solution of methyldopa in 0.1 N hydrochloric acid.
2. 0.4% w/v solution of ortho-aminophenol in alcohol.
3. 0.1% w/v solution of hydroquinone in water.
4. 0.1 M, 1 M and 4 M ammonium hydroxide solution.

Standard solution

Prepared by dissolving in distilled water 50 mg of the compound previously dried for 2 hours at 105°C. To this, add 1 ml of 0.1 N sodium hydroxide to clear the solution, followed by 1 ml of glacial acetic acid to preserve the solution. The volume is made to 250 ml with distilled water to give 200 mcg/ml of riboflavin. Ten ml of the stock solution is further diluted with water to 100 ml to give 20 mcg/ml.

Sample solution

The sample solution is prepared by dissolving and diluting the sample with water to give a concentration of 20 mcg/ml. The colour coating in the case of tablets is removed by rubbing the tablet with cotton wetted with water and/or organic solvent.

Procedure

(a) **Methyldopa :** In clean, dry 10 ml graduated test tubes, 3 ml each of standard and sample solutions are taken separately. 5 ml of 0.4 M ammonia and 0.5 ml of the reagent are added and diluted to the mark with water. Absorbance is measured at about 445 nm against reagent blank after about 10 minutes and results calculated by comparison.

(b) **Ortho-aminophenol :** In 10 ml graduated test tubes, 3 ml each of standard and sample solutions are taken. Add 1.5 ml of reagent, 2 ml of 4 M ammonia and dilute to the mark with water. Absorbance is measured at about 440 nm against a reagent blank after about 10 minutes and results calculated by comparison.

(c) **Hydroquinone :** 3 ml each of standard and sample solutions are mixed with 0.6 ml of the reagent and 5 ml of 0.1 M ammonia. The volume is made to 10 ml with water and absorbance measured against reagent blank at about 450 nm after about 5 minutes.

The following compounds do not interfere up to the minimum folds indicated in brackets.

Thiamine (8), Niacinamide (2), Pyridoxine (5), Calcium pantothenate (3), Ascorbic acid (33), Calcium glycerophosphate (65), Magnesium oxide (15), Manganese sulphate (1), Phosphorus (6), Copper sulphate (1), Zinc sulphate (0.5), Vitamin B_{12} (0.004), Folic acid (1), Calcium phosphate (25), Manganese glycerophosphate (8).

METHOD 2

In preparations containing diastase, papain, pepsin, vitamin B_1, B_6, niacinamide, choline dihydrogen citrate, the following method gives reliable results.

Standard solution

To 100 mg of accurately weighed vitamin B_2, add 2 ml of glacial acetic acid and dilute to 500 ml with water.

Sample solution

Weigh accurately sample equivalent to 200 mcg of vitamin B_2, add 0.2 ml of 5 N sodium hydroxide and 0.5 ml of glacial acetic acid. Heat on boiling water-bath, cool and extract with 20 ml of n-butanol, shaking vigorously. Allow the layers to separate and measure extinction of alcoholic layer at 445 nm. Treat the standard similarly and calculate the results by comparison.

METHOD 3

This method is based on chromatographic separation over a column of talc, followed by colorimetric measurements. Talc is one of the weakest adsorbents, but has sufficient adsorption affinity for riboflavin, whereas other constituents pass freely. This is the general method for removal of interfering substances and riboflavin so eluted can be estimated by any of the suitable methods such as fluorometric.

Reagents

1. Talc, purified, IP.
2. Dioxane : Its absorbance at 267, 374 and 445 nm (usual wavelength used for measurements of vitamin B_2) should not exceed 0.03.
3. 10% v/v and 20% v/v dioxane in 0.01 N hydrochloric acid.
4. Glass column : 200 mm × 10 mm (i.d.), fitted with G_0 sintered disc.

Talc : Although the mesh size of the talc is not very critical but to maintain a reasonable flow rate, finer particles have to be removed. About 50-75 g of talc is suspended in 500-700 ml of water, shake and allow to settle for about 2 min. Decant off unsettled portion and repeat the process till supernatant liquid is almost free from fine particles. After this treatment, the talc is found to have size of 25-50 μm.

Procedure

The aqueous slurry of the talc is poured into the column to get 8-10 cm working bed. The column is repeatedly washed with water till washings are colourless. The sample equivalent to 50 mcg of vitamin B_2 contained in about 5-10 ml of water is poured on the top of the column and is allowed to be absorbed. Then wash the column with 0.01 N hydrochloric acid, followed by 10% dioxane in order to elute other constituents adsorbed on talc column. Washings are continued till the eluate is colourless. Finally elute the yellow coloured band of riboflavin with 20% dioxane. The absorbance of yellow solution is measured at 445 nm (to maintain a flow rate of 80-100 drops per minute, the use of slight suction may be required). The above column chromatographic separation has been tried on several liquid samples containing various vitamin B group, glycerophosphates, liver extract, caffeine, panthenol etc.

successfully. It is possible to eluate the entire band of riboflavin in about 3-4 ml of solvent and the method gives excellent results with recovery of more than 95%.

The above method has also been tried on yeast tablets, with satisfactory results.

Note : Change the receiver when yellow band of vitamin B_2 is near the tip of the column.

METHOD 4

Reagents

1. 0.1 N sodium hydroxide.
2. Phosphate buffer (1 M), pH 6.0.
3. Glacial acetic acid.
4. 2% w/v solution of potassium permanganate.
5. Hydrogen peroxide (30%).

Standard solution

150 mcg/ml of riboflavin in 0.1 N hydrochloric acid.

Sample solution

Weigh accurately a quantity of the sample equivalent to 15 mg of riboflavin, extract with 0.1 N hydrochloric acid to make 100 ml.

Procedure

To 2 ml each of sample and standard solutions, add 1 drop of phenolphthalein solution and neutralize with 0.1 N sodium hydroxide. Add 10 ml of buffer solution followed by 2 ml of acetic acid, 1 ml of potassium permanganate solution. Allow to stand for 2 minutes, neutralize pink colour with 1 ml of hydrogen peroxide. Shake vigorously and dilute to 25 ml with water.

Measure the absorption of both the solutions at about 444 nm and calculate the results by comparison.

Note : The method is applicable to most of the vitamin combinations and gives good results.

METHOD 5

Reagents

1. Acetate buffer, pH 4.00 : Prepared by mixing 10 ml of glacial acetic acid and 30 ml of 1 N sodium hydroxide.
2. 1% w/v solution of potassium permanganate in water.
3. Hydrogen peroxide 30%.
4. Concentrated sulphuric acid.

Procedure

Accurately weighed quantity of the powdered sample equivalent to 1 mg of riboflavin was extracted with 1 ml of concentrated sulphuric acid. Add 30 ml of acetate buffer (pH 4) and keep in water-bath for 30 min, cool and filter. Add potassium permanganate solution till pink colour persists for 30 seconds. Add hydrogen peroxide to remove the excess colour and finally dilute to 100 ml with buffer solution. Measure the extinction at 444 nm using acetyl buffer pH 4 as blank (prepared by adding 20 mg of sodium dihydrogen sulphide to 5 ml of above solution and measuring the extinction at 444 nm within 5 seconds). Calculate the results taking 323 as value of A 1%, 1 cm at maximum, i.e., 444 nm.

Note : 1. Initial with sulphuric acid removes all the impurities.

2. Various ingredients of multivitamin formulations including minerals (iron, calcium, manganese, phosphorus, magnesium) did not interfere.

METHOD 6

Reagents

1. 1 N sodium hydroxide.
2. Glacial acetic acid.
3. Sodium dithionate.

Standard solution

Weigh accurately 100 ml of riboflavin, add 30 ml of 1 N sodium hydroxide and 5 ml of glacial acetic acid. Heat on boiling water-bath and dilute to 100 ml with water. 5 ml of this solution is finally diluted to 500 ml with water (10 mcg/ml).

Sample solution

Sample equivalent to 1 mg of riboflavin is suspended in 3 ml of 1 N sodium hydroxide and 5 ml of glacial acetic acid; solution is effected by heating on water-bath, add 5 mg of sodium dithionate, shake well and measure at 444 nm against reagent blank and calculate the contents of riboflavin by comparing with standard.

METHOD 7

This method is based on oxidation of riboflavin with periodate. Due to presence of $-CH(OH)CH_2OH$ group in the side chain. One mole of formaldehyde is produced during periodate oxidation and the resulting formaldehyde reacts with chromotropic acid to produce complex with absorption maxima at about 570 nm. However, the chromotropic acid reagent being very corrosive this method is no more popular. Further vitamin C or any other substance having $-CH(OH)CH_2OH$ grouping will interfere.

Pyridoxine hydrochloride (Vitamin B$_6$)

METHOD 1

The method based on pH induced spectral change is suitable for estimation of vitamin B$_6$ in presence of vitamin B$_1$ and B$_{12}$.

Prepare solution of 10 mcg/ml of the vitamin in acidic and alkaline solution. For details, see method 2 for vitamin B$_1$. Read absorbance of alkaline solution at 300 and 310 nm using acidic solution in reference cell. The difference between the absorbance of alkaline solution at 300 and 310 nm is linear to the concentration of B$_6$ in range of 4-30 mcg/ml.

METHOD 2

Refer to method 3 for estimation of vitamin B$_1$ which is based on simultaneous spectrophotometric determination of both vitamin B$_1$ and vitamin B$_6$.

METHOD 3

Reagents

1. Buffer solution, pH 7.0 : Dissolve 11.876 g of disodium hydrogen phosphate, monohydrate in sufficient distilled water to produce 1000 ml, solution A. Dissolve 9.078 g of potassium dihydrogen phosphate in sufficient distilled water to produce 1000 ml, solution B. Transfer 1000 ml of the solution A to a beaker and add sufficient quantity of the solution B to get a pH of 7.0 as measured with a glass electrode (about 500 ml of the solution B is usually needed).

2. 0.1% w/v diethyl-p-phenylenediamine solution : Dissolve 100 mg of diethyl p-phenylenediamine sulphate (p-aminoaniline diethyl sulphate) in sufficient distilled water to produce 100 ml. Prepare fresh for every estimation. This solution is sensitive to light.

3. 1% w/v potassium ferricyanide solution in water, prepare fresh.

4. 5% w/v boric acid solution in water.

5. 0.1 N and 1 N hydrochloric acid.

6. 1 N sodium hydroxide.

7. Benzene.

Standard solution

Dissolve 100 mg of pure pyridoxine hydrochloride in 1000 ml of 0.1 N hydrochloric acid. This stock solution can be stored in the refrigerator for 1 to 2 months. Shortly before use, pipette 5 ml of the stock solution (pre-warmed to 25°C) into a 100 ml volumetric flask and dilute to volume with distilled water. Each ml of this standard solution contains 5 mcg of pyridoxine hydrochloride.

Sample solution

The sample solution should have a pH of 7.0 and contains approximately 5 mcg of pyridoxine hydrochloride per ml.

(a) **Solid preparations :** Finely powder the sample and weigh accurately a quantity equivalent to about 1 mg of pyridoxine hydrochloride, into a 150 ml beaker. Add 80 ml of distilled water and 10 ml of 1 N hydrochloric acid. Heat on a steam-bath for 10 minutes, agitating occasionally. Cool to room temperature and adjust the pH to 7.0 with 1 N sodium hydroxide, using glass electrode. Transfer quantitatively to a 200 ml volumetric flask with distilled water and dilute to volume. This is the sample solution, containing approximately 5 mcg of pyridoxine hydrochloride per ml.

(b) **Liquid preparations :** Transfer sample equivalent to about 1 mg of pyridoxine hydrochloride, to a 150 ml beaker. Add 80 ml of distilled water and adjust to pH 7.0 with 1 N sodium hydroxide or 1 N hydrochloric acid, using glass electrodes. Transfer quantitatively to a 200 ml volumetric flask with distilled water and dilute to volume. This is the sample solution containing approximately 5 mcg of pyridoxine per ml.

Procedure

Pipette into seven glass-stoppered centrifuge tubes (capacity about 35 ml) the following reagents :

	A1 (ml)	A2 (ml)	A3 (ml)	B1 (ml)	B2 (ml)	B3 (ml)	Blank (ml)
Distilled water	—	—	—	—	—	—	2
Sample solution	—	—	—	2	2	2	—
Pyridoxine standard solution	2	2	2	—	—	—	—
Buffer solution, pH 7.0	10	10	10	10	10	10	10
Benzene	10	10	10	10	10	10	10
Diethyl-p-phenylene-diamine solution	1	1	1	1	1	1	1

Proceed successively with each of these mixtures as follows : Rapidly add 1 ml of potassium ferricyanide and immediately mix by shaking for 30 seconds (delayed mixing yields low assay values). Centrifuge the seven tubes for 5 minutes in order to separate the layers. Pipette 4.5 ml of the clear blue benzene layer of each sample and standard preparations into a dry 1 cm cell and measure the absorption at 605 nm against benzene layer of the blank preparation and calculate the results by taking average absorption of three samples and three standard solutions.

Note : Interference due to presence of foreign substances which are soluble in benzene and which exhibit some absorption at 605 nm can be eliminated by following method : Shake 5 ml of benzene layers of the sample preparations and of the blank preparation for one minute with 5 ml of boric acid solution and centrifuge. Measure absorption of the benzene layers again as described above and subtract their mean value from the average absorption of the original determinations. If the benzene solution in the cells show some haziness or turbidity, this can be eliminated by slight mixing with a thin glass rod. Benzene layer should not come in contact with moisture.

Note : 1. Ascorbic acid will reduce potassium ferricyanate. It is advisable to increase the amount of potassium ferricyanate if ascorbic acid is present in the formulation.

2. This reaction is pH sensitive. It is essential to adjust the pH to 7.0. Multivitamin preparations containing significant amount of ascorbic acid may have pH below 7.0, hence, adjust the pH to 7.0 before determination.

3. Phenolic compounds interfere in the method as they produce violet colour with absorption maxima at 580 nm.

4. Pyridoxine reacts with boric acid to give a compound which no longer reacts with the reagent. This is the basis of the blank preparation as it will differentiate pyridoxine from other phenolic substances and from other analogues of pyridoxine such as pyridoxal and pyridoxane as these analogues do not possess hydroxy methylene (CH_2CH) grouping at position 4.

METHOD 4

Reagents

1. 20% w/v solution of sodium acetate in water.
2. 5% w/v solution of boric acid in water.
3. 1 N sodium hydroxide in water.
4. Chlorimide reagent (Gibbs reagent) : Dissolve 20 mg of 2,6-dichloroquinone chlorimide in 50 ml of isopropyl alcohol. Store in refrigerator.
5. Ammonia-ammonium chloride buffer : Dissolve 8 g of ammonium chloride in 5 ml of water, add 8 ml of strong ammonia solution, dilute to 50 ml with water.

Standard solution

(a) Stock solution : 200 mcg/ml of pyridoxine hydrochloride in 0.1 N hydrochloric acid.
(b) Dilute solution : Dilute 5 ml of solution to 100 ml with water (10 mcg/ml).
(c) Working standard : Dilute 10 ml of dilute solution to 50 ml with isopropyl alcohol.

Sample solution

Weigh accurately powdered sample equivalent to 2.5 mg of pyridoxine, add 5 ml of hydrochloric acid and 100 ml of water. Digest in boiling water-bath for 45 min, cool and adjust to 250 ml with water. Filter, and to 10 ml of the filtrate, add 4 ml of 1 N sodium hydroxide and make up the volume to 50 ml with isopropyl alcohol. Shake well and filter.

Procedure

To 2.5 ml each of sample and standard solutions, taken separately in 2 test tubes each, add the following in succession :

	Sample		Standard	
	(A) ml	(B) ml	(A) ml	(B) ml
Ammonium chloride buffer	1	1	1	1
Sodium acetate	1	1	1	1
Water	1	—	1	—
Boric acid	—	1	—	1

Shake well, add 1 ml of chlorimide reagent to the respective blanks of sample and standard marked (B) and adjust the instrument to 100% transmittance at 650 nm exactly 1 min after addition of the reagent. Then add 1 ml of the chlorimide reagent to the sample and standard (marked A) and absorbances are measured at maximum at about 650 nm.

Note :   As there is small progressive change within blank, the reading for sample and standard should also be taken exactly one minute after addition of the reagent and no further adjustment of the instrument should be made with the blank.

1 mole of boric acid reacts with 2 moles of pyridoxane to give a compound which no longer reacts with chlorimide reagent, hence serves as blank and also increases the sensitivity of the method. Other analogues of vitamin B_6 such as pyridoxamine and pyridoxal do not react with boric acid as they do not possess hydroxy methylene group (CH_2OH) at position 4.

Nicotinamide

ESTIMATION

METHOD 1

Reagents

1. Sulphanilic acid buffered solution : To 2.5 g sulphanilic acid, add 15 ml water and 2 ml dilute ammonia solution. Mix, add with stirring more dilute ammonia solution if necessary to dissolve the substance, adjust pH of the solution to pH 4.5 with dilute ammonia to 100 ml with water.
2. 10% w/v solution of cyanogen bromide in water.
3. Dilute ammonia solution : Dilute 2 ml strong ammonia solution to 100 ml with water.

Standard solution

100 mcg/ml of nicotinamide in water.

Sample solution

Weigh powdered sample accurately equivalent to 10 mg of the substance, suspend in water to make 100 ml, stir and filter.

Procedure

To 2 ml each of sample and standard solutions, add 2 ml of sulphanilic acid buffered solution, 5 ml water, shake well and add 2 ml of cyanogen bromide solution. Measure the extinction of both sample and standard solutions at 450 nm after 2 min against reagent blank and calculate the contents of nicotinamide by comparison.

METHOD 2

The sample is extracted with acetone. After evaporating the acetone on water-bath, the residue is taken up in glacial acetic acid and titrated with 0.1 N perchloric acid using crystal violet as indicator. Each ml of 0.1 N perchloric acid is equivalent to 12.31 mg of nicotinic acid.

Note : This method is suitable for solid dosage forms whereas in liquid preparations, dextrose and sucrose interfere.

Cyanocobalamine (Vitamin B$_{12}$)

ESTIMATION

The method is based on isolating vitamin B$_{12}$ by passing through a column of weekly acidic ion-exchange resin. There is no loss of vitamin in this process. Since vitamin B$_{12}$ is eluted as a narrow band, enrichment of the solution also occurs. This is followed by spectrophotometric measurements for quantitative determination.

Reagents

1. Ion-exchange resin CG-50 (type-II) or XE-97.
2. Tetrahydrofuran-hydrochloric acid : 60 ml of tetrahydrofuran, 10 ml of 1 N hydrochloric acid and 30 ml of water are mixed.
3. Dioxane-hydrochloric acid mixture : 60 ml of freshly distilled dioxane is mixed with 10 ml of 1 N hydrochloric acid and 30 ml of water.
4. Buffer solution, pH 4 : 65 g of sodium citrate and 60 g of citric acid are dissolved in water to produce 1000 ml. The solution is adjusted to pH 4 with sodium hydroxide or citric acid.
5. 1% w/v solution of ferric chloride in water.
6. 1% w/v solution of potassium ferricyanide in water.
7. 5% w/v solution of potassium cyanide in water.
8. 50% w/v solution of potassium cyanide in water.
9. Aqueous acetone, 85% v/v.

Glass column

2 cm (i.d.) × 20 cm fitted with glass stopcock and a sintered glass disc of zero porosity.

Activation of ion-exchanger

The resin is shaken with water and mixture allowed to stand at least for 2 hours. The turbid supernatant liquid is decanted and resin is again shaken with water. After 10 minutes, it is again decanted and the process is repeated till supernatant liquid is practically clear. After the last portion is decanted, 1 N sodium hydroxide solution is added and is allowed to act on the resin for 1 hour, and then poured off. The resin is washed with water till washings are neutral to litmus. The water is decanted and the resin is kept under buffer solution of pH 4 for 1 hour. The material is now ready for use.

Preparation of ion-exchange column

Sufficient resin suspension is poured into the column having a plug of glass wool on the sintered disc, to give a column height of about 10 cm on setting. The liquid is drained off and buffer is further added. The tube is closed and tilted to mix the resin with the solution and then column is allowed to settle slowly. Wash the column with buffer till the pH of the eluate is 4.0. Cover the top of the column with glass wool and drain the solvent to level of 1 cm above the glass wool.

Procedure

The sample containing at least 100 mcg of vitamin B_{12} is accurately weighed and suspended in 50-80 ml of water. This solution is passed through the prepared column. After the entire sample solution is passed through the column, wash the column with 100 ml of 0.1 N hydrochloric acid. Collect two 5 ml aliquots of the eluate in two separate test tubes. In one tube, add few drops of ferric chloride solution, brown colour should be absent (confirms removal of vitamin B_6); to the other tube, add 5 ml of 2 N sodium hydroxide, 10 ml of potassium ferricyanide solution and 5 ml of isobutyl alcohol, shake, alcoholic layer exhibits no fluorescence (confirms removal of vitamin B_1). When the washing of the column is complete, it is eluted with dioxane-hydrochloric acid mixture and the enriched red colour is collected in 5 ml volumetric flask until the dripping liquid is colourless. Adjust the volume with dioxane-hydrochloric acid mixture, filter and measure the extinction at 548 nm and 361 nm against water as blank. The absorbance ratio at 361 and 548 nm should be between 3.0 and 3.5.

Note : 1. The same column can be used several times on the same day but after every use, it should be washed with buffer solution, pH 5 and it may be ensured that the washings has pH 4 before using the column again.

2. After the experiment is complete, the resin is removed into a clean beaker and washed with water till the washings are practically neutral. Add 1 N hydrochloric acid and keep it for at least 1 hour. Decant the supernatant liquid and wash the resin with water till washings are neutral. Preserve the resin in water. This material can again be used for estimation of vitamin B_{12}.

Total Vitamin B12

To estimate total vitamin B_{12} contents as cyanocobalamin in liver extract or in vitamin B_{12} solution, which may contain aquo- or hydroxycobalamin, the cobalamins are first converted into cyanocobalamin by treating with potassium cyanide. The sample solution containing about 100-150 mcg of vitamin B_{12} is treated with 2 ml of potassium cyanide solution and the pH is adjusted to between 4 and 6 with citric acid (make use of pH meter as indicator paper imparts its colour to the solution which may get eluted by the solvent). Keep the solution in fume hood for 15-20 minutes, the solution is then poured onto the prepared ion-exchange column.

Tablets, Capsules

The tablets and capsules containing equivalent to 100 mcg of vitamin B_{12} are powdered and suspended in 30-35 ml of water. The solution is then treated with potassium cyanide and chromatographed as above.

Feeding Stuff

The extraction and potassium cyanide treatment is done as above. After addition of potassium cyanide, the mixture is heated on water-bath for about 30 minutes. Potassium cyanide treatment not only converts B_{12} to 'cyano' form but also liberates the vitamin from proteins.

Very Dilute Solutions

Very low levels of vitamin B_{12} are usually encountered in the form of drop or syrups for oral use. Because of their relatively high viscosity, filtration through column is difficult. In such cases, the vitamin can be enriched by extraction with chlorophenol before proceeding with ion-exchange separation. Such samples are diluted with water and then treated with 2 drops of potassium cyanide.

The above solution is extracted with three 10 ml portions of chlorophenol solution. To the combined extract, add 10 ml of carbon tetrachloride and 20 ml of n-butanol. The resulting mixture is shaken with two 5 ml portions of water. The aqueous layer is used for ion-exchange separation.

Note :   1.   While carrying out the estimation of vitamin B_{12} in foodstuff, it is recommended that after the column has been washed with 0.1 N hydrochloric acid, the column should be treated with 50-100 ml of aqueous acetone before proceeding with elution by dioxane-hydrochloric acid mixture.

2.   Allowances for losses in extraction with p-chlorophenol should be made in calculations. Usually 5-10% of vitamin is lost in above purification procedure.

Eluting mixtures

It has been seen that after the column has been washed, reddish colour of adsorbed vitamin B_{12} is mainly confined to upper part of the column. If the washing has been complete, there should be no other foreign coloration on the exchanger.

(a)   **Dioxane-hydrochloric acid mixture :** This is used when the vitamin B_{12} left on the upper part of the column has characteristic colour, no other brownish substances being observed on the column. This is the case with simple pharmaceutical preparations containing sufficiently large amount of vitamin B_{12}.

(b)   **Tetrahydrofuran-hydrochloric acid mixture :** Elution with this solvent is essential while analysing the vitamin in feeding stuff. In the analysis of some pharmaceutical specialities, certain brown colour material cannot be removed in spite of repeated washings. These substances behave like vitamin B_{12} and get eluted with the vitamin. In such cases purification by chlorophenol extraction is advisable after chromatography.

Note :   If the determinations cannot be completed in a single day, it can be interrupted before elution of the vitamin if the column is filled with 0.1 N hydrochloric acid (acetone if used must be completely displaced with hydrochloric acid).

The solution of vitamin B_{12} in hydrochloric acid is stable until the following day. It is not stable in solutions containing dioxane or tetrahydrofuran.

Formulation 6

Ascorbic acid (Vitamin C)

ESTIMATION

METHOD 1

Reagents

1. 10% v/v sulphuric acid in water.
2. 10% w/v solution of ammonium molybdate in water.

Standard solution

100 mcg/ml of ascorbic acid in water.

Sample solution

Dilute or extract the sample with water to get 100 mcg/ml concentration.

Procedure

To 2 ml of the sample and standard solutions, add 2 ml of sulphuric acid and 4 ml of ammonium molybdate solution. Keep at room temperature for 60 minutes and dilute with water to 25 ml. Measure the absorbance of both the sample and standard solutions at maximum at about 650 nm against reagent blank. The method obeys Beer's law in the concentration range of 2-10 mcg/ml. Since the colour starts fading after 1 hour, reading must be taken within this period.

Note : 1. This method has been tried on different liquid and solid formulations containing water and fat soluble vitamins, rutin, cysteine, reducing sugars and different iron salts and found to give reliable results.

2. Analgin, if present in the formulations, was found to interfere in this method.

METHOD 2

Reagents

1. 0.01 M chloramine-T reagent : Solution prepared by dissolving 2.81 g of sodium N-chloro-4-toluene sulphonamide, trihydrate in 1000 ml of water. The solution can be standardized iodometrically.
2. 0.025 M sodium tetrathionate solution : This solution is prepared freshly by titrating 100 ml of 0.1 M sodium thiosulphate with 0.05 M iodine to the first appearance of iodine colour which is bleached by dropwise addition of 0.01 M sodium thiosulphate. This solution is stored in amber coloured bottle.
3. 1% w/v solution of 2-furfuraldehyde.
4. 0.01% w/v solution of methyl red in alcohol.

Procedure

A. Accurately weighed quantity of powdered tablets/capsules is stirred with 30 ml of water containing 1 ml of glacial acetic acid. After 15 minutes, the residual solid is filtered and washed with water. To the filtrate (test solution) add :

(a) 0.5 g of potassium iodide, 1 ml of 0.5% w/v starch solution and 2 ml of 0.1 N sulphuric acid, or

(b) 0.5 g of potassium bromide, 2-3 drops of methyl red and 2 ml of 1 N sulphuric acid and the resultant solution is titrated with 0.01 M chloramine-T to the appearance of a blue colour of starch-iodide or to the sharp bleaching of the red colour of methyl red.

B. If the preparation contains sulphite along with vitamin C, then to the 10 ml of test solution as obtained under method A, add 5 ml of furfuraldehyde solution and allow to stand for 15 minutes. The mixture is diluted to 20 ml, then mixed with 0.5 g of potassium iodide, 1 ml of 0.5% w/v starch solution and 2 ml of 0.1 N sulphuric acid. Vitamin C is then titrated with 0.01 M chloramine-T to the appearance of a blue colour. Each ml of 0.01 M chloramine-T is equivalent to 0.8806 mg of vitamin C.

Note : Vitamin B_1, B_2, B_6, B_{12}, folic acid, calcium pantothenate, nicotinamide, ferrous fumarate, ferrous gluconate, calcium lactate, rutin and acetylsalicylic acid do not interfere in this method.

Folic acid

ESTIMATION

METHOD 1

This method is based on the reaction of folic acid with formaldehyde to yield a coloured product having absorption maximum at 360 nm.

Standard solution

100 mcg/ml of folic acid in 0.01 N sodium hydroxide.

Sample solution

Weigh a quantity of powdered tablets accurately equivalent to 5 mg of folic acid and extract with 25 ml of 0.01 N sodium hydroxide by shaking for 15 minutes, filter and dilute to 50 ml with water.

Procedure

To 10 ml each of sample and standard solutions, add 13 ml of 1 N sulphuric acid and 3 ml of formaldehyde solution. Close the tube with rubber stopper in which a hypodermic needle has been inserted. Heat on a boiling water-bath for 1 hour, cool and dilute to 25 ml with water. Measure the absorbance of sample and standard solutions at maximum at about 360 nm against a reagent blank prepared by adding 13 ml of 1 N sulphuric acid to 10 ml of sample solution and diluting to 25 ml with water.

METHOD 2

This method is based on reduction of folic acid to 2,4,5-triamino-6-hydroxypyrimidine which gives colour with ninhydrin.

Reagent

1. 3% w/v solution of ninhydrin in 2-methoxy ethanol, to be freshly prepared.

Standard solution

1 mg/ml of folic acid in 0.1 N sodium hydroxide. It is stable for 4 days if stored in dark under toluene.

Sample solution

Extract accurately weighed quantity of powdered material equivalent to 20 mg of folic acid with 0.1 N sodium hydroxide to produce 1 mg/ml.

Procedure

To 10 ml each of sample and standard solutions, add 10 ml of water and 20 ml of 4 N hydrochloric acid and 2 g of zinc dust. Maintain at 35°C ± 0.5°C for 45 minutes, filter and dilute to 100 ml with water. To 1 ml of the above solutions (sample and standard), add 10 ml of isopropyl alcohol, 2 ml of ninhydrin solution and dilute to 25 ml with isopropyl alcohol. Keep at room temperature and after 10 minutes, but not later than 30 minutes, after addition of ninhydrin reagent, measure the absorbance of both the solutions at about 550 nm and calculate the results.

Note : 1. Vitamin B_1, B_6, vitamin C, ferrous sulphate and ferrous gluconate do not interfere.
2. Vitamin B_2 interferes and leads to low assay value.
3. If niacin is also present in the formulation, measure the colour exactly after 10 minutes after addition of ninhydrin.
4. The method obeys Beer's law in the range of 5-45 mcg/ml.

METHOD 3

Reagents

1. 0.1% w/v solution of sodium nitrite in water.
2. 0.5% w/v ammonium sulphamate in water.
3. 0.1% w/v solution of N-(1-naphthyl)-ethylenediamine dihydrochloride (NED) in water.
4. 5% w/v solution of sodium edetate in water.

Procedure

Weigh or measure aliquot of the sample equivalent to 5 mg of folic acid and dilute to 100 ml with water. To 10 ml of the above solution, add 5 ml of edetate solution and 10 ml of 4 N hydrochloric acid. Dilute to 100 ml with water, this is called unreduced solution (URS).

To about 75 ml of 'URS' solution, add 1 g of zinc dust, shake for 10 minutes and filter. This is called reduced solution (RS).

To each of two test tubes, marked 'RT' and 'RB', add 2 ml of reduced solution. In another two test tubes, marked 'URT' and 'URB', add 2 ml of unreduced solution. Store all the tubes in ice-bath (15°C), add 0.5 ml of 4 N hydrochloric acid to each tube. Add 1 ml of sodium nitrite solution to tubes marked 'RT' and 'URT' and keep in ice-bath for 2 minutes. Take out of ice-bath and add 1 ml of ammonium sulphamate solution, keep at room temperature for 3 minutes, add 1 ml of 'NED' solution to each tube and allow to stand for 10 minutes and finally adjust the volume of each tube to 10 ml with water. Measure the absorbance at about 550 nm. The calculations are based on the net absorbance due to reduced molecule of folic acid. Treat the standard solution of folic acid similarly and calculate the contents of folic acid by comparison.

METHOD 4

Reagents

1. 0.1% w/v solution of sodium nitrite in water.
2. 0.5% w/v solution of ammonium sulphamate in water.
3. 0.1% w/v solution of phloroglucinol in water.
4. 15% w/v solution of sodium hypochlorite in water.
5. 6% w/v solution of phenol in water.
6. 0.1% w/v solution of p-dimethylaminocinnamaldehyde (PDCA) in alcohol.
7. 4 N hydrochloric acid.
8. 2 N sodium hydroxide.

Procedure for reduction of folic acid

Weigh accurately either pure compound or the formulation equivalent to 100 mg of folic acid. Add 10 ml of 4 N hydrochloric acid and 1.2 g of zinc dust. Allow to stand for 1 hour at room temperature and filter through a plug of cotton wool. Wash the residue with three 5 ml portions of alcohol and adjust the total filtrate to 100 ml with alcohol.

Procedure

(a) To an aliquot of reduced folic acid solution equivalent to 100 mcg, add 0.5 ml of p-dimethylaminocinnamaldehyde solution, 2 ml of 4 N hydrochloric acid and dilute to 10 ml with alcohol. Measure the absorbance of the purple colour at 520 nm after 2 minutes. The results are calculated by comparison with the standard. The method obeys Beer's law in the concentration range of 2.5-20 mcg/ml.

(b) To an aliquot of reduced folic acid solution equivalent to 200 mcg, add 5 ml of 4 N hydrochloric acid and 5 ml of sodium nitrite solution. Wait for 5 minutes and add successively 5 ml of ammonium sulphamate solution, 5 ml of phloroglucinol solution and dilute to 50 ml with water. Measure the absorbance of the orange-red coloured complex at 450 nm against reagent blank and calculate the results by comparison with the standard. The method obeys Beer's law in the concentration range of 0.5-5 mcg/ml.

(c) To an aliquot of reduced folic acid solution equivalent to 1.5 mg, add 2 ml of 2 N sodium hydroxide, 2 ml of phenol solution, 1 ml of sodium hypochlorite solution and dilute to 10 ml. After 10 minutes, measure the absorbance of greenish blue complex at 610 nm against reagent blank. Compute the results by comparison with the standard. The method obeys Beer's law in the concentration range of 25-175 mcg/ml.

Vitamins and excipients commonly present in formulation do not interfere in above method.

Note : Ferrous sulphate-folic acid is one of the most common formulation encountered for analysis. It has been observed that while removing the ferrous sulphate by precipitating as phosphate, folic acid usually gets trapped in cheesy precipitates and recovery of folic acid is usually 70-80%. Recovery (%) by adding internal standard is usually recommended in such cases.

Formulation 8

Calcium pantothenate, Panthenol

ESTIMATION

Removal of interferences by solvent extraction

Purification of panthenol

To the sample equivalent to 5-10 mg of panthenol, in water, add 7 g of ammonium sulphate. Shake for 5-10 min, add 20 ml of benzyl alcohol and again shake mechanically for 10-15 min. Centrifuge to separate the layer. To 10 ml of benzyl alcohol layer (upper) add 10 ml of toluene and 20 ml of water, shake for 15 min and centrifuge. The lower aqueous layer will contain panthenol which can be used for any of the methods described below. (In the presence of ammonium sulphate, the compound is extracted with benzyl alcohol layer and re-extracted with aqueous layer with the use of toluene).

Purification of calcium pantothenate

To 10 ml of aqueous solution of the sample containing 3-5 mg of calcium pantothenate, add 13 g of sodium dihydrogen phosphate, shake vigorously for 15 min, add 20 ml of benzyl alcohol. Shake for 15 min, centrifuge to separate the layer. To 15 ml of organic layer (upper) add 10 ml of toluene and 12 ml of boric acid solution (5%). Shake for 15 min and centrifuge. The lower boric acid layer containing calcium pantothenate is appropriately diluted.

Removal of decomposition product, β-alanine

A. Prepare slurry with 5 g of the talc and pour over filtration funnel. Pass 5 ml of the sample solution obtained above through the slurry and let it drain. Wash the slurry with two 5 ml portions of water to complete the elution.

   Talc being weak adsorbent is capsule of retaining amino acid and riboflavin, but calcium pantothenate is not adsorbed.

B. Suspend prepared florisil in water and add to the glass column (250 mm × 12 mm, i.d., fitted with G_2 sintered disc) under suction. Pass the solution of the sample and standard as obtained above through column and elute with water.

Prepared florisil

50-100 g of the florisil is taken in beaker and covered with sufficient volume of solvent (glacial acetic acid-pyridine-water; 02 : 20 : 78 v/v). Boil gently for several minutes and allow to settle. Remove the supernatant liquid and repeat the washing process twice. Finally wash it with hot water till there is no perceptible smell of pyridine. Florisil thus treated is dried at 110 ± 10°C and stored in close container to be used for preparatory column for purification of sample.

METHOD 1

This method is based on hydrolytic cleavage of the substance in acid medium with the formation of pantoyl lactone. The lactone reacts with hydroxylamine in alkaline medium to form hydroxamic acid of pantoyl lactone. Hydroxamic acid derivative so produced yields a purple coloured complex on acidification in presence of ferric chloride.

Reagents

1. 1% w/v solution of ferric chloride in water.
2. Hydroxylamine-sodium hydroxide reagent : Prepared by dissolving 7.5 g of hydroxylamine hydrochloride in 100 ml of 1 N sodium hydroxide. Prepare the solution fresh.

Standard solution

1.5 mg/ml of calcium pantothenate or panthenol in water.

Sample solution

After purification, as discussed above, appropriate dilution with water to get solution of 1.5 mg/ml.

Hydrolysis

To 5 ml each of the sample and standard solutions, add 3 ml of 1 N hydrochloric acid. Cap the flask loosely and heat the mixture for 5 hrs at $69 \pm 1°C$ for effecting the hydrolysis. Cool to room temperature and to each of the hydrolysed solution add 2 ml of hydroxylamine reagent, followed by 5 ml of 1 N sodium hydroxide. Allow to stand for 5 min, adjust the pH to $2.7 \pm 0.1°C$ (pH meter) with 1 N hydrochloric acid and make up the volume to 50 ml with water.

Procedure

To 5 ml of hydrolysed solutions each of the sample and standard, add 1 ml of ferric chloride solution, mix and tap the tubes against table top to remove air bubbles and measure the absorbance of purple colour so developed at about 500 nm against blank and calculate the results by comparison.

Blank : Prepared by heating 5 ml each of the sample and standard solutions in the same manner except hydrolysis procedure in acid medium. Blank so prepared will eliminate interference due to any pre-formed pantoyl lactone.

Note : 1. Pantoyl lactone has melting point of 92°C, some decomposition might occur at temperature higher than 70°C.
2. pH 2.7 is critical as excess of hydrochloric acid results in marked decrease in colour intensity.
3. As alkaline medium is necessary for formation of hydroxamic acid of pantoyl lactone, there is possibility of formation of some pantoic acid. It is therefore advisable that after addition of sodium hydroxide the solution should be brought to pH 2.7 immediately after 5 min, longer exposure to alkali gives lower assay values.

METHOD 2

This method involves alkaline hydrolysis of panthenol or calcium panthenol and β-alanol or β-alanine so formed reacts with naphthoquinone reagent to give brownish-yellow coloured complex having absorption maxima at 465 nm.

Hydrolysis : To aliquot of the sample and standard containing 2-5 mg of the substance in 40 ml of water as purified by the method described above, add 3 ml of 2.5 N sodium hydroxide solution and heat in boiling water-bath for 1 hr to ensure complete cleavage of the molecule, cool, adjust the volume to 50 ml with water.

Reagents

1. 0.04 M formaldehyde prepared by diluting 3 ml of 40% formaldehyde to 1000 ml with water.
2. Acidic formaldehyde : 0.3 N hydrochloric acid in 0.04 M formaldehyde.
3. 0.05 M sodium thiosulphate in water.
4. 0.5% w/v solution of 1,2-naphthoquinone-4-sulphamate, sodium salt in water, prepare fresh.

Procedure

5 ml each of hydrolysed sample and standard solution is adjusted to pH 9.3 with 0.1 N sulphuric acid. Add 1 ml of naphthoquinone reagent and heat for 10 min in boiling water-bath, cool to room temperature, add 1 ml of acidic formaldehyde followed by 1 ml of thiosulphate solution. Allow to stand at room temperature for 10 min and dilute to 25 ml with methanol. Measure the absorbance of both sample and standard solutions at 465 nm against respective blank prepared with hydrolysed sample without naphthoquinone reagent.

METHOD 3

Reagents

1. 0.2 M citrate buffer, pH 5 : Dissolve 21 g of citric acid in 200 ml of 1 N sodium hydroxide and dilute to 500 ml with water. Check pH 5.0 ± 0.1.
2. 0.2% w/v solution of stannous chloride dihyride, in citrate buffer.
3. 2% w/v solution of ninhydrin in methanol.
4. Ninhydrin-stannous chloride reagent : Mix equal volume of reagents 2 and 3.

Procedure

After alkaline hydrolysis, the solution is made distinctly acidic with 1 N sulphuric acid. Add 50 ml of methanol and dilute to 100 ml with water. To 2 ml aliquot of the above solution add 1 ml of citrate buffer and 1 ml of ninhydrin reagent. Heat in water-bath at 95-100°C for 5 min, cool and adjust to 10 ml with 60% methanol. The absorbance of both sample and standard solutions is measured at about 570 nm against reagent blank and results calculated by comparison.

Formulation 9

Cyproheptadine hydrochloride, Lysine monohydrochloride, Dried Yeast, Tricholine citrate

ESTIMATION

Cyproheptadine hydrochloride

METHOD 1

Reagent

1. Citric acid-acetic anhydride reagent : Dissolve 2 g of citric acid (monohydrate) in 5 ml of methanol (anhydrous) and dilute to 100 ml with acetic anhydride.

Standard solution

100 mcg/ml of cyproheptadine hydrochloride in chloroform.

Sample solution

Weigh accurately a quantity of the sample equivalent to 10 mg of the substance, extract with four 20 ml portions of chloroform, filter through sintered funnel. Wash the residue with chloroform and make up the volume to 100 ml (100 mcg/ml). Retain the residue for estimation of lysine monohydrochloride.

Procedure

Evaporate 1 ml each of sample and standard solutions to dryness, add 1 ml of citric acid reagent and immerse in water-bath for 30 min. Cool and dilute to 10 ml with acetic anhydride. Measure the absorption of both the solutions at about 570 nm against reagent blank and calculate the results by comparison. Alternatively, the residue is dissolved in methanol to produce 100 ml, filtered and extinction measured at maximum at about 286 nm and contents of cyproheptadine hydrochloride calculate by taking 355 value of A 1%, 1 cm.

METHOD 2

To accurately weighed quantity of sample (syrup), add 20 ml of sodium bicarbonate solution (0.1%) and extract with iso-octane (2 × 25 ml). Wash the combined iso-octane layer with 50 ml of sodium bicarbonate solution, discard the aqueous layer. Iso-octane layer is extracted with 0.1 N sulphuric acid (3 × 25 ml). The acidic layer is combined and diluted to 100 ml. Filter and measure the extinction at maximum at about 286 nm using 0.1 N sulphuric acid as blank. Calculate the contents of cyproheptadine hydrochloride taking 355 as value of A 1%, 1 cm.

Lysine monohydrochloride

METHOD 1

Reagents

1. 0.1% w/v solution of copper sulphate in methanol.

2. 0.5% w/v solution of ninhydrin in methanol-pyridine mixture.
3. Methanol-pyridine mixture (1 : 1) v/v.

Standard solution

50 mcg/ml of lysine monohydrochloride in water.

Sample solution

Extract the accurately weighed quantity of the sample with water to get a concentration of 50 mcg/ml of the substance.

Procedure

To 2 ml each of the sample and standard solutions, add 5 ml of ninhydrin solution. Keep in water-bath for 10 min, cool and dilute to 25 ml with copper sulphate solution. Measure the absorption of both the solutions at about 530 nm against reagent blank. Calculate the results by comparison.

Alternatively, dissolve the residue retained in estimation of cyproheptadine in water to get a concentration of 50 mcg/ml of lysine monohydrochloride and follow the above method.

METHOD 2

Reagents

1. 0.2% w/v solution of ninhydrin in ethyl alcohol.
2. 50% w/v solution of copper nitrate in water. Dilute 0.5 ml to 100 ml with water just before use.
3. 10% v/v n-propanol in water.
4. TLC plates (glass) 20 × 20 cm, coated with silica gel G (0.25 mm). After coating, the plates are allowed to dry in air overnight (do not activate in the oven).
5. Mobile phase : n-propanol-water-glacial acetic acid (7 : 3 : 1) v/v.

Standard solution

(a) Stock solution : 1 mg/ml of lysine monohydrochloride in aqueous propanol.
(b) Working standard : Dilute stock solution appropriately to get 200 mcg/ml. To be prepared freshly on the day of use.

Sample solution

Extract the sample with 10% n-propanol to get a concentration of 200 mcg/ml.

Procedure

Line the chromatographic chamber with filter paper on 3 sides. Spot 100 µl each of sample and standard solutions as streaks. Dry and develop the plate up to a distance of 10 cm. Remove and dry in oven at 90°C for 10 min. Cool and spray evenly with ninhydrin reagent, again heat in oven at 90°C for 30 min. The coloured spots (Rf 0.45) corresponding to sample and standard are scrapped and transferred quantitatively to stoppered centrifuge tube. Add 10 ml of dilute copper nitrate solution, shake vigorously and centrifuge to get clear solution. Measure the absorption of both the solutions at about 520 nm using dilute copper nitrate solution as blank. Calculate the results by comparison.

Dried yeast

Estimate the nitrogen contents and calculate the amount of protein. The yeast can also be analysed for various vitamins preferably for B_1 and B_2, calcium pantothenate.

Riboflavin (vitamin B$_2$)

METHOD 1

Reagents

1. 2% w/v solution of potassium permanganate in water.
2. Hydrogen peroxide (30%) solution.
3. Phosphate buffer, pH 6.0.

Standard solution

30 mcg/ml of riboflavin in phosphate buffer.

Sample solution

Take appropriate quantity of the sample. Add 60-70 ml of phosphate buffer, pH 6.00, boil under reflux for 30 min, cool and adjust to 100 ml with buffer. Final solutions in buffer should contain 30 mcg/ml of riboflavin.

Procedure

To 10 ml each of the standard and sample solutions, add 2 ml of glacial acetic acid and 1 ml of potassium permanganate solution. Keep for 2 min, add 1 ml of hydrogen peroxide, shake vigorously and dilute to 25 ml with water. Measure the absorption of both the solutions at about 445 nm and calculate the results by comparison.

METHOD 2

Chromatographic separation through a column of talc gives satisfactory results. For details, refer to the method 3 for estimation of riboflavin under formulation 2 of this chapter.

Tricholine citrate

To the sodium bicarbonate layer obtained during estimation of cyproheptadine hydrochloride, add 10 ml of freshly prepared ammonium reineckate. The precipitates are dried at 105°C, weighed and multiplied by 0.397 to give the weight of tricholine citrate present in the volume of the sample taken for analysis. For further details refer to formulation 24 of this chapter.

$$\boxed{\text{Formulation 10}}$$

Inositol, N-Hydroxymethyl nicotinamide, Vitamin B$_{12}$

ESTIMATION

Inositol

Reagents

1. Borate buffer : Dissolve 4 mg of boric acid in 200 ml of water and adjust the pH to 8.0 with 1 N sodium hydroxide solution.
2. Potassium periodate solution : Weigh about 120 mg of potassium periodate and dissolve in water to produce 100 ml.
3. 2% w/v solution of potassium iodide in water, prepare fresh.
4. 1 N sodium hydroxide.

Standard solution

20 mcg/ml of inositol in water.

Sample preparation

Weigh accurately powdered sample equivalent to 100 mg of the substance and dissolve in water to produce 100 ml. Shake, filter and dilute 5 ml of the filtrate to 250 ml with water (20 mcg/ml).

Procedure

Transfer 10 ml each of standard and sample solutions to two different tubes, add 10 ml of water and 2 ml of potassium periodate solution. Shake and keep at 50°C for 2 hrs and cool. Take 2 ml each of the above solutions, add 15 ml of borate buffer and 8 ml of potassium iodide solution. Shake and dilute to 50 ml with borate buffer. Measure the extinction of both the solutions after 5 minutes at 352 nm and calculate the results.

N-hydroxymethyl nicotinamide (pyridine-3 carboxylic acid hydroxymethylamide)

Reagents

1. Citrate buffer : 0.2 N solution of sodium acid citrate is prepared in boiled water, cooled and adjusted to pH 6. Alternatively, 25 g of citric acid is dissolved in 75 ml of water and pH adjusted to 6 with 40% w/v sodium hydroxide solution.

Standard solution

500 mcg/ml of the substances in water.

Sample solution

Shake an accurately weighed portion of the sample equivalent to 100 mg of the substance with 70 ml of water for 20-25 min. Dilute to 200 ml and filter.

Procedure

To 5 ml each of sample and standard solutions, add 10 ml of citrate buffer, pH 6 and dilute to 100 ml with water. Measure the extinction of both the solutions at 262 nm and deduce the results by comparison.

Vitamin B$_{12}$

Weigh accurately powdered material equivalent to 200 mcg of vitamin B$_{12}$ and add 50 ml of distilled water. Shake and add 30 g of ammonium sulphate and 100 ml of isobutyl alcohol. Shake well and collect the separated isobutyl alcohol layer. Shake the alcoholic layer with 5 ml of water and use aqueous layer for estimation by ion-exchange method described under general assay methods for vitamin B$_{12}$. However, microbiological assay is the method of choice.

Ascorbic acid, Menadione, Ferrous gluconate, Calcium lactate, Citrus bioflavonoid compound

ESTIMATION

Ascorbic acid

Reagents

1. Dilute sulphuric acid.
2. 0.1 N iodine.
3. Starch solution.

Procedure

Dissolve the accurately weighed sample equivalent to 150 mg of ascorbic acid in 25 ml of dilute sulphuric acid and add 60 ml of water. Titrate with 0.1 N iodine using starch solution as indicator. Each ml of 0.1 N iodine is equivalent to 0.008806 g of ascorbic acid.

Citrus bioflavonoid compound (CFC)

This method is based on estimation of hespiridin contents.

Reagents

1. Methanol AR.
2. 0.04% w/v solution of copper sulphate in water.
3. 0.1 N hydrochloric acid.

Standard solution

Heat 150 mg of 'CFC' standard in 50 ml of methanol, cool and make up to 100 ml with methanol.

Sample solution

Heat the sample equivalent to 150 mg of 'CFC' in 50 ml of methanol, cool, make up to 100 ml with methanol and filter.

Procedure

To 5 ml each of the standard and sample solutions, add 1 ml of copper sulphate solution, 1 ml of 0.1 N hydrochloric acid and dilute to 100 ml with methanol. Measure the extinction of the resulting solutions at the maximum at about 283 nm and deduce the results by comparison.

Calcium lactate

Reagents

1. Ammonia-ammonium chloride buffer solution.
2. 0.05 M EDTA solution.

3. 10% w/v solution of potassium cyanide.
4. Solochrome black T solution.

Procedure

Dissolve an accurately weighed sample equivalent to 150 mg of calcium lactate, in about 100 ml of water, add 2 ml of potassium cyanide solution and 5 ml of buffer. Titrate the above solution with 0.05 M EDTA solution using solochrome black T solution as indicator. Each ml of 0.05 M EDTA solution is equivalent to 0.01542 g of calcium lactate. Alternatively estimate (Ca^{++}) by flame photometric method described in formulation 34 of the chapter on alimentary drugs.

Ferrous gluconate

Reagents

1. Nitric acid.
2. Hydrochloric acid.
3. Dilute sulphuric acid.
4. 10% w/v solution of ammonium thiocyanate.

Standard solution

40 mcg/ml solution of Fe^{++} (as ferrous sulphate).

Sample solution

To accurately weighed sample equivalent to 50 mg of ferrous gluconate, add 1 ml of nitric acid and 5 ml of hydrochloric acid. Heat on water-bath till there are no fumes of nitrous acid. Dilute to 250 ml with water and filter.

Procedure

To 2 ml each of the sample and standard solutions, add 5 ml of ammonium thiocyanate solution, dilute to 25 ml with dilute sulphuric acid. Measure the absorption of the sample and standard solutions at about 520 nm and deduce the results by comparison.

Menadione

Reagents

1. Chloroform.
2. 0.2% w/v solution of 2,4-dinitrophenyl hydrazine in hydrochloric acid-alcohol (1 : 5 v/v) mixture.
3. Ammonia-alcohol (1 : 1) mixture.

Standard solution

5 mcg/ml solution of menadione in chloroform.

Sample solution

Suspend an accurately weighed sample equivalent to 300 mcg in 5 ml of water and extract with three 10 ml portions of chloroform, make up to 50 ml with chloroform and filter.

Procedure

To 5 ml each of standard and sample solutions, add 2 ml of 2,4-dinitrophenyl hydrazine solution. Heat on water-bath to almost dryness, add 15 ml of ammonia-alcohol mixture and dilute to 50 ml with alcohol. Measure the extinction of the standard and sample solutions at about 635 nm and deduce the results by comparison.

Ascorbic acid, Ferrous gluconate, Calcium lactate, Rutin, Adrenochrome monosemicarbazone, Menadione sodium bisulphite, Methyl hespiridin

ESTIMATION

For estimation of ascorbic acid, calcium lactate, ferrous gluconate follow the method described under formulation 11 of this chapter.

Rutin

Reagents

1. 0.1 M aluminium chloride : Weigh and dissolve 2.41 g of aluminium chloride in water to produce 100 ml.
2. 1 M potassium acetate : 9.81 g in water to produce 100 ml.
3. 1 N hydrochloric acid.

Standard solution

100 mcg/ml of rutin in alcohol.

Preparation of sample

Accurately weigh powdered sample equivalent to 10 mg of rutin, add 80 ml of ethyl alcohol. Heat on water-bath to boil, cool to room temperature, make up to 100 ml with ethyl alcohol.

Procedure

Carry out the colour development as follows :

	Std	Std blank	Sample	Sample blank
Prepared solutions	2 ml	2 ml	2 ml	2 ml
Aluminium chloride reagent	3 ml	—	3 ml	—
Potassium acetate solution	5 ml	5 ml	5 ml	5 ml
1 N hydrochloric acid	1 ml	1 ml	1 ml	1 ml
Distilled water	—	3 ml	—	3 ml

Allow to stand at room temperature for about 20 minutes, make up to 25 ml. Measure the absorbance of the sample against sample blank and standard against standard blank at about 420 nm. Calculate the results by comparison.

Menadione sodium bisulphite (MSB)

METHOD

Weigh the powdered sample accurately equivalent to 60 mg of MSB, add 25 ml of water and 2-3 pellets of sodium hydroxide and saturate with sodium chloride. Shake and extract with three 50 ml portions of chloroform. Combine all the chloroform extracts, pass through anhydrous sodium sulphate, wash the sodium sulphate layer with additional 20 ml of chloroform. Evaporate combined chloroform layer to dryness.

Treat the residue by any one of the following two methods for estimation.

(a) Dissolve the residue in 10 ml of glacial acetic acid followed by 10 ml of dilute hydrochloric acid. Add 3 g of zinc dust and the flask is shaken. Allow the flask to stand in the dark with intermittent shaking (every 10 minute) for one hour. Filter the solution through cotton plug wetted with water. Wash the reduction flask with three 10 ml portions of water (CO_2 free). To the combined filtrate, add 2-3 drops of orthophenanthroline solution and titrate with 0.02 N cerric ammonium sulphate or cerric sulphide. Each ml of 0.02 N cerric ammonium sulphate is equivalent to 3.03 mg of menadione sodium bisulphite.

Or

(b) Dissolve the residue obtained after evaporation of chloroform layer in 10 ml of glacial acetic acid. Add 5 ml of 10% w/v solution of sodium potassium tartrate and 4 g of anhydrous sodium carbonate. Immediately titrate with 0.2 N titanous chloride using few drops of 0.1% solution of indigo carmine as indicator. Each ml of 0.2 N titanous chloride is equivalent to 3.03 mg menadione sodium bisulphite.

Adrenochrome monosemicarbazone (AMS)

Reagents

1. 0.5% w/v solution of sodium nitrite in water.
2. 0.5% v/v hydrochloric acid.
3. 13.25% w/v solution of sodium carbonate in water.

Standard solution

Weigh the analyte mixture as prepared under preparative TLC, accurately equivalent to 2 mg of AMS. Add 80 ml of water, shake continuously for 2 hours and centrifuge. Transfer the supernatant liquid to 100 ml volumetric flask wash the residue with 2 × 5 ml water, centrifuge again, transfer clear liquid to volumetric flask and make up to 100 ml with water (20 mcg/ml in respect of AMS).

Sample solution

Weigh the powdered sample accurately equivalent to about 2 mg of AMS and extract with 80 ml of water, proceed further as described under standard preparation.

Procedure

To 2 ml each of standard and sample solutions, add 2 ml each of 0.5% hydrochloric acid and of 0.5% sodium nitrite solution. Shake gently till colourless. Then add 3 ml of 1.25 M (13.25 w/v %) sodium carbonate solution and 3 ml of water. Measure the absorbance of both sample and standard solutions at about 430 nm using mixture of 2 ml each of water, 0.5% hydrochloric acid, 0.5% sodium nitrite, 3 ml of 1.25 M sodium carbonate and 3 ml of water as blank.

Adrenochrome monosemicarbazone (AMS) and Methyl hespiridin (MH) by preparative TLC

Absorbent layer : Silica gel GF$_{254}$
TLC plates : Precoated plates, 20 × 20 cm (0.2 mm thickness)
Solvent system : Ethyl acetate-formic acid (85%)-acetic acid-water (100 : 11 : 11 : 27) v/v
Volume used : 20 ml

Chamber saturation : Chamber lined on three sides with filter paper and saturated for 60 minutes.

Preparation of analyte mixture : The pure samples of various ingredients as present in the tablet (adrenochrome monosemicarbazone, methyl hespiridin, ascorbic acid, rutin, menadione bisulphite representing 10 tablets = 10 mg of AMS) were weighed and mixed.

(The analyte mixture stored in air-tight amber coloured bottle may be used for further analysis of sample).

Preparation of standard solution

Analyte mixture was weighed accurately and shaken with methanol to produce 5 ml (200 mcg/ml of AMS).

Preparation of sample solution

Weigh accurately powdered sample equivalent to 1 mg of AMS. Add sufficient methanol to produce 5 ml. Shake vigorously for 10-15 minutes, centrifuge and use clear supernatant liquid for spotting.

Procedure

Apply 100 µl (0.1 ml) each of sample and standard solutions as bands (about 7.5 cm long) with the help of graduated microcapillary and current of air, drying after each application. Dry the plate and transfer to pre-saturated developing chamber. Develop the plate to a distance of about 15-17 cm. Remove the plate and allow the solvent to evaporate. Examine the plate under visible light for (AMS) and UV (for methyl hespiridin) to locate the compounds. Scrap the relevant portions representing sample and standard separately. MH gives three bands; all the three bands are scrapped and the material mixed together for analysis.

Adrenochrome monosemicarbazone

Extract the scrapped material of both sample and standard separately with methanol to produce 5 ml. Filter and measure the absorbance of clear filtrates of both sample and standard solutions at 444 nm and calculate the results by comparison.

Methyl hespiridin

Extract the combined scrapped material of three bands of both sample and standard with methanol to produce 100 ml, filter and measure the extinction of both sample and standard solutions at maxima at about 283 nm.

Blank : Scrap the silica gel of similar area from similarly developed plate, extract with 5 ml of methanol, filter and use as blank.

Ferrous fumarate/Ferrous gluconate, Folic acid, Calcium phosphate dibasic, Ascorbic acid, Vitamin B$_{12}$

ESTIMATION

Ferrous fumarate/Ferrous gluconate

METHOD 1

Reagents

1. 1 N sodium hydroxide.
2. 0.1 N cerric ammonium sulphate.
3. Ortho-phenanthroline solution (indicator).
4. Concentrated sulphuric acid.

Procedure

Transfer accurately weighed quantity of the sample equivalent to 300 mg of ferrous fumarate. Add 200 ml of water and 20 ml of 1 N sodium hydroxide. Mix, filter and transfer the precipitates (iron hydroxide) quantitatively to filter paper with the aid of water. Wash the precipitates with water till the filtrate is almost colourless. (Use the filtrate for estimation of folic acid). Pierce the filter paper with a glass rod and wash the precipitates to a 250 ml conical flask with the aid of water. Add slowly through sides with stirring concentrated sulphuric acid till the precipitates just dissolve, add 2-5 ml more of sulphuric acid. Add about 1 g of zinc dust, plug the flask loosely with cotton and allow it to stand at room temperature for 30 min. Filter, wash the flask and residue with small volume of water and filter. Titrate the combined filtrate and washings with 0.1 N cerric ammonium sulphate using orthophenanthroline solution as indicator. Each ml of 0.1 N cerric ammonium sulphate is equivalent to 0.017167 g of ferrous fumarate or 0.02061 g of ferrous gluconate.

METHOD 2

Reagents

1. Nitric acid.
2. Hydrochloric acid.
3. Dilute sulphuric acid.
4. 10% w/v solution of ammonium thiocyanate in water.

Standard solution

40 mcg/ml of Fe^{++} (as ferrous sulphate).

Sample solution

To accurately weighed quantity of the sample equivalent to 50 mg of ferrous fumarate or gluconate, add 1 ml of nitric acid and 5 ml of hydrochloric acid. Heat on a water-bath till there are no fumes of nitrous acid. Dilute to 250 ml and filter.

Procedure

To 2 ml each of sample and standard solutions, add 5 ml of ammonium thiocyanate solution, dilute to 25 ml with dilute sulphuric acid. Measure the absorption of both the solutions at about 520 nm against reagent blank. Calculate the results by comparison.

METHOD 3

Reagents

1. Acetate buffer, pH 4.7 : To 2.9 ml of acetic acid, glacial, add 6.805 g of sodium acetate and dilute to 1000 ml with water. Adjust the pH to 4.7 with sodium acetate solution or with glacial acetic acid as required.
2. 5% w/v solution of sodium metabisulphite in water.
3. 3% w/v solution of 2,2é-bipyridyl in water.
4. 10% v/v sulphuric acid in water.

Standard solution

To 50 mg of ferrous fumarate accurately weighed, add 20 ml of 10% sulphuric acid, heat on water-bath for about 30 min, shake, cool and dilute to 100 ml with water. Dilute 2.5 ml of the resulting solution to 50 ml with water.

Sample solution

Weigh accurately quantity of the sample equivalent to 50 mg of the substance and proceed for sample preparation as under standard solution.

Procedure

To 5 ml each of sample and standard solutions, add 5 ml of buffer solution and 2.5 ml of sodium metabisulphite solution. Allow to stand at room temperature for 15 min, add 2.5 ml of bipyridyl solution, shake and adjust to 25 ml with water. Measure the absorbance of both sample and standard solutions at about 510 nm against reagent blank and calculate the results by comparison.

Ascorbic acid

Follow the method described in formulation 11 of this chapter.

Folic acid

Follow the method 3 described under formulation 7 of this chapter.

Note : Precipitation of iron with alkali results in low recovery of folic acid as it gets trapped in creamy precipitates of iron hydroxide. Standard solution should also be treated similarly after addition of appropriate amount of ferrous fumarate.

Vitamin B$_{12}$

Follow microbiological method. However in such formulations initial extraction should be done with 25% alcohol to enhance the solubility of vitamin, thus complete extraction. Stock solution may be diluted with buffer or water as necessary.

Calcium phosphate, dibasic

Reagent

1. Vanadate-ammonium molybdate solution : To 20 g of ammonium molybdate and 1 g of ammonium vanadate, add about 500 ml of water and warm. Add 140 ml of concentrated nitric acid to dissolve, dilute to 1000 ml with water.

Standard solution

200 mcg/ml of calcium phosphate, dibasic in 1 N hydrochloric acid.

Sample solution

Weigh sample accurately equivalent to 100 mg of the substance, add 50-60 ml of 1 N hydrochloric acid, warm on water-bath for 30 min to dissolve the substance. Make the volume to 100 ml with the acid and further dilute appropriately with 1 N hydrochloric acid to get 200 mcg/ml.

Procedure

To 5 ml of sample and standard solutions, add 5 ml of vanadate molybdate solution, mix, allow to stand for 10 min, and measure the absorbance at about 450 nm against reagent blank. Deduce the results by comparison.

Ergometrine maleate, Adrenochrome monosemicarbazone, Rutin, Dicalcium phosphate, Menadine sodium bisulphite

ESTIMATION

Rutin, Adrenochrome monosemicarbazone and Menadine sodium bisulphite

Follow the method described in formulation 12 of this chapter.

Dicalcium phosphate

Follow the method described in formulation 13 of this chapter.

Ergometrine maleate

Reagents

1. 1% w/v solution of p-dimethylaminobenzaldehyde (PDAB).
2. Brine solution.

Standard solution

20 mcg/ml of the substance in tartaric acid.

Sample solution

Weigh accurately quantity of powdered sample equivalent to 4 mg of substance, suspend in 15 ml of brine solution and make alkaline with ammonia. Extract with 5 × 25 ml portions of diethyl ether (anaesthetic). Wash the combined ether extract with 3 × 5 ml portions of brine and reject the brine layer. Extract the ether layer with tartric acid to get final concentration of 20 mcg/ml.

Procedure

To 5 ml each of sample and standard solutions, add 10 ml of PDAB solution and measure the absorbance of both the solutions at 550 nm against reagent blank and calculate the results by comparison.

Cyproheptadine hydrochloride, L-lysine hydrochloride, Peptone

ESTIMATION

Cyproheptadine hydrochloride

Follow the method 2 described in formulation 9 of this chapter.

L-lysine hydrochloride

Follow the colorimetric method described in formulation 9 of this chapter.

Peptone

Digest the sample with sulphuric acid, basify and carry out ammonia distillation by Kjeldahl method. From the total nitrogen, subtract the amount of nitrogen equivalent to both the other ingredients.

Peptone (mg/ml) = $[N_T - (N_C + N_2)] \times 6.7843$

where N_T (total nitrogen) = $T_R \times N \times 35.025$

$$N_C = a \times 0.399$$

$$N_L = b \times 0.1534$$

a = contents of cyproheptadine determined in 5 ml of the sample

b = contents of L–lysine determined in 5 ml of the sample

T_R = Titre value (blank) – Titre value (back titration)

Haemoglobin, Ferric ammonium citrate, Folic acid, Cyanocobalamin

ESTIMATION

Haemoglobin

This method is based on oxidation of haemoglobin into methaemoglobin and subsequent conversion to cyanmethaemoglobin which is coloured.

METHOD 1

Reagents

1. Ferricyanide-cyanide reagent : Dissolve 0.2 g of potassium ferricyanide, 0.05 g of potassium cyanide and 0.14 g of potassium and phosphate in water to produce 1000 ml, pH should be between 7.0 and 7.4 (adjacent if necessary).

Transfer accurately measured quantity of the sample equivalent to 200 mg of haemoglobin to 250 ml volumetric flask, add about 100 ml of water, shake well and add 10 ml of ferricyanide-cyanide reagent and dilute to 250 ml with water. Allow to stand for 10 min, filter and measure the absorbance of the solution at 540 nm against blank and calculate the results. If solution is hazy it may be centrifuged.

$$\text{Haemoglobin (g)/15 ml} = \frac{A_U}{11} \times \frac{16114.5}{1000} \times \frac{200}{1000} \times \frac{15}{10} \times \frac{\text{S.G.}}{1}$$

where A_U = absorbance of the sample; 11 = factor of A 1%, 1 cm; S.G. = specific gravity of the preparation.

Alternatively, use standard haemoglobin for comparison.

METHOD 2

Take sample equivalent to about 3 g of haemoglobin, heat in a crucible on a burner to char the sample completely. Cool and moisten with 1 ml of concentrated sulphuric acid and again heat till all fumes are expelled out. Transfer the contents to furnace and heat at 450-500°C till ashing is complete. Cool, moisten with little water, add about 20 ml of concentrated hydrochloric acid, warm on water-bath till ash dissolves. Transfer the extract to 250 ml conical flask with the aid of water. Now add strong ammonia solution drop by drop till slight brown precipitate appears in solution (the pH at this stage is about 4). Add about 0.25 g of salicylic acid, warm on water-bath at about 60°C and titrate the hot solution with 0.05 M disodium edetate, end point being change of deep violet colour (colour of iron salicylate) to bright yellow, indicating the complete titration of iron. Each ml of 0.05 M disodium edetate is equivalent to 0.8502 g of haemoglobin.

Note : Haemoglobin contains 0.34% of elemental iron.

METHOD 3

Weigh sample equivalent to 500 mg of the substance and transfer to Kjeldahl flask, add 1 g of copper sulphate and 10 g of sodium sulphate. Add 20 ml of sulphuric acid. Heat until solution is clear blue (this will ensure conversion of nitrogen into ammonium sulphate). Cool, add water and 100 ml of 40% odium hydroxide. Collect the distillate with 50 ml of 0.1 N sulphuric acid. Titrate the excess of the acid with 0.1 N sodium hydroxide using methyl red as indicator (A ml). Perform the blank (B ml). Each ml of 0.1 N sulphuric acid is equivalent to 1.4 mg of nitrogen.

From the total nitrogen (mg), calculate the content of haemoglobin.

$$\text{Glycerrinated haemoglobin} = \frac{B \times A \times N \times 1.4 \times 6.38 \times W \times 100}{0.1 \times W_1 \times 35}$$

where B = blank reading; A = volume consumed by the sample; N = normality of sodium hydroxide; W = average fill of the capsule; W_1 = weight of the sample taken for analysis.

Ferric ammonium citrate (FAC)

METHOD 1

Reagents

1. 20% w/v solution of citric acid.
2. Strong ammonia solution.
3. 80% thioglycollic acid.
4. Concentrated hydrochloric acid.
5. Strong ammonia solution.

Standard solution

Accurately weighed sample equivalent to 200 mg of ferric ammonium citrate, add 10 ml of concentrated hydrochloric acid and dilute to 100 ml with water. Further dilute 5 ml to 100 ml with water.

Sample solution

To appropriate quantity of the sample, add 10 ml of concentrated hydrochloric acid and then dilute with water.

Procedure

To 10 ml each of sample and standard solutions, add 2 ml of citric acid solution, 0.1 ml of thioglycollic acid and 5 ml of strong ammonia, dilute to 25 ml with water. Measure the absorbance of both the solutions at 525 nm against reagent blank. This will give total quantity (mg) of iron in the sample.

Note : 100 mg of ferric ammonium citrate contains 21.5 mg of elemental iron.

METHOD 2

Digest accurately weighed quantity of the sample with 4-5 ml of concentrated hydrochloric acid. Transfer to 250 ml flask with the help of water. Add 15 ml of potassium iodide solution (10% w/v). Keep in the dark for 5 min and titrate the liberated iodine with 0.1 N sodium thiosulphate using starch paste as indicator, added near the end of titration. Each ml of 0.1 N sodium thiosulphate is equivalent to 5.585 mg of iron. Calculate the contents of FAC in the sample considering each 100 mg of FAC is equivalent to 21.5 mg of iron.

Folic acid

Follow the methods described in formulation 7 of this chapter.

Cyanocobalamin

Follow the microbiological method.

Thiamine hydrochloride, Riboflavin, Nicotinamide, Pyridoxine hydrochloride, Folic acid, Calcium pantothenate, Ascorbic acid, Zinc sulphate, Vitamin B$_{12}$, Glutamic acid, Lactobacillus sporogenes, Sodium selenite, Copper sulphate, Manganese sulphate

ESTIMATION

Ascorbic acid

Accurately weighed quantity of powdered sample equivalent to 150 mg of ascorbic acid is diluted in 300 ml of water and 20 ml of dilute sulphuric acid and titrated with 0.1 N cerric ammonium sulphate using ferric sulphate as indicator. Each ml of 0.1 N cerric ammonium sulphate is equivalent to 8.8806 mg of ascorbic acid.

For estimation of thiamine hydrochloride (B$_1$), riboflavin (B$_2$), pyridoxine hydrochloride (B$_6$), nicotinamide, calcium pantothenate and vitamin B$_{12}$, follow the general methods described under each vitamin in this chapter.

Zinc sulphate

Follow the method described in formulation 18 of this chapter, which is based on titration with EDTA.

Selenium (Sodium selenite)

To 5 ml of 1 mmol solution of sodium selenite, add 10 ml of dilute hydrochloric acid and 5 ml of potassium iodide (10%), shake for 2 min, add 10 ml of water and 2 ml of chloroform. Mixture was titrated with 1 mmol (0.176%) of l-ascorbic acid using starch as indicator.

$$\text{Selenium (µg)} = V \times C \times \frac{\text{Atomic weight of selenium}}{\text{Molecular weight of ascorbic acid} \times 2}$$

$$= V \times C \times \frac{78.96}{176 \times 2}$$

$$= V \times C \times 0.23$$

where V = volume of standard ascorbic acid

C = concentration (mg or µg/ml) of l–ascorbic acid

1 ml of 0.004 N ascorbic acid $\equiv$ 78.96 µg of selenium

1 ml of 0.1 N ascorbic acid $\equiv$ 4.325 mg of sodium selenite

Copper sulphate

Accurately weighed quantity of the sample equivalent to 1.25 mg of copper sulphate is ignited at 450°C, add 5 ml of hydrochloric acid and evaporate to dryness, add 2.5 ml of nitric acid and evaporate. **Extract** the residue with three 5 ml portions of hot hydrochloric acid, combine the acid extract and dilute to 25 ml with water.

To 1 ml of this solution, add 10 ml of edetate-citrate solution, 0.1 ml of thymol blue solution **and** sufficient dilute ammonia solution to produce green to blue-green colour. Add 10 ml sodium diethyldithiocarbamate solution and extract the yellow colour with four 5 ml portions of carbon tetrachloride. Combine the organic extracts and dilute to 20 ml with carbon tetrachloride. Measure the absorption at maxima at about 435 nm. Use standard solution of copper sulphate for comparison.

Manganese sulphate

METHOD 1

To 2 ml of the solution obtained during estimation of copper sulphate add 2.5 ml of dilute sulphuric acid, evaporate to dryness. To the residue, add 3 ml of phosphoric acid, 6 ml of water and 0.5 g of sodium periodate and dissolve by aid of heat. Heat in a water-bath for 30 min, cool, dilute to 10 ml with water. Measure the absorption of the resulting solution at the maximum at about 526 nm. The result can be calculated from a standard curve prepared by diluting 1, 2, 3, 4, 5 ml of 0.005% w/v solution of potassium permanganate to 10 ml with water. Each mg of potassium permanganate is equivalent to 1.4114 mg of $MnSO_4 \cdot 4H_2O$.

METHOD 2

Reagents

1. 0.002% w/v solution of rhodamine B.
2. 0.015 N solution of potassium periodate.
3. 0.5 M solution of sodium fluoride.
4. 0.025% w/v solution of 1,10-phenanthroline in 10% alcohol.
5. 0.5 M acetic acid-sodium acetate buffer (pH 3.8).

Standard solution

0.1 mcg/ml of manganese (Mn^{++}).

Sample solution

Containing equivalent to 0.1 mcg/ml of manganese (Mn^{++}).

Procedure

To 0.4 ml of rhodamine B solution, add 1.6 ml of mixture of 1,10-phenanthroline, potassium iodate, sodium fluoride and buffer solution (1 + 1 + 1 + 7). Then add 0.2 ml each of sample and standard solutions, adjust the volume to 4 ml with water. Heat at 60°C for 8.5 min, cool quickly to terminate the reaction. Measure the absorbance of sample and standard solutions against reagent blank. Oxidation of rhodamine B by potassium periodate in acidic medium results in decoloration of the dye. This oxidation reaction is accelerated by 1,10-phenanthroline and minute quantity of manganese. The decrease in colour intensity is proportional to the amount of manganese. Other elements such as Co, Ni, Cu^{++}, chromium (III), Zn, Fe^{+++}, Fe^{++}, Ca^{++}, Mg^{++}, Al^{+++} have insignificant interference.

Glutamic acid

Reagents

1. 0.5% w/v solution of ninhydrin in methanol.
2. 1% w/v solution of copper sulphate in water.
3. Pyridine.
4. Methanol.

Standard solution

60 mcg/ml of glutamic acid in water.

Sample solution

Accurately weighed quantity of sample is extracted with water (treat with charcoal if colour is present).

Procedure

To 5 ml each of sample and standard solutions, add 5 ml of ninhydrin solution and 5 ml of pyridine and heat in water-bath for 15 min. Cool, add 1 ml of copper sulphate solution and dilute to 50 ml with methanol. Measure the absorbance of both the solutions at 500 nm against reagent blank and calculate the contents of glutamic acid by comparison.

Lactobacillus sporogenes

Determine the viable spore count and lactic acid producing capacity.

Formulation 18

Microcrystalline hydroxyapatite (Calcium orthophosphate), L-lysine monohydrochloride, Zinc sulphate

ESTIMATION

Phosphate

Reagents

1. Ammonium molybdate reagent : Introduce drop by drop 13.9 ml of concentrated sulphuric acid in 80 ml of ice-cooled water, cool and add 3.3 g of ammonium molybdate, dissolve and dilute to 100 ml with water, filter before use.
2. 2 N sulphuric acid.
3. Nitric acid.
4. Ammonia solution.
5. Reducing reagent : Dissolve 3 g of ferrous sulphate in 10 ml of water, add 5 ml of 2 N sulphuric acid, dilute to 100 ml with water and filter. Reducing solution should always be freshly prepared.

Standard solution

Weigh accurately 50-60 mg of sodium or potassium acid phosphate and dissolve in water to produce 100 ml. Dilute further 10 ml of this solution to 100 ml with distilled water.

Sample solution

Take sample equivalent to 20 mg of phosphorus, evaporate to dryness on steam-bath in a silica dish and ignite the contents to almost white ash. Cool, weigh and calculate the concentration of the ash. Dissolve the ash in a mixture of 15 ml water and 10 ml nitric acid. Boil for 3-5 min, cool, neutralize the solution with ammonia solution. Then, acidify with 2 N sulphuric acid and add 35 ml of 2 N sulphuric acid in excess. Transfer to 250 ml volumetric flask, rinse silica dish with water, add the washings to volumetric flask and dilute to 250 ml with water. 20 ml of the resultant solution is further diluted to 100 ml (sample solution).

Procedure

To 5 ml each of sample and standard solutions, add 2 ml of ammonium molybdate reagent and then 2 ml of reducing agent. Shake well and measure the absorbance of both the solutions at about 660 nm after 10 minutes against reagent blank.

Note : This method was experimentally checked on number of formulations and found to give excellent results. The method is simpler than official methods. Commonly used glycerophosphate can be estimated by this method for phosphate contents.

Zinc sulphate

Weigh accurately sample equivalent to 100 mg of zinc sulphate and dissolve in 100 ml of water. Filter and add 5 ml of strong ammonia-ammonium chloride solution and 0.1 ml of eriochrome black-T solution and titrate with 0.05 M EDTA until deep blue colour. Each ml of 0.05 M EDTA is equivalent to 14.38 mg of zinc sulphate.

Lysine monohydrochloride

Follow the method described in formulation 9 of this chapter.

Calcium (Ca^{++})

Weigh sample accurately equivalent to 100 ml of calcium (Ca^{++}), dissolve in dilute hydrochloric acid to make 100 ml. To 25 ml of this solution, add 25 ml of ammonium oxalate solution (saturated) and heat on water-bath for 1 hr. Filter through 42 Whatman filter paper. Wash the precipitates with hot water till precipitates are free from oxalate ions. Dissolve the precipitates along with filter paper in warm dilute sulphuric acid and titrate while still warm with 0.1 N potassium permanganate until faint pink colour persists for 15 seconds. Each ml of 0.1 N potassium permanganate is equivalent to 2.004 mg of calcium (Ca^{++}).

Microcrystalline hydroxyapatite (Calcium orthophosphate), Zinc sulphate, Ferrous fumarate, Folic acid, Vitamin B$_{12}$

ESTIMATION

Phosphate of calcium

Follow the method described in formulation 18 of this chapter.

Zinc sulphate

Follow the method described in formulation 18 of this chapter.

Ferrous fumarate

Weigh accurately sample equivalent to 1.5 g of ferrous fumarate and dissolve in 15 ml of dilute sulphuric acid with with the aid of gentle heat. Cool, add 50 ml of water, filter and titrate the whole filtrate with 0.1 N ceric ammonium sulphate using ferrous sulphate as indicator. Each ml of 0.1 N ceric ammonium sulphate is equivalent to 16.99 mg of ferrous fumarate.

Folic acid

Follow the general method described for folic acid in this chapter.

Vitamin B$_{12}$

Follow the microbiological method as per I.P. or the method described in this chapter under vitamin B$_{12}$.

Starch Digesting Enzymes

The starch digesting enzymes are being used by pharmaceutical manufacturers in their digestive preparations. Depending on the mode of action, starch digesting enzymes, biochemically known as amylases, are fundamentally of two types :

(a) Dextrinogenic

(b) Saccharogenic.

The first type of enzymes, dextrinogenic, degrade starch only up to a stage of dextrins and not below it, the end product being dextrins. The second type of enzymes, saccharogenic, degrade starch right down to reducing sugars, the end product being predominantly maltose. These saccharogenic enzymes are mainly useful for digestive aid formulations.

Diastase from *Aspergillus oryzae* contains primarily α-amylase which is known to liquefy starch paste by reducing viscosity. In order to arrive at some meaningful idea of the comparative activity of enzymes, it is necessary that a standard way of expression is used. This is all the more important considering that there is proliferation of the ways of this expression.

Amylases are of animal or plant origin. Animal amylases are termed as α-amylases, whereas plant amylases are termed as β-amylases; pancreatin contains α-amylases.

For α-amylases of bacterial origin, a buffer of pH 6.0 and for α-amylases of fungal origin, acetate buffer of pH 5.3 is used for estimation of diastase activity. For β-amylases, buffer solution of pH 5.6 may be used.

Note :   It is absolutely essential that the type of diastase added in the formulation is correctly indicated on the label to enable the analyst to use buffer of appropriate pH.

Number of methods are available for measurement of starch digesting capacity of amylases, the important of them are :

1. Starch-iodine colouration method.

2. Estimation making use of fall in viscosity of starch solution.

3. Estimation of reducing sugars formed by the enzymic action on starch.

Diastase activity

METHOD 1

The method determines the diastase activity in term of starch hydrolysed to a stage when it gives no blue colour with iodine.

Reagents

1. Freshly prepared normal saline solution (0.9%), pH 5.0—use dilute acetic acid to adjust the pH.

2. Soluble starch having about 15% moisture content—BDH grade starch is most suitable.

3. Buffer solution, pH 5.0 (0.1 N sodium acetate) : Weigh accurately 2.05 g of sodium acetate, dissolve in sufficient quantity of water and make the volume to 250 ml. When 5.9 ml of 0.1 N acetic acid is mixed with 14 ml of 0.1 sodium acetate, solution will attain pH 5.0.

4. Iodine solution, 0.1 N (stock solution) : Weigh accurately, 1.276 g of iodine and dissolve in 15 ml of water containing 4 g of potassium iodide and make the volume to 100 ml. Standardise this solution to get a solution of exactly 0.1 N.

5. Iodine solution, 0.02 N : Dilute 20 ml of the stock solution (0.1 N) with 80 ml of water to obtain 0.02 N iodine solution. Prepare 0.02 N iodine solution just before use, and use 1 drop of this solution, per tube.

6. 10 N hydrochloric acid, to arrest the enzymatic reaction.

7. Substrate : Weigh 200 mg of soluble starch accurately (on dry weight basis) and transfer into 200 ml measuring flask with little quantity of water. Boil the suspension till it gets into solution, constantly shaking the flask while boiling. Cool under tap water, add 5.9 ml of 0.1 N acetic acid, 14 ml of 0.1 N sodium acetate and finally make the volume to 200 ml with normal saline, pH 5.0. Dispense this solution in 5 ml aliquot to each tube. Thus each tube contains 5 mg of soluble starch.

Dilution of sample (enzyme dilution) : All dilutions are to be made with normal saline, pH 5.0. The sample is diluted so that the final solution contains 200 mcg/ml of 1 in 50 enzyme. This solution is used as test enzyme solution in graded amounts of 0.1 ml to 1.0 ml per tube.

Procedure

Dispense substrate (starch solution) and saline solution as shown in the following table, and pre-incubate the tubes for 5 min in a water-bath at 37°C (± 0.5°C). Then, add graded amount of diluted enzyme solution, shake to mix well and incubate for one hour at 37°C. At the end of incubation period, stop the enzyme action by adding 5 drops of 10 N hydrochloric acid. Shake the tube well after adding hydrochloric acid. Add to each tube 1 drop of 0.02 N iodine and shake well. Note the change of colour in the tubes. With increasing concentration of enzyme, there will be fall in the intensity of the colour from light purple, red to colourless. The tube showing no colour on the addition of iodine is to be taken as the end point.

It is assumed that amount of enzyme present in the tube showing no colour on the addition of iodine solution has fully digested the quantity of starch present, viz. 5 mg.

	Tube No.										
	1	2	3	4	5	6	7	8	9	10	11
Substrate, starch solution (ml) 1 mg/ml	5.0	5.0	5.0	5.0	5.0	5.0	5.0	5.0	5.0	5.0	5.0
Saline, pH 0.5 (ml)	0.9	0.8	0.7	0.6	0.5	0.4	0.3	0.2	0.1	0.0	1.0
Diluted enzyme solution (ml) 200 mcg/ml	0.1	0.2	0.3	0.4	0.5	0.6	0.7	0.8	0.9	1.0	0.0

Calculations

Each tube contains 5 mg of starch. At the end of incubation period, stop the reaction and add solution of iodine. Let us assume that tube No. 5 shows no colour with iodine. Thus 100 mcg of enzyme digests 5 mg of starch in one hour.

$$\text{Diastase activity} = \frac{5 \times 1000}{100} = \frac{5000}{100} = 50 \text{ units (1 in 50)}$$

Claimed : 50 (1 in 50)

i.e. the ratio = 1 : 50

Note : The starch-iodine complex has a change of colour from blue → violet purple → reddish brown → colourless, depending upon the degradation of starch to lower molecular weight products; dextrin showing reddish brown colour. This test only ensures that the starch is degraded to below the stage of dextrins, but this does not necessarily mean that starch is digested to the stage of reducing sugars, maltoses.

METHOD 2

Undigested starch reacts with iodine to give blue colour having absorption maximum at about 610 nm.

Reagents

1. Soluble starch (BDH) solution, substrate : Boil 80 ml of water and into this pour 1 g of starch previously suspended in 5 ml of water, stir till a clear solution is obtained. Cool and dilute to 100 ml with water.
2. Phthalate buffer (0.2 M), pH 5.4.
3. 0.5 M solution of sodium chloride.
4. Stock solution of iodine, 0.1 N : To be prepared as described under method 1 above.
5. 0.01 N iodine solution : Dilute 10 ml of the stock solution to 100 ml with water.
6. 2 N hydrochloric acid.

Standard enzyme solution

Weigh accurately standard diastase of known enzymatic activity and dilute with water to produce concentration similar to the sample.

Sample solution

Take appropriately weighed or measured aliquot of the sample equivalent to 50 mg of diastase (1 in 400) and extract or dilute with water to produce 100 ml.

Procedure

Take two tubes of 50 ml each. To each, add 10 ml of substrate, 6 ml of buffer solution, pH 5.4 and 2 ml of sodium chloride solution, mixing after each addition. Place them in water-bath maintained at $40°C \pm 0.5°C$. Add 1 ml of sample and 1 ml of water to the sample and blank tubes and note the starting point. Shake the tubes and keep in water-bath (40°C) for 15 minutes. Then, add 1 ml of 2 N hydrochloric acid to arrest the reaction. Transfer contents of both the tubes to 100 ml volumetric flask and dilute to 90 ml with water. Then, add accurately 1 ml of 0.01 N iodine and make up the volume with water. Dilute 5 ml of the digested mixtures (sample and blank) further to 25 ml with water and measure the absorbance of blue colour of sample and blank solutions at about 610 nm. Calculate the activity; amount (g) of starch digested by the enzyme. Repeat the procedure with the standard enzyme solution.

Amount (g) of starch digested by enzyme present in each tablet =

$$= \frac{A_s - A_u}{A_s} \times C \times \frac{\text{Average weight of tablets}}{\text{Weight of the sample (g) taken}} \times d_f$$

where A_s = absorbance of blank; A_u = absorbance of sample; C = quantity of starch used as substrate for digestion (0.1 g); d_f = dilution factor.

METHOD 3

By this method, liquefying power of the enzyme is determined. Two methods are proposed to determine this activity.

(a) This is based on the measurement of outflow time of liquefied starch. The outflow time decreases with the fall in viscosity of the substrate.

Reagents

1. Potato starch, BDH grade.
2. Sodium chloride.
3. 1 N sodium hydroxide.
4. Acetate buffer solution : Mix 16.4 g of anhydrous sodium acetate and make up the volume to 500 ml with water.

5. Starch solution, substrate : Weigh 25 g of potato starch (BDH) and make a paste with 50 ml of water in a 150 ml beaker. In a 1000 ml beaker having a 500 ml mark, dissolve 2 g of sodium chloride in 450 ml water and heat this to boiling. Add the above starch suspension to the boiling water in 1000 ml beaker with continuous stirring and transfer any residue of starch suspension with minimum quantity of water. Note the time when boiling commences throughout the entire mass and continue boiling for 5 minutes. Remove the source of heat, cool, add 5 ml of acetate buffer solution. Mix thoroughly by pouring and make up the volume to 500 ml with water.

Procedure

Set a thermostatically controlled water-bath at a temperature of $40 \pm 1°C$. Take five 150 ml beakers, each with a stirring rod, and to each of the beakers, add 100 ml of starch solution. Mark three beakers as A_1, A_2, A_3 and other two beakers as B_1, B_2. Put the beakers containing the starch solution in the water-bath and allow them to attain the temperature of the bath ($40°C$). When the starch solution inside the beakers has attained the temperature of $40 \pm 1°C$, add 0.25 ml of the sample to each of the three beakers marked A_1, A_2, A_3. At the same time, add 0.25 ml of water to each of two beakers marked B_1, B_2. Immediately after addition, stir thoroughly the solution in the beaker for one minute and allow them to remain in the bath for 10 minutes after addition of the sample. Take out the beakers and while stirring, add 1 ml of 1 N sodium hydroxide solution to each of the beakers and stir for 30 seconds more. Allow 2-3 minutes time interval between operation of successive beakers for proper manipulation of the experiment.

Allow the contents of the beaker to cool to room temperature. Measure the outflow time with the help of a 100 ml pipette and record the time taken by each of three samples marked A_1, A_2, A_3 and take mean of three readings. Also measure the time taken by the solutions in B_1, B_2 and take mean. Express the liquefying power by the mean time taken by the sample against the mean time taken by the blank solution.

(b) In this method, liquefying power is estimated by fuchsin colour test.

Reagents

1. Starch suspension : 10 g of potato starch (moisture-free basis) is suspended in 10 ml of 0.1 M acetate buffer solution, pH 6.0 and made to 100 ml with distilled water.
2. Fuchsin solution : 0.2 g of fuchsin is dissolved in 1.5 ml alcohol and made to 200 ml with distilled water.

Enzyme solution

The enzyme preparation is mixed with an appropriate amount of distilled water, allowed to stand for 30 minutes at $30°C$ with occasional shaking and filtered.

Procedure

10 ml of starch suspension is placed in each of ten test tubes. Add 0.1, 0.2, ..., 1.0 ml of the enzyme solution and 0.9, 0.8, ..., 0.0 ml of distilled water to each of these test tubes respectively (the final content of each tube should be (11 ml). These test tubes are heated at successive time intervals in a boiling water-bath with vigorous shaking to keep starch suspension homogeneous. As soon as the content is gelatinised, the test tube is transferred to a water-bath kept at $40°C$ and incubated for 10 minutes exactly. Then, the tube is heated in a boiling water-bath for 5-7 minutes to destroy amylase and cooled in a water-bath at $20°C$ for 3 minutes. To each tube, add 1 ml fuchsin solution. The tube is stoppered, turned upside down gently twice, and the colour distribution is observed. Among the tubes, whose contents are uniformly coloured, the one to which has been added the least amount of test enzyme solution, is picked up. The activity of unknown enzyme in the sample is calculated by comparing with the standard.

Formulation 21

Cellulase and Hemicellulase

Cellulase and Hemicellulase activity

METHOD 1

Cellulases and hemicellulases split hydrated cellulose. The reducing groups released by this process are determined iodometrically.

Reagents

1. Cellulose suspension, substrate : Moisten 50 g of thin picked cellulose with 450 ml of concentrated hydrochloric acid in a 5 litre flask and keep for 3 hours under frequent swirling. Dilute the mass with 2.5 litres of water, shake well and let hydrated cellulose to settle. Remove the supernatant solution as completely as possible and suspend the sediment again in 2.5 litres of water. Repeat this procedure till the supernatant liquid is free of chloride ions. Transfer the precipitate to a suction filter and suspend the residue homogeneously in 500 ml of water. Then determine the content of cellulose in this suspension by drying 5 ml to constant weight at 105°C. Dilute the rest of the suspension with water so that 10 ml of the cellulose substrate suspension contains 320 mg of hydrated cellulose.
2. Buffer solution (0.04 M), pH 4.5 : Dissolve 2.4 ml of glacial acetic acid and 5.44 g of crystalline sodium acetate, trihydrate in water and make up to 1000 ml with water, check pH.
3. Starch solution : Dissolve 1.0 g of soluble starch (BDH) in 100 ml of water and heat the mixture under swirling just to boiling.
4. 0.02 N iodine solution.
5. 0.02 N sodium hydroxide solution.
6. 0.02 N sodium thiosulphate solution.
7. Dilute sulphuric acid.

Enzyme suspension

Suspend the finely powdered sample homogeneously in 100 ml of water and use 5 ml of the previously well stirred suspension for the test.

Procedure

A blank value is necessary for every test. The blank test distinguishes itself from the analysis test by the fact that immediately after addition of the enzyme suspension, the enzymes are inactivated by boiling the whole mixture for a few minutes.

Scheme of the reactions

Solutions	Sample	Blank
Cellulose substrate suspension	10.0 ml	10.0 ml
Buffer solution, pH 4.5	4.0 ml	4.0 ml
Enzyme suspension	5.0 ml	5.0 ml

Immediately after addition of the enzyme suspension, boil the blank only for 5 minutes and then incubate both the blank and the sample for 8 hours in a thermostatic water-bath at 30°C ± 0.5°C. Cool and proceed with addition of other reagents to each tube as below :

0.02 N iodine solution	20.0 ml	20.0 ml
0.02 N sodium hydroxide	40 ml	40 ml

(To be added slowly with swirling)

After 15 minutes, proceed with the addition of other reagents as given below :

Dilute sulphuric acid (3 N)	10.0 ml	10.0 ml
Starch solution	2.0 ml	2.0 ml

Titrate both sample and the blank with 0.02 N sodium thiosulphate from a microburette till the blue colour disappears. Record the volume (ml) of 0.02 N sodium thiosulphate used for sample (a) and blank (b).

Calculation

The unit is defined as the amount of enzyme which splits during 8 hours at a pH of 4.5 and temperature of 30°C amount of hydrated cellulose (320 mg) present in 20 ml at a rate which is equivalent to an increase of iodine consumption of 2 ml of 0.02 N iodine solution.

Then calculate the activity as follows :

$$(\text{Grassmann units}) = \frac{(b-a) \times F \times \text{Average weight of the tablet}}{2 \times 60}$$

where F is the normality factor of the 0.02 N sodium thiosulphate solution.

METHOD 2

Reagents

1. 1 N hydrochloric acid.
2. 0.1 N iodine solution.
3. 0.1 N sodium thiosulphate.
4. 0.1 N sodium hydroxide.
5. 0.5 N sodium chloride solution.
6. 20% v/v sulphuric acid.
7. 1% solution of soluble starch : 1 g of soluble starch is stirred in 20 ml of water and poured into boiling water, boiled for 2 min and made up to 100 ml.
8. Phosphate buffer, pH 5.3 : Prepared by mixing 21.5 ml of 0.1 N disodium hydrogen phosphate dihydrite and 978.5 of potassium dihydrogen phosphate.
9. Enzyme solution : To 300 mg of mass (after removal of coating, if any), add 9 ml of water and shake for about 30 min, separate the undissolved portion by centrifuging at high speed and use the supernatant solution for assay.

Procedure

In a 250 ml iodine flask add 25 ml of (7) and 10 ml of buffer solution (8) and 1 ml of (5). Keep in a thermostatic water-bath at 37°C for 15 min, and then add 3 ml of enzyme solution. After exactly 2 hrs, stop the enzyme reaction by addition of 2 ml of (1) and then 15 ml of iodine solution (2) and then 45 ml of (4) is added slowly and drop by drop while shaking. After 15 min, the entire reaction mixture as obtained above is acidified with 5 ml of (6) and excess iodine is extracted with thiosulphate (3) using 1 ml of solution (7) as indicator.

Blank : Blank titration is performed as main titration except 2 ml of (1) is added before the addition of enzyme solution.

Results

Difference between the sample and the blank titration should not be less than 2 ml of 0.1 N iodine for each 30 mg of tablet mass.

Note : We may use 1% solution of lichenin (stir 1 g of lichenin with 20 ml of water, pour into boiling water, boil for 1-2 min and make up to 100 ml with water) instead of soluble starch as substrate.

Pepsin

ESTIMATION

Proteolytic activity of pepsin

METHOD 1

Reagents

1. Acidified water : Dilute 65 ml of 1 N hydrochloric acid to 1000 ml with distilled water.
2. Coagulated egg albumin : Hen's eggs, preferably of country side, 5-10 days old are selected. Boil the eggs for 5 minutes, cool to room temperature, separate the white. At once, rub through sieve No. 40.

Note :   1.   Fresh eggs give erratic results.

2. Eggs are generally boiled for 5 minutes and allowed to cool to room temperature. Prolonged heating is not desirable as it produces hard coagulation.

Sample solution

Dilute accurately measured aliquot of the sample with acidified water to produce approximately 0.5 mg of the pepsin per ml. If the sample is in powder form, triturate with acidified water and dilute with the same solvent to contain about 0.5 mg of pepsin per ml.

Procedure

Triturate 12.5 g or 15 g of freshly prepared coagulated egg albumin, depending upon the activity of pepsin i.e. 1 in 2500 or 1 in 3000, in a small mortar with 50 ml of acidified water until reduced to uniform paste. Transfer to a 250 ml flask, rinse the mortar with 60 ml of acidified water and add the rinsing to the contents of the flask. Immerse the flask in a water-bath maintained at 50-52°C, its contents being on a lower level than water in the bath. When the contents of the flask have attained the temperature of the bath, add 10 ml of assay preparation and dilute the contents of the flask to 125 ml with acidified water. Cover the flask with butter paper and digest for 4 hrs, shaking at interval of fifteen minutes. Centrifuge the content of the flask and pour out the greater portion of the clear liquid. Wash remainder into a 10 ml graduated cylinder and allow to stand for 30 minutes. Measure the volume of the undissolved albumin residue.

Note :   One can either repeat the experiment using different amount of albumin (7.5 g to 15.0 g) or different volume of assay preparations (6-10 ml) and find out the minimum amount of assay preparation for which residue left after digestion is not more than 2 ml.

Working example

Suppose a flask containing 15 g of egg albumin and 8 ml of sample solution (0.5 mg/ml) leaves 1.8 ml of sedimentation, the pepsin activity is 4 mg of pepsin I.P. digests 15 g of egg albumin. However, as per claim (1 in 3000), it should digest 12 g of egg albumin.

Amount of pepsin present in 8 ml aliquot of the sample $= \dfrac{15}{12} \times 4 = 5$ mg.

Net content (mg) of pepsin (1 in 3000) = 5 × dilution factor.

METHOD 2

Reagents

1. 0.1 N sodium hydroxide.
2. 1 N sodium hydroxide.
3. 1 N hydrochloric acid.
4. 20% w/v solution of sodium sulphate in water.
5. Acidic sodium chloride solution : 0.01 1% solution of sodium chloride in 0.065 N hydrochloric acid.
6. Formaldehyde.
7. 5% caseine solution, substrate : Triturate 50 g of caseine with little water, then add 50 ml of 1 N sodium hydroxide and dilute to 1000 ml with water. Heat on boiling water-bath for 30 minutes, cool and again adjust the volume to 1000 ml. Filter through glass wool.

Enzyme solution

The sample of enzyme solution is prepared in acidified sodium chloride solution and pH of the substrate is adjusted to 2 to 2.8.

METHOD

To 100 ml of caseine solution, add 12 ml of 1 N hydrochloride acid and known quantity of pepsin. Mix and incubate for 1 h at 40°C ± 0.5°C. Then, add sufficient sodium sulphate solution to produce 400 ml. Filter to remove undigested caseine. To 100 ml of the filtrate, add 10 ml of neutralized (phenolphthalein) formaldehyde and titrate with 0.1 N sodium hydroxide using undigested caseine as blank. Prepare the standard curve for volume of 0.1 N sodium hydroxide required in titration against the concentration of pepsin taken for the test. Pepsin concentrations varying from 5-100 mg are usually employed for this purpose. The sample is subjected to above method and amount of pepsin in the sample calculated from the standard curve.

Note : Papain, if present, interferes in this test. In such cases, pepsin is assayed by egg albumin method and papain by casein digestion method at pH 7 at which pepsin will not interfere as it gets inactivated at higher pH.

Papain

ESTIMATION

Proteolytic activity of papain

METHOD 1

Reagents

1. Solution of cysteine hydrochloride : Dissolve 0.5 g of cysteine hydrochloride accurately weighed in 10 ml of water, adjust to pH 7.0 with solution of sodium hydroxide. It should be freshly prepared.
2. Solution of caseine, substrate : Dissolve 4.0 g of purified caseine (Hammerstan grade) accurately weighed by shaking with 90 ml of water. Adjust to pH 7.0 with 1 N sodium hydroxide and dilute to 100 ml with water.

Assay preparation

(a) For liquid preparation : Mix an aliquot of the sample with 10 ml solution of cysteine hydrochloride and dilute to 100 ml with water to get 1 mg/ml of papain.
(b) For tablet and powder : Triturate an aliquot of the sample with 10 ml of solution of cysteine hydrochloride and dilute to 100 ml with water to get 1 mg per ml of papain.

Procedure

To 10 ml of water in each of two flasks, add 15 ml accurately measured solution of caseine and maintain at 60°C by heating on water-bath. To the first flask, add 25 ml of accurately measured assay preparation and to the second flask, add 25 ml accurately measured same assay solution previously boiled for 3 minutes and cooled. Maintain the solution at 60°C for 30 minutes, cool rapidly to room temperature and add to each flask 10 ml of solution of formaldehyde previously neutralised to phenolphthalein. Titrate both solutions with 0.1 N sodium hydroxide to pH 8. The difference between the two titrations is not less than 4.5 ml.

Note : 1. Ordinary grade of caseine does not give satisfactory results.
2. It has been experienced that boiling of liquid sample solution for 3 min is often not adequate to destroy completely the enzyme due to buffering property of the sample and lower pH (3.5-5.5) as papain is highly stable in buffered medium. Longer heating time may be required while handling oral liquid samples.

METHOD 2

Reagents

1. Buffer solution, pH 7.6.
   (a) Weigh 11.41 g of potassium phosphate diabasic and make up to 500 ml with distilled water.
   (b) Weigh 6.804 g of potassium phosphate monobasic and make up to 500 ml with distilled water. Adjust solution (a) to pH 7.6 with solution (b).

2. Caseine solution, substrate : Dissolve 1 g of caseine in pH 7.6 buffer solution and make up to 100 ml with the same buffer.
3. 5% w/v trichloroacetic acid in water.

Standard preparation

Weigh 50 mg of standard papain, add 5 ml of 0.1 N hydrochloric acid and make up to 100 ml with water. Take 100 ml, add 1 ml of 0.1 N hydrochloric acid and make up to 100 ml with water.

Sample preparation

Take sample powder equivalent to 25 mg of papain. Add 10 ml of distilled water, followed by 5 ml of 0.1 N hydrochloric acid, make up to 100 ml with distilled water and filter. Pipette 20 ml, add 1 ml of 0.1 N hydrochloric acid and make up to 100 ml with distilled water.

Procedure

Take 1 ml of the sample solution in one test tube and 1 ml of the standard solution in two test tubes, one of which serves as a blank. Add to all test tubes, 1 ml of buffer solution, pH 7.6 and then, add 2 ml of caseine solution except in blank. Add 6 ml of trichloroacetic acid in blank only and maintain all the tubes at 37°C for 20 minutes. Then, add 6 ml of trichloroacetic acid to the sample and the standard. Keep for one hour at room temperature, filter and measure the extinction at 280 nm of both sample and standard solutions against blank and calculate the results by comparison. This method is based on spectrophotometric measurement of amino acid-tyrosine released as result of proteolytic action of papain on caseine.

Pepsin, Papain, Diastase, Choline dihydrogen citrate, Tricholine citrate, Methionine

ESTIMATION

Pepsin

Follow the method 1 described for pepsin using appropriate aliquots of egg albumin and enzyme preparations.

Papain

Use caseine as substrate in pH 7.0 buffer and determine the contents of papain by formol titration method. For details, refer to method 1 for determination of proteolytic activity of papain in this chapter.

Diastase

Follow the method 1 described under determination of diastase activity. This method determines, diastase activity in term of starch hydrolysed to a stage when it gives no blue colour with iodine. Calculate the diastase activity as per example explained under method 1 for estimation of diastase activity.

Note : Type of diastase (fungal or bacterial) must be indicated on the label to enable the analyst to use buffer of correct pH, refer to formulation 1 of this chapter.

Choline dihydrogen citrate

Wash solution

Prepared by diluting 2 ml of saturated aqueous ammonium reineckate solution to 1000 ml with water.

Procedure

Transfer an accurately weighed portion of the sample equivalent to 100 mg of choline dihydrogen citrate to a beaker and dissolve in 40 ml of water. Filter and to the filtrate, add carefully 10 ml of freshly prepared saturated reineckate solution from a pipette, allowing it to run down the side of the beaker so that it forms a layer under the sample solution without producing turbulence. Mix by rotating the beaker gently and allow to stand in a refrigerator for one hour. Filter, collect the precipitates in 30 ml low form sintered glass crucible of medium porosity using gentle suction. Rinse the beaker with three 10 ml portions of wash solution previously cooled to 5°C and pass through the crucible containing the precipitates. Remove most of the water by suction, then dry in an oven at 105°C for an hour. Cool in desiccator and weigh as choline reineckate. The weight of the choline reineckate multiplied by 0.6988 gives the weight of choline dihydrogen citrate.

In case of tricholine citrate, each g of the residue (as reineckate) is equivalent to 0.4114 g of tricholine citrate :

$$0.6988 \times \frac{295.29}{501.63} = 0.4114 \text{ g}$$

Methionine

Reagents

1. Bentonite.
2. 10% w/v solution of sodium nitroprusside in water.
3. 20% v/v hydrochloric acid.
4. 1% w/v solution of glycine in water.

Standard solution

1 mg/ml of methionine, in water.

Sample solution

1 mg/ml of methionine, in water.

Sample solution

Weigh accurately a quantity of powdered sample equivalent to 50 mg of methionine. Add 50 ml of water, 1 g of bentonite, 0.5 g of sodium chloride, shake for 15 minutes and dilute to 100 ml with water.

Procedure

To accurately measured volume of sample and standard solutions, representing 2 mg of methionine, add water to produce 6 ml. Add 1 ml of 5 N sodium hydroxide, 1 ml of glycine solution and 0.5 ml of sodium nitroprusside solution. Shake for 15-20 seconds and keep on water-bath (40°C) for 10 minutes. Cool and add 2 ml of hydrochloric acid. Shake well and measure the extinction of both the sample and standard solutions at about 530 nm against reagent blank and calculate the results by comparison.

Note : The sample can be subjected to paper chromatography or thin layer chromatography. For details regarding chromatographic separation and colour development, refer to the method described for estimation of lysine monohydrochloride in formulation 10 of the chapter on vitamins and minerals.

Pancreatin, Bromelain, Ox-bile

ESTIMATION

Pancreatin

Estimate the proteolytic, lipolytic and amylolytic activities of pancreatin as per methods described in standard Pharmacopoeias, i.e., I.P., B.P., U.S.P.

Bromelain

Unit of enzyme activity is defined as that quantity of enzyme which under the test conditions as described below releases the amount of compounds which react positively with Folin-ciocalteaus-phenol reagent which correspond to 1 μm of tyrosine in depth of colour.

Reagents

1. Folin-ciocalteaus-phenol reagents : 100 g of sodium tungstate, 25 g of sodium molybdate and 50 ml of phosphoric acid (85%) are refluxed with 800 ml of water for 3 hrs. This reagent is quite stable and sensitive.
2. Haemoglobin, substrate.
3. Sodium chloride.
4. 0.5 N sodium hydroxide.
5. 1 N sodium hydroxide.
6. 0.2 N hydrochloric acid.
7. 1 N hydrochloric acid.
8. 5% w/v trichloroacetic acid solution in water.
9. L-tyrosine
10. Boric acid solution : 4.12 g of boric acid and 0.195 g of sodium chloride are dissolved in water by slight warming and adjusted with water to 100 ml.
11. Folin-ciocalteaus (FC) solution : Mix 1 part of the reagent with 2 parts of water. Prepare fresh as and when required.
12. Solution of haemoglobin, substrate : Suspend 2 g of haemoglobin in 150 ml beaker with 25 ml of water, add 36 g of urea and 80 ml of 1 N sodium hydroxide. Stir for 50-60 minutes, add 15 ml of boric acid solution and adjust the pH to 6.0 with 1 N hydrochloric acid. Make up the volume to 100 ml with water.
13. Buffer solution, pH 4.0 : Dissolve 22.6 g of diammonium hydrogen citrate in 900 ml of water, adjust the pH to 4.0 with 1 N hydrochloric acid and dilute to 1000 ml with water, mix well.
14. Buffer solution, pH 6.0 : Dissolve 22.6 g of diammonium hydrogen citrate in 900 ml of water, adjust the pH to 6.0 with 1 N hydrochloric acid and dilute to 1000 ml with water.

Tyrosine standard solution

Weigh accurately 18.12 mg of 1-tyrosine and dilute to 100 ml with 0.2 N hydrochloric acid. 0.5 ml of the resulting solution is further diluted to 25 ml with 0.2 N hydrochloric acid.

Tyrosine standard curve

Take 1, 2, 3, 4, 5 ml of tyrosine standard solution in separate tubes, adjust to 5 ml where necessary with 0.2 N hydrochloric acid. To each tube, add 10 ml of 0.5 N sodium hydroxide, mix and add 3 ml of Folin-ciocalteaus solution and mix. Measure the absorbance of different solutions at maximum at about 750 nm against reagent blank. Plot the graph of absorbance against quantities of tyrosine. Above quantities of tyrosine correspond to 0.2 to 1 µm of 1-tyrosine.

Sample solution

Bromelain coating is usually done over the protective cellulose acetate coating. Therefore pancreatin which is present in lower coating of the tablet will not interfere in this assay. Take whole tablet equivalent to 750 units of bromelain, add 50 ml of buffer solution, pH 4.0 and stir for 10-15 minutes. Care should be taken not to damage inner layer while extracting bromelain. 5 ml of above suspension is diluted to 50 ml with buffer solution, pH 6.0.

Procedure

Add 1 ml of sample solution to 5 ml of the substrate (previously maintained at 35°C ($\pm$ 0.5°C) for 15 minutes. Incubate exactly for 10 minutes and then, add 10 ml of trichloroacetic acid. After 20 minutes, filter and to 5 ml of the filtrate, add 10 ml of 0.5 N sodium hydroxide and 3 ml of Folin's solution. After 5 minutes, measure the absorbance of the sample solution at 750 nm against blank, prepared by adding 1 ml of sample solution after addition of 10 ml of trichloroacetic acid. Calculate the amount of bromelain from the standard curve.

Calculation

Units/tablet : $E \times 3.2 \times d_f$

From the absorbance of sample (E), calculate the µm of tyrosine from the standard curve.

3.2 = ratio value (16 : 5)

Total digesting volume comes to 16 ml (1 + 5 + 10) and out of this, 5 ml is taken for colour development.

Bile constituents (Cholic acid)

Reagents

1. 60% v/v acetic acid.
2. Solution of furfural (1 in 100) : Measure 1 ml of freshly distilled furfural and make to 100 ml with water. This solution is prepared fresh every time.
3. Dilute sulphuric acid : Mix cautiously, 50 ml of sulphuric acid with 65 ml of water and cool.

Standard cholic acid solution

Dissolve 25 mg of cholic acid, accurately weighed in 10 ml of 60% acetic acid and make up the volume to 50 ml with acetic acid (0.5 mg/ml).

Sample solution

Weigh accurately about 700 mg of finely powdered tablets and suspend them in 20 ml of alcohol. Shake well and make the volume to 50 ml with alcohol. Shake again for about 10 minutes and filter. This solution should contain about 0.5 mg/ml of cholic acid.

Procedure

Pipette exactly 1 ml each of standard and sample solutions into two test tubes. To each tube, add exactly 1 ml of furfural solution and place the tubes at once in an ice-bath for 5 minutes. Then, add to each tube exactly 18 ml of dilute sulphuric acid. Thoroughly mix the contents of the tubes and place them in water-bath maintained at 70°C for 10 minutes. At the end of this period, place the tube immediately in ice water for 2 minutes and determine the absorbance of each solution at about 650 nm. A blank is taken by omitting the addition of furfural. Calculate the results by comparison.

Pancreatin, Sodium tauroglycocholate

ESTIMATION

Pancreatin

Estimate amylase, lipase and protease activities as per method described in I.P.

Sodium tauroglycocholate

Weigh sample accurately equivalent to 500 mg of the substance, add 30 ml of sodium hydrochloride solution (15% w/v) and 1 ml of methanol. Filter, wash the flask and filter paper with hot water. Cool to 10°C and acidify the combined filtrate and washing with dilute sulphuric acid, cool and extract with 4×50 ml portions of ether. Wash the combined ether extract with 2×10 ml portions of ether. Evaporate the ether extract and dry at 105°C to a constant weight. The weight represents the amount of tauroglycocholic acid in the sample taken for analysis.

L-ornithine-L-aspartate, Pancreatin

ESTIMATION

Pancreatin

Follow the method described in formulation 25 of this chapter for proteolytic, amylolytic and lipolytic activities.

L-ornithine-L-aspartate

METHOD 1

This method is based on post-derivatisation preparative thin layer chromatography.

Standard solution (30 mg/ml)

Dissolve 300 mg of L-ornithine-L-aspartate working standard in water sufficient to produce 10 ml.

Sample solution

Weigh 20 tablets and take powder equivalent to 300 mg of L-ornithine-L-aspartate and shake vigorously with 10 ml of water for about 15 minutes and centrifuge. Use supernatant as sample solution.

Stationary phase

Silica gel $60F_{254}$ pre-coated on aluminium back.

Mobile phase

h-butanol : glacial acetic acid : water (50 : 25 : 25) v/v

Derivatising agent

1% ninhydrin solution in acetone.

Development, derivatisation and elution procedure

Saturate the chamber with mobile phase for 20 minutes. Wash the silica gel plate in methanol and activate it. Apply 100 μl of standard and sample solution in form of band. Run the plate up to 150 mm and air dry. Spray ninhydrin solution and heat it for 10 minutes at 110°C. Violet purple spots (two) appear on the plate for L-ornithine-L-aspartate. Cut out both the bands carefully for standard and sample separately. (In sample some extra spot appears for pancreatin, so take care while cutting the bands for sample). Extract both the bands with 5 ml of methanol and centrifuge for 10 minutes. Prepare the blank in similar manner using silica gel from the same plate. Measure the absorbance of both sample and standard solutions at about 595 nm against reagent blank and calculate the results by comparison.

Note : The above sample was also analysed by HPTLC using the same mobile phase. L-ornithine and L-aspartate could be estimated separately. The spot with lower Rf value corresponds to ornithine.

METHOD 2

L-ornithine-L-aspartate can be estimated by non-aqueous titration. 100 mg of the substance is dissolved in 2 ml of formic acid (98%), add 50 ml of glacial acetic acid and titrate with 0.1 N perchloric acid using α-napthol benzein as indicator. Each ml of 0.1 N perchloric acid is equivalent to 8.842 mg of l-ornithine-l-aspartate.

Index

Quantitative Analysis of Drugs in Pharmaceutical Formulations
Third Edition

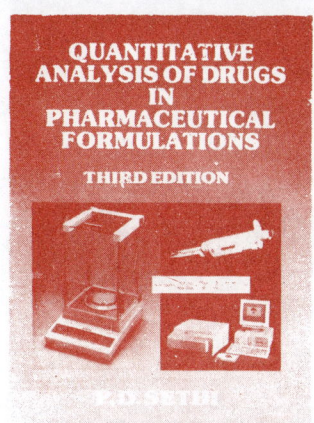

Dear Analysts

Just because someone has developed the method and has claimed to have validated it in respect of various analytical parameters, does not simply imply that the method is reliable and can be directly applied. It has been found that most of the original research papers or their abstracts often do not provide adequate experimental details on LOD, LOQ, precision, accuracy, analytical range, reagents preparation and their storage, possible interference, or application of the described method in presence of other drug substances likely to be present in a multi-component formulation. Thus the reported method may have several weak spots which can give the method a kind of metastatic state. It may work one day but not the next. Although the analytical chemistry is based on reproduction of the method from written protocols as long as all the variables that can influence the reproducibility of the method are precisely controlled. However, skill obtained during development of the method cannot be simply transmitted via written description of the method. It is always preferable that you learn through your own experience as every described method may need some degree of optimisation. It is therefore desirable that any shortcoming in the method·as and when observed or any practical suggestion about the method must be promptly brought to the notice of person authorized to make suitable changes in the method instead of wasting your time and your employer's resources collecting useless and unreliable analytical data.

Analytical procedures for currently available multi-component formulations included in this book have been described in sufficient details to be reproduced without difficulty, but some degree of optimization may be needed in certain procedures. It is my earnest feeling that with the sound knowledge of chemistry (inorganic/organic), equipped with special skill needed for analytical work and the information available in this book, you will be able to carry out the analysis of any viable combination of drugs either inadvertently escaped my attention or you may encounter in your analytical career. **Be determined that the method can and shall be devised, no analytical problem will ever defy solution.** You may even find better alternative method for your analytical problem than the one described in this book. If there is a better method of analysing your sample, follow it, it will give you considerable personal satisfaction. Without continuous improvement in skill you will become obsolete, most important thing to do is to develop life-time learning habit. However, if you are ever confronted with any analytical problem defying solution, discussion with the author will be rewarding and in mutual interest, as perfection for anyone is impossible to achieve. Your constructive criticism, comments and suggestions have always been source of inspiration to me. I shall feel obliged for sharing your practical experience with me.

Address :
B-140, Shivalik Enclave,
New Delhi - 110 017 (India)

Sincerely yours,

(P.D. SETHI)

"An analyst has to be in love with analysis without which it is virtually impossible to pass on the knowledge and experience one has to those wanting to learn "

The book has been published by :

CBS Publishers & Distributors,
4596/1A, 11-Darya Ganj, New Delhi - 110 002 (India)